# Principles and Practice of Regional Anaesthesia

## Third Edition

*Commissioning Editor:* Paul Fam
*Project Development Manager:* Aoibhe O'Shea
*Project Manager:* Alan Nicholson
*Designer:* Andy Chapman

# Principles and Practice of Regional Anaesthesia

## Third Edition

*Edited by*

**J.A.W. Wildsmith** MD FRCA FRCPEd
Foundation Professor of Anaesthesia, University of Dundee, Honorary Consultant Anaesthetist,
Tayside University Hospitals Trust, Ninewells Hospital and Medical School, Dundee, UK

**Edward N. Armitage** MB BS DObstRCOG FRCA
Honorary Consultant Anaesthetist, The Royal Sussex County Hospital, Brighton, East Sussex, UK

**John H. McClure** BSc(Hons) MB ChB FRCA
Consultant Anaesthetist and Honorary Senior Lecturer, Edinburgh Royal Infirmary,
University of Edinburgh, Department of Anaesthesia, Critical Care & Pain Medicine,
Edinburgh, UK

*Ilustrated by*
**Patrick Elliott**
BA(Hons) ATC MMAA MIMI RMIP

*Photographs by*
**Ken Crowe**  Publicity Manager,
SIMS Portex Ltd, Hythe, Kent

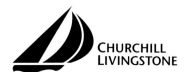

CHURCHILL
LIVINGSTONE

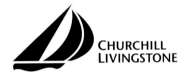

CHURCHILL LIVINGSTONE
An imprint of Elsevier Science Limited

First edition 1987
Second edition 1993
Third edition 2003
Reprinted 2003

ISBN 0 44306 2269

**British Library Cataloguing in Publication Data**
A catalogue record for this book is available from the British Library

**Library of Congress Cataloging in Publication Data**
A catalog record for this book is available from the Library of Congress

**Note**
Medical knowledge is constantly changing. As new information becomes available, changes in treatment, procedures, equipment and the use of drugs become necessary. The authors and the publishers have taken care to ensure that the information given in this text is accurate and up to date. However, readers are strongly advised to confirm that the information, especially with regard to drug usage, complies with the latest legislation and standards of practice.

 your source for books,
journals and multimedia
in the health sciences
www.elsevierhealth.com

Typeset by RDC Tech
Printed in China

The
publisher's
policy is to use
**paper manufactured
from sustainable forests**

# Contents

List of Contributors                                              vii

Foreword                                                           ix

Preface                                                            xi

Acknowledgements                                                  xiii

**PART 1 General principles**

**History and development of local anaesthesia**                    1
J A W Wildsmith

**The features of regional anaesthesia**                            9
N B Scott and A R Absalom

**Anatomy and physiology of pain**                                 21
L A Colvin and J H McClure

**Peripheral nerve and local anaesthetic drugs**                   35
J A W Wildsmith and G R Strichartz

**Local anaesthetic kinetics**                                     49
G T Tucker

**Clinical use of local anaesthetic drugs**                        65
J A W Wildsmith

**Preoperative considerations**                                    77
M R Checketts and J A W Wildsmith

**Managing the block**                                             91
J E Charlton

**PART 2 Anatomy and technique**

**Anatomy and physiology of the vertebral canal**                 111
M Brockway and W A Chambers

**Spinal anaesthesia**                                            125
A P Rubin

**Lumbar and thoraic epidural block**                             139
E N Armitage

**Sacral epidural (caudal) block**                                169
L V H Martin and E Doyle

**Regional anaesthesia of the trunk**                             177
A Lee

**Upper limb blocks**                                             193
H B J Fischer

**Lower limb blocks**                                             213
W A Macrae and D M Coventry

**Head, neck and airway blocks**                                  229
N G Smart and S Hickey

**Eye blocks**                                                    241
A P Rubin

**Regional anaesthesia in obstetrics**                            251
J H McClure

**Regional anaesthesia in children**                              269
A R Lloyd-Thomas

**Postoperative pain and audit**                                  283
J D R Connolly and G A Mcleod

**Pain and autonomic nerve block**                                293
D M Justins

**Regional anaesthesia for day-care surgery**                     313
H B J Fischer

**Regional anaesthesia in the elderly patient**                   323
B T Veering

Index                                                             333

v

# Contributors

**Anthony R Absalom** MB ChB, FRCA, ILTM
Consultant Anaesthetist
Department of Anaesthesia
Norfolk and Norwich University Hospital
Norwich
United Kingdom

**Edward N Armitage** MB BS, DObstRCOG, FRCA
Honorary Consultant Anaesthetist
Royal Sussex County Hospital
Brighton
United Kingdom

**Michael Brockway** MB ChB, FRCA
Consultant in Anaesthesia and Intensive Care
Department of Anaesthesia and Intensive Care
St John's Hospital
Livingstone
West Lothian
United Kingdom

**William A Chambers** MD, MEd, FRCA, FRCPEd
Consultant in Anaesthesia and Pain Management
Department of Anaesthesia
Aberdeen Royal Infirmary
Aberdeen
United Kingdom

**J. Edmond Charlton** MB BS, FRCA
Consultant in Pain Medicine and Anaesthesia
The Royal Victoria Infirmary
Newcastle-upon-Tyne
United Kingdom

**Matthew R Checketts** MB ChB, FRCA
Consultant Anaesthetist
University Department of Anaesthesia
Ninewells Hospital and Medical School
Dundee
United Kingdom

**Lesley A Colvin** BSc, MB ChB, PhD, FRCA
Consultant in Anaesthesia and Pain Medicine
Department of Anaesthesia, Critical Care and Pain
Medicine
Western General Hospital
Edinburgh
United Kingdom

**James D Connolly** MB ChB, FFARCSI
Consultant Anaesthetist and Medical Director
Green Park Healthcare Trust
Belfast
Northern Ireland
United Kingdom

**David M Coventry** MB ChB, FRCA
Consultant Anaesthetist
Department of Anaesthetics
Ninewells Hospital and Medical School
Dundee
United Kingdom

**Edward Doyle** MD, FRCA
Consultant Paediatric Anaesthetist
Department of Anaesthesia
Royal Hospital for Sick Children
Edinburgh
United Kingdom

**H B J Fischer** MB ChB, FRCA
Consultant Anaesthetist
Department of Anaesthesia
The Alexandra Hospital
Worcestershire
United Kingdom

**Stephen Hickey** MB ChB, FRCA
Consultant and Honorary Clinical Senior Lecturer in
Anaesthesia
Department of Anaesthesia
Glasgow Royal Infirmary
Glasgow
United Kingdom

**Douglas Justins** MB BS, FRCA
Consultant in Pain Management and Anaesthesia
Department of Anaesthesia
St Thomas' Hospital
London
United Kingdom

**Alistair Lee** BSc, MB ChB FRCA
Consultant in Anaesthesia and Critical Care
Edinburgh Royal Infirmary
Edinburgh
United Kingdom

**Adrian R Lloyd-Thomas** MB BS, FRCA
Clinical Chair, Division of Anaesthesia and Surgery
Hospital for Sick Children
London
United Kingdom

**William A Macrae** MB ChB, FRCA
Consultant Anaesthetist and Pain Specialist
The Pain Service
Ninewells Hospital
Dundee
United Kingdom

**Lawrence V H Martin** MB ChB, FRCA, DA, DObstRCOG
Honorary Senior Lecturer
University of Edinburgh
Edinburgh
United Kingdom

**John H McClure** BSc(Hons), MB ChB, FRCA
Consultant Anaesthetist and Honorary Senior Lecturer
Department of Anaesthesia, Critical Care and
Pain Medicine
Edinburgh Royal Infirmary and University of Edinburgh
Edinburgh
United Kingdom

**Graeme A McLeod** MB ChB, MRCGP, FRCA
Consultant and Part-time Senior Lecturer
Department of Anaesthesia
Ninewells Hospital and Medical School
Dundee
United Kingdom

**Anthony P Rubin** MB ChB, FRCA
Consultant Anaesthetist
Royal National Orthopaedic Hospital
Stanmore
Middlesex
United Kingdom

**Nicholas B Scott** MB ChB, FFARCSI, FRCSEd
Director of Pain Services
HCI International Medical Centre
Glasgow
United Kingdom

**Neil G Smart** BSc(Hons), MB ChB, FFARCSI
Department of Anaesthesia
Glasgow Royal Infirmary
Glasgow
United Kingdom

**Gary R Strichartz** BS, AM(Hon), PhD
Professor of Anesthesia (Pharmacology),
Department of Anesthesiology Perioperative
and Pain Medicine
Director, Pain Research Center
Brigham and Women's Hospital
Boston
USA

**Geoffrey T Tucker** B Pharm, PhD, FRCPEd, FRCA, FFPM
Professor of Clinical Pharmacology
Academic Unit of Molecular Pharmacology and
Pharmacogenetics
Clinical Sciences Divisions
University of Sheffield
Royal Hallamshire Hospital
Sheffield
United Kingdom

**Bernadette Th. Veering** MD, PhD
Staff Anaesthesiologist
Department of Anaesthesiology
Leiden University Medical Centre
Leiden
The Netherlands

**J A W Wildsmith** MD, FRCA, FRCPEd
Foundation Professor of Anaesthesia
University of Dundee
Honorary Consultant Anaesthetist
Tayside University Hospitals Trust
Ninewells Hospital and Medical School
Dundee
United Kingdom

# Foreword

The continued upsurge in interest in regional anaesthesia has several explanations. Firstly, undesirable intra- and post-operative organ dysfunctions such as impairment in pulmonary function, increased cardiac demand, ileus and pain may all be reduced by regional anaesthetic techniques. These effects have translated into the demonstration of improved postoperative recovery and outcome in well-designed studies over the last decade. Secondly, educational programmes and textbooks on the procedural principles of regional anaesthesia have been offered in order to optimise the balance between the benefits, risks and safety of regional anaesthetic techniques.

In this context, *Principles & Practice of Regional Anaesthesia*, edited by Tony Wildsmith, Edward Armitage and John McClure, and now in its 3rd edition, has shown proven survival value over 20 years. The editors and their collaborative authors have provided a completely updated and easily readable description of the various regional anaesthetic techniques to be applied under different surgical conditions, and in a way which can be adopted easily by the practising clinician.

Being a surgeon, I felt both honoured and surprised to be asked to write a foreword for this fine textbook, previously introduced by the late D.B. Scott. Having been a non-anaesthetist pupil of Bruce Scott, I was introduced early to the principles and potential of regional anaesthetic techniques to optimise perioperative outcome. It is therefore with great pleasure that I recommend this excellent textbook on the principles and practice of regional anaesthesia, which undoubtedly will support the increased use and quality of the practice of these techniques in order to improve care and outcome in our surgical patients.

Prof. Henrik Kehlet,
MD, PhD,
Hvidovre University Hospital
Denmark
June 26, 2002

# Preface

It is now twenty years since the first edition of this text was conceived. In the interim much has changed in regional anaesthetic practice, and we hope that our efforts have contributed in some degree to that change. When we began there were many centres where regional methods were never used; now they are an integral part of the competency based training programmes of the Royal College of Anaesthetists in the United Kingdom and equivalent organisations elsewhere. Thus, whereas the second edition was simply a revision of the first, this one has been expanded to take into account recent research and modern practice, albeit within a basic structure which remains the same: we still aim to give an indication of the scope and potential place of regional methods in anaesthetic practice, as well as providing instruction in their use.

Our prescription for the successful use of regional anaesthesia remains unchanged also: it requires a thorough knowledge of anatomy, and skill in the appropriate technique of needle insertion, but much more besides these. The anaesthetist must be able to determine which patients will and will not benefit. This requires a full understanding of the effects of the techniques and the ways in which these differ from those of general anaesthesia. Having decided that a block would be beneficial, the anaesthetist must then choose, from the several techniques and drugs available, the most suitable combination for the particular patient and surgical procedure. Finally, the needs of the patient, both during and after the operation, must be recognised and catered for.

The aim of this book is to help the specialist anaesthetist learn about, and understand, the use of regional anaesthesia. The book is divided into two parts: the first outlines the general principles for safe, effective practice; and the second describes anatomy and technique. Some aspects are considered in both sections. The main reason for this is to allow each chapter to stand on its own, but we have tried to avoid extensive repetition. We have adhered to the convention of expressing drug dosage in milligrams of a specified percentage concentration of solution, but in an attempt to eliminate arithmetical error, we have given, in brackets, the volume which such dosage represents. Also, we have bowed to the inevitable and adopted the internationally agreed nomenclature of lidocaine for lignocaine, and epinephrine for adrenaline.

We have confined ourselves to those methods which our authors find useful in routine clinical practice, and we have made no attempt to describe every known block. Few anaesthetists can expect to master the whole range of regional techniques to a level at which they can instruct others and we are grateful to our authors for contributing material on subjects in which they have special expertise. In an attempt to produce a uniform appearance and a cohesive style all the illustrations were prepared by the same artist or photographer and every script has been subjected to editorial changes.

No text can provide all the necessary information in such a practical subject – clinical training and experience are essential. Neither can anatomy be learnt entirely from a book because there is no substitute for a visit to the dissecting or autopsy room, or for asking a surgical colleague to demonstrate relevant structures exposed during surgery. We believe that regional anaesthesia has much to offer our patients, but it requires just as much attention to detail as general anaesthesia. Regional anaesthesia is *not* an excuse for taking short cuts in patient care – it is a very satisfying way of making patient care better.

J.A.W.W.
E.N.A.
J.H.McC.

# Acknowledgements

The first two editions of this book were very well received and we are grateful to everyone who helped in their production, and to all those who commented favourably upon them. We are also grateful to those who suggested improvements, every one of which has been taken into account when preparing this new edition.

A very special word of thanks must go to Smiths Medical (SIMS-Portex Ltd) for their very generous contribution to the production costs of this edition, and to Ken Crowe, Smiths Marketing and Communications Manager, who once again has been responsible for all the clinical photography. Equally important are Patrick Elliott's illustrations, and we are most grateful to both Ken and Patrick for their expertise and continued involvement.

Inevitably, there has not been the same continuity of authorship. Retirement or changes in interest have necessitated some changes among our authors, and we thank both the 'old' and the 'new' for their help and acceptance of editorial decisions, large and small. In anticipation of the same 'rules' applying eventually to the original editors, John McClure has joined the team for future continuity. In spite of the many changes in the industry we have, technically at least, the same publishers – Churchill Livingstone. We thank Maria Khan for persuading us to start again; Miranda Bromage, Serena Bureau and Francesca Lumkin for their support; and Paul Fam, Aoibhe O'Shea and Alan Nicholson for seeing the project through to publication.

Editorial working has been much facilitated by computers and the internet. The three of us owe thanks to too many individuals to mention for our education in these techniques, but specific reference should be made to Marie Thomson (secretary to the University Department of Anaesthesia in Dundee), and to Hannah and Helen Armitage who, having outgrown their role as paediatric models for the earlier editions, have dragged their father into the electronic age. In addition, we thank the patients and staff at Brighton General Hospital, The Royal Infirmary of Edinburgh, the Princess Alexandra Hospital, Redditch, and the Portland Hospital, London, for their help with the production of new clinical photographs.

Last, but far from least, we thank our families for their support, and tolerance of the many long editorial sessions which were necessary.

J.A.W.W.
E.N.A.
J.H.McC.

# 1. History and development of local anaesthesia

## J A W Wildsmith

### The first steps

*The possible production of local anaesthesia by this or by other means, is certainly an object well worthy of study and attainment. Surgeons everywhere seem more and more acknowledging the facility, certainty, and safety with which the state of general anaesthesia can be produced at will before operating, as well as the moral and professional necessity of saving their patients from all requisite pain. But if we could by any means induce a local anaesthesia, without that temporary absence of consciousness, which is found in the state of general anaesthesia, many would regard it as a still greater improvement in this branch of practice. If a man, for instance, could have his hand so obtunded that he could see, but not feel, the performance of amputation upon his own fingers, the practice of anaesthesia in surgery would, in all likelihood, advance and progress even still more rapidly than it has done.*

This striking appreciation of the benefits of local anaesthesia was published in 1848, decades before local anaesthesia became a practical possibility. The paper from which it is taken was by James Young Simpson (Fig. 1.1) in which he also described his own (unsuccessful) experiments with the topical application of various liquids and vapours (Simpson 1848). Because it was published less than 2 years after Oliver Wendell Holmes had suggested the word 'anaesthesia' to William Morton, it probably represents the first use of the term 'local anaesthesia'. However, Simpson was aware that his were far from being the first attempts to produce peripheral insensibility, for he refers to some ancient methods (which he considered 'apocryphal') and also to Moore's method of nerve compression (Fig. 1.2). Some success had been achieved with the

latter towards the end of the 18th century and there are even earlier reports of its use.

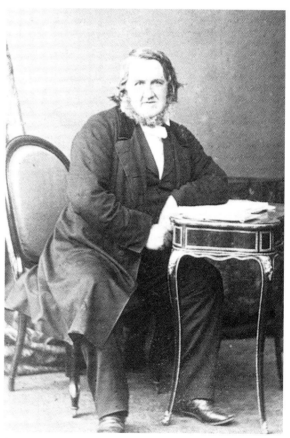

**Fig 1.1** James Young Simpson. Photograph courtesy of the Royal Medical Society

Another eminent Victorian who became interested in the possibility of producing local anaesthesia, and who appreciated its potential advantages over general anaesthesia, was Benjamin Ward Richardson (Fig. 1.3). He experimented with electricity before turning his attention to the effect of temperature. As with nerve compression, reports of the numbing effect of cold go back to antiquity, the best known being by Napoleon's surgeon, Baron Larrey. Richardson's interest in this method (Richardson 1858) culminated in his introduction of the ether spray (Fig. 1.4), which worked by evaporation and was the only practical method of local anaesthesia until the local action of cocaine was fully appreciated. Ethyl chloride supplanted ether as the cooling agent after 1880.

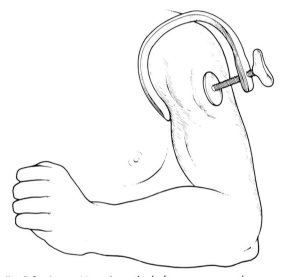

**Fig 1.2** James Moore's method of nerve compression

The development of the hypodermic syringe and needle was an important prerequisite for the use of cocaine for anything but topical application. They both evolved over many years and their introduction cannot be ascribed to any one person, but Alexander Wood

(Fig. 1.5), a contemporary of Simpson, was, in 1853, the first to combine these items for hypodermic medication (Fig. 1.6). Wood was a physician interested in the treatment of neuralgia and he reasoned that morphine might be more effective if it were injected close to the nerve supplying the affected area (Wood 1855). Although morphine may have some peripheral actions, the effect of Wood's morphine was probably central, but he was nevertheless the first to think of the possibility of producing nerve block by drug injection and he has been called the 'father-in-law' of local anaesthesia – all he lacked was an agent which worked locally.

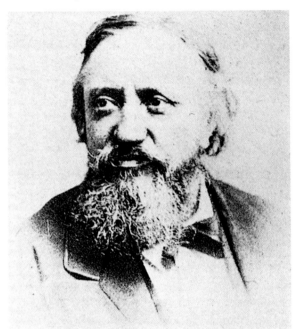

**Fig 1.3** Benjamin Ward Richardson. Photograph from Disciples of Aesculapius

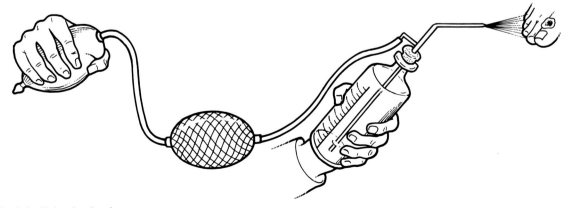

**Fig 1.4** Richardson's ether spray

## The introduction of cocaine

The sequence of events leading to the introduction of cocaine, the alkaloid derived from the leaves of *Erythroxylon coca*, into clinical practice began shortly after Wood's experiments with local morphine injection. Sporadic reports of the systemic effects of chewing the leaves had reached Europe from the time of the Spanish conquest, but it was not until 1857 that Montegazza gave the first detailed description of these actions. Prior to that, Gaedke had extracted some reddish crystals, but it was Niemann in 1860 who produced pure white crystals which he named cocaine. Niemann noted that these crystals produced numbness of the tongue, an observation subsequently confirmed by several other workers. Alexander Hughes Bennett was the first to demonstrate in animals that *injection* of cocaine produces sensory block but, as with the work of others, the significance of his observation was not appreciated (Wildsmith 1983).

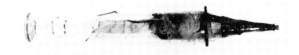

Fig 1.6  Syringe devised by Wood. Photograph courtesy of the Royal College of Surgeons of Edinburgh

During this time cocaine came to be looked upon as a universal panacea and was even used to treat morphine addiction. A report of this latter use attracted the attention of Sigmund Freud, who reviewed the literature and started a programme of research. In this research he enlisted the assistance of his friend Carl Koller (Fig. 1.7) who, like Freud then, was a young graduate of the Vienna medical school spending a portion of his time in Stricker's research laboratories. Koller wished to become an ophthalmologist and, having heard from his teacher – Ferdinand Arlt –

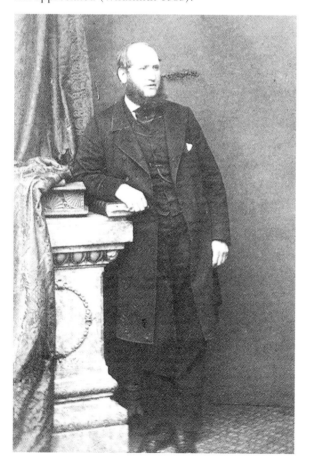

Fig 1.5  Alexander Wood. Photograph courtesy of the Royal Medical Society

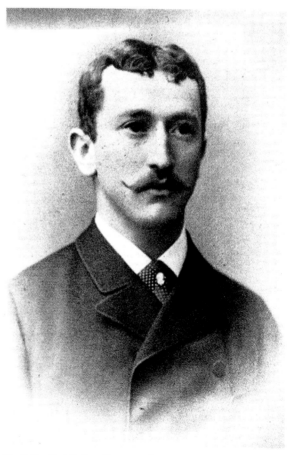

Fig 1.7  Carl Koller. Photograph courtesy of Mrs Hortense Koller Becker

3

of the disadvantages of general anaesthesia for eye surgery, had applied a variety of agents to the conjunctiva without success (Wildsmith 1984). Koller was aware of the reports of cocaine's ability to produce local insensibility, but not even he appreciated the significance of this at first. It was only a chance comment from a colleague that made him realise that he had in his possession the local anaesthetic agent for which he had been searching (Becker 1963). Experiments, firstly with animals, then on himself and colleagues, led on to clinical trials during the summer of 1884. A preliminary communication was read (by a former colleague – Joseph Brettaur – because Koller could not afford the trip) at the Heidelberg meeting of the German Ophthalmological Society on 15 September 1884 and from there the news spread with amazing speed.

## Immediate developments

The full account of his own work (Koller 1884) appeared shortly after, and many others reported their experience before the end of the year. Although there is evidence (Faulconer & Keys 1965) that William Burke may have absolute priority for the first nerve block (performed before the end of November 1884), credit is usually given to William Halsted and Richard Hall of New York. Before the end of 1885 they had blocked virtually every peripheral somatic nerve, including the brachial plexus, and had demonstrated the effectiveness of such methods (Boulton 1984).

Central neural block may be considered to have been introduced almost as soon. We will never know for certain whether the New York neurologist, Leonard Corning, produced epidural or subarachnoid block in 1885, but there is no doubt that at that early stage he deliberately injected cocaine between the posterior spinous processes of both a dog and a patient and produced block of the lower half of the body. Although he suggested that it might be used in surgery, no further development of the method took place until nearly the end of the century. In 1891, Quincke in Kiel, Germany, had shown that lumbar puncture was a practical procedure, and it was in the same centre that August Bier performed the first spinal blocks for surgery in 1898. However, Bier abandoned the technique before he had gained much experience with it and it was Tuffier, working independently in Paris, who was responsible for popularising the method in Europe. In the USA Tait, Caglieri and Matas were the early pioneers.

## Pharmacological advances

The major factor in Bier's decision to abandon spinal anaesthesia was the toxicity of cocaine. It was also difficult to sterilise, brief in duration of action and had exacted a terrible price from pioneers like Halsted and Hall who became addicted to it as a result of experimenting on themselves. Because of these factors the early use of cocaine was largely limited to topical application. Later, Schleich in Germany and Reclus in France developed safe dose regimens for, and popularised, infiltration anaesthesia. Braun increased its duration and reduced its toxicity, first by the use of a tourniquet and later by adding epinephrine to the solution.

Widespread use of local methods had to await the introduction of safer drugs. Niemann, in his pioneer work, had hydrolysed benzoic acid from cocaine and it was the search for other benzoic acid esters that produced new local anaesthetics. Amylocaine (Stovaine) was introduced in 1903 and was popular for spinal anaesthesia until it was shown to be irritant, but it was the development of procaine by Einhorn in 1904 that was the really significant advance. Its low toxicity, lack of addictive properties and relative stability ensured its popularity for the techniques already in use, and made feasible the development of new techniques for which larger doses of drug were required.

Procaine is still far from ideal because it hydrolyses when heated in solution, does not have a particularly long duration of action and may induce allergic reactions. Many other drugs were tried, but in the first 50 years after Koller's introduction of cocaine the only ones to become established were amethocaine and cinchocaine. Both are potent and toxic, but were well suited to spinal anaesthesia for which they became standard agents. Choroprocaine is the only ester-type drug to be developed successfully in more recent times, but even it is of relatively limited availability.

The 1930s saw the start of the next major advance. Working in Stockholm on the structure of the alkaloid gramine, Erdtman, an organic chemist believing in the importance of the senses in analysis, tasted one of the substances which had been produced as a precursor of gramine. The significance of the ensuing numbness was appreciated immediately and the search for a clinically useful derivative was started by Erdtman and continued by Nils Lofgren, who synthesised lidocaine in 1943. Perhaps almost as important as the synthesis of lidocaine was Lofgren's systematic study of a whole range of compounds

(Lofgren 1948), so laying the foundations for all subsequent studies of local anaesthetic drugs. From these studies have come derivatives of lidocaine such as mepivacaine, prilocaine, bupivacaine, etidocaine and ropivacaine.

While the introduction of these agents has considerably widened the scope of local anaesthesia, they are essentially variations on a theme. Since the development of lidocaine the most important work has been in the field of membrane physiology. Many workers have contributed to this, the most notable being Hodgkin and Huxley. Use of apparatus such as the voltage clamp has produced major advances in our knowledge of the mechanism of nerve conduction and its block by drugs at the molecular level. This has yet to lead to the development of new drugs, but a number of alternative approaches continue to be investigated (Kendig & Courtney 1991).

Concurrent studies of the pharmacokinetics of local anaesthetic drugs have made a more practical contribution to our knowledge because they have indicated the most appropriate doses and agents for the various techniques. They have thus played an important part in basing clinical local anaesthesia on sound scientific principles. In more recent years, pharmaceutical research has led to the development of novel ways of delivering local anaesthetics. The first local anaesthetic preparation to be effective on application to intact skin (EMLA – the eutectic mixture of local anaesthetics) is a classic example, and depot preparations (such as liposomal local anaesthetics) continue to be evaluated.

## Developments in technique

As has been mentioned, most local techniques had been described by 1900, even if they were not widely used. In 1906, Sellheim introduced paravertebral and intercostal block, and 2 years later Bier, taking advantage of the low toxicity of procaine, developed his technique for intravenous regional anaesthesia. Another important development at about this time was Barker's description of the way in which the curves of the lumbar spine and gravity interact to affect the spread of intrathecally injected solutions.

Epidural block is very much a product of the 20th century. The sacral approach, described independently by Sicard and Cathelin in 1901, was used by Stoeckel for analgesia during vaginal delivery in 1909. The lumbar approach is considered to have been first described by Pages in Spain in 1921, but he died soon afterwards

and the technique was 'rediscovered' and popularised by Dogliotti in Italy a decade later. He used the loss of resistance technique to identify the epidural space. The lumbar approach was first used in labour in 1938 by Graffagnino and Seyler. Massey Dawkins performed the first epidural in Britain in 1942.

Most other subsequent advances in technique may be looked upon as being refinements or rediscoveries of techniques which had been described previously. This is not to deny the importance of these latter authors because they did a great deal to improve and popularise the practice of local anaesthesia. One important technical development which does deserve mention is the introduction of continuous methods of local anaesthesia. Continuous spinal anaesthesia was introduced by Lemmon in the USA in 1940. He left the spinal needle in situ (projecting through a gap in the operating table) and connected it to a length of rubber tubing through which repeated injections of procaine were made. In 1945, Tuohy described his needle for the insertion of a catheter into the subarachnoid space. This was adapted by Curbelo in 1949 to produce continuous lumbar block, although the first continuous epidural blocks are attributed to Hingson and Edwards, who used the caudal approach in 1942.

## The popularity and use of local anaesthesia.

Ever since Koller's original work, the popularity of local anaesthesia has waxed and waned, like that of many other medical developments. The announcement of his work produced a massive wave of enthusiasm, which was tempered as the problems of cocaine became appreciated. The first resurgence of interest came with the introduction of safer drugs at the beginning of the century, and the second as a result of the efforts of Labat, Lundy, Maxson, Odom and Pitkin in the USA in the years between the two World Wars.

In Britain, general anaesthesia has traditionally been administered by qualified doctors (though not always by specialists who practised anaesthesia exclusively). Because the conduct of general anaesthesia has been their entire responsibility, standards have usually been high. By contrast, local and regional techniques, if they were used at all, were performed by the surgeon, whose interest and attention were divided between anaesthetic and operation. Regional anaesthesia was not seen to best advantage under such circumstances. Nevertheless, when the examination for the Diploma in Anaesthesia was instituted in 1935, the curriculum included local anaesthesia. This, together with the establishment of anaesthesia as an independent speciality within the British National Health Service in 1948, did much to encourage local techniques.

Unfortunately, the years between 1950 and 1955 saw a sharp decrease in the use of local, particularly spinal, anaesthesia in Britain. The many advances in general anaesthesia then taking place were partly responsible, since they encouraged the belief that a local technique was unnecessary. More important though was the fear of severe neurological damage. The report entitled 'The grave spinal cord paralyses caused by spinal anesthesia ' written in 1950 in New York by a British-trained neurologist, Foster Kennedy (Kennedy et al 1950), was followed by the Woolley and Roe case (Cope 1954, Hutter 1990), and the use of local anaesthesia all but died out. That it did not do so entirely was due to anaesthetists such as Macintosh, Gillies, Massey Dawkins, Lee and Scott who were prepared to advocate, use and teach local techniques. Subsequently, many reports (Lee & Atkinson 1978) appeared describing very large numbers of cases without neurological sequelae, and local anaesthesia became re-established in British practice during the 1980s, although concerns about sequelae remain current.

There were more positive influences. The advantages of lidocaine and its derivatives – potent, predictable, heat-resistant and virtually free of allergic side-effects – should not be underestimated. The introduction of bupivacaine was particularly important because its long duration of action allows repeated injection with relatively little risk of cumulative toxicity. This was a major factor in the increased use of continuous epidural techniques in labour. Local techniques are very appropriate for the obstetric patient because they are effective and exert minimal effects on the child. Anaesthetists observing these benefits were encouraged to try them in other branches of practice, especially as they became aware that general anaesthesia cannot provide the ideal answer to every anaesthetic problem.

Local anaesthetic techniques are of value in blocking afferent stimuli even in very major surgery because of the reduction in the pain and stress suffered by the patient. This approach is now extending even to cardiac surgery, but the concept is far from new. As early as 1902, Harvey Cushing was advocating the combination of local with general anaesthesia to reduce surgical 'shock', a concept which was developed by Crile into 'Anoci-association'. The term 'balanced anaesthesia' is very common today, and implies a triad of sleep produced by either inhalational or intravenous route, profound analgesia with opioid drugs and muscle relaxation by neuromuscular block. In fact, when Lundy first used the term in 1926 he intended that the second and third parts of the triad would be produced by a local anaesthetic block.

There have been other advances which, although more difficult to quantify, have directly or indirectly helped the cause of local anaesthesia. For example, developments in the field of medical plastics have resulted in safe and reliable syringes, catheters and filters; and the anaesthetist can select from a wide variety of sedative and anxiolytic drugs which, carefully used, can greatly improve the patient's acceptance of a nerve block. Of great importance has been the understanding of the effects, and treatment, of sympathetic block. Ephedrine became available in 1924 and was first used to treat hypotension during spinal anaesthesia in 1927, but readily available intravenous fluids and equipment for their administration are more recent developments.

It is not inappropriate to conclude by mentioning the organisations which seek to promote the use of local anaesthetic techniques. The American Society of Regional Anesthesia was formed in 1975 and became firmly established. Its European counterpart is younger, but is now equally well established, and similar societies are flourishing in other parts of the world. The fundamental aim of them all is to ensure that properly managed local anaesthesia is an essential part of the armamentarium of the specialist anaesthetist.

## Further Reading

Rushman GB, 1999 Lee's synopsis of anaesthesia, 12th edn. Butterworth Heinemann, London

Ellis ES 1946 Ancient anodynes: primitive anaesthesia and allied conditions. Heinemann, London

Keys TE 1963 The history of surgical anesthesia, 2nd edn. Dover, New York

Liljestrand G 1971 The historical development of local anesthesia. International encyclopedia of pharmacology and therapeutics, vol 1, pp 1–38. Pergamon Press, Oxford

# References

Becker HK 1963 Carl Koller and cocaine. Psychoanalytic Quarterly 32: 309–373

Boulton TB 1984 Classical file. Survey of Anesthesiology 28: 150–152

Cope RW 1954 The Woolley and Roe case. Anaesthesia 9: 249–270

Faulconer A, Keys TE 1965 Foundations of anesthesiology, vol II, pp 769–845. Charles C Thomas, Springfield

Hutter CDD 1990 The Woolley and Roe case. A reassessment. Anaesthesia 45: 859–864

Kendig JJ, Courtney KR 1991 Editorial: New modes of nerve block. Anesthesiology 74: 207–208

Kennedy FG, Effron AS, Perry G 1950 The grave spinal cord paralyses caused by spinal anesthesia. Surgery, Gynecology and Obstetrics 91: 385–398

Koller C 1884 On the use of cocaine for producing anaesthesia of the eye. Lancet ii: 990–992

Lee JA, Atkinson RS 1978 Sir Robert Macintosh's lumbar puncture and spinal analgesia: intradural and extradural, 4th edn. pp 179–181. Churchill Livingstone, Edinburgh

Lofgren N 1948 Studies on local anesthetics: xylocaine, a new synthetic drug. Morin Press, Worcester [reprinted]

Richardson BW 1858 On local anaesthesia and electricity. Medical Times and Gazette i: 262–263

Simpson JY 1848 Local anaesthesia, notes on its production by chloroform etc in the lower animals, and in man. Lancet ii: 39–42

Wildsmith JAW 1983 Three Edinburgh men. Regional Anesthesia 8: 1–5

Wildsmith JAW 1984 Carl Koller (1857–1944) and the introduction of cocaine into anesthetic practice. Regional Anesthesia 9: 161–164

Wood A 1855 New method of treating neuralgia by the direct application of opiates to the painful points. Edinburgh Medical Journal 82: 265–281

# 2. The features of regional anaesthesia

## N B Scott and A R Absalom

Local and regional anaesthetic techniques have much to offer patients, surgeons and anaesthetists. The simplicity of administration of topical, infiltration and minor nerve block anaesthesia has ensured, and will continue to ensure, their popularity for casualty work, dentistry and minor surgery. General anaesthesia in these situations is usually unnecessary, and regional methods preserve consciousness and thus the patient's protective reflexes. Single-handed practitioners may be working in situations where there are limited resources for the purchase of expensive drugs and the maintenance of modern general anaesthetic equipment. They can perform a local block, observe its onset and then operate in relative safety. The lower cost of regional anaesthesia can be a considerable advantage in countries where health care is developing or facilities are limited.

Regional block has also been advocated as a means of avoiding the morbidity and mortality associated with general anaesthesia. It has been argued that this would not necessarily reduce the number of anaesthesia-related deaths, since unskilled use of spinals and epidurals might be at least as dangerous (Rosen 1981). However, complications of general anaesthesia such as failure to intubate the trachea and aspiration of gastric content are much more difficult to manage than hypotension of sympathetic origin, no matter how skilled the anaesthetist. The reduction in the number of maternal deaths due to 'anaesthetic' factors seen in both the UK and the USA with the progressive change to central nerve block for Caesarean section supports this analysis (Hawkins et al 1997, Reports on Confidential Enquiries, 1952 to 1998).

However, general anaesthesia tends to be preferred where there are the staff and facilities to provide it safely, but even where a high standard of care is available it is increasingly apparent that there are other reasons for using local blocks. Many of the minor sequelae and complications of general anaesthesia can be minimised or avoided altogether. The conditions required for a particular operation may be provided simply and without polypharmacy. There is an increasing body of evidence to show that the physiological 'stress' to which the patient is exposed during and immediately after surgery is considerably decreased by local anaesthesia. Neither general anaesthesia nor the opioids reduce significantly the endocrine response to surgery and trauma, whereas effective regional anaesthesia ablates it (Scott 1991). As a result the morbidity, and perhaps even the mortality, of anaesthesia and surgery have been reduced by the use of local blocks, even for major operations (see below).

This is not to deny that there are potential drawbacks to the wider use of local blocks by the specialist anaesthetist. One very practical objection is that they may prolong significantly the operation list. This may be true for the occasional and inexperienced user because the block may take longer to perform than the induction of general anaesthesia, and this is particularly true if the theatre staff are not familiar with the routine of these procedures. Such delays may be quite justifiable in the interests of a particular patient, but soon become unacceptable if lists are prolonged repeatedly. However, proficiency, speed of induction and success rate increase when blocks are practised regularly, and recovery time is usually decreased because the patient recovers consciousness rapidly and free of pain. If consecutive patients are to have local blocks it is possible, given the right circumstances (skilled assistance and careful planning), to save time by performing the second block while the first operation is being finished.

The major complications of regional anaesthesia are related to systemic toxicity; either from the injected drugs (the local anaesthetic and adjuvants such as a vasoconstrictor) or from the effects of the block itself. Drug toxicity is usually due to accidental intravascular injection or, more rarely, to the administration of an overdose. Both mishaps are avoidable. Careful technique and the correct choice of drug, concentration and volume should virtually eliminate them as causes of complications. Arterial hypotension due to sympathetic paralysis is the commonest 'systemic' effect of central blocks. Choice of an appropriate technique should minimise unwanted spread of local anaesthetic solution to the upper thoracic dermatomes, but if this should occur, or if it is necessary for a particular case, clear guidelines for management are available (see Chapter 8).

Hypotension is a good example of a feature of regional anaesthesia which is traditionally considered undesirable, but which can be an advantage during certain surgical procedures. Conversely, preservation of consciousness – commonly considered an advantage – may be unacceptable to the anxious patient undergoing anything more than the most minor procedure. When choosing an anaesthetic for a particular patient and operation, the anaesthetist should be able to assess the advantages and disadvantages of all techniques, local and general, and decide which is the most appropriate. The aim of this chapter is to suggest why, where, how and when local anaesthesia may be of benefit.

## Simplicity of administration

Local anaesthesia is a safe simple technique for the non-specialist anaesthetist undertaking relatively minor surgery. For the specialist involved with more major surgery, regional anaesthesia may also simplify the procedure. A single intrathecal injection of one drug will produce excellent conditions for many procedures – complete anaesthesia, muscle relaxation and a reduction in blood loss. The patient's life is less dependent on the proper functioning and constant monitoring of complex general anaesthetic equipment. Moreover, simplicity of administration means that the practitioner with a good knowledge of anatomy can easily become proficient in these methods.

The ease of administration, particularly of infiltration and topical anaesthesia, does produce problems. Minimal training or complacency may result in lack of awareness of, or an inability to treat, complications. Systemic toxicity due to drug overdosage, cardiorespiratory arrest due to poorly managed high spinal or epidural block, and pneumothorax after supraclavicular brachial plexus block are all potentially fatal complications. It is important to be aware that the combination of sympathetic block with even a minor degree of hypovolaemia (from whatever cause) will cause more hypotension than will general anaesthesia in the same circumstances. Thus, knowledge of the pharmacology of drugs, of the complications of the techniques to be used, and training in appropriate methods of resuscitation are essential.

## Preservation of consciousness

By its nature, uncomplicated regional anaesthesia will preserve consciousness, a desirable end in itself for the patient who wishes to remain awake. However, it is the avoidance of the secondary effects of unconsciousness that is important for the majority of patients. For example, the obstetric patient receiving regional analgesia is aware of her surroundings and the birth of her child, is able to maintain and protect her own airway and can co-operate with her attendant staff. There is also minimal fetal depression. These factors add up to a major argument for the use of local techniques.

The ability of the conscious patient to maintain and protect the airway and to co-operate is also of great value in dental practice, a field where airway obstruction during general anaesthesia is an ever present risk. Minor orthopaedic trauma is often dealt with under general anaesthesia, although it is recognised that gastric emptying is delayed in such patients. The majority of these injuries are peripheral and eminently suitable for local techniques.

In some circumstances general anaesthesia may be preferred even though the risk of pulmonary aspiration is high, as for example in emergency surgery for gastrointestinal obstruction. The general condition of these patients tends to be poor because of the effects of the obstruction, particularly dehydration leading to hypovolaemia, and the presence of intercurrent disease. If a spinal or an epidural is to be used, a block to the mid-thoracic region is required because the extent of surgery is unpredictable in this setting and blood loss may lead to severe hypotension. Nevertheless, an epidural sited at the time of surgery, but activated later when the patient's physiology has been stabilised, can be invaluable.

A conscious, co-operative patient is an advantage in other situations. Surgery for varicose veins on the back of the legs or for pilonidal sinus requires the patient to be prone. If a local technique is used, patients can help to position themselves, indicate that the position is comfortable and confirm that respiration is unimpeded. A spinal anaesthetic can be used very effectively, although a full understanding of the factors which influence block height is particularly important, so a solution which will not spread to the upper thoracic dermatomes is used. Treatment of a high block in a prone patient is difficult. Further, the conscious or lightly sedated patient may be able to warn of the subjective effects of complications at an early stage. The diabetic patient may recognise and report the initial symptoms of hypoglycaemia, and patient agitation or distress during transurethral surgery may arouse suspicion that bladder irrigation fluid has entered the circulation.

Most of the problems of regional anaesthesia due to preservation of consciousness relate to patients' anxiety about being aware during the performance of the block and the surgical procedure. The majority of British patients expect to be asleep and it is at least arguable that, although many European and North American patients expect to be awake during their operations, they might prefer to be asleep. To undergo major surgery under regional anaesthesia alone is an unpleasant experience and patients subjected to this may faint, *even* in the supine position. This may be mistaken for other causes of hypotension. Finally, because most operating tables are uncomfortable, the conscious patient may become restless and unable to remain still – one of the few situations where the surgeon may be justifiably upset by an anaesthetic technique.

Explanation and reassurance can help, but the more nervous the patient and the longer and more extensive the surgery, the greater is the need for some kind of sedation. Oral premedication is rarely contraindicated, and intravenous or inhalational sedation can both be used to produce amnesia while preserving the benefits of consciousness. However, some patients may be so frightened that they will not tolerate surgery with anything but complete loss of consciousness and then of course these benefits may be lost.

## Analgesia

The most outstanding advantage of even *single-shot* local anaesthetic techniques is the excellent analgesia (without central depression) which is produced. For the patient this means a period of complete postoperative analgesia during which the administration of oral or parenteral analgesics can be timed so that they become effective before the block wears off. This results in a gradual, rather than a sudden, awareness of pain and reduces the requirement for subsequent analgesic therapy. As a consequence, the side-effects of both opioids and non-steroidal anti-inflammatory drugs (NSAIDs) are reduced. For example, the use of caudal block for haemorrhoidectomy results not only in much greater patient comfort, but also in an earlier return of bowel function because of reduced opioid requirements (Berstock 1979).

*Catheter techniques* may be used to maintain analgesia after major surgery for as long as is necessary, and certainly until all painful procedures, such as surgical drain removal, have been completed. In practice, this may mean continuing the block for up to 5 days after surgery. Continuous epidural infusions make the post-operative period considerably less unpleasant and allow the patient to co-operate fully during nursing procedures, chest physiotherapy and mobilisation.

The analgesia produced by local blocks may also simplify certain general anaesthetics as well as providing greater comfort for the patient. This is best seen in surgery for a number of minor, but extremely painful, operations such as nail-bed ablation, distal orthopaedic procedures (e.g. Mitchell's osteotomy), Lord's anal dilatation and circumcision. Opioids are best avoided in ambulant patients because of their sedative and emetic effects. A local technique will provide very useful post-operative analgesia, even if the block is, in itself, insufficient for the surgery. A lighter plane of general anaesthesia can then be used, so recovery time is shorter and the patient can mobilise sooner.

## Sympathetic block

Until recently sympathetic block was widely considered to be a disadvantage of regional anaesthesia, but there is increasing evidence that it is beneficial, particularly after major surgery. Because of improved outcome in cardiac patients receiving β-adrenoceptor blocking agents, Roizen (1988) has advocated that they should be used routinely for surgery. Virtually all regional anaesthetic techniques produce sympathetic, as well as somatic, block so that many of the same effects are produced. The influence of these will depend not only on the site and level of the block, but also on the dose of local anaesthetic, the dose of vasoconstrictor (if used), the presence of intercurrent disease and the pre-existing state of the circulation. The detailed effects of sympathetic block produced by epidural injection have been reviewed by Bowler and colleagues (1988), but a sound knowledge of the autonomic control of the circulation (Mason 1965) is also needed because the balance between sympathetic and parasympathetic nerve activity is particularly important.

Before the effects of sympathetic block can be appreciated it is important to understand that increased sympathetic activity occurs after all types of surgical trauma. Organ dysfunction after surgery is to a large degree influenced by this increased activity and the pain which gives rise to it. However, a sympathetic response is inappropriate after elective surgery, because it is not a 'fight, flight or fright' situation, and the effects are largely deleterious.

### Pathophysiology of increased sympathetic activity

**Cardiovascular effects** The physiological effects of norepinephrine, epinephrine and dopamine on the heart and circulation are well known, but in summary, tachycardia and increased contractility both result in increased myocardial work and oxygen consumption. In the presence of increased systemic vascular resistance these may cause myocardial ischaemia and infarction, especially if there is pre-existing disease. Decreased organ blood flow, most notably to the liver and kidneys, may also result in ischaemia and cell necrosis. Epinephrine has been shown, in animal studies, to increase pulmonary arterio-venous admixture by producing non-uniform vasodilatation/constriction within the pulmonary vasculature. Both $\alpha$ and $\beta$ block can reduce this (Berk et al 1973, 1976). During cardiac catheterisation there is a close correlation between pulmonary vascular resistance and pulmonary artery catecholamine concentrations in the presence of pulmonary arterial hypertension. Local neurogenic stimuli have also been shown to contribute to the pulmonary platelet trapping seen in shock (Thorne et al 1980).

**Respiratory effects** For many years it has been known that reflexes mediated through sympathetic nerves result in substantial inhibition of normal breathing patterns, particularly after abdominal and thoracic procedures (Guenter 1984). Furthermore, studies have demonstrated that, even in the virtual or complete absence of pain, pulmonary function remains depressed for many days following surgery (Benhamou et al 1983). Among other factors known to influence pulmonary function are diaphragmatic contractility, abdominal distension,

secondary ileus, age, obesity, type of surgery and incision, personality, pre-existing lung disease, smoking habits, neuromuscular disease and muscle weakness, changes in thoracoabdominal blood volume and, of considerable importance, the position of the patient (Hedenstierna 1988).

Pain itself leads to a reduction in both static and dynamic lung parameters, most notably functional residual capacity (FRC) and peak flow rate (Craig 1981). Basal atelectasis occurs rapidly and results in hypoxia, hypercapnia and venous admixture. Pain also decreases tidal volume and the ability to breathe deeply and cough effectively (Bromage 1978). Thus secretions are retained and airways collapse so providing an ideal environment for sepsis. This further enhances the metabolic response to trauma, which in turn increases catecholamine synthesis.

**Gastrointestinal effects** Catecholamines have potentially harmful effects on gastrointestinal blood flow and function. In hypovolaemic states, splanchnic blood flow is greatly decreased and healing may be compromised in patients with gastrointestinal anastomoses (Tagart 1981). The gastrointestinal tract plays a central role in protein catabolism after injury (Wilmore 1983). Mucosal cell atrophy may occur secondary to ischaemia and hypoxia, resulting in breakdown of the gut barrier to micro-organisms and endotoxin, and further stimulating the glucocorticoid response and immunosuppression. Intestinal secretions and sphincter tone are increased, while motility is decreased. Gastric dilatation and paralytic ileus are believed to be caused by local sympathetic inhibitory reflexes both within the gut wall and the spinal cord (Hedenstierna 1988). A similar state occurs within the genitourinary tract resulting in acute retention of urine.

**Renal effects** The postoperative effects of circulating catecholamines, adrenergic stimulation, hypotension, hypoxia and the neuroendocrine response (i.e. renin, angiotensin II, aldosterone and antidiuretic hormone) on renal function are well recognised (Ganong 1985). In addition, enkephalins, kinins and prostaglandins $PGE_2$ and $PG_1$ (prostacyclin) have important vasodilator actions. $PGE_2$ is further stimulated by antidiuretic hormone, atrial natriuretic hormone and angiotensin II, making the overall extrinsic control of renal vessels complex. Although intrinsic autoregulation is more important than these extrinsic factors in maintaining renal blood flow, care must be taken in the postoperative period to maintain arterial blood pressure and minimise these effects.

***Metabolic effects*** Catecholamines, particularly epinephrine, promote the catabolic state, increasing blood sugar, plasma lactate and free fatty acid levels. In addition, epinephrine contributes to the retention of sodium and water and the excretion of potassium, while fluid shifts from the extracellular to vascular and intracellular compartments are also mediated partly by catecholamines. By inhibiting pancreatic release of insulin and antagonising its peripheral effects on glucose utilisation, epinephrine inhibits anabolism and promotes a negative nitrogen balance (Frayn 1986, Little & Frayn 1985, Wilmore et al 1988).

In addition to the catecholamines, several other substances are released in response to trauma, the most important being cortisol, glucagon, histamine and interleukin-1. Some of their actions may be beneficial, but they are also known to have potentially detrimental effects. In the presence of severe trauma or sepsis their actions can lead to rapid depletion of lean body mass and organ failure (Kehlet 1998). Although these changes are well documented, little is known about the trigger mechanisms. Pain is *not* one of them, but it will amplify the effects. In addition, haemorrhage, acidosis, hypoxia, infection, anxiety and heat loss further amplify the response (Kehlet 1998). Histamine, serotonin, bradykinin and substance P are released locally in response to nociceptive stimuli. Prostaglandins and interleukins can also modulate many of the observed responses (Dinarello 1984). However, in modern elective surgery where the contributions of the above should be minimal, afferent stimuli travelling through nociceptive and autonomic pathways play a predominant role.

***Immunofunction*** Current understanding of the mechanisms which initiate postoperative immunosuppression is poor, but the magnitude of the 'stress response' correlates directly with both serum cortisol and the degree of immunosuppression. Indeed this suppression has also been implicated in the formation of tumour metastases and postoperative sepsis. After tumour resection there is down-regulation of the cellular immune system, and T-helper lymphocytes are decreased, causing an imbalance between these and the suppressor lymphocytes (Hole & Bakke 1984). After major surgery both helper and suppressor cells are suppressed, and the numbers of circulating natural killer (NK) cells,

which have a wide range of cytotoxic activity particularly against tumour cells, are reduced also (Tonnesen et al 1984). Thus, cellular immunity is disturbed for up to 7 days postoperatively, and changes in the plasma concentrations of the mediators persist for much longer (Lennard et al 1985).

Histamine may initiate some of these changes because release of interleukin-II, itself pivotal in the activation of both lymphocyte subpopulations and humoral responses (Fletcher & Goldstein 1987), has been shown to involve the $H_2$ receptors present on macrophages (Beer & Rocklin 1987). Indeed, ranitidine has been shown to have beneficial effects on the postoperative decrease in delayed cutaneous hypersensitivity which is a manifestation of lymphocyte suppression (Nielsen 1989).

***Psychological effects*** Pain, while difficult to define, is readily understood by all who experience it, but its effects on the individual patient's psyche will be determined by many factors. These include race, religion, age, sex, social circumstance, upbringing, fear, anxiety and neurosis, time of day, marital status, the presence or absence of relatives and friends, the expectations of the patient prior to operation, and the nature, site and extent of the surgery performed. Philips and Cousins (1986) highlighted the need to relieve anxiety in the perioperative period and to maintain normal sleep patterns. Premedication with benzodiazepines, such as temazepam and lorazepam, is said to cause least disruption to sleep, which can be disturbed by many factors, especially pain, for up to 48 hours after surgery. Few would deny that the psychology of pain is largely neglected in the perioperative period. Various therapies have been used to reduce psychological trauma, particularly manipulating the placebo effect and patient counselling before and after surgery.

### Results of sympathetic block

***Cardiovascular system*** In supine, healthy volunteers block up to, and including, the upper thoracic segments may have remarkably little effect on arterial pressure. Cardiac output and limb and organ blood flow are maintained, or even increased. Studies in normovolaemic patients without pain tend to confirm this except that hypotension is more likely to be seen as the block extends above $T_5$, when the sympathetic innervation to the heart is interrupted. Peripheral flow is usually increased in spite of the hypotension.

When a block is performed in a patient in pain, cardiac output and arterial pressure decrease, but this is usually only to 'normal' levels because pain causes an increase in sympathetic activity. Sympathetic block may result in cardiovascular collapse in the sitting or hypo-volaemic patient, because the circulation has been maintained by the increased sympathetic activity. The patient with severe valvular heart disease may be less able to compensate for peripheral vasodilatation, because cardiac output may be relatively 'fixed'. Sympathetic block may also cause an unexpected degree of hypotension in the anxious patient, because the accompanying parasympathetic overactivity is then unopposed, and the patient simply faints.

The effects of an epidural block may be different from those of a spinal of similar extent. Very high systemic concentrations of local anaesthetic may be produced by the former and may contribute to circulatory depression, but it is usually considered that epidural block is less likely to cause hypotension. This may be because an epidural block usually spreads more slowly than a spinal so that there is more time for auto-compensation to occur. However, hypotension may be more marked when a local anaesthetic solution containing epinephrine is used for an epidural (Kennedy et al 1966) because the dose absorbed is only sufficient to produce β-adrenergic effects. A comparison of the cardiovascular effects of epidurals and spinals was carried out by Ward and colleagues (1965).

Moderate hypotension improves the surgical field and decreases blood loss by a combination of arterial *and* venous hypotension (Modig 1988). Even in the cardiac patient, a moderate degree of hypotension will improve performance because it is accompanied by reductions in preload, afterload and heart rate (Merin 1981). Thoracic epidural techniques have also been shown to improve endocardial blood flow (Klassen et al 1980). Sympathetic block produces an increase in lower limb blood (and arterial graft) flow and this may be partly responsible for the reduction in thrombo-embolic disease reported after regional anaesthesia (Thorburn et al 1980). This anti-thrombotic effect may also be related to a direct pharmacological action of the local anaesthetic drug on blood coagulability and fibrinolysis (Modig et al 1983a,b).

*Respiratory system* Sympathetically mediated reflexes result in substantial inhibition of normal breathing patterns for many days after surgery (Guenter 1984).

This may partially explain the beneficial effect of high spinal or epidural block on postoperative respiratory function (Spence & Smith 1971). However, these techniques also block the sympathetic supply to the lungs and airways. In theory, this may precipitate bronchospasm in the asthmatic patient because of un-opposed parasympathetic activity. In practice, few problems arise and, paradoxically, there are even reports of epidural block proving therapeutic in cases of status asthmaticus (Bromage 1978). Nevertheless, the anaesthetist must be aware of this possible complication. Bronchospasm may also develop during general anaesthesia, and regional anaesthesia may help prevent this complication by removing the need for airway instrumentation and by blocking afferent stimuli (both potent causes of reflex bronchospasm).

*Gastrointestinal system* Because of unopposed parasympathetic activity, sympathetic block leads to an increase in gastrointestinal motility and relaxation of many sphincters, although oesophageal sphincter tone is preserved (Thoren et al 1988). Large bowel incontinence is a theoretical consequence, but occurs no more often than during general anaesthesia. Bowel rupture may be more likely if there is an obstruction, and this is another reason why spinal and epidural blocks should be used with great caution, if at all, in such cases, and certainly not until the obstruction has been relieved. However, in elective bowel surgery regional anaesthesia has very definite benefits (Aitkenhead 1984). The sympathetic block may increase colonic blood flow (Johansson et al 1988), and use of a regional technique to provide muscle relaxation avoids the need to administer neostigmine, which may increase the incidence of anastomotic breakdown. However, if neostigmine is used to reverse neuromuscular block in a patient who also has a central nerve block, atropine, if given well in advance, reduces bowel motility.

If the block is continued into the postoperative period, distension and anastomotic leakage secondary to opioid-induced ileus can be minimised.

## The neuroendocrine response

Physiological measurements have indicated that the metabolic and hormonal changes which have been noted when surgery is performed under general anaesthesia are reduced when regional techniques are employed. General anaesthesia does not, in itself, seem to induce a 'stress response' and the evidence suggests that the trauma of surgery is responsible for most of the changes observed.

These changes include an increased rate of catabolism, a negative nitrogen balance and salt and water retention. Plasma levels of cortisol, glucose, catecholamines and antidiuretic hormone increase soon after the start of surgery (Gordon et al 1973), and the increases are maintained well into the postoperative period. In clean, uncontaminated surgery the response is generated by noxious stimuli being transmitted from the operative site to the central nervous system. The part played by somatic and sympathetic afferent, and by sympathetic efferent, impulses to the pancreas and adrenal medulla in the generation of the response has long been appreciated. More recently, it has been recognised that humoral factors, such as the interleukins and tumour necrosis factor, are also involved. General anaesthesia may do little more than reduce the response intraoperatively (Roizen et al 1981).

Complete block can be achieved more easily for many types of surgery with local anaesthetic techniques. The reduction in response has been shown most convincingly during and after lower abdominal surgery and the effect is more marked if the regional block extends from $T_4$ to $S_5$ (Engquist et al 1977). During upper abdominal surgery, epidural block, even when combined with vagal nerve block, may be insufficient to prevent some rise in the plasma levels of stress-related hormones (Traynor et al 1982). After cardiac surgery the catecholamine response is completely obtunded by continuous thoracic epidural analgesia.

## The immune response

Changes in immunocompetence parallel the endocrine response which follows major surgery, and they have been implicated in the formation of tumour metastases and postoperative sepsis (Lennard et al 1985). The changes involve non-specific humoral and cellular elements, are proportional to the degree of 'trauma', are unaffected by general anaesthesia and may be exacerbated by opioids (Scott 1991). Specific indicators have been studied: after major surgery depression of lymphocyte transformation has been shown to be reduced by regional anaesthesia (Cullen & van Belle 1975); and the ratio of 'T' helper 1 to 'T' helper 2 cells was higher after transurethral resection of the prostate under spinal compared to general anaesthesia (LeCras et al 1998).

These findings suggest that use of central blocks may result in less immunosuppression, but, as with hormonal and metabolic changes, there is still relatively little objective evidence to indicate whether such effects influence outcome. Even if the patient does benefit it must be remembered that a very extensive block is required when major surgery is performed, and that it must be continued well into the postoperative period. Unless this is so, the changes seen will be the same as if no block had been used.

## Muscle relaxation

Local techniques produce motor as well as sensory block. This means that for the majority of patients undergoing even major surgery the need to use muscle relaxants is virtually abolished, thereby avoiding all their side-effects and the risk of developing postoperative pulmonary complications (Berg et al 1997). The muscle relaxation which results from regional anaesthesia has the specific advantage of being confined to the operative field (unlike that due to neuromuscular-blocking drugs), so the patient can continue to breathe spontaneously. Spinal and epidural block may result in impairment of the nerve supply to some respiratory muscles, but unless a very high block is produced this is of little clinical consequence. Blocks to the level normally required for abdominal surgery produce only a slight decrease in expiratory reserve volume and expulsive ability (Bowler et al 1988). However, these latter effects may be more important in patients with respiratory disease, although the effect of the block in preventing pain and reducing the requirement for opioid drugs will more than compensate for any decrease in muscle power. The latter will in any case be minimised by careful choice of local anaesthetic and use of an appropriate concentration.

Weakness of the legs may be relatively prolonged after spinal anaesthesia, because the highest concentration of local anaesthetic in the cerebrospinal fluid will be around the lumbar and sacral nerve roots. Provided patients are warned in advance that motor block is likely, they should not become very concerned about it, although some patients may prefer an alternative, albeit less effective, analgesic technique which preserves more motor power and mobility than an epidural infusion of local anaesthetic.

## Side-effects and sequelae

In addition to its effect on postoperative pain, regional anaesthesia may also reduce the incidence of other less major sequelae of anaesthesia and surgery, although freedom from wound pain may make the patient more aware of other sources of discomfort such as a venepuncture site or a nasogastric tube. Few controlled studies have been performed of the relative incidence of these sequelae, but Table 2.1 shows data from two reasonably comparable groups of patients having surgery with either spinal or general anaesthesia. All but one of the symptoms occurred less frequently after spinal anaesthesia, the exception being headache, although the proportion of patients who graded this as 'severe' was the same in each group.

**Table 2.1** Total incidence (%) of minor postoperative complications after spinal and general anaesthesia (from Dempster 1984). The incidence of complications graded 'severe' by the patient is also shown

| Complications | Spinal anaesthesia | | General anaesthesia | |
|---|---|---|---|---|
| | Total | Severe | Total | Severe |
| Nausea | 9 | 0 | 40 | 6 |
| Vomiting | 15 | 2 | 43 | 6 |
| Headache | 34 | 6 | 23 | 6 |
| Sore throat | 2 | 0 | 30 | 0 |
| Muscle pains | 4 | 0 | 9 | 0 |
| Backache | 28 | 2 | 32 | 6 |
| Urinary difficulty | 6 | 0 | 30 | 0 |

However, Lanz and colleagues (1982) have suggested that differences in minor sequelae are not quite so clearly in favour of regional anaesthesia, although in their study the patient was responsible for the choice of anaesthetic technique. Patients who have suffered severe nausea and vomiting after previous general anaesthetics are particularly appreciative of regional techniques which minimise the requirement for opioids. However, no method can prevent certain patients from reacting to the psychological stress of surgery by becoming nauseated or even vomiting, particularly if they are given little in the way of perioperative sedation. Untreated hypotension and bradycardia are themselves potent causes of nausea and vomiting during central blocks.

In addition, there are some disadvantages to the extension of the effects of these techniques into the postoperative period. Some patients find prolonged lack of feeling, especially in the legs, unpleasant and urinary retention may occur, notably if large volumes of intravenous fluids have been used in an attempt to maintain blood pressure. A high standard of medical and nursing care will minimise these complications and in the obstetric unit the staff/patient ratio is high enough for this to be provided. In the general ward the routine use of continuous epidurals requires careful appraisal of the staff available.

Finally, there will always be concern about the major sequelae of continuous blocks such as haematoma and abscess formation (see Chapter 8). In a review of 505 000 obstetric epidurals there were two cases of epidural haematoma and one abscess, with two of the patients suffering permanent sequelae (Scott & Hibbard 1990). Only constant vigilance and early diagnosis and treatment can minimise the effects on the patient.

## Effect on morbidity and mortality

Given the beneficial effects of regional anaesthesia in controlling pain, suppressing adverse cardiovascular reflexes, reducing pulmonary dysfunction and minimising the factors contributing to thromboembolic disease, it is reasonable to expect a consequent decrease in the incidence of some of the major complications of surgery. In an attempt to show whether the clear physiological benefits translate into a demonstrable effect on outcome, a large number of workers have studied a variety of its aspects. This work has been reviewed in detail by Kehlet (1994) and is summarised below.

*Cardiac morbidity* A number of studies, mostly in relatively healthy patients, have shown a statistically insignificant reduction in the incidence of ischaemic electrocardiographic changes with regional anaesthesia compared to general anaesthesia. More positive results have been obtained in higher risk patients. Reiz and colleagues (1982) found that epidural block resulted in significantly better intraoperative stability than general anaesthesia in patients undergoing major vascular surgery within 3 months of a myocardial infarction, and Yeager and colleagues (1987) found that the incidence of cardiovascular failure after major surgery in high-risk patients was reduced. Subsequent, larger studies failed to show such clear-cut benefits, but a recent overview has concluded that there is growing evidence of better outcome when regional anaesthesia and analgesia are used (Buggy & Smith 1999).

*Pulmonary morbidity* Regional anaesthesia has long been known to reduce the degree of both pulmonary dysfunction (Spence & Smith 1971) and hypoxia (McKenzie et al 1980) after surgery. These effects are presumably produced by the reduced incidence of atelectasis shown in a number of studies (Kehlet 1994). However, the significance of atelectasis as such is questionable, the important postoperative complication being infection. More recently three studies have shown that the incidence of infection is reduced (Cushieri et al 1985, Cook et al 1986, Yeager et al 1987). A meta-analysis of all published studies has shown a clear and important advantage of regional anaesthesia in reducing pulmonary morbidity (Ahn et al 1986).

*Gastrointestinal morbidity* The effects of regional anaesthesia, or perhaps of the reduction in use of drugs such as neostigmine and morphine, on the minor sequelae of surgery have been considered above. The same factors might be expected to influence more major complications, and the duration of ileus after both hysterectomy (Ahn et al 1986) and colonic surgery (Thoren et al 1988) has been shown to be reduced. A more recent study confirmed the more prompt return of gastrointestinal function after colonic resection using regional anaesthesia (Liu et al 1995). There is also some retrospective evidence that regional anaesthesia may decrease the incidence of breakdown of bowel anastomoses (Aitkenhead et al 1978), although a follow-up prospective study did not confirm this (Worsley et al 1988).

*Blood loss* Although spinal anaesthesia was one of the earlier techniques of induced hypotension, the relationship between blood pressure and blood loss is far from clear. Notably, it has been shown that artificial maintenance of blood pressure does not increase blood loss (Thorburn 1985), and other studies have suggested that the main effect of the blocks is to diminish venous oozing (Modig 1988). Controlled studies show that a consistent decrease in bleeding with regional anaesthesia occurs, but that the effect is only statistically significant in surgery to the lower half of the body (Scott 1991).

*Thromboembolism* A large number of studies have now shown that regional anaesthesia has a significant impact on the incidence of thromboembolic complications of surgery to the lower half of the body. Fewer studies have been performed on patients undergoing surgery to the upper half of the body and they have tended to show that regional anaesthesia makes little difference. However, one study did find that epidural block was as effective as low-dose heparin (Hjortso et al 1985).

*Convalescence* By controlling pain, regional anaesthesia has a profound effect on well-being and ease of mobilisation in the early postoperative period. As a result, Yeager and colleagues (1987) were able to show a marked reduction in the duration of intensive care after major surgery in high-risk patients. There is now growing support for the early ambulation and enteral feeding of patients and the need to reduce the use of surgical drains, which hinder patient mobility. The use of regional anaesthesia may also influence events later in the postoperative period and even decrease the length of hospital stay, although statistically significant data to support this view have yet to be published.

*Regional versus general anaesthesia* In 1988, Scott and Kehlet reviewed the then current data from controlled clinical studies comparing the morbidity of surgery performed under regional or general anaesthesia. They found good statistical support for the use of regional anaesthesia for procedures below the umbilicus, but the choice between regional and general anaesthesia did not seem to have a clear influence on the outcome of surgery above that level. The study performed by Yeager and colleagues (1987) provided statistically significant evidence in favour of regional anaesthesia in more extensive surgery and the later work of Tuman and colleagues (1991) confirmed this. Although subsequent studies have not always produced such definitive support (Buggy & Smith 1999), the meta-analysis carried out by Rodgers and colleagues (2000) showed a decrease in early morbidity and mortality in favour of regional anaesthesia (see Ch. 20).

There are several reasons why it is more difficult to demonstrate objectively the benefits of regional anaesthesia in more extensive surgery. It is more difficult to block completely the neuroendocrine response to such surgery: this requires a very extensive block, which introduces potential risks. Because of concerns about these risks, many previous workers may not have provided a block which was extensive or profound enough, or may not have continued it for long enough. It is, none the less, worth noting that no study has found regional anaesthesia to cause *more* morbidity than general anaesthesia. The benefits of regional anaesthesia may be easier to demonstrate when the advantages which it confers (e.g. early mobilisation and oral feeding) become a routine part of postoperative care (Kehlet 1994).

However, it must be recognised that regional procedures are associated with the risk of certain complications that would not occur if 'traditional' methods of anaesthesia and analgesia were used. It may be argued that these complications are very often the result of a failure of proper care, but this only serves to emphasise that clinicians must learn how to perform and manage regional anaesthesia properly if the potential benefits are to accrue to the patient (Wildsmith 1990). It does seem that there is benefit to be gained, but more data are needed (Buggy & Smith 1999). However, randomised comparisons may not be the most appropriate way to generate such data (Wildsmith 1999).

## Benefits to the anaesthetist

A most important benefit to the specialty as a whole is the way in which local techniques have enabled anaesthetists to extend their practice beyond the operating theatre. The provision of epidural services in the labour wards and the staffing of chronic pain clinics are two good examples, and the wider use of these methods in the management of acute pain is an area of continuing interest. An additional benefit of these activities is that the anaesthetist maintains and improves both communication skills and, perhaps more importantly, professional identity with the patient.

The anaesthetist who is prepared to learn and practise regional anaesthesia has a larger armamentarium with which to deal with the many clinical problems which present in routine practice. Those who use these methods successfully obtain considerable satisfaction, not only from the technical skill required, but also from the benefits which accrue to their patients, particularly in the period immediately after surgery. If, by the use of a single technique, it is possible to offer complete neural block which results in control of pain, abolition of the stress response, efferent sympathetic block with increased regional blood flow, early ambulation, DVT prophylaxis, reduced susceptibility to infection, and reductions in nausea and vomiting, respiratory depression and hypoxia, then such a technique should be more expertly taught and more widely advocated. At the same time significant efforts should be made to overcome its avoidable side-effects. Today, neural block makes it possible to provide a quality of recovery and convalescence after major surgery which was undreamed of a decade or more ago.

## Further Reading

Hall GM 1985 The anaesthetic modification of the endocrine and metabolic response to surgery. Annals of the Royal College of Surgeons of England 67: 25–29

Kehlet H 1994 Post-operative pain relief – what is the issue? British Journal of Anaesthesia 72: 375–378

Scott NB 1991 The effects of pain and its treatment. In: McClure JH, Wildsmith JAW (eds). Mechanisms and management of conduction blockade for postoperative analgesia, pp 78–110. Arnold, London

## References

Ahn H, Lindhagen J, Bronge A, Ygge H 1986 The effect of postoperative epidural local anaesthetics on gastrointestinal motility. Proceedings of the 5th Annual Meeting, Malmö, Sweden. European Society of Regional Anaesthesia [abstract]

Aitkenhead AR 1984 Anaesthesia and bowel surgery. British Journal of Anaesthesia 56: 95–101

Aitkenhead AR, Wishart HY, Peebles-Brown DA 1978 High spinal nerve block for large bowel anastomosis: a retrospective study. British Journal of Anaesthesia 50: 177–183

Ballantyne JC, Carr DB, deFerranti S, Suarez T, Lau J, Chalmers TC, Angelillo IF, Masteller F 1998 The comparative effects of postoperative analgesic therapies on pulmonary outcome: cumulative meta-analyses of randomized, controlled trials. Anesthesia and Analgesia 86: 598–612

Beer DJ, Rocklin RE 1987 Histamine-induced suppressor-cell activity. Journal of Allergy and Clinical Immunology 72: 439–452

Benhamou D, Samii K, Noviant Y 1983 Effect of analgesia on respiratory muscle function after upper abdominal surgery. Acta Anaesthesiologica Scandinavica 27: 22–25

Berg H, Viby-Mogensen J, Roed J, Mortensen CR, Engbaek J, Skovgaard LT, Krintel JJ 1997 Residual neuromuscular block is a risk factor for postoperative pulmonary complications. A prospective, randomised, and blinded study of postoperative pulmonary complications after atracurium, vecuronium and pancuronium. Acta Anaesthesiologica Scandinavica 41: 1095–1103

Berk JL, Hagen JF, Koo R 1973 Pulmonary insufficiency caused by epinephrine. Annals of Surgery 178: 423–434

Berk JL, Hagan JF, Koo R 1976 Effect of alpha and beta adrenergic blockade on epinephrine induced pulmonary insufficiency. Annals of Surgery 183: 369–376

Berstock DA 1979. Haemorrhoidectomy without tears. Annals of the Royal College of Surgeons of England 61: 51–54

Bowler GMR, Wildsmith JAW, Scott DB 1988 Epidural administration of anesthetics. Clinics in Critical Care Medicine: acute pain management 8: 187–235

Bromage PR 1978 Epidural analgesia. WB Saunders, Philadelphia

Buggy DJ, Smith G 1999 Editorial: Epidural anaesthesia and analgesia: better outcome after major surgery? Growing evidence suggests so. British Medical Journal 319: 530–531

Cook PT, Davis MJ, Cronin KD, Moran P 1986 A prospective randomised trial comparing spinal anaesthesia using hyperbaric cinchocaine with general anaesthesia for lower limb vascular surgery. Journal of Anaesthesia and Intensive Care 14: 373–380

Craig DB 1981 Postoperative recovery of pulmonary function Anesthesia and Analgesia. 60: 46–52

Cullen BF, van Belle G 1975 Lymphocyte transformation and changes in leukocyte count: effects of anesthesia and operation. Anesthesiology 43: 563–569

Cushieri RJ, Morran CG, Howie JC, McArdle CS 1985 Post-operative pain and pulmonary complications: comparison of three analgesic regimes. British Journal of Surgery 72: 495–498

Dempster S 1984 The sequelae of spinal analgesia as opposed to general anaesthesia. Undergraduate prize essay: Association of Anaesthetists of Great Britain and Ireland.

Dinarello CA 1984 Interleukin-l. Reviews of Infectious Diseases 6: 51–94

Engquist A, Brandt MR, Fernandes A, Kehlet H 1977 The blocking effect of epidural anaesthesia on the adrenocortical responses to surgery. Acta Anaesthesiologica Scandinavica 21: 330–335

Fletcher M, Goldstein AL 1987 Recent advances in the understanding of the biochemistry and clinical pharmacology of interleukin-2. Lymphokine Research 6: 45–57

Frayn KN 1986 Hormonal control of metabolism in trauma and sepsis. Clinical Endocrinology 24: 577–599

Ganong WF 1985 Review of Medical Physiology, 12th edn. Lange Medical Publications, Los Altros, California

Gordon NH, Scott DB, Percy-Robb IW 1973 Modification of plasma corticosteroid concentrations during and after surgery by epidural blockade. British Medical Journal 1(853): 581–583

Guenter CA 1984 Toward prevention of postoperative pulmonary complications. American Review of Respiratory Diseases 130: 4–5

Hawkins JL, Koonin LM, Palmar SK, Gibbs CP 1997 Anesthesia-related deaths during obstetric delivery in the United States, 1979–1990. Anesthesiology 86: 277–284

Hedenstierna G 1988 Mechanisms of postoperative pulmonary dysfunction. Acta Chirurgica Scandinavica Supplement 550: 152–158

Hjortso NC, Andersen T, Frosig F 1985 A controlled study of the effect of epidural analgesia with local anaesthetics and morphine on morbidity after abdominal surgery. Acta Anesthesiologica Scandinavica 29: 790.

Hole A, Bakke O 1984 T-lymphocytes and the subpopulations of T-helper and T-suppressor cells measured by monoclonal antibodies (T11, T4 and T8) in relation to surgery under epidural and general anaesthesia. Acta Anaesthesiologica Scandinavica 28: 296–300

Johansson K, Ahn H, Lindhagen J, Tryselius U 1988 Effect of epidural anaesthesia on intestinal blood flow. British Journal of Surgery 75: 73–76

Kehlet H 1994 Post-operative pain relief – what is the issue? British Journal of Anaesthesia 72: 375–378

Kehlet H 1998 Modification of responses to surgery by neural blockade: clinical implications. In: Cousins MJ, Bridenbaugh PO (eds). Neural blockade in clinical anesthesia and management of pain, 3rd edn, pp129–178. Lippincott-Raven, Philadelphia

Kennedy WF, Bonica JJ, Ward RJ, Tolas AG, Martin WE, Grinstein A 1966 Cardiorespiratory effects of epinephrine when used in regional anesthesia. Acta Anaesthesiologica Scandinavica Supplement 26: 320–333

Klassen GA, Bramwell RS, Bromage PR, Zborowska-Sluis D 1980 Effect of acute sympathectomy by epidural anesthesia on the canine coronary circulation. Anesthesiology 52: 8–15

Lanz E, Theiss D, Emmerich EA, Emmerich M 1982 Regional versus general anaesthesia: attitudes and experiences of patients. Regional Anaesthesia 7: S163–171

LeCras AE, Galley HF, Webster NR 1998 Spinal but not general anesthesia increases the ratio of T helper 1 to T helper 2 cell subsets in patients undergoing transurethral resection of the prostate. Anesthesia and Analgesia 87: 1421–1425

Lennard TW, Shenton BK, Bortotta A, Donnelly PK, White M, Gerrie LM, Proud G, Taylor RM 1985 The influence of surgical operation on components of the immune system. British Journal of Surgery 72: 771–776

Little RA, Frayn KN (eds) 1985 The scientific basis for the care of the critically ill. Manchester University Press, Manchester

Liu S, Carpenter RL, Mackey DC, Thirlby RC, Rupp SM, Shine TSJ, Feinglass NG, Metzger PP, Fulmer JT 1995 Effects of perioperative analgesic technique on rate of recovery after colon surgery. Anesthesiology 83: 757–765

McKenzie PJ, Wishart HY, Dewar KMS, Gray I, Smith G 1980 Comparison of the effects of spinal anaesthesia and general anaesthesia on postoperative oxygenation and perioperative mortality. British Journal of Anaesthesia 52: 49–53

Mason DT 1965 The autonomic nervous system and regulation of cardiovascular performance. Anesthesiology 29: 670–680

Merin RG 1981 Local and regional anesthetic techniques for the patient with ischaemic heart disease. Cleveland Clinic Quarterly 48: 72–74

Modig J 1988 Beneficial effects on blood loss in total hip replacement when performed under lumbar epidural anaesthesia versus general anaesthesia: an exploratory study. Acta Chirurgica Scandinavica Supplement 550: 95–103

Modig J, Borg T, Bagge L, Saldeen T 1983a Role of extradural and of general anaesthesia in fibrinolysis and coagulation after total hip replacement. British Journal of Anaesthesia 55: 625–629

Modig J, Borg T, Karlstrom G, Maripuu E, Sahlstedt B 1983b Thromboembolism after total hip replacement: role of epidural and general anesthesia. Anesthesia and Analgesia 62:174–180

Nielsen HJ 1989 Ranitidine for prevention of postoperative suppression of delayed hypersensitivity. American Journal of Surgery 157: 291–294

Philips GD, Cousins MJ 1986 Neurological mechanisms of pain and the relationship of pain anxiety and sleep. In: Cousins MJ, Philips GD (eds) Acute pain management, pp 21–48 Churchill Livingstone, Melbourne

Reiz S, Balfors E, Sorensen MB, Haggenmark S, Nyhman H 1982 Coronary hemodynamic effects of general anesthesia and surgery. Modification by epidural analgesia in patients with ischemic heart disease. Regional Anesthesia 7: S8–S18

Reports on Confidential Enquiries into Maternal Deaths in England and Wales 1952–54 (1957); 1955–57 (1960); 1958–60 (1963); 1961–63 (1966); 1964–66 (1969); 1967–69 (1972); 1970–72 (1975); 1973–75 (1979); 1976–78 (1982); 1979–81 (1986); 1982–84 (1989); 1985–87 (1991); 1988–90 (1994); 1991–93 (1996); 1994–96 'Why Mothers Die' (1998). HMSO & TSO

Reports on Confidential Enquiries into Maternal Deaths in the United Kingdom, 1985–87 (1991); 1988–90 (1994); 1991–93 (1996); 1994–96 (1998). HMSO & TSO

Rodgers A, Walker N, Schug S, McKee A, Kehlet H, van Zundert A, Sage D, Futter M, Savuille G, Clark T, MacMahon S 2000 Reduction of postoperative mortality with epidural or spinal anaesthesia: results from overview of randomised trials. British Medical Journal 321: 1493–1497

Roizen MF 1988 Should we all have a sympathectomy at birth? Or at least preoperatively? Anesthesiology 68: 482–484

Roizen MF, Horrigan RW, Frazer BM 1981 Anesthetic doses blocking adrenergic (stress) and cardiovascular responses to incision – MAC BAR. Anesthesiology 54: 390–398

Rosen M 1981 Editorial comment. Anaesthesia 36: 36–37

Scheinin B, Asantila R, Orko R 1987 The effect of bupivacaine and morphine on pain and bowel function after colonic surgery. Acta Anaesthesiologica Scandinavica 31: 161–164

Scott DB, Hibbard BM 1990 Serious non-fatal complications associated with extradural block in obstetric practice. British Journal of Anaesthesia 64: 547–541

Scott NB 1991 The effects of pain and its treatment. In: McClure JH, Wildsmith JAW (eds) Mechanisms and management of conduction blockade for postoperative analgesia, pp 78–110. Arnold, London

Scott NB, Kehlet H 1988 Regional anaesthesia and surgical morbidity. British Journal of Surgery 75: 299–304

Spence AA, Smith G 1971 Postoperative analgesia and lung function: a comparison of morphine with extradural block. British Journal of Anaesthesia 43: 144–148

Tagart REB 1981 Colorectal anastomosis: factors influencing success. Journal of the Royal Society of Medicine 74: 111–118

Thorburn J 1985 Subarachnoid blockade and total hip replacement: effect of ephedrine on intraoperative blood loss. British Journal of Anaesthesia 57: 290–293

Thorburn J, Louden JR, Vallance R 1980 Spinal and general anaesthesia in total hip replacement: frequency of deep vein thrombosis. British Journal of Anaesthesia 52: 1117–1121

Thoren T, Carlsson E, Sandmark S, Watwil M 1988 Effects of thoracic epidural analgesia with morphine or bupivacaine on lower oesophageal sphincter pressure: an experimental study in man. Acta Anaesthesiologica Scandinavica 32: 391–394

Thorne LJ, Kuenzig M, McDonald HM, Schwartz SI 1980 Effect of denervation of a lung on pulmonary platelet trapping associated with traumatic shock. Surgery 88: 208–214

Tonnesen E, Huttel MS, Christensen NJ, Schmitz O 1984 Natural killer cell activity in patients undergoing upper abdominal surgery: relationship to the endocrine stress response. Acta Anaesthesiologica Scandinavica 28: 654–660

Traynor C, Paterson JL, Ward ID, Morgan M, Hall GM 1982 Effects of extradural analgesia and vagal blockade on the metabolic and endocrine response to upper abdominal surgery. British Journal of Anaesthesia 54: 319–323

Tuman KJ, McCarthy RJ, March R, Ivankovich D 1991 Epidural anesthesia/analgesia improves outcome after major vascular surgery: a hypothesis reconfirmed. Anesthesia and Analgesia 72: S302

Ward RJ, Bonica JJ, Freund FG, Akamatsu TJ, Danziger F, Engelson S 1965 Epidural and subarachnoid anesthesia: cardiovascular and respiratory effects. Journal of the American Medical Association 191: 275–278

Wildsmith JAW 1990 Regional anaesthesia must be properly managed. Anaesthesia 45: 984

Wildsmith JAW 1999 Correspondence: Regional anaesthesia for carotid endarterectomy. British Journal of Anaesthesia 83: 688

Wilmore DW 1983 Alterations in protein, carbohydrate and fat metabolism in injured and septic patients. Journal of the American College of Nutrition 2: 3–13

Wilmore DW, Smith RJ, O'Dwyer ST, Jacobs DO, Ziegler TR, Wang XD 1988 The Gut: a central organ after surgical stress. Surgery 104: 917–923

Worsley MH, Wishart HY, Peebles-Brown DA, Aitkenhead AR 1988 High spinal nerve block for large bowel anastomosis. A prospective study. British Journal of Anaesthesia 60: 836–840

Yeager MP, Glass DD, Neff RK, Brinck-Johnsen T 1987 Epidural anesthesia and analgesia in high-risk surgical patients. Anesthesiology 66: 729–736

# 3. Anatomy and physiology of pain

## L A Colvin and J H McClure

Pain is defined by the International Association for the Study of Pain (1986) as '*an unpleasant sensory and emotional experience associated with actual or potential tissue damage, or described in terms of such damage*', and so it encompasses much more than the simple reflex response to a noxious stimulus. Sensory impulses arising from noxious stimuli undergo considerable processing at all levels in the central nervous system before finally resulting in the conscious perception of pain. In the biological situation pain prevents further damage by leading to the removal of injured tissue from the stimulus, and promotes wound healing by discouraging movement. This type of pain has been termed *physiological* because it serves a purpose (Woolf 1989). However, in some situations pain may persist for much longer than would be expected from the severity of the original injury so that it actually interferes with recovery of function. Abnormal processes may result in long-term alterations in the central response to peripheral stimuli, so that conventional treatment is no longer effective. This chronic syndrome has been termed *pathological* pain (Woolf 1995), and any consideration of pain physiology must explain how such changes occur.

Even relatively modern views, such as Melzack and Wall's *Gate control theory of pain* (Nathan, 1976), assumed a system with fixed neuronal connections (a 'hard-wired' system) which conducted impulses directly from the periphery to the brain. The theory recognised that some modulation of the original input could occur in both the spinal cord and brain, but it is now known that the actual situation is even more complex with functional, and even anatomical, changes occurring in neurones in response to pain. Prolonged stimulation, particularly, can induce alterations in neuronal phenotype, with 'up' or 'down' regulation of a variety of genes leading to changes in the type and pattern of neurotransmitter release, altered neuronal response characteristics and recruitment of previously inactive neurones. Both peripheral and central nervous systems may respond to noxious stimuli in the environment by changing their connections, and nerve fibres in both systems can 'sprout' to make new ones – the phenomenon of *plasticity* (Besson & Chaouch 1987).

Fibres involved in the transmission of pain have long been known to project widely and, in turn, to receive multiple inputs. The phenomenon of plasticity means that these can be changing all the time. As a result, there is no single pain pathway because the system is actually very complex. However, it is possible to outline the basic components of the systems involved in the transmission and modulation of pain (Fig. 3.1), and to recognise functional components within these:

1. The primary afferent neurones in the peripheral nerves.
2. Signal transduction by neurotransmitters in the spinal cord.
3. Modulation by supraspinal systems.
4. Peripheral and central sensitisation mechanisms.

## THE PERIPHERAL NERVES

A peripheral nerve may contain any combination of sensory (primary afferent), motor and autonomic fibres, the exact anatomical arrangement depending on the particular nerve. For example, the femoral nerve contains fibres serving all three broad functions, but its most distal continuation, the saphenous nerve, contains mainly sensory fibres (Willis & Coggeshall 1991). If a mixed peripheral nerve is stimulated adequately, an electrode placed some distance away will record the resulting electrical activity (Fig. 3.2). The latencies of the various peaks in this *compound action potential* indicate the

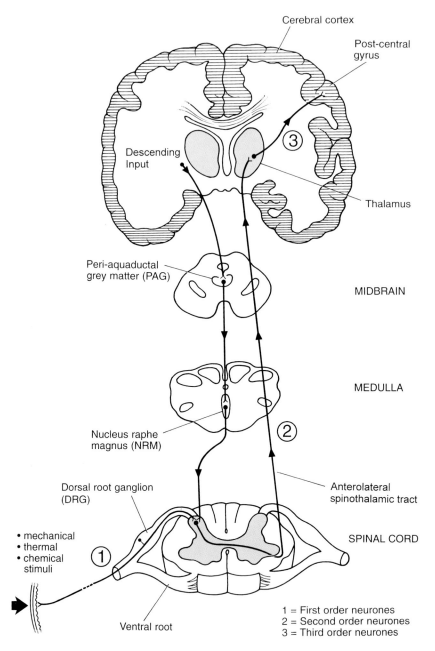

**Fig 3.1** An outline of the pain pathway

conduction velocities of the different fibre types, and the amplitudes of those peaks relate to the number of fibres of that type. Several classifications of nerve fibres have been proposed, but the one most commonly used relates the function subserved by the fibre, and to its diameter and conduction velocity (Table 3.1).

The physical structure of peripheral nerve, the physiology of axonal conduction and the pharmacology of its block are considered in Chapter 4.

## Nerve distribution

Specific segmental nerves are formed in the vertebral canal by the joining of dorsal (sensory) and ventral

**Table 3.1** Classification of nerve fibres. (Adapted from Erlanger & Gasser 1937)

| Fibre type | Function | Diameter (μm) | Conduction velocity (m s⁻¹) |
|---|---|---|---|
| **Large, myelinated**<br>Aα | Proprioception, motor | 12–20 | 70–120 |
| Aβ | Light touch, pressure | 5–12 | 30–70 |
| Aγ | Motor to muscle spindles | 3–6 | 15–30 |
| **Small, myelinated**<br>Aδ | *Pain*, cold, touch | 2–5 | 12–30 |
| B | Preganglionic autonomic | <3 | 3–15 |
| **Unmyelinated**<br>C | *Pain*, temperature, postganglionic sympathetics | 0.4–1.3 | 0.5–2 |

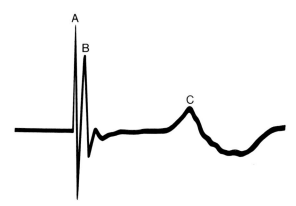

**Fig 3.2** Compound action potential recorded from a peripheral nerve

(motor) roots after they emerge from the spinal cord (Fig. 3.1). The course which these nerves take towards the periphery is determined during development and is regulated by growth factor substances (Stoeckli 1997). In general, distribution of both motor and sensory neurones follows a well-defined pattern, with the sensory component of each segmental nerve innervating a specific area of skin known as a dermatome (Fig. 3.3). The distribution of these varies among individuals and there is some degree of overlap between adjacent dermatomes, possibly related to local connections within the spinal cord. In addition, contributions from afferent autonomic fibres to the viscera can result in pain perception in areas distant from those that would be expected. Thus, block of cutaneous sensation does not necessarily imply block of either underlying visceral sensation or motor function.

Pain originating in the thoracic and abdominal viscera is transmitted by afferent sympathetic fibres through the sympathetic chain to segmental nerves ($T_1$–$L_2$) and by parasympathetic vagal (X) fibres. Other parasympathetic fibres transmit deep pain from structures in the pelvis ($S_2$–$S_3$) and the head and neck (cranial nerves III, VII and IX). Referred pain, such as shoulder tip pain secondary to diaphragmatic irritation, indicates the common embryonic origin of the nerve supply to the two structures involved. Stimulation of sympathetic and parasympathetic afferent fibres which transmit nociceptive information to the spinal cord results in pain, which tends to be diffuse and poorly localised in nature.

## Primary afferent (sensory) neurone

A typical primary afferent neurone consists of:

1. Peripheral nerve ending(s) and any associated receptor(s);
2. The axon (nerve fibre) connecting centrally;
3. The cell body in the dorsal root ganglion; and
4. Its central termination(s) in the dorsal horn of the spinal cord.

### Peripheral nerve endings

Many sensory nerve endings are associated with specialised receptors (e.g. Merkel disks, Pacinian corpuscles) for stimulus transduction, but nociceptors tend to consist of fine branches of the nerve fanning out through the dermis and, sometimes, the epidermis. Signal transduction is by the generation of action

23

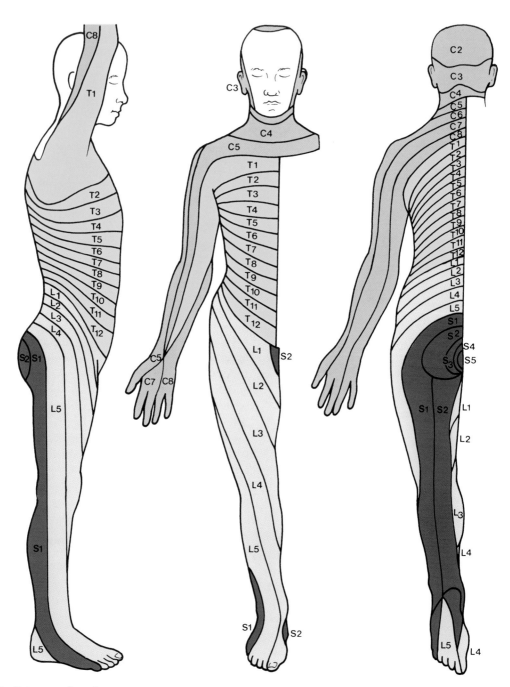

**Fig 3.3** Cutaneous dermatomes

potentials, although the nerve endings contain neuro-active substances, the release of which may modify their own responsiveness, particularly after tissue damage has occurred. The type of stimulus to which each neurone responds tends to be highly specific, so that thermal receptors, for example, are not activated by mechanical or chemical stimuli. Additionally, the intensity of the stimulus required to activate a peripheral receptor varies: light touch will only activate low threshold mechanoreceptors, whereas a much more severe stimulus is needed to activate nociceptors.

If these nociceptors are related to Aδ fibres, rapid impulse transmission occurs, with immediate perception of relatively well localised pain. However, the majority of neurones concerned with nociceptive transmission are small, unmyelinated, slowly conducting C-fibres, with receptors which respond to a variety of high intensity stimuli. Their activation results in perception of a more diffuse and persistent pain which is poorly localised. The initial activation of the peripheral receptor is responsible for encoding the type of stimulus, but further information about its exact nature is transmitted proximally by alterations in the frequency and pattern of impulse generation. For instance, a 'firing' rate of less than 5Hz in a C-fibre does not result in the perception of pain (Wiesenfeld & Lindblom 1980).

### Axonal functions

Until recently the only significant function of the axon was thought to be the electrical transmission of the nerve impulse (see Ch. 4), but recent studies have demonstrated that axoplasmic transport (both peripheral and central) is also important. This provides a slower method of communication whereby structural components and transmitter substances produced in the cell body are transported distally to maintain the neuronal phenotype or (after release peripherally) to modulate impulse generation. There is also evidence that peripherally derived growth factor substances (neurotrophins) are transported centrally to the dorsal root ganglia to regulate neurotransmitter synthesis (DiStefano & Curtis 1994, Bhattacharyya et al 1997, Bonni & Greenberg, 1997). In addition, recent studies have shown that the Schwann cells, previously thought to be important only for their electrical 'insulating' properties, have a much more dynamic interaction with the neurone itself. They produce neurotrophic substances and cytokines, particularly in response to injury (Friedman et al 1995). These substances may be transported retrogradely or anterogradely, and produce significant effects in both the periphery and the cell body of the neurone. It is thus apparent that the axons and the surrounding glial cells have a much more active role than was previously thought, and that there is the potential for longer-term modulation by neuroactive compounds, as well as control of the rate and direction of neuronal growth.

### The cell body and its central terminations

The cell bodies of primary sensory neurones lie in the dorsal root ganglia, situated within the confines of the vertebral canal. The neurone dies if the cell body is damaged because it contains the nucleus of the cell, its DNA and the systems which manufacture cell components, including the neurotransmitters which are essential for survival. In general, the diameter of the cell body correlates well with the diameter of its nerve fibre. Thus, small diameter cells in the dorsal root ganglia are thought to be concerned mainly with the transmission of nociceptive information, whereas large diameter cells are related to their fibres' discriminatory functions such as light touch or pressure. Transmission of information within neurones occurs by electrical conduction of action potentials (see Ch. 4), but at the 'synapse' in the dorsal horn of the spinal cord, chemicals (neurotransmitters) are released to activate the secondary neurone.

One of the characteristic differences between the dorsal root ganglia cell bodies is in the neurotransmitters synthesised and 'packaged' in them (Bean et al 1994). The small diameter cells synthesise peptides which are stored in large dense core vesicles (LDCVs), whereas the larger cells do not produce significant amounts of such peptides under normal conditions (Zhang et al 1995). Other neurotransmitters, such as amino acids and purines, are also produced and, although common to many other neuronal subtypes, they are often stored in the same LDCVs. The transmitters are released at the first central synapse in the dorsal horn of the spinal cord, a point with great potential for manipulation of the pain signal because of the significant degree of impulse modulation which takes place there.

## TRANSMISSION IN THE SPINAL CORD
### Neural connections

The circuitry in the dorsal horn is complex, with many neurones converging and diverging at the synapse. There are many influences, both pre- and post-synaptic, on the pain signal at the termination of the primary afferent neurone, before it is transmitted onwards in the spinothalamic tracts. The incoming afferent volley may be modulated by the actions of intrinsic dorsal horn neurones, as well as by fibres descending from supraspinal systems (Fig. 3.4). Equally, the initial afferent stimulus can act, not only on neurones in the precise area where the primary neurone terminates, but may also have effects spreading to proximal and distal segments of the cord.

The concept that there are specific areas and pathways in the spinal cord is an old one, there being obvious

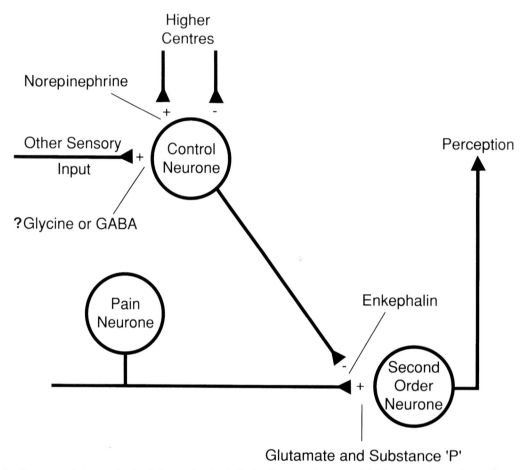

**Fig 3.4** Gate control theory of pain. Release of enkephalin by the control neurone inhibits transmitter release. Exogenous opioids have the same effect

distinctions between motor and sensory systems, and between sensory information which is noxious and innocuous. Previous work has shown some correlation between neuronal type and area of termination in the spinal cord (Brown 1982), although this may be altered in certain abnormal situations, such as after nerve injury. Additionally, it is possible to correlate peripheral receptive fields within each area of the cord with central terminations (Handwerker et al 1975, Brown & Fyffe 1981). This has also been demonstrated at supraspinal levels.

The spinal cord, in cross-section, has been divided into various areas according to their characteristic histological appearances: Rexed's laminae (Fig. 3.5). There is some slight species variation (Molander et al 1984), but lamina II, also known as the substantia gelatinosa,

is the area of the cord thought to be concerned with nociceptive transmission. This is where the majority of C and $A\delta$ fibres terminate, although some $A\delta$ fibres also terminate more deeply at lamina V. The larger, $A\beta$ fibres terminate in laminae III/IV (Willis & Coggeshall 1991), and large proprioceptive fibres terminate deeper still, in laminae VI/VII.

Many neurotransmitters and their receptors can be located in the dorsal horn, with a particularly high density in the superficial layers. This reflects the major degree of modulation which can be applied to the incoming signal in these areas. The complexity of the systems is outside the scope of this book, but a brief summary of the major neurotransmitters considered important in the processing of nociception at spinal cord level is appropriate.

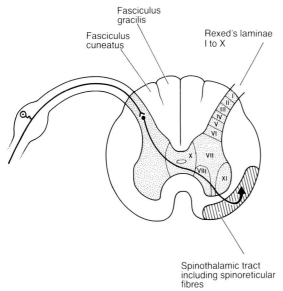

Fasciculus gracilis

Fasciculus cuneatus

Rexed's laminae I to X

Spinothalamic tract including spinoreticular fibres

**Fig 3.5** Transverse section of the spinal cord to show Rexed's laminae

## Neurotransmitters

### Amino acids

The 'classical', fast-acting neurotransmitters include amino acids, which may be either excitatory (glutamate and aspartate) or inhibitory (γ-amino-butyric acid (GABA) and glycine) (Aanonsen et al 1990). Characteristically, their release, reuptake and metabolism are rapid, and the major site of action very close to the site of release, usually within the synaptic cleft. Each of these transmitters acts on several subtypes of receptor, allowing a whole series of actions to be initiated. If, in the future, it is possible to develop highly specific agonists or antagonists, each able to target the actions of a specific receptor subtype and so minimise side-effects, some very useful analgesic drugs would be available (Dickenson 1995).

Glutamate is one of the main excitatory amino acids involved in pain transmission, and acts at two different groups of receptors. The *ionotropic* receptors, which include N-methyl-D-aspartate (NMDA), amino-3-hydroxy-5-methylisoxazole-4-propionic acid (AMPA) and kainate receptors have rapid response times. They activate ligand-gated ion channels and thus produce changes in intracellular ionic concentrations (e.g. an increase in intraneuronal calcium in the case of NMDA receptor stimulation). The NMDA receptor, at which glutamate acts, is thought to be important in the development of central sensitisation (Davis & Lodge 1987; see below also), as well as the rapid transmission of nociceptive information. In contrast to the receptors associated with ion channels, the *metabotropic* glutamate receptors (mGluRs) are G-protein coupled, and have effects on a variety of intracellular second messenger systems. At least seven subtypes, some of which are involved in pain processing, have been identified. There is recent evidence that mGluRs may facilitate NMDA receptor function and prove to be important in pain transmission (Budai & Larson 1998).

### Neuropeptides

Normally, neuropeptides are synthesised by the majority of primary afferent neurones involved in nociception, but many of the neurones intrinsic to the dorsal horn, and some of those in the descending systems, also contain neuropeptides. Unlike amino acids, the majority of the neuropeptides do not act at ligand-gated ion channels, but at G-protein coupled receptors. There is no evidence of rapid reuptake systems for neuropeptides, their termination of action being determined by rate of metabolism. Thus, they may diffuse beyond the synaptic zone to act at distant sites, an effect which has been termed *volume transmission* (Fuxe & Agnati 1991) and which reflects the possible 'paracrine' action of these neurotransmitters.

Substance P, a member of the tachykinin family, is synthesised by primary afferent neurones and is thought to play a major role in pain transmission (Duggan et al 1988, Levine et al 1993, Otsuka & Yoshioka 1993). Its predominantly excitatory action (at the neurokinin-1 receptor) is in contrast to the opioid peptides (e.g. enkephalins, endorphins and dynorphin) which have predominantly inhibitory actions and normally act as endogenous analgesics. Opioid peptides are synthesised and released by intrinsic dorsal horn neurones and also by neurones which form part of descending modulatory systems (Morton et al 1990). There is a high density of opioid receptors in the superficial dorsal horn, approximately 70% of them being of the μ subtype, 20% δ and 10% κ. Opioids acting in this area may have both pre- and post-synaptic effects.

The classification of opioid receptors has been revised recently following their genetic cloning, and now includes the recently identified 'orphan' opioid receptor (Table 3.2). When it was originally cloned it was found to have a high degree of sequence homology with the μ receptor, but it was named 'orphan' because none of

**Table 3.2** Classification of opioid receptors

| Original classification | New classification |
| --- | --- |
| Mu ($\mu$) | OP3 |
| Delta ($\delta$) | OP1 |
| Kappa ($\kappa$) | OP2 |
| Orphan | ORL1 |

the known opioid peptides activated it, and naloxone did not antagonise its activation. However, an endogenously produced peptide, nociceptin (or orphanin FQ), which acts on this receptor, has since been identified (Henderson & McKnight 1997). It is of interest that insults (traumatic or surgical), causing either inflammation or nerve injury, dramatically alter neuropeptide synthesis in primary afferent neurones (Hokfelt et al 1994, Calza et al 1998). Although the functional significance of these changes is not fully understood, it is likely that the neuropeptides play a major role in the response to such stimuli.

It is relatively common for neurones to release more than one type of neurotransmitter in response to a specific stimulus. In some primary afferent neurones, amino acids, catecholamines and neuropeptides may be stored and released together, there being some evidence that the type and quantity of neurotransmitter released may vary with the character of the incoming signal (De Potter et al 1997).

## Ascending pathways

Some of the neurones with which primary afferent neurones synapse project to adjacent segments. The remainder join the anterolateral spinothalamic tract (STT), from which some fibres separate at the brainstem (the spinoreticular tract) to terminate in the reticular formation. The STT neurones display certain characteristics which allow their identification in functional studies. They have small receptive fields, respond maximally to noxious or thermal stimulation at the periphery, receive convergent inputs from deep and visceral structures, and are able to code for threshold and intensity of stimulation. Although the majority of these fibres cross to the contralateral side before ascending, a small proportion ascend ventrally on the same side of the spinal cord.

The STT is the major ascending pathway involved in nociceptive processing. The monosynaptic connection of each of its fibres has allowed anatomical studies using antidromic activation and retrograde tracers to determine the termination of specific neurones (Bolton & Tracey 1992). Within the thalamus are groups of nuclei – ventral, posterior, medial and lateral – each with further subdivisions. Their function varies between species and the relative contribution of each nucleus to nociceptive processing has been reviewed (Hodge & Apkarian 1990). From the thalamus the tertiary neurones of the pain pathway project widely throughout the brain.

## DESCENDING MODULATION

Pathways descending from the brainstem play a significant role in modulating the level of tonic excitability of the spinal cord. This has been termed *diffuse noxious inhibitory control*, because cord transection results in a marked increase in basal excitability at the spinal level (Morgan et al 1994). Stimulation of certain areas of the brainstem, including the nucleus raphe magnus and the locus coeruleus, has been shown to result in release of neurotransmitters in the spinal cord and behavioural signs of decreased pain perception (Mokha et al 1985). The neurotransmitters released include catecholamines, such as norepinephrine and serotonin (5-hydroxytryptamine, 5-HT). It may be that analgesics such as tramadol act through this system, as well as the more unconventional agents, such as antidepressants, used in the treatment of chronic pain. Neuropeptides, including endogenous opioids and substance P, also play a role in this descending control (Stamford 1995).

## Supraspinal systems

The conscious perception of pain has never been localised to any specific part of the brain, although it seems that many areas are involved. Several parts of the brainstem are thought to be of particular importance including the periaqueductal grey (PAG) matter, where the locus coeruleus is situated, the nucleus raphe magnus and the surrounding reticular formation. The hypothalamus, the amygdala and the PAG are thought to make major contributions to nociceptive processing, and are involved in the integration of the responses to a noxious stimulus, including activation of the autonomic, endocrine and motor elements of these responses (Giesler et al 1994).

Modern imaging methods are providing much useful information on both the brain's acute response to a noxious stimulus and the modification of this response after tissue injury (Casey et al 1995, Iadarola et al 1995, Hsieh et al 1996). Thus, clinical and volunteer studies have confirmed the involvement of many areas of the brain, reflecting the multifaceted nature of pain perception (Hsieh et al 1996, Logothetis et al 1999). The acute response has been shown to involve the PAG, the hypothalamus, the prefrontal, insular, anterior cingulate and posterior parietal areas of the cerebral cortex, the primary motor and sensory areas, the supplementary motor area, and the cerebellum. Interestingly, imaging studies in chronic pain patients have demonstrated activation of quite different areas of the brain in response to noxious stimuli. This may reflect altered spinal processing, but could also indicate plasticity at supraspinal levels (Iadarola et al 1995, Liaw et al 1998).

## SENSITISATION MECHANISMS
### Peripheral sensitisation

Normally, a high intensity noxious stimulus is required to activate peripheral nociceptors. This results in the central transmission of action potentials which encode the site and character of the pain, but after tissue injury peripheral 'sensitisation' may occur. This lowers the threshold for activation of nociceptors, so that previously innocuous stimuli generate action potentials in nociceptive neurones. This may result in hyperalgesia, which is an exaggerated response to a painful stimulus, or allodynia, which is perception of a previously innocuous stimulus as painful. An additional feature may be recruitment of larger myelinated Aβ fibres, normally concerned with light touch transmission, to become involved in pain transmission. The development of allodynia has been reviewed (Cervero & Laird 1996).

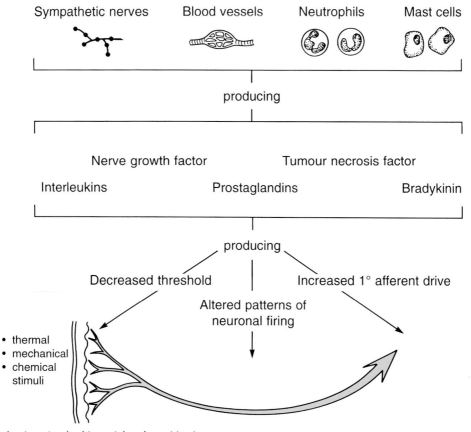

**Fig 3.6** Mechanisms involved in peripheral sensitisation

Peripheral sensitisation involves mast cells, neutrophils, the surrounding vascular bed, the autonomic nervous system and the primary afferent neurones themselves. A complex series of processes is activated, the exact mechanisms of which are not yet fully understood (Woolf 1995). One effect of the activation of these inter-linked cascades is the development of what has been termed an *inflammatory soup*, an alteration in the milieu of the peripheral nerve endings that lowers their activation threshold (Fig. 3.6).

Other peripheral changes may result in alterations in primary afferent 'drive', the final result of which is increased peripheral sensitivity. After peripheral nerve damage, the injured fibres start to generate action potentials spontaneously at sites other than the noci-ceptors. Increased 'mechanosensitivity' occurs at the site of injury, and impulses also arise *de novo* at the cell bodies in the dorsal root ganglia. These 'ectopic dis-charges' may correlate with the generation of spontaneous pain because clinical microneurography studies have demonstrated a correlation between its severity and the rate of ectopic discharge (Devor 1991). The factors causing these ectopic discharges are unclear, but they may be related to peripherally produced mediators, such as tumour necrosis factor (Sorkin et al 1997).

The end result of peripheral sensitisation is an amplification of peripheral sensory input so that there is an increase in the transmission of impulses to the spinal cord.

## Central sensitisation

The process of central sensitisation begins in the spinal cord, initially as a response to increased excitatory input from the injured tissue, and may be associated with changes in the transport from the periphery of substances involved in maintenance of neuronal phenotype. There are several components to the central response.

1. The acute response to repeated noxious stimulation, the phenomenon known as *wind up*, is an increase in the responsiveness of the secondary neurone. The end result is amplification of the response to a defined peripheral stimulus, with an increase in neuronal firing rate and summation of action potentials. One of the principal excitatory amino acids in the spinal cord, glutamate, acting through both NMDA (Woolf & Thompson 1991) and mGlu receptor subtypes (Baranauskas & Nistri 1998), appears to be important in the development of central sensitisation.

2. In addition to the rapid change in firing pattern mediated by glutamate receptor activation, there are rapid alterations in the dorsal horn cell bodies. Increases in the activity of *immediate early genes* and in their protein products (e.g. c-fos and c-jun), can be detected within hours of intense noxious stimulation. Potentially, these can produce rapid alterations in neuronal phenotype and function (Munglani & Hunt 1995).

3. There are major changes in neurotransmitter concentrations in both the dorsal root ganglia and the spinal cord, their specific nature being dependent on the type and severity of tissue damage. For example, synthesis of substance P is increased in primary afferent neurones in response to inflam-mation, but is reduced after peripheral nerve injury. After nerve injury, there may also be preferential damage to inhibitory neurones (Sugimoto et al 1990), with decreases in both glycine and GABA concen-trations within the dorsal horn (Satoh & Omote 1996, Ibuki et al 1997). A corresponding increase in spontaneous (Sotgui et al 1995) and evoked (Colvin et al 1996) activity within the dorsal horn has been found.

4. In the longer term, anatomical connections within the dorsal horn may alter. For example, after peri-pheral nerve injury large myelinated Aβ fibres, which normally terminate in the deeper dorsal horn, sprout into the substantia gelatinosa where they may actually make functional connections with intrinsic neurones which synapse there (Woolf et al 1992, 1995). Addition-ally, sprouting of sympathetic fibres around dorsal root ganglia has been found, with evidence of cross excitation between these fibres and primary afferent neurones (McLachlan et al 1993, Devor et al 1994).

## CONDUCTION BLOCK

The pain pathway may be interrupted at many points along its course. Opioids and other analgesic drugs affect pain receptors or the synaptic transmission of pain, while local anaesthetics have the advantage of producing a complete, yet reversible block of axonal transmission. In addition, local anaesthetics may be used at many points along the pain pathway (Fig. 3.7), although the anaesthetist must consider carefully the deep and super-ficial innervation of the operative field when choosing the point of block. The standard methods of local anaesthetic administration are as follows:

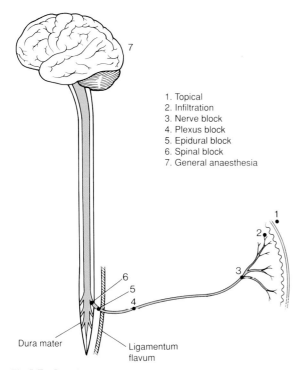

1. Topical
2. Infiltration
3. Nerve block
4. Plexus block
5. Epidural block
6. Spinal block
7. General anaesthesia

**Fig 3.7** Possible sites (1–7) of local anaesthetic action. Other analgesic drugs act at some of these points: opioids at 1, 2 and 5–7; $\alpha_2$-agonists and ketamine at 5–7; and NSAIDs at 1, 2 and 7

*Topical* Local anaesthetics may be applied directly to the mucous membranes of the nose, mouth, throat and urethra, and also to the external surfaces of the eye. Standard preparations will penetrate these surfaces, but until relatively recently intact skin presented an almost impermeable barrier to drug diffusion. The development of the eutectic mixture (lidocaine and prilocaine) of local anaesthetics (EMLA) in a cream formulation, and of a 4% tetracaine (amethocaine) gel, has overcome this difficulty.

*Infiltration* The extent of infiltration will depend on the area of anaesthesia required. Large volumes of dilute local anaesthetic solution are commonly used.

*Peripheral nerve block* Many small peripheral nerves are readily accessible and easily blocked, given a reasonable knowledge of the distribution and anatomical relations of the peripheral nerves.

*Proximal nerve block* Accessibility is the essential prerequisite for a proximal nerve block. The brachial plexus is easily located at a number of points by reference to anatomical landmarks, by eliciting paraesthesiae or by electrical stimulation. The lumbosacral plexus is not so easily identified and the sciatic nerve is deeply placed in the buttock and upper leg. Paravertebral somatic block involves injecting local anaesthetic close to the vertebral column where the segmental nerves emerge from the intervertebral foramina. (This technique had been virtually superseded by epidural block, which anaesthetises several nerves with a single injection, but it has recently increased in popularity again.)

*Epidural block* Ease of identification of the epidural space and unimpeded spread of the local anaesthetic solution make this a most useful technique. Continuous block can be produced with catheter techniques.

*Spinal (subarachnoid) block* This is a simpler technique than the epidural approach because identification of cerebrospinal fluid (CSF) is an unambiguous end-point. It is usually performed in the lumbar region to avoid needle damage to the spinal cord.

*General anaesthesia* Local anaesthetic drugs stabilise *all* excitable membranes. Procaine infusion has been used to produce general anaesthesia, but the technique is rarely used now.

## SUMMARY

It is apparent that the 'pain pathway' is not a static, hard-wired component of the nervous system, but is part of a much more dynamic system. Both the nature of the peripheral stimulus and the degree of tissue damage can influence the level of neuronal activity and even the actual phenotype of the primary sensory neurone. This in turn can have major effects on signal processing at spinal level, initiating long-term changes within the spinal cord which alter all subsequent processing of sensory information. Any attempt to produce analgesia with local anaesthetics or other agents which act at the various accessible points in the pathway (Fig. 3.7) must therefore take account of the changes which may already have occurred, and also of the possibility of preventing the development of detrimental long-term changes.

Clinical implementation of the theory of 'pre-emptive analgesia', that is, inducing impulse block prior to injury to prevent the initiation and development of peripheral and central sensitisation, is controversial. Much of the work from animal studies supports the effectiveness of

31

pre-treatment, but the results from clinical studies have been disappointing (Niv 1996). This may be due to the complexity and plasticity of the system being manipulated. It is now clear that a multiplicity of neurotransmitters are involved at a variety of sites so that use of a single agent is almost bound to fail. It seems more likely, therefore, that optimal analgesia will be obtained only by using a 'balanced' approach, that is, non-specific analgesics (e.g. opioids and NSAIDs) combined with site-directed local anaesthetics.

## Further Reading

Basbaum AI, Dubner R, Fields HL, McMahon SB, Mendell LM, Woolf CJ 1999 A tribute to Patrick D Wall. Pain Supplement 6: S1–S152.

## References

Aanonsen, LM, Sizheng L, Wilcox GL 1990 Excitatory amino acid receptors and nociceptive neurotransmission in rat spinal cord. Pain 41: 309–321

Baranauskas G, Nistri A 1998 Sensitisation of pain pathways in the spinal cord: cellular mechanisms. Progress in Neurobiology 54: 349–365

Bean AJ, Zhang X, Hökfelt T 1994 Peptide secretion: What do we know? FASEB Journal 8: 630–638

Besson JM, Chaouch A 1987 Peripheral and spinal mechanisms of nociception. Physiological Reviews 67: 67–186

Bhattacharyya A, Watson FL, Bradlee TA, Pomeroy SL, Stiles CD, Segal RA 1997 Trk receptors function as rapid retrograde signal carriers in the adult nervous system. Journal of Neuroscience 17: 7007–7016

Bolton PS, Tracey DJ 1992 Spinothalamic and propriospinal neurons in the upper cervical cord of the rat – terminations of primary afferent-fibers on soma and primary dendrites. Experimental Brain Research 92: 59–68

Bonni A, Greenberg ME 1997 Neurotrophin regulation of gene expression. Canadian Journal of Neurological Sciences 24: 272–283

Brown AG 1982 The dorsal horn of the spinal-cord. Quarterly Journal of Experimental Physiology and Cognate Medical Sciences 67: 193–212

Brown AG, Fyffe REW 1981 Form and function of dorsal horn neurons with axons ascending the dorsal columns in cat. Journal of Physiology, London 321: 31–47

Budai D, Larson AA 1998 The involvement of metabotropic glutamate receptors in sensory transmission in dorsal horn of the rat spinal cord. Neuroscience 83: 571–580

Calza L, Pozza M, Zanni M, Manzini CU, Manzini E, Hokfelt T 1998 Peptide plasticity in primary sensory neurons and spinal cord during adjuvant-induced arthritis in the rat: an immunocytochemical and in situ hybridization study. Neuroscience 82: 575–589

Casey KL, Minoshima S, Morrow TJ, et al 1995 Imaging the brain in pain: Potentials, limitations and implications. In: Bromm B, Desmedt JE (eds) Advances in pain research and therapy, vol 22, pp 201–211. Raven Press, New York

Cervero F, Laird JMA 1996 Mechanisms of touch-evoked pain (allodynia): a new model. Pain 68: 13–23

Colvin LA, Mark MA, Duggan AW 1996 Bilaterally enhanced dorsal horn postsynaptic currents in a rat model of peripheral mononeuropathy. Neuroscience Letters 207: 29–32

Davis SN, Lodge D 1987 Evidence for involvement of N-methyl-D-aspartic acid receptors in 'wind up' of class 2 neurons in the dorsal horn of the rat. Brain Research 424: 402–406

De Potter WP, Partoens P, Schoups A, Llona I, Coen EP 1997 Noradrenergic neurons release both noradrenaline and neuropeptide Y from a single pool: the large dense cored vesicles. Synapse 25: 44–55

Devor M 1991 Neuropathic pain and injured nerve: peripheral mechanisms. British Medical Bulletin 47(3): 619–630

Devor M, Janig W, Michaelis M 1994 Modulation of activity in dorsal root ganglion neurons by sympathetic activation in nerve-injured rats. Journal of Neurophysiology 71: 38–47

Dickenson AH 1995 Spinal pharmacology of pain. British Journal of Anaesthesia 75: 193–200

DiStefano PS, Curtis R 1994 Receptor mediated retrograde axonal transport of neurotrophic factors is increased after peripheral nerve injury. Progress in Brain Research 103: 35–45

Duggan AW, Hendry IA, Morton CR, Hutchison WD, Zhao ZQ 1988 Cutaneous stimuli releasing immunoreactive substance P in the dorsal horn of the cat. Brain Research 451: 261–273

Erlanger J, Gasser HS 1937 Electrical signs of nervous activity, University of Pennsylvania Press, Philadelphia

Friedman B, Wong V, Lindsay RM 1995 Axons, Schwann Cells and Neurotrophic Factors. The Neuroscientist 1(4): 192–198

Fuxe K, Agnati LF 1991 Two principal modes of electrochemical communication in the brain: volume versus wiring transmission. In: Fuxe, K (ed) Volume transmission in the brain, pp 1–9. Raven Press, New York.

Giesler GJ Jr, Katter JT, Dado RJ 1994 Direct spinal pathways to the limbic system for nociceptive information. Trends in Neuroscience 17: 244–250

Handwerker HO, Iggo A, Zimmermann M 1975 Segmental and supraspinal actions on dorsal horn neurons responding to noxious and non-noxious skin stimuli. Pain 1: 147–165

Hendersen G, McKnight AT 1997 The orphan opioid receptor and its endogenous ligand-nociceptin/orphan FQ. Trends in Pharmacological Sciences 18: 293–300

Hodge CJ, Apkarian AV 1990 The spinothalamic tract. Critical Reviews in Neurobiology 5, 363–397

Hokfelt T, Zhang X, Wiesenfeld-Hallin Z 1994 Messenger plasticity in primary sensory neurons following axotomy and its functional implications. Trends in Neuroscience 17: 22–29

Hsieh JC, Stahle-Backdahl M, Hagermark O, Stone-Elander S, Rosenquist G, Ingvar M 1996 Traumatic nociceptive pain activates the hypothalamus and the periaqueductal gray: a positron emission tomography study. Pain 64: 303–314

Iadarola MJ, Max M., Berman KF, Byas-Smith MG, Coghill RC, Gracely RH, Bennett GJ 1995 Unilateral decrease in thalamic activity observed with positron emission tomography in patients with chronic neuropathic pain. Pain 63: 55–64

Ibuki T, Hama AT, Wang X-T, Pappas GD, Sagen J 1997 Loss of GABA-immunoreactivity in the spinal dorsal horn of rats with peripheral nerve injury and promotion of recovery by adrenal medullary grafts. Neuroscience 76: 845–858

Levine JD, Fields HL, Basbaum AI 1993 Peptides and the primary afferent nociceptor. Journal of Neuroscience 13: 2273–2286

Liaw MY, You DL, Cheng PT, Kao PF, Wong AM 1998 Central representation of phantom limb phenomenon in amputees studied with single photon emission computerized tomography. American Journal of Physical and Medical Rehabilitation 77: 368–375

Logothetis NK, Guggenberger H, Peled S, Pauls J 1999 Functional imaging of the monkey brain. Nature Neuroscience 2: 555–562

McLachlan EM, Janig W, Devor M, Michaelis M 1993 Peripheral nerve injury triggers noradrenergic sprouting within dorsal root ganglia. Nature 363: 543–545

Mokha SS, McMillan JA, Iggo A 1985 Descending control of spinal nociceptive transmission. Actions produced on spinal multireceptive neurones from the nuclei locus coeruleus (LC) and raphe magnus (NRM). Experimental Brain Research 58: 213–226

Molander C, Xu Q, Grant G 1984 The cytoarchitectonic organization of the spinal cord in the rat. I. The lower thoracic and lumbosacral cord. Journal of Comparative Neurology 230: 133–141

Morgan NM, Gogas KR, Basbaum AI 1994 Diffuse noxious inhibitory controls reduce the expression of noxious stimulus-evoked fos-like immunoreactivity in the superficial and deep laminae of the rat spinal cord. Pain 56: 347–352

Morton CR, Hutchison WD, Duggan AW, Hendry IA 1990 Morphine and substance P release in the spinal cord. Experimental Brain Research 82: 89–96

Munglani R, Hunt SP 1995 Molecular biology of pain. British Journal of Anaesthesia 75: 186–192

Nathan PW 1976 The gate-control theory of pain. A critical review [109 refs]. Brain 99: 123–158

Niv D 1996 Intraoperative treatment of post-operative pain In: Pain 1996 – an up-dated review Campbell JN (ed) pp 173–187 IASP Press, Seattle.

Otsuka M, Yoshioka K 1993 Neurotransmitter functions of mammalian tachykinins [1459 refs]. Physiological Reviews 73: 229–308

Satoh O, Omote K 1996 Roles of monoaminergic, glycinergic and GABAergic inhibitory systems in the spinal cord in rats with peripheral mononeuropathy. Brain Research 728: 27–36

Sorkin LS, Xiao WH, Wagner R, Myers RR 1997 Tumour necrosis factor-alpha induces ectopic activity in nociceptive primary afferent fibres. Neuroscience 81: 255–262

Sotgui ML, Biella G, Riva L 1995 Poststimulus afterdischarge of spinal WDR and NS units in rats with chronic nerve constriction. Neuroreport 6: 1021–1024

Stamford JA 1995 Descending control of pain. British Journal of Anaesthesia 75: 217–227

Stoeckli ET 1997 Molecular mechanisms of growth cone guidance: stop and go? Cell and Tissue Research 290: 441–449

Sugimoto T, Bennett GJ, Kajander KC 1990 Transsynaptic degeneration in the superficial dorsal horn after sciatic nerve injury: effects of a chronic constriction injury, transection and strychnine. Pain 42: 205–213

Wiesenfeld Z, Lindblom U 1980 Behavioural and electro-physiological effects of various types of peripheral nerve lesions in the rat: a comparison of possible models for chronic pain. Pain 8: 285–298

Willis WD, Coggeshall RE 1991 Sensory Mechanisms of the Spinal Cord, 2nd edn. Plenum Press, New York and London

Woolf CJ 1989 Recent advances in the pathophysiology of acute pain [comment] [65 refs]. British Journal of Anaesthesia 63: 139–146

Woolf CJ 1995 Somatic pain – pathogenesis and prevention. British Journal of Anaesthesia 75: 169–176

Woolf CJ, Thompson SWN 1991 The induction and maintenance of central sensitisation is dependent on N-methyl-D-aspartic acid receptor activation; Implications for the treatment of post-injury pain hypersensitivity states. Pain 44: 293–299

Woolf CJ, Shortland P, Coggeshall RE 1992 Peripheral nerve injury triggers central sprouting of myelinated afferents. Nature 355: 75–78

Woolf CJ, Shortland P, Reynolds M, Ridings J, Doubell T, Coggeshall RE 1995 Reorganization of central terminals of myelinated primary afferents in the rat dorsal horn following peripheral axotomy. The Journal of Comparative Neurology 360: 121–134

Zhang X, Aman K, Hokfelt T 1995 Secretory pathways of neuropeptides in rat lumbar dorsal root ganglion neurons and effects of peripheral axotomy. The Journal of Comparative Neurology 352: 481–500

# 4. Peripheral nerve and local anaesthetic drugs

## J A W Wildsmith and G R Strichartz

Local anaesthetics are drugs which block reversibly the conduction of impulses in the peripheral nervous system. By definition, the latter comprises the roots, rami and distal branches of both cranial and spinal nerves, and includes components of the autonomic nervous system. The peripheral nervous system may be distinguished from the central component on both gross and micro-anatomical grounds, both aspects having some relevance to local anaesthesia. The gross anatomical arrangement of the nerves governs the distribution of block once an agent has been applied at a particular site, with this impulse block having the same functional significance whatever factor (drug, temperature, surgery, etc.) is used to produce it. By contrast, micro-anatomical, in addition to neurophysiological, circumstances affect the action of drugs, because they must be able to penetrate the often considerable coverings of a nerve before its function can be interrupted.

## STRUCTURAL COMPONENTS OF NERVE

A considerable part of the substance of a peripheral nerve is connective tissue. Structurally and functionally, this may be divided into three separate layers (Fig. 4.1). Bundles of nerve fibres – the fasciculi – are embedded in *endoneurium*. This consists mainly of longitudinally arranged collagen fibrils, with some condensation of the collagen around both the nerve fibres and the capillaries which supply them. Each fasciculus is surrounded by layers of flattened, overlapping or interdigitating fibroblasts, which are the major component of the *perineurium* (Shanthaveerappa & Bourne 1962). The larger the fasciculus, the thicker is this layer of cells. Finally, there is a condensation of areolar connective tissue around the perineurium that comprises the *epineurium*. Collagen and elastic fibrils are arranged

longitudinally and this layer also contains lymphatics and blood vessels. The epineurium attaches the nerve only loosely to surrounding structures, so that it is mobile except where branches and blood vessels tether it.

These structural components serve to bind the fibres together and to protect them. Peripheral nerves have considerable longitudinal strength, mainly a property of the epineurium, and the collagen in the perineurium is arranged in a lattice-work pattern to help prevent kinking when the nerve bends. Some nerves, particularly the human sciatic, contain a considerable amount of fat and this may help to cushion the nerve in the sitting position. The cellular component of the perineurium acts as a perifascicular diffusion barrier, preventing or slowing the diffusion of many substances, including local anaesthetics, into the nerve (Feng & Liu 1949). In combination with the permeability properties of the endoneurial capillaries, this diffusion barrier maintains the composition of the extracellular fluid around the nerve fibres (Shanthaveerappa & Bourne 1962). Blood vessels enter the nerve at intervals and form anastomotic plexuses in both epineurium and perineurium. Within the endoneurium there are only capillaries but, as in the other layers, these are arranged longitudinally.

### Nerve root structure

The connective tissue components of the spinal nerve roots are essentially the same as those of the mixed peripheral nerves, although there is much less collagen. The endoneurium continues to the point of attachment of the root to the spinal cord, where there is a clearly defined transitional area, the Obersteiner–Redlich zone. In this zone the Schwann cell sheaths (see below) are replaced by sheaths produced by oligodendrocytes, the supporting cells of the central

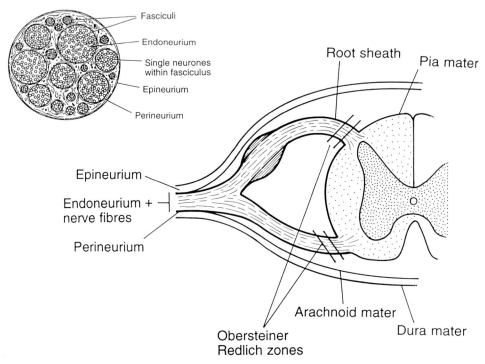

**Fig 4.1** Cross-section (top) and structural components (below) of peripheral nerve. (Redrawn with permission from *British Journal of Anaesthesia* 1986; 5 8: 692–700)

nervous system. Perineural tissue is much thinner in the spinal roots and is present only as a thin root sheath. In fact, the mixed nerve perineurium divides to be continuous with both the arachnoid mater and the root sheath, while the epineurium merges into the dura mater (Fig. 4.1). The nerve roots are thus less well protected by connective tissue than are the peripheral nerves, but they are of course bathed in cerebrospinal fluid and contained within the protection of the vertebral canal. The cell bodies of the sensory fibres are situated towards the periphery of the dorsal root ganglia and the fibres run uninterrupted through its centre.

## FUNCTIONAL COMPONENTS OF PERIPHERAL NERVE

The functional unit of peripheral nerve is the *nerve fibre*. This term may be defined solely as the axon emanating from the cell body situated in the dorsal root ganglion or spinal cord, but it is more useful to widen the definition to include the Schwann cell sheath which surrounds every axon. This sheath has some structural and supportive roles, but its most significant effect is on the mode of impulse transmission in myelinated fibres. Recent research has shown that it has some 'metabolic' functions also (see Ch. 3).

Two distinct arrangements are recognised (Fig. 4.2). In the simpler situation, projections from a single Schwann cell surround several axons, which are described as being *unmyelinated*. At junctions, the Schwann cells, which have a maximum length of 500 µm, simply overlap each other. The other arrangement is for the projection from each Schwann cell to wind itself many times around a single axon. Thus the axon is surrounded by a 'tube' formed of multiple double layers of phospholipid cell membrane, the *myelin sheath*. Each Schwann cell extends for 1 mm or more, but at junctions between them (the nodes of Ranvier) the myelin is absent (Fig. 4.2). However, there is close interdigitation between processes of the adjacent cells, so that the axonal membrane still has considerable coverings. Fibres less than 1 µm total diameter are almost always unmyelinated (so called 'C-fibres'), while those greater than 1 µm are myelinated.

Nerve axoplasm contains the usual organelles, such as mitochondria and endoplasmic reticulum, which are

UNMYELINATED                    MYELINATED

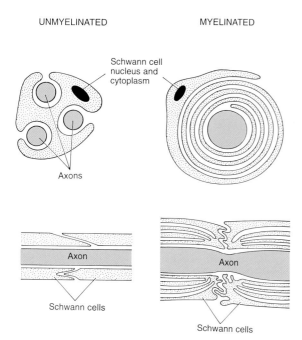

**Fig 4.2**  Types of Schwann cell sheaths. (Redrawn with permission from *British Journal of Anaesthesia* 1986; 5 8: 692–700)

required for normal cellular metabolism, but the most important structure for the transmission of nerve impulses is the axonal plasma membrane. Its basic structure (Fig. 4.3) is a double layer of phospholipid arranged so that the polar, hydrophilic, phosphate-containing head groups are in contact with the interstitial or intracellular fluid. The hydrophobic, lipid groups are opposed to one another in the centre of the membrane. Embedded in the membrane are large protein molecules, many of which function as enzymes, active transport 'pumps', receptors for hormones (and drugs) or as 'channels' for the passive movement of ions both into and out of the cell.

In the present context the most important of these proteins are the ion channels. Each has a 'pore' through which the ions pass, and most have some type of 'filter' which makes the channel selective for one ion (Fig. 4.3). This selectivity may depend on the diameter, or the electrostatic properties of the ion, or both. Many channels also have a 'gate' which regulates the passage of ions through them. Associated with such a gate is a sensor mechanism which responds to changes in the membrane's electric field or potential (Stuhmer et al 1989). Such changes produce conformational changes in the protein,

causing the gate to open or close. Channels which respond in this way are described as *voltage-gated*.

## THE NERVE IMPULSE

If a micro-electrode is inserted into the axoplasm of a single nerve fibre it records a transmembrane potential in the region of –70 mV, the inside of a cell being negative relative to the outside. This is known as the *resting potential*. When the nerve is stimulated the electrode will record a transient *depolarisation* to approximately +40 mV. This is quickly followed by repolarisation back to the resting value. The entire process, which occupies 1–2 ms, is known as the *action potential* (Fig. 4.4) and is associated with the longitudinal propagation of the nerve impulse.

## Generation of the resting potential

The resting potential is the net result of many factors. The most important are the marked differences in ionic concentrations between intracellular and extracellular fluid, and the factors which tend to maintain those differences, particularly the semipermeable nature of the intervening membrane. For instance, sodium would normally diffuse down its concentration gradient into the cell, but cannot do so because the membrane is normally impermeable to it. Conversely, potassium can diffuse down its concentration gradient more easily, almost certainly utilising specific channels in the membrane to do so. This outward diffusion of potassium leaves an excess of anions over cations within the cell and this imbalance produces the negative intracellular potential. The electrical gradient so generated retards the further movement of positively charged potassium ions out of the axon and eventually an equilibrium is established between the concentration gradient (causing outward movement of potassium) and the electro-chemical gradient (causing inward movement). If any factor causes the membrane potential to decrease, more potassium will diffuse out, but if the membrane tends to hyperpolarise, potassium will diffuse in. In each case the resting potential is restored, as long as the potassium gradient is maintained across the membrane.

## Basis of the action potential

Depolarisation (the steep, rising phase of the action potential) is caused by the movement into the axon of

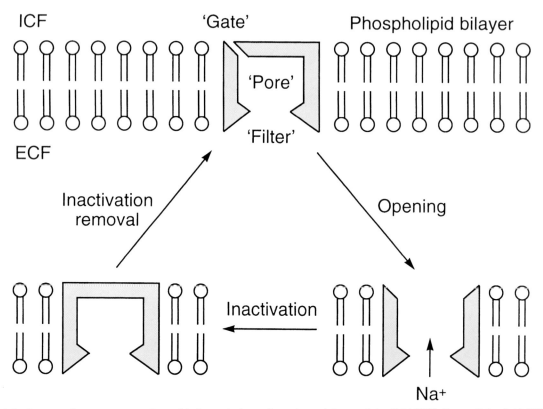

**Fig 4.3** Functional components and possible 'states' of a sodium channel. Intracellular fluid (ICF), Extracellular fluid (ECF) (Redrawn with permission from *British Journal of Anaesthesia* 1986; 5 8: 692–700)

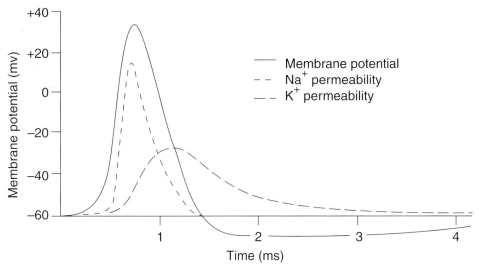

**Fig 4.4** Relationship of the phases of a single action potential to the changes in membrane permeability to sodium and potassium associated with the opening and closing of their respective channels. The figures for, and changes in, membrane potential shown are less than those quoted in the text because of damage to the nerve during preparation of the specimen for the experiment. (Personal communication: Sir Andrew Huxley. Redrawn with permission from *Journal of Physiology* 1952; 1 1 7: 500–544)

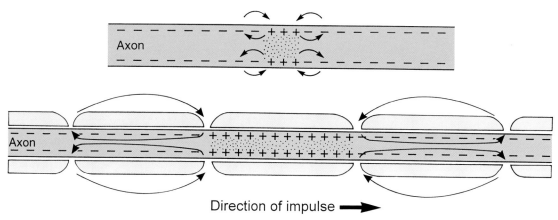

**Fig 4.5**  Local current flows around depolarised segment (stippled area) in unmyelinated (top) and myelinated (bottom) axons. (Redrawn with permission from *British Journal of Anaesthesia* 1986; 5 8: 692–700)

positive charge in the form of sodium ions, and re-polarisation (the falling phase) by the outward movement of an equivalent amount of positive charge in the form of potassium ions. The essential element of this 'regenerative' process is a sudden increase in the permeability of the membrane to sodium (Hodgkin & Huxley 1952). Specific channels in the membrane open (Fig. 4.3), so allowing sodium ions to diffuse down both concentration and electrical gradients (Hille 1984, Moorman 1998). This influx, which swamps the tendency for potassium diffusion to maintain the resting potential, stops when the membrane potential reaches about +40 mV because of three factors: (i) the inward concentration gradient for sodium is almost balanced by the outward electrical gradient; (ii) the open sodium channels slowly 'inactivate' (close) at depolarised potentials; and (iii) a subset of voltage-gated potassium channels opens slowly (see below), leading eventually to a larger current of potassium outward than sodium inward. A small amount of potassium then diffuses out until the membrane potential is re-established.

Potassium can pass through the membrane by several routes. Voltage independent (sometimes called *leakage*) channels, which are probably open at all times, are responsible for the background permeability to potassium that generates the resting potential. In addition, specific voltage-gated potassium channels open during depolarisation. The sequence of depolarisation followed by repolarisation is produced because these gated channels open and close more slowly than those for sodium (Fig. 4.4). Relative to the total number of ions present, the number of ions involved in the ex-

change during one action potential is very small. The distribution of these ions across the membrane is restored during the resting phase by the sodium–potassium coupled pump, another membrane situated protein. The use of ATP to power this active transport process is the only point where energy is required to support impulse activity. By contrast, the ion fluxes that occur when channels open are examples of passive, facilitated diffusion.

## Impulse propagation

When a segment of an axon is depolarised a potential difference exists between it and the adjacent sections. This causes a *local circuit current* (Fig. 4.5) to flow into the adjacent segment, making its membrane potential less negative. This actuates the *voltage sensors* on the gates of the sodium channels there, and it is this local current which thus causes some channels in the adjacent segment of the fibre to open. Sodium permeability increases, and the resulting inward sodium current further depolarises the axon, spreading the action potential to the adjacent undepolarised region. Thus the impulse is propagated along the axon (Hodgkin & Huxley 1952).

Local currents also flow 'backwards' along the axon to the segment of nerve that has just repolarised, but it cannot fire an impulse again immediately for two reasons. First, the delay in closure of the voltage-dependent potassium channels (Fig. 4.4) ensures that any tendency for depolarisation of the membrane potential is immediately counterbalanced by further outward movement of potassium. Second, the inherent properties of sodium channels act against further immediate depolarisation. During an initial depolarisation the channels change in *state* from 'closed' to 'open', but then (and at a slower rate) they close again – this time to an *inactivated* state from which spontaneous opening cannot occur (Fig. 4.3). Only when the membrane has repolarised does a further transition from the *closed-inactivated* to the *closed-resting* state take place, so eventually restoring the conditions present before the impulse. Thus nerve conduction is normally unidirectional.

An impulse in a non-myelinated fibre spreads almost like a continuous 'ripple' along the axon, but in a myelinated nerve this is not so because its sodium channels are situated almost exclusively in the region of the nodes of Ranvier. Thus the local currents have to flow from node to node, passively depolarising the intervening section of axon. In fact, the local current from one node of Ranvier will affect more than the immediately adjacent one, and the length of axon depolarised by the action potential extends over several nodes. This *saltatory conduction* is much more rapid and accounts for the faster rate of impulse transmission in myelinated than in unmyelinated fibres.

## Initiation of the action potential

Action potentials are initiated at peripheral nerve endings in much the same way that they are propagated, but with appropriate physiological stimuli producing the initial depolarisation. Relatively little is known about the nature of the receptors that cause this, but it is obvious that each must be able to respond specifically to one of a range of stimuli as diverse as mechanical deformation, temperature and neuro-active chemicals. Prostaglandins have an integral relationship with the endings of pain fibres and may have a role in maintaining certain classes of sodium channels in the activatable state, so that they respond to amines or peptides, such as bradykinin, released by tissue damage. The action of non-opioid analgesics, such as aspirin, is probably related to their 'anti-prostaglandin' action in decreasing receptor sensitivity. The initial opening of non-specific cation channels associated with the receptors allows some depolarisation of the membrane. If the stimulus is inadequate, potassium leakage will stop the membrane from depolarising sufficiently, but with an adequate stimulus the membrane potential will reach the threshold value

which triggers the opening of other, voltage-sensitive channels, leading to the generation and propagation of a definitive action potential.

Centrally, most nerves have connections to others that may cause excitation or inhibition by the release of transmitter substances. Membrane receptors for these transmitters are associated with ion channels which are activated either directly by transmitter release (they are *ligand-gated*), or indirectly by intracellular *second messengers* such as 'G' proteins. Excitatory transmitters are usually associated with non-selective cation channels which open under their influence and catalyse primarily sodium influx, thus leading to a degree of local depolarisation. Inhibitory transmitters are usually associated with potassium or chloride channels, the opening of which will cause local hyperpolarisation or at least maintain the membrane potential near its resting value. An action potential will only be generated when the effects of excitatory transmitters predominate to yield a net inward depolarising current.

## CONDUCTION BLOCK

The transmission of nerve impulses is dependent upon a wave of depolarisation, followed by repolarisation, passing along the nerve membrane. Theoretically at least, the process could be interrupted in several ways, but it is obvious that the initial increase in sodium permeability produced by the opening of ion-specific channels is the key factor. Agents that interfere with the processes which underlie the other, subsequent phases of the action potential are known, but they do not have the same immediate effect on impulse transmission as sodium channel block.

A wide range of substances can be shown to block sodium channels when they are applied directly to neurophysiological preparations *in vitro*. They include many biotoxins (e.g. tetrodotoxin, saxitoxin), the phenothiazines, β-adrenergic blocking agents and some opioids, in addition to the traditional local anaesthetic agents. Only the last are widely used clinically to block nerve conduction because they also have the ability to penetrate nerve coverings and are relatively free from local and systemic toxicity (Strichartz 1986). Fundamental to their mode of action is the chemistry of their behaviour in solution (Strichartz et al 1990). All the clinically useful local anaesthetics have a common basic structure with an aromatic ring attached to an

**Table 4.1** Physicochemical properties of some local anaesthetics measured at 37 °C

| Drug | Mol wt | $pK_a$ | Distribution coefficient[a] | % protein bound |
|---|---|---|---|---|
| PROCAINE | 236 | 8.9 | 3.1 | 5.8 |
| LIDOCAINE | 234 | 7.7 | 110 | 64 |
| PRILOCAINE | 220 | 7.7 | 25[b] | 55 |
| MEPIVACAINE | 260 | 7.7 | 42 | 77 |
| ROPIVACAINE | 288 | 8.1 | 115[b] | 95 |
| BUPIVACAINE | 302 | 8.1 | 560 346[b] | 95 |
| ETIDOCAINE | 276 | 7.9 | 1853 | 94 |

[a] Between water and octanol at pH 7.4; [b] at 25 °C.

amine group by an intermediate chain (Table 4.1). In common with general anaesthetics, they are more soluble in organic solvents than in aqueous ones. To allow them to be administered by injection they are usually prepared as an acid solution of the hydrochloride salt in water. In this combination the amine

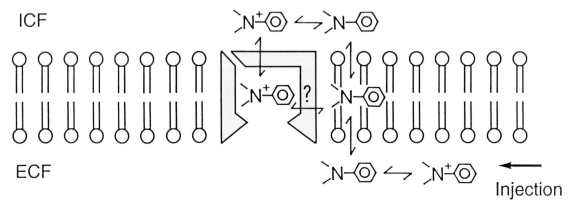

**Fig 4.6**  Access path of local anaesthetics to sodium channel. Intracellular fluid (ICF), Extracellular fluid (ECF) (Redrawn with permission from *British Journal of Anaesthesia* 1986; 58: 692–700)

group becomes protonated, albeit reversibly, the water solubility of the drug is increased considerably, and a preparation suitable for injection results.

The molecular mechanism of action of local anaesthetic drugs has still to be elucidated, but present views may be summarised as follows (Fig. 4.6). After injection, tissue buffers increase the pH of the solution around the drug and some of the more lipid-soluble, base form of the drug is released. This is able to diffuse through tissue barriers (the perineurial sheath, etc.) to penetrate the nerve (Bernards & Hill 1992). Eventually, it passes through the lipid nerve cell membrane and into the axoplasm, from which it enters the sodium channel pore. Simplistically, it may be thought of as obstructing the pore of the channel, although it is more likely that it combines with a *receptor* related to the gating mechanism of the sodium channel (Butterworth & Strichartz 1990). The most convincing mechanistic evidence of this comes from *in vitro* experiments in which permanently ionised (and thus less lipid soluble) analogues of local anaesthetics have been applied to either the inside or the outside of the axon of single nerve fibre preparations (Narahashi et al 1970). Applied to the outside, these drugs have little effect because they cannot penetrate the cell membrane, but when perfused through the inside of the axon they have a potent action.

However, the above does not explain the action of benzocaine, which does not ionise at all. Either this agent enters the membrane and causes it to expand (and 'compress' the channel) in a way similar to the now archaic theory put forward to explain the action of general anaesthetics, or it reaches the receptor by diffusing into the sodium channel directly from the membrane. Such mechanisms may also be relevant to the action of the other, tertiary amine drugs acting in their neutral base forms.

## Use-dependent block

The structural relationship between local anaesthetic drug and sodium channel receptor is the subject of much current research, centred mostly on a combination of site-directed mutagenesis (Ragsdale et al 1994) and the phenomenon known as *use-dependent block* (Courtney 1980). If an nerve preparation *in vitro* is stimulated at a very low frequency (<0.1 Hz) and exposed to a low concentration of a local anaesthetic, a minor decrease in impulse transmission develops. An increase in the stimulus frequency (to >5 Hz) will then appear to increase the degree of block (Fig. 4.7), but a brief period of rest allows conduction to recover again (Schwarz et al 1977).

The most likely explanation of the difference between *tonic* (or *resting*) block and *phasic* (*use-* or *frequency-dependent*) block is that the binding affinity of local anaesthetics differs among the various states of the sodium channels. Binding is weak to the resting state and stronger to open and inactivated states. Use-dependent block arises from this selective affinity, because depolarisations increase the population of open and inactivated channels. It would appear that at least a part of local anaesthetic action is to prolong the period which sodium channels spend in the inactivated state.

Whether or not this phenomenon has any significant clinical relevance for nerve block is, at best, not proven, if only because the conditions of such experiments are

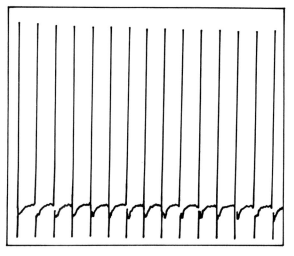
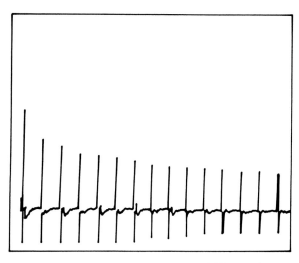

Control                                                                    Plus drug

**Fig 4.7** Use-dependent block. 'A' fibre compound action potentials from rabbit vagus nerve stimulated at 30 Hz for 0.5 s before and after the application of tetracaine at 0.02 mmol l⁻¹ . The decrease in 'spike' height between the control trace and the first spike of the second trace represents the degree of 'resting' block. The subsequent decrease in trace height is caused by 'phasic' block. Repetition of the stimulus train after a few seconds of rest would produce an identical trace. (Redrawn with permission from *British Journal of Anaesthesia* 1986; 58: 692–700)

so artificial. By contrast, the therapeutic actions of local anaesthetic-like Class 1 antiarrhythmic agents on cardiac impulses probably depend critically on this use-dependent mechanism. Recent concern over the cardiotoxicity of bupivacaine, coupled with the fact that drugs vary in the degree to which they produce phasic block, has led to suggestions that the two may be related, but the evidence of a clear relationship is poor.

## STRUCTURE–ACTIVITY RELATIONSHIPS

Local anaesthetics vary in their clinical profiles and these differences may be related to their chemical structures (Strichartz & Berde 1994). Because certain physicochemical properties are related to activity, it is possible to quantify the differences between drugs. The factors usually quoted are $pK_a$, partition coefficient (an index of lipid solubility) and the degree of protein binding (Strichartz et al 1990, Table 4.1). It is important to appreciate that these features are not independent of one another, and even correlate with other pharmacological actions of the drugs, so that when two drugs with several structural differences are compared the relationship of physicochemical property with clinical feature may not appear to be a direct one. The true relationship is only seen when a strictly homologous drug series is examined (Wildsmith et al 1989, Lee-Son et al 1992).

The local anaesthetic drugs in current use are classified into two groups according to the nature of the bond in the chain between the aromatic ring and the amine group. This may be either an ester linkage (procaine and its derivatives) or an amide linkage (lidocaine and its derivatives). These bonds have notable effects on the route of metabolism and the chemical stability of the compounds. Most esters are metabolised rapidly by plasma cholinesterase, so their systemic toxicity is less, but they have relatively short shelf-lives when stored in solution without preservatives. The amides are very stable and cannot be hydrolysed by cholinesterase; therefore, they rely on hepatic detoxification mechanisms for breakdown.

The other important difference between the two groups is that the $pK_a$ values of the esters are greater than those of the homologous amides. This means that the proportion of the lipid-soluble, un-ionised form of the drug present in solution at physiological pH is greater with amides. These differences in $pK_a$ affect the overall rate of axonal membrane penetration and binding to sodium channels because the base form penetrates to the site more rapidly, yet the charged form stays there longer (Schwartz et al 1977) (Fig. 4.6). In addition, the coverings of nerves are essentially lipid

43

membranes (Strichartz 1977) and the un-ionised, lipid-soluble form of the drug is required to penetrate them as well. Thus drugs with $pK_a$ nearer to 7.4 may have a noticeably faster onset than those with $pK_a$ greater than 8 when applied to nerves with considerable barriers to diffusion around them. Lidocaine has only a marginally lower $pK_a$ than bupivacaine, but it is also a smaller molecule and this may aid its membrane penetrance. In addition, being less potent, it is applied at higher concentrations and therefore has a higher molecular gradient driving its diffusion into the nerve.

Addition of side chains to the basic local anaesthetic drug structure increases lipid solubility and sodium channel affinity, and this is related directly to potency (compare lidocaine with bupivacaine, procaine with tetracaine) (Courtney 1980, Wildsmith et al 1989). The third important physicochemical property, protein binding, also increases as side chains are added to the molecule. This measurement is related to the reaction with serum proteins, not with membrane targets, and any correlation between protein binding and duration of action is largely fortuitous.

Prilocaine presents an apparent contradiction to these rules. It is less lipid-soluble and less protein-bound than lidocaine, yet the two are equipotent in clinical use, and prilocaine has a longer duration of action. The apparent inconsistency relates to a difference in vasoactivity. Prilocaine does not have the vasodilator action of lidocaine, so it is removed from the site of in-jection more slowly. This more than compensates for its physicochemical disadvantage, because vascular flow removes more than 95% of the injected dose of local anaesthetic before it even enters the peripheral nerve. Similar factors may account for the finding that ropivacaine and bupivacaine produce almost equal degrees of sensory block.

## Chirality and local anaesthetics

Chirality is derived from the Greek word, *chiros*, meaning 'handed'. A chiral compound is one that contains at least one atomic centre (usually a carbon atom) to which four different atoms or chemical groups are attached. If a molecule contains one such 'asymmetric' atom, two distinct, three-dimensional, mirror-image arrangements of the components, known as 'stereo-isomers', are possible. Although such isomers have identical atomic composition and chemical properties, the different spatial arrangement of the atoms means that, like our

hands, they cannot be superimposed one upon the other. Matching stereo-isomers are called enantiomers, and a substance containing equal amounts of the two enantiomers is known as a 'racemate', or 'racemic' mixture. Enantiomers have identical physicochemical properties, and have the same $pK_a$ and lipid solubility values (Tucker 1997), but there may be differences, qualitative and quantitative, in their pharmacokinetic and pharmacodynamic properties (Sidebotham & Schug 1997). This is because of stereoselective interactions (those due to differences in the three dimensional structure) at drug receptors sites.

Stereo-isomers may be described and identified in a number of ways, with the current standard being the use of the 'Sequence Rule Notation' (Cahn et al 1956). In this, the smallest of the four groups attached to the asymmetric atom is identified, and the molecule 'positioned' with this group directed away from the 'viewer', that is, on the 'far' side of the molecule. If the sequence of the sizes of the other three groups is 'clockwise' from smallest to largest, it is defined as an 'R' (from the Latin *rectus* – right) isomer, whereas if the sequence is 'anticlockwise' it is defined as an 'S' isomer (*sinister* – left) (Fig. 4.8). These terms are described as the '*absolute* descriptors', although the best known

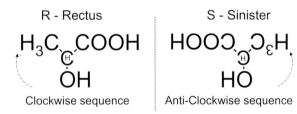

**2-dimensional formula**

COOH

$CH_3$-$\dot{C}$-H

$\dot{O}H$

**3-dimensional formulae**

R - Rectus        S - Sinister

$H_3C$  COOH        HOOC  $CH_3$

OH        HO

Clockwise sequence        Anti-Clockwise sequence

**Fig 4.8** Chemical formulae of lactic acid to illustrate absolute descriptor methodology. The smallest atom (–H) attached to the asymmetric carbon atom is positioned 'away' from the viewer. If the sequence of the other three atoms, from largest to smallest (here –OH, –COOH, –$CH_3$), is clockwise, then it is an 'R' isomer. If the sequence is anticlockwise, it is an 'S' isomer. If, as is the case here, two of the atoms attached to the asymmetric carbon are the same, it is the next one in the sequence of each side chain that decides the rule

method of identifying isomers relates to their property of rotating plane-polarised light in equal degree, but in opposite directions, either clockwise (+) or anticlockwise (−). These are known as the '*relative* descriptors'. Unfortunately, there is no consistency between the absolute and relative descriptors and, within an homologous series of compounds, the S/R notation may change as the length of a particular side chain alters. This is seen in the 'bupivacaine' series of local anaesthetics where S-mepivacaine has the same spatial arrangement of atoms as R-bupivacaine. To deal with these complications it is common to quote both descriptors (e.g. S(−) bupivacaine) of a chiral compound.

With the exception of lidocaine, all the currently used amide local anaesthetics are chiral, and differences in the pharmacokinetic and pharmacodynamic properties of the isomers of each drug have been recognised for many years. Prilocaine was the first agent to be studied (Åckerman et al 1967), but the differences between its isomers are of relatively little clinical impact. The local anaesthetic and toxic effects of the enantiomers of bupivacaine were first described by Aberg (1972), who showed that the S(−) enantiomer is less toxic than the R(+) form. However, the full significance of the difference was not apparent at that time, and it was not possible to produce a single isomer preparation in commercial quantities. It was only when clinical concerns about the cardiotoxicity of racemic bupivacaine became apparent that further development took place. The first single isomer local anaesthetic to reach clinical practice was ropivacaine, the 'S(−)' isomer of the propyl analogue of bupivacaine, chosen initially because it has a longer duration of action than the R(+) version (Åckerman et al 1988). It was only later that it was shown that R(+)bupivacaine is the more cardiotoxic of the two isomers (Vanhoutte et al 1991), a finding which led eventually to the development of S(−) bupivacaine, now known as levobupivacaine.

The stereoselectivity of the interactions of local anaesthetics at sodium channels is weak, but is probably of more significance when the channel is in the inactivated state (Nau et al 1999), something that would explain the greater cardiotoxicity of the 'R' forms of bupivacaine and ropivacaine (see 'Use-dependent block' above). However, the issue is complicated by differences in vasoactivity, with both ropivacaine and levobupivacaine having a greater vasoconstrictor effect than their matching 'R' isomers. Thus, in a parallel to the differences between lidocaine

and prilocaine (see 'Structure–activity relationships' above), ropivacaine appears, in clinical use at nerve blocking concentrations, to be equipotent to racemic bupivacaine even though its lipid solubility is less. For the same reason, levobupivacaine may be slightly more potent than the racemate, and there is some controversy about the relative potencies of the three agents (Whiteside & Wildsmith 2001), small though the differences may be. Unfortunately, clinical comparisons are further complicated by the 'weight per unit volume' method used to describe local anaesthetic drug concentrations in commercial preparations. Ropivacaine and bupivacaine are presented as $mg\,ml^{-1}$ of the hydrochloride salt, but levobupivacaine as $mg\,ml^{-1}$ of the local anaesthetic base, a result of recent changes in the regulations governing labelling of new (but not older) drugs. Because the base has a lower molecular weight, levobupivacaine has about 11% more molecules of local anaesthetic than the racemic bupivacaine preparations of superficially the same concentration. This is a significant difference.

## DYNAMICS OF NERVE BLOCK

The effect of physiological factors on the performance of any particular drug is also seen in the way in which its clinical profile varies between injection sites. Each technique of local anaesthesia (spinal, epidural, plexus, major and minor nerve blocks) has its own particular rate of onset, duration and risk of systemic toxicity (Winnie et al 1977). These may be clearly related to the thickness of the coverings of the nerve at that point and the blood supply to the area of injection. The faster onset and lower dose requirement of spinal compared with epidural anaesthesia may be explained simply in terms of the considerable difference in the coverings of the nerves in the two spaces (Cohen 1968). After they have passed through the intervertebral foramina, the segmental nerves acquire further coverings, especially if they are involved in the formation of a plexus. These coverings become thinner as the nerve passes more peripherally so the rate of onset of block becomes faster.

The difference in diffusion barriers may also explain the greater susceptibility to chemical damage of nerves in the subarachnoid space. Reports of permanent neurological damage after the use of chloroprocaine for epidural block seem to have been related to the effects of the metabisulphite preservative which was once included in the solution. When injected correctly in the epidural space this preservative has minimal effect because it cannot penetrate the dural sheath, but accidental intrathecal injection of large quantities 'bypasses' that protection.

The pattern of onset of nerve block is further affected by the arrangement of fibres within the mixed nerve. Fibres to and from the most distal structures supplied by it are arranged at its core and those joining it more proximally are on the outside. As local anaesthetic diffuses into a nerve it affects the fibres innervating the periphery last (Winnie et al 1977). This is one reason why anaesthesia of the hand may be slow to develop during brachial plexus block, but this will, of course, depend also on the particular technique chosen and on gross anatomical factors such as which component (root, cord, trunk, branch) of the plexus is closest to the point of injection.

## Differential nerve block

It is a common clinical observation that different modalities of nerve function are not blocked at the same rate (Catterall & Mackie 1996). The sequence depends on the site of injection and the drug used, but a typical order of development of block is sympathetic function first, followed by pin-prick sensation, touch, temperature, and finally motor. This phenomenon may be manipulated clinically. Adjustment of drug concentration and volume injected during continuous epidural techniques may produce sympathetic afferent block, with minimal sensory and motor block. The subarachnoid injection of increasing concentrations of procaine has been used to produce differential blocks in the diagnosis and treatment of chronic pain (but see Hogan & Abram 1997).

Peripheral nerve fibres are classified according to both the modality they subserve and their physiological properties. The most important of the latter is velocity of impulse transmission and this depends on both axon diameter and degree of myelination. These various factors may be correlated (Table 3.1). Early laboratory work and clinical observations were often misinterpreted to conclude that the smallest nerve fibres were the most sensitive to local anaesthetic block and the largest the least sensitive (Raymond & Gissen 1987). However, there is now a large amount of evidence against this simplification. Laboratory studies *in vivo* on single functionally identified fibres show that B-fibres are most sensitive, followed by Aγ (motor) and Aδ (sensory) fibres, then Aβ (sensory) and Aα (motor) fibres and finally C-fibres, which are the most resistant to block.

Clinically, loss of function is assessed rather than block of impulse transmission, and these two results may not be equivalent. For example, a reduction in the average frequency of C-fibre discharge in response to pin-prick may fall from 10 Hz to 4 Hz due to use-dependent block by a local anaesthetic, but the perceived stimulus intensity would drop from noticeable to sub-liminal, because a minimal impulse frequency of about 5 Hz is required for this perception. In another example, partial block of small myelinated Aγ efferents will relax muscle spindles and thus attenuate firing of Ia-sensory fibres (muscle spindle afferents). This results in flaccid paralysis through the myotonic stretch reflex circuitry of the spinal cord. Clinicians often equate such paralysis or paresis with block of the large motor Aα fibres, although this is not required for 'motor block'. Thus, functional block observed clinically can arise for many reasons and it may not be directly apparent exactly which fibres are blocked.

## FUTURE DEVELOPMENTS

The currently available local anaesthetic drugs meet most requirements for local anaesthetic block during surgery, especially when their flexibility is extended by the use of catheter techniques for prolonged effect. What problems there are relate more to systemic toxicity than inadequacies in blocking characteristics, although a drug which could penetrate thick sheaths rapidly (as around the brachial plexus) and have a long duration of action would be extremely useful. The greater need is for an agent which specifically provides analgesia without affecting the other modalities of nerve function, so that the benefits of regional nerve block can be extended simply and safely into the post-operative period. The great wave of enthusiasm, which followed the introduction to clinical practice of the spinal application of opioid drugs, is clear evidence that many anaesthetists are aware of this need.

Possibly, the manipulation of physicochemical properties may allow variations on the traditional local anaesthetic drug theme to fill these requirements, but different classes of 'local anaesthetic' are also being sought, including derivatives of substances which produce sodium channel block in different ways. The biotoxins, tetrodotoxin and saxitoxin, for instance, act by forming complexes with sites at the outer end of the sodium channel. They are very potent, and may yet hold promise for clinical application.

Sodium channel block is a relatively non-specific property of many classes of chemical. An equally necessary property is the ability to reach the membrane rapidly and in such amounts that the action is effective for a useful period of time (Popitz-Bergez et al 1994). The synapse between the first and second order pain neurone is, as has been outlined in Chapter 3, the subject of considerable interest in the search for a peripheral modulator of painful stimuli. This chapter's focus has been on impulse block produced by in-

hibition of sodium channels, but traditional local anaesthetics block both calcium channels (Coyle & Speralakis 1987) and many receptors for neuro-transmitters, both the ligand-gated and G-protein-coupled varieties (Butterworth & Strichartz 1990). At their peripheral and central terminations, therefore, peripheral nerve actions can be inhibited by local anaesthetics acting on targets other than sodium channels. Such mechanisms may be essential con-tributors to infiltration anaesthesia and central nerve block. In the future these may become explicit targets for the design of newer structures of 'local anaesthetics'.

# References

Aberg G 1972 Toxicological and local anaesthetic effects of optically active isomers of two local anaesthetic compounds. Acta Pharmacologica et Toxicologica 31: 444–450

Åckerman B, Persson H, Tegner C 1967 Local anaesthetic properties of the optically active isomers of prilocaine (Citanest®) Acta Pharmacologica et Toxicologica 25: 233–241

Åckerman B, Hellberg I-B, Trossvik C 1988 Primary evaluation of the local anaesthetic properties of the amino amide agent ropivacaine (LEA 103). Acta Anaesthesiologica Scandinavica 32: 571–578

Bernards CM, Hill HF 1992 Physical and chemical properties of drug molecules governing their diffusion through the spinal meninges. Anesthesiology 77: 750–756

Butterworth JF, Strichartz GR 1990 Molecular mechanism of local anesthetics: a review. Anesthesiology 72: 711–720

Cahn RS, Ingold CK, Pelog V 1956 The specification of asymmetric configuration in organic chemistry. Experentia 12: 81–124

Catterall W, Mackie K 1996 Local anesthetics. In: Hardman JG, Limbird LE, Molinoff PB, Ruddon RW, Goodman AG (eds), Goodman and Gilman's The Pharmacological Basis of Therapeutics, 9th edn, pp 331–347. McGraw Hill, New York

Cohen, EN 1968 Distribution of local anesthetic agents in the neuraxis of the dog. Anesthesiology 29: 1002–1005

Courtney KR 1980 Structure–activity relations for frequency-dependent sodium channel block in nerve by local anesthetics. Journal of Pharmacology and Experimental Therapeutics 213: 114–119

Coyle DE, Speralakis N 1987 Bupivacaine and lidocaine blockade of calcium mediated slow action potentials in guinea pig ventricular muscle. Journal of Pharmacology and Experimental Therapeutics 242: 1001–1005

Feng TP, Liu YM 1949 The connective tissue sheath of the nerve as effective diffusion barrier. Journal of Cellular and Comparative Physiology 34: 1–16

Hille B 1984 Ionic channels of excitable membranes. Sinauer Associates, Sunderland, Mass.

Hodgkin AL, Huxley AF 1952 A quantitative description of membrane current and its application to conduction and excitation in nerve. Journal of Physiology 117: 500–544

Hogan QH, Abram SE 1997 Neural blockade for diagnosis and prognosis. A review. Anesthesiology 86: 216–241

Lee-Son S, Wang GK, Concus A, Crill E, Strichartz GR 1992 Stereoselective inhibition of neuronal sodium channels by local anesthetics: evidence for two sites of action? Anesthesiology 77: 324–335

Moorman JR.1998 Sodium Channels. In: Yaksh TL, Lynch C, Zapol WM, Maze M, Biebuyck JF, Saidman LJ (eds) Anesthesia: biologic foundations, Ch 11, pp 145–162. Lippincott-Raven, Philadelphia and New York

Narahashi T, Frazier D, Yamada M 1970 The site of action and active form of local anesthetics, 1. Theory and pH experi-ments with tertiary compounds. Journal of Pharmacology and Experimental Therapeutics 171: 32–44

Nau C, Wang S-Y, Strichartz GR, Wang GK 1999 Point mutations at N434 in D1-S6 of mu-1 Na$^+$ channels modulate binding affinity and stereoselectivity of local anesthetic enantiomers. Molecular Pharmacology 56: 404–413.

Popitz-Bergez FA, Lee-Son S, Thalhammer JG, Strichartz GR 1994 Intraneural lidocaine uptake and distribution during sciatic nerve block neurologically assessed in the rat. Regional Anesthesia 19S: 20

Ragsdale DS, McPhee JC, Scheuer T, Catterall WA 1994 Molecular determinants of state-dependent block of Na$^+$ channels by local anesthetics. Science 265: 1724–1730

Raymond SA, Gissen, AJ 1987 Mechanisms of differential block. In: Strichartz GR (ed.) Handbook of experimental pharma-cology, Vol. 81, Ch 4, pp 95–164. Springer-Verlag, Berlin and Heidelberg

Schwarz W, Palade PT, Hille B 1977 Local anesthetics: effect of pH on use-dependent block of sodium channels in frog muscle. Biophysics Journal 20: 343–368

Shanthaveerappa TR, Bourne GH 1962 The 'perineural epithelium', a metabolically active, continuous, protoplasmic cell barrier surrounding peripheral nerve fasiculi. Journal of Anatomy, London 96(4): 527–537

Strichartz GR 1977 The composition and structure of excitable nerve membrane. In: Jamieson GA, Robinson DM (eds) Mammalian cell membranes, vol 3, pp 173–205. Butterworths, London

Sidebotham DA, Schug SA 1997 Stereochemistry in Anaesthesia. Clinical and Experimental Pharmacology Physiology 24: 126–130

Strichartz GR (ed.) 1986 Handbook of Experimental Pharmacology, Vol 68, Local anesthetics. Springer-Verlag, Berlin and Heidelberg

Strichartz GR, Berde CB 1994 Local anesthetics. In: Miller R. (ed.) Anesthesia, 4th edn, pp 489–521. Churchill Livingstone, New York

Strichartz GR, Sanchez V, Arthur GR, Chafetz R, Martin D 1990 Fundamental properties of local anesthetics, II. Measured octanol:buffer partition coefficients and pKa values of clinically-used drugs. Anesthesia and Analgesia 71: 158–170

Stuhmer W, Conti F, Harukazu S, Wang X, Noda M, Yahagi N, Kubo H, Numa S 1989 Structural parts involved in activation and inactivation of the sodium channel. Nature 339: 597–603

Tucker GT 1997 Ropivacaine: human pharmacokinetics. American Journal of Anesthesiology 24(Suppl 5): 8–13

Vanhoutte F, Vereecke J, Verbeke N, Carmeliet E 1991 Stereoselective effects of the enantiomers of bupivacaine on electro-physiological properties of the guinea-pig papillary muscle. British Journal of Pharmacology 103: 1275–1281

Whiteside J, Wildsmith JAW 2001 Developments in local anaesthetic drugs. British Journal of Anaesthesia; 87: 27–35

Wildsmith JAW, Brown DT, Paul D, Johnson S 1989 Structure–activity relationships in differential nerve blockade at high and low frequency stimulation. British Journal of Anaesthesia 63: 444–452

Winnie AP, Tay C-H, Patel KP, Ramamurthy S, Durrani Z 1977 Pharmacokinetics of local anesthetics during plexus blocks. Anesthesia and Analgesia 56: 852–861

# 5. Local anaesthetic kinetics

## G T Tucker

Knowledge of the factors influencing the plasma drug concentration–time profiles (pharmacokinetics) of local anaesthetics (Fig. 5.1) underpins their safe and effective use. The plasma drug concentration provides information not only on the margin of systemic safety, but also, indirectly, on the amount of dose yet to be absorbed and still available locally for anaesthetic effect. The relevant pharmacokinetic properties are determined by the physicochemical and structural features of the compounds. The former, in particular lipid solubility, have a major influence on systemic absorption rate and hence duration of activity. In concert with chemical structure, they determine how and at what rate the compound is removed from the body. In addition, stereochemical features (see Ch. 4) can also modulate pharmacokinetic properties.

The key physicochemical properties of the main local anaesthetics are shown in Table 4.1. Of the amides, only lidocaine is achiral, the rest have an asymmetric carbon atom, giving rise to the possibility of two stereoisomers. Prilocaine, mepivacaine and etidocaine are available as racemates (50:50 mixtures of the two isomers), ropivacaine as the single S-isomer, and bupivacaine as either the racemate or the single S-isomer (levobupivacaine).

Consideration of the pharmacokinetics of local anaesthetic agents can be divided into three aspects: local disposition, systemic absorption, and systemic disposition.

## LOCAL DISPOSITION

Physiological and biochemical factors affecting the dispersion and distribution of local anaesthetics at and near the site of administration have been reviewed by Tucker and Mather (1998), and include bulk flow of the injected solution, regional blood flow and its distribution, and diffusion and binding of the agent. Local metabolic breakdown seems less important. There appears to be no stereoselectivity in the local membrane permeability of anaesthetics, as demonstrated by similar diffusion of the isomers of bupivacaine across excised monkey dura (Bernards et al 2000). Clement and colleagues (1999), using microdialysis, found that access of lidocaine to the cerebrospinal fluid after epidural injection in rabbits was about three times greater than that of bupivacaine. This probably reflects much greater sequestration of bupivacaine in epidural fat (Tucker & Mather 1998).

Of considerable current interest is the possibility that the pharmaceutical formulation of local anaesthetics can be manipulated in order to prolong the duration of action. For example, liposomal encapsulation provides a depot from which drug is released slowly. Compared to the use of equivalent doses in aqueous media, it has

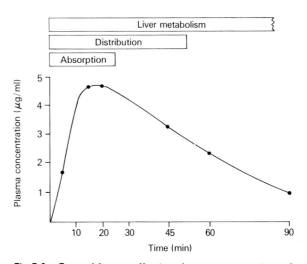

**Fig 5.1**  General factors affecting plasma concentrations of a local anaesthetic after injection

been shown to prolong duration of action and lower the risk of systemic toxicity when injected perineurally, epidurally or intrathecally in experimental animals, and epidurally in man (Grant & Bansinath 2001). If lack of neurotoxicity from such vehicles can be guaranteed, they offer the promise of ultra-long-lasting local effect.

## SYSTEMIC ABSORPTION

Knowledge of the rates of systemic absorption of local anaesthetics helps to set confidence limits on the likelihood of systemic toxic reactions after different regional nerve block procedures. Indirectly, these rates give some indication of the relationship between neural block and the amount of drug remaining at or near the site of injection.

## Plasma drug concentration and toxicity

To assess safety margins, blood or plasma drug concentrations measured after perineural injection are compared with estimates of the threshold values associated with the onset of significant CNS toxicity. The latter are available from controlled studies involving intravenous infusion of the agents into healthy volunteers (Tucker & Mather, 1998). Figures range from 5 to $10\,\mu g\,ml^{-1}$ of plasma for lidocaine, and from 2 to $4\,\mu g\,ml^{-1}$ for bupivacaine. Such intravenous tolerance studies have indicated that ropivacaine causes fewer CNS symptoms and cardiovascular changes than racemic bupivacaine, and is about 25% less toxic with regard to the maximum tolerated dose. At equal plasma concentrations ropivacaine is less toxic than bupivacaine (Scott et al 1989, Knudsen et al 1997).

Although 'threshold' levels associated with toxicity are useful guidelines for safe perineural dosage, they refer to the mythical 'average patient', and they should be interpreted in the light of a number of considerations. These include whether measurements are made of plasma or blood, total or unbound drug, ionised or un-ionised species, enantiomers, active drug metabolites and, most importantly, the rate of drug administration. The values are most relevant when concentrations are not changing rapidly and there is time for equilibration between drug concentrations in plasma and tissue. The site of blood sampling (artery or vein) is critical for interpretation when drug concentrations are changing rapidly (Tucker 1986).

## Determinants of systemic absorption

Because local anaesthetics are relatively lipid-soluble compounds, diffusion across the capillary endothelium is unlikely to limit their rates of absorption. Hence these will primarily be related directly to local blood flow, and inversely to local tissue binding. Important determinants of these variables include the physico-chemical and vasoactive properties of the agent, the site of injection, dose, the presence of additives such as vasoconstrictors, other formulation factors intended to modify local drug residence and release, the influence of nerve block, and pathological features of the patient (Tucker & Mather 1998).

### Agent

The extensive data on peak blood and plasma concentrations ($C_{max}$) of the amide local anaesthetics, and the times at which $C_{max}$ occurs ($t_{max}$) after various routes of injection, have been tabulated elsewhere (Tucker & Mather 1979, 1988). For example, after single-dose epidural injection of plain solutions, the whole blood drug concentration reaches a peak of about 0.9 to $1.0\,\mu g\,ml^{-1}$ for every 100 mg injected for lidocaine and mepivacaine, slightly less for prilocaine, and approximately half as much for bupivacaine and etidocaine. The figure for ropivacaine appears to be similar to that for bupivacaine (Katz et al 1990).

Values of $C_{max}$ and $t_{max}$ for the isomers of mepivacaine and bupivacaine after epidural administration of the racemates are shown in Table 5.1. The enantiomeric differences reflect differences in systemic disposition rather than absorption. Sequestration in the epidural fat of the more lipid-soluble bupivacaine has a rate-limiting effect on its systemic uptake and these factors account for its much longer half-life. This has been confirmed by direct measurement of residual drug concentrations in the epidural fat of sheep (Tucker & Mather 1998), and by estimation of the time-course of systemic absorption from the epidural space in humans using the mathematical technique of deconvolution analysis (Tucker & Mather 1979, Burm et al 1987). The latter calculations show that systemic drug uptake after epidural injection is a biphasic process, the contribution of the initial rapid phase being greater for short-acting agents than for long-acting ones. In the case of ropivacaine a correlation has been noted between the duration of sensory block and the slower absorption half-life (Emanuelsson et al 1997).

**Table 5.1** Mean pharmacokinetic parameters describing plasma concentration – time profiles of the R and S isomers of mepivacaine (460 mg) and bupivacaine (114 mg) after epidural injection of the racemates (Groen et al 1997)

| | Mepivacaine | | | Bupivacaine | | |
|---|---|---|---|---|---|---|
| | R(–) | S(+) | R/S | R(+) | S(–) | R/S |
| $C_{max}$ (ng ml$^{-1}$) | 1350 | 1740 | 0.77* | 389 | 449 | 0.87* |
| $Cu_{max}$ (ng ml$^{-1}$) | 485 | 460 | 1.00 | 20 | 15 | 1.36* |
| $T_{max}$ (min) | 18 | 18 | 1.00 | 8 | 8 | 1.00 |
| $t_{1/2,z}$ (h) | 2.0 | 2.2 | 0.96 | 7.3 | 6.9 | 1.05 |

$C_{max}$ = peak total plasma drug concentration; $Cu_{max}$ = peak unbound drug concentration; $t_{max}$ = time to $C_{max}$; $t_{1/2,z}$ = terminal half-life; R/S = ratio of the two; *indicates statistically significant difference from unity

Differences in the absorption rates of the various agents after epidural injection have implications for their accumulation during repeated or continuous administration. Whereas systemic accumulation is most marked with the short-acting amides, extensive local accumulation is predicted for the longer-acting compounds despite their longer dosage intervals (Tucker & Mather 1975, Tucker et al 1977, Inoue et al 1985). The slow absorption phase will determine the terminal plasma half-life and hence the rate of systemic accumulation.

The relatively low (in comparison to its toxic threshold) plasma concentrations of prilocaine after brachial plexus block (Fig. 5.2) and intravenous regional anaesthesia support the claim that this compound should be the agent of choice for such single-dose procedures (Wildsmith et al 1977). In this case, however, high systemic clearance, rather than slow absorption, is mainly responsible for the relatively low plasma drug concentrations.

Although the rate of systemic absorption of local anaesthetics is controlled largely by the extent of local binding, their intrinsic vasoactive properties may also modulate local perfusion and hence uptake. Thus, the greater vasoconstrictor potency of the S-isomers of amide agents may explain why they are longer acting than their 'R' equivalents after subcutaneous injection, despite lower intrinsic nerve blocking potency (Aps & Reynolds 1978).

## Site of injection

Vascularity and the presence of tissue and fat that can bind local anaesthetic are primary influences on their rate of uptake from specific sites of injection. In general, and independent of the agent used, absorption rate decreases in the order: intercostal block > caudal block > epidural block > brachial plexus block > sciatic and femoral nerve block (Tucker & Mather 1988).

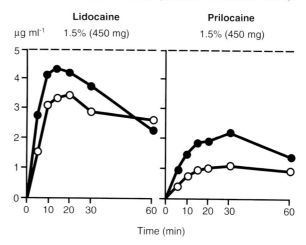

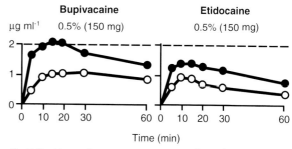

**Fig 5.2** Mean plasma concentrations of amide-type local anaesthetics after interscalene brachial plexus block. Thirty millilitres of agent, with (○) or without (●) epinephrine, were injected. The broken lines indicate the putative thresholds for the onset of signs of toxicity. (From Wildsmith et al 1977, with permission)

Variations in anatomical approach or site of injection within particular block techniques are not associated with significant differences in local anaesthetic absorption rate (Vester-Andersen et al 1981, Maclean et al 1988, Yokoyama et al 2001).

The greatest risk of producing excessive plasma drug concentrations is associated with intercostal nerve block, especially when supplementary bolus injections are superimposed on a continuous infusion (Safran et al 1990), and with interpleural block, where large doses are applied to a relatively large surface area permitting rapid absorption (van Kleef et al 1990, Kastrissios et al 1991).

A pharmacokinetic analysis of plasma lidocaine concentrations after cuff-release during intravenous regional anaesthesia indicated that only about 20–30% of the dose is released immediately into the general circulation. About 50% still remains in the arm after 30 minutes, and longer application of the cuff further delays washout of drug from the arm (Tucker & Boas, 1971).

Deconvolution analysis has shown significant differences in the pattern of systemic drug absorption after subarachnoid and epidural injection, and confirms that there is a slower net absorption of bupivacaine compared to lidocaine (Burm et al 1987, 1988). Slower initial uptake from the subarachnoid space may reflect delay imposed by dural diffusion. The similarity of the slower phases of uptake after subarachnoid injection of bupivacaine (and the overall monoexponential uptake of subarachnoid lidocaine) to the corresponding slow phases of uptake after epidural bupivacaine suggests a common rate-limiting removal from epidural fat.

By far the largest doses of local anaesthetics are administered by subcutaneous infiltration as a component of the anaesthetic technique for liposuction. Klein (1990) considers that 35 mg kg⁻¹ is a conservative estimate of the safe maximum dose of lidocaine, based on the observation that peak plasma drug concentrations are well below the toxic threshold 10–15 hours after injection. He emphasises the importance of using a dilute solution with added epinephrine, and injecting slowly over 45 minutes. Injection of larger doses over less than 5 minutes results in dangerously rapid drug absorption. About 30% of the injected dose of lidocaine is removed with the subcutaneous fat.

### Epinephrine

The degree to which epinephrine will decrease the systemic absorption rate of local anaesthetic is a complex function of the type, dose and concentration of local anaesthetic, and of the characteristics of the injection site (Tucker & Mather 1998). Although peak plasma concentrations of local anaesthetics are lowered by epinephrine after most of the common regional blocks, it does not always prolong the time to peak (Tucker & Mather 1988). In general, the greatest effects of epinephrine are seen after intercostal block, and with short-acting rather than long-acting agents. This suggests that the greater local binding of the latter drugs has more influence on their duration of action than the vasoconstriction caused by epinephrine. In addition, the inherent vasoactivity of the local anaesthetic may modulate the effects of epinephrine. For example, addition of epinephrine to ropivacaine not only has no effect on plasma concentrations after brachial plexus injection, but results in tendency towards a *shorter* duration of nerve block (Hickey et al 1990). Thus ropivacaine may actually be exerting an antagonistic, 'anti-epinephrine' effect.

### Physical and pathophysiological factors

After nerve block, plasma concentrations of local anaesthetics are rather poorly correlated with body weight and height (Moore et al 1976a, b, Scott et al 1972, Tucker et al 1977, Pihlajamäki 1991). Increasing age (22–81 years) has been associated with an increase in the rate of the late phase of bupivacaine absorption after subarachnoid block, although no change was noted with epidural block (Veering et al 1987, 1991, 1992). Thus, these findings reinforce the view that an increased duration of analgesia in elderly patients has a pharmacodynamic rather than a pharmacokinetic basis. Limited data in children indicate a somewhat faster systemic absorption of local anaesthetics than in adults (Eyres et al 1978, 1983, Ecoffey et al 1984, Takasaki 1984, Rothstein et al 1986). Pregnancy appears to have little influence on the plasma concentration–time profile of local anaesthetics after epidural injection (Pihlajamäki et al 1990). Acute hypovolaemia slows lidocaine absorption after epidural injection in dogs (Morikawa et al 1974). The hyperkinetic circulation associated with chronic renal failure does not appear to enhance the systemic uptake of local anaesthetic and does not, therefore, explain the decreased duration of brachial plexus block in these patients (Rice et al 1991).

## SYSTEMIC DISPOSITION

Systemic disposition refers to all processes occurring after absorption from the site of injection, and comprises distribution to other tissues (including placental transfer) and elimination, which is the combination of metabolic breakdown and excretion of unchanged drug.

## Role of the lung

The lung is strategically placed to receive the entire dose of drug entering the systemic circulation. By acting as a 'capacitor', temporarily sequestering drug, it modulates the initial arterial drug concentration reaching the target organs of local anaesthetic toxicity, the brain and the heart (Tucker & Boas 1971, Lofström 1978, Jorfeldt et al 1979). Lung uptake is dependent on binding within its tissues, and ion-trapping due to the pH gradient between plasma and the more acidic lung (Post et al 1979, Post & Eriksdotter-Behm 1982, Palazzo et al 1991). Thus, it may be altered by acid–base changes or by competition for uptake with other basic drugs (Rothstein et al 1987). No stereoselectivity was observed in a study of the lung uptake of bupivacaine isomers in man (Sharrock et al 1998).

Administration of local anaesthetics to patients with 'right to left' cardiac shunts (Bokesh et al 1987), or inadvertent injection into the carotid or vertebral artery during attempted block of adjacent nerves, will by-pass this 'first-pass' lung uptake, and increase the probability of CNS toxicity.

## Plasma binding

The extent of binding to plasma protein, principally to $\alpha_1$-acid glycoprotein, is greater for the long-acting, more lipid-soluble agents (Table 5.2). Significant increases in the plasma levels of $\alpha_1$-acid glycoprotein, accompanied by increased drug binding, occur postoperatively and in association with many disease states, including cancer and arthritis (Jackson et al 1982, Routledge et al 1982). Conversely, low levels of the protein, and decreased drug binding, occur in neonatal plasma (Tucker et al 1970).

The implications of changes in plasma binding, either because of disease or drug–drug interactions, are widely misunderstood (Tucker 1986, 1994). It is essential to appreciate the difference between a change in the *fraction* bound or unbound, and a change in *unbound*

**Table 5.2** Mean plasma unbound fractions (FU) of amide-type local anaesthetics (Burm et al 1994, 1997, Emanuelsson et al 1995, Tucker & Mather 1998, van der Meer et al 1999)

| Drug | Isomer | Fu |
|------|--------|-----|
| Prilocaine | R(−) | 0.70 |
| | S(+) | 0.73 |
| Mepivacaine | R(−) | 0.36 |
| | S(+) | 0.25 |
| Lidocaine | Achiral | 0.30 |
| Ropivacaine | S(−) | 0.06 |
| Bupivacaine | R(+) | 0.07 |
| | S(−) | 0.05 |
| Etidocaine | Racemate | 0.05 |

drug concentration. A change in the former is rarely accompanied by change in the latter, and it is the unbound concentration which generally affects pharmacological activity. Thus, it is important to allow for plasma binding when interpreting measurements of total (bound plus free) plasma drug concentrations. For example, there is marked accumulation of the total amount of local anaesthetic in plasma postoperatively, because the 'stress response' to surgery produces an increase in the concentrations of binding proteins, and therefore in the fraction of bound drug (Tucker & Mather 1975, Tucker 1986, Erichsen et al 1996, Burm et al 2000). However, unbound concentrations, which are likely to be a better index of systemic effects, are relatively constant.

When systemic drug absorption is gradual, as after perineural injection, distribution of the dose is spread over time, and the large extravascular distribution space and extensive tissue binding ensure that only a small percentage remains in the blood at any time. In this situation, any changes in plasma binding are buffered effectively by a high volume of distribution. Also, for drugs with relatively low hepatic extraction ratios, like bupivacaine and ropivacaine, any transient change in free drug concentration will be compensated rapidly by an increase in net plasma clearance.

In theory, plasma binding could limit the first-pass uptake of local anaesthetic into the brain and myocardium after rapid, inadvertent intravenous injection, and could thereby modulate toxicity. However, it is probable that a toxic dose would initially produce sufficiently high plasma drug concentrations to overwhelm the limited binding capacity of $\alpha_1$-acid glycoprotein during the first-pass through these organs (Tucker & Mather 1998, Tucker 1994). Although it is important to distinguish events during first-pass through an organ from those occurring after several recirculations, in neither case should it be assumed that plasma binding modulates tissue drug uptake and 'protects' against toxicity.

## Tissue distribution

After passage through the lungs, local anaesthetics are distributed preferentially to those organs with a high blood supply, including the brain, heart and liver (Fig. 5.3). Concentrations in muscle and fat equilibrate with those in the blood more slowly. The time to reach distribution equilibrium will be inversely proportional to tissue blood flow, and directly related to the capacity of the organ or tissue to take up the drug. In turn, the latter will depend on the volume of the organ and the affinity of drug for the tissue. Net tissue binding is reflected in the steady-state volume of distribution based on measurement of unbound drug in plasma ($Vu_{ss}$). The value of this parameter for amide-type local anaesthetics varies over a five-fold range, being greatest for the more lipid-soluble agents and exhibiting little or no stereoselectivity. Distribution volumes based on total plasma drug concentration ($V_{ss}$) vary less between

agents, reflecting the balance between plasma and tissue binding (Table 5.3).

It is well established that the systemic toxicity of local anaesthetics is enhanced by acidosis and hypercapnia (Englesson 1974, Englesson & Grevsten 1974). In theory, increased brain and myocardial concentrations of free, un-ionised drug could be produced by haemodynamic changes and ion trapping. However, during metabolic acidosis of the type associated with convulsions there is no significant increase in the brain:blood partition coefficients of local anaesthetic, presumably because blood and tissue pH are lowered equally (Simon et al 1984, Nancarrow et al 1987). Nevertheless, data from rat studies suggest that treatment of convulsions by paralysis and artificial ventilation will actually tend to *promote* entry of local anaesthetic into the brain, because correction of the systemic acidosis promotes ion trapping of drug in the organ unless the cerebral acidosis is also corrected (Simon et al 1984).

## Excretion

As local anaesthetics are relatively lipid-soluble compounds, extensive passive tubular reabsorption limits the renal excretion of unchanged drug to less than 1–6% of the dose under normal conditions (Tucker & Mather 1979). Although recovery of drug from the urine can be augmented by acidification of the urine to

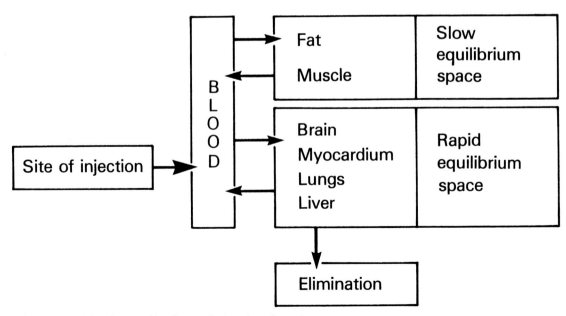

**Fig 5.3** Pattern of distribution of local anaesthetics after absorption

**Table 5.3** Mean parameters describing the kinetics of amide-type local anaesthetic after intravenous injection in healthy individuals (Burm et al 1994, 1997, Emanuelsson et al 1995, Tucker & Mather 1998, van der Meer et al 1999)

| | Prilocaine | | Mepivacaine | | Lidocaine | Ropivacaine | Bupivacaine | | Etidocaine |
| --- | --- | --- | --- | --- | --- | --- | --- | --- | --- |
| | R(–) | S(+) | R(–) | S(+) | achiral | S(–) | R(+) | S(–) | racemate |
| $V_{ss}$ (l) | 279 | 291 | 103 | 57* | 73 | 54 | 84 | 54* | 80 |
| $Vu_{ss}$ (l) | 402 | 401 | 290 | 232* | 253 | 900 | 1578 | 1498 | 1478 |
| CL (l min$^{-1}$) | 2.6 | 1.9* | 0.8 | 0.4* | 1.2 | 0.5 | 0.4 | 0.3* | 0.7 |
| Clu (l min$^{-1}$) | 3.5 | 2.7* | 2.2 | 1.4* | 3.7 | 7.9 | 6.6 | 8.7* | 13.4 |
| $CL_b$ (l min$^{-1}$) | 1.8 | 1.7* | 0.9 | 0.4* | 0.9 | 0.3 | 0.3 | 0.2* | 1.1 |
| $t_{1/2,z}$ (h) | 1.5 | 2.1* | 1.9 | 2.0* | 1.6 | 1.9 | 3.6 | 2.6* | 2.7 |

$V_{ss}$ = volume of distribution at steady state for total drug concentration; $Vu_{ss}$ = volume of distribution at steady state for unbound drug; CL = total drug clearance; Clu = unbound drug clearance; $t_{1/2,z}$ = terminal half-life; all figures relate to measurement of drug in plasma, except for $CL_b$ = estimated clearance from whole blood based on plasma clearance and the blood/plasma drug concentration ratio; *indicates an R/S enantiomer ratio value significantly different from unity.

increase ionisation, and thereby decrease reabsorption, the gain is insufficient to warrant using this procedure as a treatment for systemic toxicity. Similarly, gastric lavage, to remove local anaesthetic ion-trapped in the contents of the stomach, is not indicated because the percentage of dose recoverable in this way is small.

## Clearance

The amide linkage present in the commonly used local anaesthetic agents is stable in blood, and most of their clearance is due to metabolism in the liver. Mean blood clearance values vary in the order: bupivacaine < ropivacaine < mepivacaine (reflecting the size of the *N*-methyl substituent in this homologous series) < lidocaine < etidocaine < prilocaine (Tucker & Mather 1998, Table 5.3) This sequence shows no relationship to anaesthetic potency or lipid solubility. Etidocaine clearance is dependent mostly on liver blood flow, whereas that of bupivacaine and ropivacaine should be more sensitive to changes in intrinsic hepatic enzyme function (Tucker 1986). The relatively high clearance of prilocaine (which is in excess of liver blood flow) indicates that extrahepatic metabolism contributes significantly to the elimination of this agent. Significant differences in the clearance of R and S enantiomers have been observed (Table 5.3). For example, systemic exposure to unbound (active) concentrations of the intrinsically less toxic S(–)isomer of bupivacaine (levobupivacaine) is lower than that of the R form.

## Elimination half-life

The mean terminal elimination half-lives ($t_{1/2,z}$) of the amide local anaesthetics also show stereoselectivity, and vary between 1.5 and 3.6 hours, reflecting the balance between distribution and clearance characteristics (Table 5.3). Note that the figures obtained after bupivacaine is given intravenously are substantially less than after epidural injection (Table 5.1), reflecting rate-limiting absorption after the latter route of administration.

## Accumulation

During continuous administration of a local anaesthetic its plasma concentration will increase over about four terminal half-lives until a steady-state concentration ($C_{ss}$), determined by the ratio of dosage rate and the systemic clearance, is reached. When assessing the safety of continuous dosage regimens, it is important to be sure that there is no time-dependent decrease in clearance that will result in systemic accumulation of drug greater than that predicted from single-dose data. Although there will be a progressive postoperative decrease in total clearance of local anaesthetic as a result of the increased protein level and binding, unbound clearance, as has been discussed, remains relatively stable. This certainly seems to be true for ropivacaine during postoperative epidural infusions lasting up to about 70 hours (Erichsen et al 1996, Scott et al 1997,

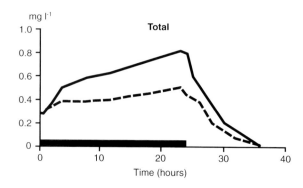

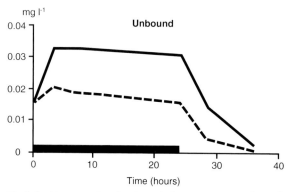

**Fig 5.4** Mean total and unbound plasma concentrations of ropivacaine during 24 h continuous epidural infusions for postoperative pain control in patients undergoing abdominal hysterectomy. Infusions were given at 10 mg h$^{-1}$ (broken lines) and 20 mg h$^{-1}$ (solid lines) in two groups of 10 patients after bolus epidural injections for surgical anaesthesia. (From Erichsen et al 1996, with permission)

**4–hydroxy–2,6–xylidine**

**Fig 5.5** Metabolic pathways for lidocaine.

Burm et al 2000) (Fig. 5.4). Beyond this time, both total and unbound ropivacaine concentrations appear to *decrease* in the face of a constant infusion, suggesting either recovery of drug metabolism after surgery and mobilisation, or enzyme induction (Wiedemann et al 2000).

## Metabolites

Identification of the biotransformation products of the amide agents in urine indicates three main sites of metabolic attack, namely aromatic hydroxylation, *N*-dealkylation and amide hydrolysis (Fig. 5.5; Table 5.4). With the exceptions of lidocaine and ropivacaine, net recoveries of the dose of drug actually administered are very low, leaving further metabolic products to be identified.

Various products have been measured in human plasma after the administration of different local anaesthetics: monoethylglycinexylidide (MEGX) and glycinexylidide (GX) from lidocaine; the 4-hydroxy products of lidocaine and bupivacaine; pipecolylxylidide (PPX) from mepivacaine, ropivacaine and bupivacaine; and the monoalkylated products of etidocaine. Significant accumulation of MEGX and PPX and, to a lesser extent of GX, occurs in the plasma during continuous epidural infusion of the relevant local anaesthetic. Such accumulation continues beyond the time when the parent drug concentration reaches a steady-state (Drayer et al 1983, Rosenberg et al 1991, Miyabe et al 1998, Kakiuchi et al 1999, Kihara et al 1999, Burm et al 2000, Fukuda et al 2000). If systemic toxicity were to occur in patients

**Table 5.4** Mean urinary recoveries (% dose) of amide-type local anaesthetics and their metabolites after intravenous or epidural administration to adults (ND = not determined). (After Halldin et al 1996, Tucker & Mather 1998, Zhang et al 1998, Burm et al 2000)

| | Unchanged | Aromatic hydroxylation | | N-dealkylation | | Amide hydrolysis | |
|---|---|---|---|---|---|---|---|
| | | 3-OH | 4-OH | Mono- | Di- | 2,6-Xylidine | 4-OH-Xylidine |
| Lidocaine | 2 | <1 | <1 | 2 | 2 | 2 | 65 |
| Mepivacaine | 4 | ND | ND | 3 | – | ND | ND |
| Ropivacaine | 1 | 10–37 | <1 | 2–10 | – | ND | ND |
| Bupivacaine | 0.3–3 | 2–4 | 2 | 5–20 | – | ~0 | ~0 |
| Etidocaine | 0.3 | 5 | 5 | 2 | – | ND | ND |

on long-term dosage of local anaesthetics, it is likely that the presence of MEGX would contribute to CNS and cardiac effects (Blumer et al 1973), whereas the unbound concentrations of PPX would probably be too low (Danielsson et al 1997).

Studies using human liver microsomes and recombinant cytochromes P450 indicate that the $N$-de-ethylation of lidocaine to MEGX is mediated by the CYP1A2 isoform at low concentrations, and by CYP3A4 at higher concentrations. 3-hydroxylation, which is a minor metabolic pathway for lidocaine and a major one for ropivacaine, is also mediated principally by CYP1A2. The $N$-dealkylation of bupivacaine and ropivacaine to PPX is mediated mainly by CYP 3A4, as is formation of the 4-hydroxy and 2-hydroxymethyl products of ropivacaine (Bargetzi et al 1989, Imaoka et al 1990, Wang et al 1999, 2000, Ekstrom & Gunnarsson 1996, Gantenbein et al 2000).

Metabolism of prilocaine to $o$-toluidine, and subsequent $N$-hydroxylation of this product, is responsible for methaemoglobinaemia at doses above 600 mg (Hjelm & Holmdahl 1965). There is concern that this effect may become clinically significant in children of less than 3 months of age receiving continuous applications of the cream containing a eutectic mixture of prilocaine and lidocaine bases (Gajraj et al 1994). Although cases of methaemoglobinaemia have also been reported after lidocaine (Deas 1956), its 2,6-xylidine metabolite is less potent in this respect than $o$-toluidine (McLean et al 1969).

## Effects of patient variables

### Weight
There appears to be no relationship between body weight, surface area or lean body mass and the disposition

kinetics of amide-type local anaesthetics in males with normal height:weight ratios (Tucker & Mather 1998). An increase in volume of distribution in obese patients of both sexes with minimal cardiac dysfunction may account for a 50% increase in the terminal elimination half-life of lidocaine (Abernethy & Greenblatt 1984a).

### Age
In healthy people, increase in the elimination half-lives of lidocaine and bupivacaine with advancing age has been related to decreases in both clearance and distribution volume (Nation et al 1977, Cusack et al 1980, Abernethy & Greenblatt 1984b, Veering et al 1987). Plasma concentration ratios of MEGX:lidocaine were found to be significantly lower in elderly patients during continuous epidural infusion of lidocaine (Fukuda et al 2000).

Elimination half-lives of the amide-type local anaesthetics are prolonged two to three times in neonates, reflecting increased volume of distribution, decreased clearance, or both (Tucker & Mather 1998). In children over the age of 1 year, differences from adults are less marked, indicating similar or higher clearances and distribution volumes (Ecoffey et al 1984, 1985, Finholt et al 1986, Mazoit et al 1988, Habre et al 2000, Hansen et al 2000, Lönnqvist et al 2000). Urinary recoveries of the known metabolites of ropivacaine were found to be similar in children and adults (Halldin et al 1996, Lönnqvist et al 2000).

### Sex
The terminal elimination half-life of lidocaine is reported to be up to 50% longer in women than men; this has been variously attributed to a difference in volume of distribution (Wing et al 1984) or clearance (Abernethy & Greenblatt 1984b).

57

### Race

White, Oriental and black subjects appear to exhibit similar disposition kinetics and plasma binding of lidocaine (Goldberg et al 1982).

### Posture

Although the clearance of lidocaine decreases on standing (Bennett et al 1982), presumably because of the fall in hepatic blood flow, prolonged recumbency appears to have no effect on its kinetics (Kates et al 1980).

### Pregnancy

A trend to lower clearance of bupivacaine has been observed in healthy parturients, accompanied by higher plasma concentrations of PPX (Pihlajamäki et al 1990). The clearance of lidocaine is decreased, but its plasma binding is unchanged in pre-eclampsia (Ramanathan et al 1986, Bottorf et al 1987).

### Disease

Studies of the kinetics of lidocaine after intravenous injection indicate that, on average, its clearance is halved in patients with heart failure and in those with severe cirrhosis of the liver. This change is accompanied by a decrease in the volume of distribution in heart failure, and an increase in cirrhosis. As a result, the terminal elimination half-life of lidocaine is prolonged significantly in cirrhosis, but less so in heart failure (Thomson et al 1973). Chronic hepatitis appears to be associated with a higher clearance of lidocaine than normal, and $V_{ss}$ is also increased secondary to a decrease in plasma binding (Huet & LeLorier 1980, Huet et al 1981).

The acute phase of viral hepatitis is accompanied by increases in lidocaine half-life and volume of distribution, with a trend to lower clearance, but no change in plasma binding (Williams et al 1976). Patients undergoing hepatectomy have a marked decrease in lidocaine clearance during continuous epidural infusion (Yokoyama et al 2001). The disposition kinetics of amide-type local anaesthetics are not influenced materially by renal disease (Thomson et al 1973), although ionised metabolites tend to accumulate more than normally (Collinsworth et al 1975). Diabetes has been associated with a 60% lower clearance of lidocaine (Peeyush et al 1992).

## Drug–drug interactions

Ideally, interpretation of pharmacokinetic data should be based on measurement of unbound drug concentration in plasma. Although displacement of local anaesthetics from plasma binding sites by other drugs alters the *unbound fraction*, theory indicates that this should have no pharmacological consequences. This is because this would be accompanied by only a transient increase in the *concentration* of unbound drug (Tucker 1994), at least for the relatively low extraction compounds (i.e. all except etidocaine and, to some extent, lidocaine).

Interactions of most concern will be those mediated through inhibition of metabolism of those compounds with relatively low hepatic extraction (mepivacaine, ropivacaine, bupivacaine), and through alteration in hepatic blood flow for those with high extraction (etidocaine). The hepatic extraction ratio of lidocaine is intermediate, and its clearance is dependent on both blood flow and enzyme activity. Tucker and Mather (1998) have summarised much of the data on kinetically based drug interactions involving local anaesthetics. For example, halothane and propranolol both lower the clearance of lidocaine by about 40%, an effect mediated by both their haemodynamic effects and inhibition of drug-metabolising enzymes.

Increasing knowledge of the specific isoforms of cytochrome P450 involved in local anaesthetic metabolism allows interactions with selective inhibitor drugs to be anticipated. For example, *in vitro* studies predicted that fluvoxamine, a potent inhibitor of CYP1A2, would decrease markedly the *in vivo* clearance of ropivacaine by blocking formation of its major 3-hydroxy metabolite, but that ketoconazole and erythromycin, selective inhibitors of CYP3A4, would have much less effect on ropivacaine clearance (Arlander et al 1998, Jokinen et al 2000). However, because these studies were carried out using small intravenous doses of ropivacaine, it is possible that at the higher and more prolonged systemic ropivacaine concentrations associated with regional anaesthesia, CYP1A2 might assume less importance with respect to net metabolism and drug interactions. Indeed, during continuous epidural infusion of ropivacaine the urinary excretion rate of its 3-hydroxy metabolite decreases while that of PPX increases, the latter being formed principally by CYP3A4 (Burm et al 2000).

## Placental transfer

The ratios of cord to maternal plasma concentrations at delivery of the amide drugs decrease in the order: prilocaine (1.0–1.1) > lidocaine ≈ mepivacaine (0.5–0.7)

> ropivacaine, bupivacaine, etidocaine (0.2–0.4) (Tucker & Mather 1979, Datta et al 1995). These differences reflect, and can be predicted from, differential maternal and fetal plasma binding of drug secondary to relatively low fetal concentrations of $\alpha_1$-acid glycoprotein, together with allowance for some ion trapping in the more acidic fetal plasma (Tucker et al 1970, Kennedy et al 1979, Johnson et al 1999). As such, therefore, these ratios are not direct predictors of relative fetal toxicity, because the corresponding average ratios of unbound (active) drug across the placenta are, irrespective of the drug, close to unity (other than at times when maternal concentrations are increasing or decreasing rapidly). This also indicates that passive distribution across the placenta is relatively rapid, irrespective of the lipid-solubility of the compounds (Johnson et al 1999).

In theory, a high maternal to fetal plasma binding ratio should delay equilibration of drug in fetal tissues, despite rapid equilibrium across the placenta (Dawes 1973, Hamshaw-Thomas et al 1984). However, the similar umbilical artery to umbilical vein concentration ratios observed with the various agents argue against large differences in their equilibration rates in the fetus, although this may be masked by shunting of blood in the placenta (Tucker et al 1970). As a consequence of ion trapping, fetal acidosis increases both the cord:maternal ratio of unbound drug, and the rate of placental transfer of local anaesthetic (Tucker et al 1970, Brown et al 1976, Biehl et al. 1978, Datta et al 1981, Gaylard et al 1990).

Having entered the cord, drug is delivered directly to the fetal liver. Thus, significant first-pass metabolism in this organ may modulate fetal exposure to local anaesthetic. It may also have the effect of amplifying the transplacental gradient of drug. A significant net back-transfer of bupivacaine, but not of lidocaine, from fetus to mother was observed after short intravenous infusions of the agents into ewes (Kennedy et al 1986, 1990). This might be explained by greater first-pass metabolism of lidocaine in fetal sheep liver, thereby maintaining the maternal to cord concentration gradient for longer. The extent of *in utero* metabolism of local anaesthetics in humans is unknown, but urinary metabolites have been measured in neonates after direct administration (Tucker & Mather 1998). Metabolites produced in the mother can pass across the placenta, and have been measured in fetal blood (Blankenbaker et al 1975, Kuhnert et al 1979, 1981). However, the toxicological significance of the presence of local anaesthetic metabolites in the fetus is unknown.

## References

Abernethy DR, Greenblatt DJ 1984a Lidocaine disposition in obesity. American Journal of Cardiology 53: 1183–1186

Abernethy DR, Greenblatt DJ 1984b Impairment of lidocaine clearance in elderly male subjects. Journal of Cardiovascular Pharmacology 5: 1093–1096

Aps C, Reynolds F 1978 An intradermal study of the local anaesthetic and vascular effects of the isomers of bupivacaine. British Journal of Clinical Pharmacology 6: 63–68

Arlander E, Ekström G, Alm C et al 1998 Metabolism of ropivacaine in humans is mediated by CYP1A2 and to a minor extent by CYP3A4: an interaction study with fluvoxamine and ketoconazole as *in vivo* inhibitors. Clinical Pharmacology and Therapeutics 64: 484–491

Bargetzi MJ, Aoyama T, Gonzalez FJ et al 1989 Lidocaine metabolism in human liver microsomes by cytochrome P450IIIA4. Clinical Pharmacology and Therapeutics 46: 521–527

Bennett PN, Aarons LJ, Bending MR et al 1982 Pharmacokinetics of lidocaine and its deethylated metabolite: Dose and time dependency studies in man. Journal of Pharmacokinetics and Biopharmacology 10: 265–268

Bernards CM, Ulma GA, Kopacz DJ 2000 The meningeal permeability of R- and S-bupivacaine are not different. Anesthesiology 93: 896–897

Biehl D, Shnider SM, Levinson G et al 1978 Placental transfer of lidocaine: Effects of acidosis. Anesthesiology 48: 409–412

Blankenbaker WL, Difazio CA, Berry FA 1975 Lidocaine and its metabolites in the newborn. Anesthesiology 42: 325–330

Blumer J, Strong JM, Atkinson AJ 1973 The convulsant potency of lidocaine and its N-dealkylated metabolites. Journal of Pharmacology and Experimental Therapeutics 186: 31–36

Bokesch PM, Castenada AR, Ziemer G et al 1987 The influence of right-to-left cardiac shunt on lidocaine pharmacokinetics. Anesthesiology 57: 739–744

Bottorff MB, Pieper JA, Boucher BA et al 1987 Lidocaine protein binding in preeclampsia. European Journal of Clinical Pharmacology 31: 719–722

Brown WU, Bell GC, Alper MH 1976 Acidosis, local anesthetics and the newborn. Obstetrics and Gynecology 48: 27–30

Burm AGL, Vermeulen NPE, Van Kleef JW et al 1987 Pharmacokinetics of lidocaine and bupivacaine in surgical patients following epidural administration: Simultaneous investigation of absorption and disposition kinetics using stable isotopes. Clinical Pharmacokinetics 13: 191–203

Burm AGL, Van Kleef JW, Vermeulen NPE et al 1988 Pharmacokinetics of lidocaine and bupivacaine following subarachnoid administration in surgical patients:

Simultaneous investigation of absorption and disposition kinetics using stable isotopes. Anesthesiology 69: 584–592

Burm AGL, Van der Meer AD, Van Kleef JW et al 1994 Pharmacokinetics of the enantiomers of bupivacaine following intravenous administration of the racemate. British Journal of Clinical Pharmacology 38: 125–129

Burm AGL, Cohen IMC, Van Kleef JW et al 1997 Pharmacokinetics of the enantiomers of mepivacaine after intravenous administration of the racemate in volunteers. Anesthesia and Analgesia 84: 85–89

Burm AGL, Stienstra R, Brouwer RP et al 2000 Epidural infusion of ropivacaine for postoperative analgesia after major orthopedic surgery. Pharmacokinetic evaluation. Anesthesiology 93: 395–430

Clement R, Malinovsky J-M, Le Corre P et al 1999 Cerebrospinal fluid bioavailability and pharmacokinetics of bupivacaine and lidocaine after intrathecal and epidural administrations in rabbits using microdialysis. Journal of Pharmacology and Experimental Therapeutics 289: 1015–1021

Collinsworth KA, Strong JM, Atkinson AJ et al 1975 Pharmacokinetics and metabolism of lidocaine in patients with renal failure. Clinical Pharmacology and Therapeutics 18: 59–64

Cusack B, Kelly JG, Lavan J et al 1980 Pharmacokinetics of lignocaine in the elderly. British Journal of Clinical Pharmacology 9: 293P

Danielsson BRG, Danielsson MK, Lindström BE et al 1997 Toxicity of bupivacaine and ropivacaine in relation to free plasma concentrations in pregnant rats: A comparative study. Pharmacology and Toxicology 81: 90–96

Datta S, Brown WU, Ostheimer GW et al 1981 Epidural anesthesia for Cesarean section in diabetic parturients: maternal and neonatal acid–base status and bupivacaine concentration. Anesthesia and Analgesia 60: 574–578

Datta S, Camann W, Bader A et al 1995 Clinical effects and maternal and fetal plasma concentrations of epidural ropivacaine versus bupivacaine for Cesarean section. Anesthesiology 82: 1346–1352

Dawes GS. 1973 A theoretical analysis of fetal drug equilibrium. In: Boreus L (ed.) Fetal Pharmacology, pp. 381–400. Raven Press, New York

Deas TC 1956 Severe methemoglobinemia following dental extraction under lidocaine anesthesia. Anesthesiology 17: 204–208

Drayer DE, Lorenzo B, Werns S et al 1983 Plasma levels, protein binding, and elimination data of lidocaine and active metabolites in cardiac patients of various ages. Clinical Pharmacology and Therapeutics 34: 14–22

Ecoffey C, Desparmet J, Berdeaux A, Maury M, Giudicelli JF, Saint-Maurice C 1984 Pharmacokinetics of lignocaine in children following caudal anaesthesia. British Journal of Anaesthesia 56: 1399–1402

Ecoffey C, Desparmet J, Maury M et al 1985 Bupivacaine in children: pharmacokinetics following caudal anesthesia. Anesthesiology 63: 447–448

Ekström G, Gunnarsson U-B 1996 Ropivacaine, a new amide-type local anesthetic agent, is metabolised by cytochromes P450 1A and 3A in human liver microsomes. Drug Metabolism and Disposition 24: 955–961

Emanuelsson B-M, Dusanka Z, Nydahl P-A et al 1995 Pharmacokinetics of ropivacaine and bupivacaine during 21 hours of continuous epidural infusion in healthy male volunteers. Anesthesia and Analgesia 81: 1163–1168

Emanuelsson, B-M, Persson J, Alm C et al 1997 Systemic absorption and block after epidural injection of ropivacaine in healthy volunteers. Anesthesiology 87: 1309–1317

Englesson S 1974 The influence of acid–base changes on central nervous system toxicity of local anaesthetic agents: I. An experimental study in cats. Acta Anaesthesiologica Scandinavica 18: 79–87

Englesson S, Grevsten S 1974 The influence of acid–base changes on central nervous system toxicity of local anaesthetic agents: II. Acta Anaesthesiologica Scandinavica 18: 88–103

Erichsen C-J, Sjövall J, Kehlet H et al 1996 Pharmacokinetics and analgesic effect of ropivacaine during continuous epidural infusion for postoperative pain relief. Anesthesiology 84: 834–842

Eyres RL, Kidd J, Oppenheim RC et al 1978 Local anaesthetic plasma levels in children. Anaesthesia and Intensive Care 6: 243–247

Eyres RL, Bishop W, Oppenheim RC et al 1983 Plasma bupivacaine concentrations in children during caudal epidural analgesia. Anaesthesia and Intensive Care 11: 20–22

Finholt DA, Stirt JA, DiFazio CA et al 1986 Lidocaine pharmacokinetics in children. Anesthesia and Analgesia 65: 279–282

Fukuda T, Kakiuchi Y, Miyabe M et al 2000 Plasma lidocaine, monoethylglycinexylidide, and glycinexylidide concentrations after epidural administration in geriatric patients. Regional Anesthesia and Pain Medicine 25: 268–273

Gajraj NM, Pennant JH, Watcha MF 1994 Eutectic mixture of local anesthetics (EMLA) cream. Anesthesia and Analgesia 78: 574–583

Gantenbein M, Attolini L, Bruguerolle B et al 2000 Oxidative metabolism of bupivacaine into pipecolylxylidine in humans is mainly catalysed by CYP3A. Drug Metabolism and Disposition 28: 383–385

Gaylard DG, Carson RJ, Reynolds F 1990 Effect of umbilical perfusate pH and controlled maternal hypotension on placental drug transfer in the rabbit. Anesthesia and Analgesia 71: 42–48

Goldberg MJ, Spector R, Johnson GF 1982 Racial background and lidocaine pharmacokinetics. Journal of Clinical Pharmacology 22: 391–394

Grant GJ, Bansinath M 2001 Liposomal delivery systems for local anesthetics. Regional Anesthesia and Pain Medicine 26: 61–63

Habre W, Bergesio R, Johnson C et al 2000 Pharmacokinetics of ropivacaine following caudal analgesia in children. Paediatric Anaesthesia 10: 143–47

Halldin MM, Bredberg E, Angelin B et al 1996 Metabolism and excretion of ropivacaine in humans. Drug Metabolism and Disposition 24: 962–968

Hamshaw-Thomas A, Rogerson N, Reynolds F 1984 Transfer of bupivacaine, lignocaine and pethidine across the rabbit placenta: Influence of maternal protein binding and fetal flow. Placenta 5: 61–70

Hansen TG, Ilett KF, Lim SI, Reid C, Hackett LP, Bergesio R 2000 Pharmacokinetics and clinical efficacy of long-term epidural ropivacaine infusion in children. British Journal of Anaesthesia 85: 347–353

Hickey R, Blanchard J, Hoffman J et al 1990 Plasma concentrations of ropivacaine given with or without epinephrine for brachial plexus block. Canadian Journal of Anaesthesia 37: 878–882

Hjelm M, Holmdahl MH 1965 Clinical chemistry of prilocaine and clinical evaluation of methaemoglobinaemia induced by this agent. Acta Anaesthesiologica Scandinavica 16: 161–70

Huet P-M, LeLorier J 1980 Effects of smoking and chronic hepatitis B on lidocaine and indocyanine green kinetics. Clinical Pharmacology and Therapeutics 28: 208–215

Huet P-M, Arsene D, Richter D 1981 The volume of distribution of lidocaine in chronic hepatitis: relationship with serum alpha1-acid glycoprotein and serum protein binding. Clinical Pharmacology and Therapeutics 29: 252–258

Imaoka S, Enomoto K, Oda Y et al 1990 Lidocaine metabolism by human cytochrome P-450s purified from hepatic microsomes: Comparison of those with rat hepatic cytochrome P-450s. Journal of Pharmacology and Experimental Therapeutics 255: 1385–1391

Inoue R, Suganuma T, Echizen H et al 1985 Plasma concentrations of lidocaine and its principal metabolites during intermittent epidural infusion. Anesthesiology 63: 304–310

Jackson PR Tucker GT, Woods HF 1982 Altered plasma binding in cancer: Role of alpha1-acid glycoprotein and albumin. Clinical Pharmacology and Therapeutics 32: 295–302

Johnson RF, Cahana A, Olenick M et al 1999 A comparison of the placental transfer of ropivacaine versus bupivacaine. Anesthesia and Analgesia 89: 703–708

Jokinen MJ, Ahonen J, Neuvonen PJ et al 2000 The effect of erythromycin, fluvoxamine, and their combination on the pharmacokinetics of ropivacaine. Anesthesia and Analgesia 91: 1207–1212

Jorfeldt L, Lewis DH, Lofström B et al 1979 Lung uptake of lidocaine in healthy volunteers. Acta Anaesthesiologica Scandinavica 23: 567–574

Kakiuchi Y, Kohda Y, Miyabe M et al 1999 Effect of plasma a1-acid glycoprotein concentration on the accumulation of lidocaine metabolites during continuous epidural anesthesia in infants and children. International Journal of Clinical Pharmacology and Therapeutics 37: 493–498

Kastrissios H, Triggs EJ, Mogg GAG et al 1991 The disposition of bupivacaine following a 72 h interpleural infusion in cholecystectomy patients. British Journal of Clinical Pharmacology 32: 251–254

Kates RE, Harapat SR, Keefe DLD et al 1980 Influence of prolonged recumbency on drug disposition. Clinical Pharmacology and Therapeutics 27: 624–628

Katz JA, Bridenbaugh PO, Knarr DC et al 1990 Pharmacodynamics and pharmacokinetics of epidural ropivacaine in humans. Anesthesia and Analgesia 70: 16–21

Kennedy RL, Erenberg A, Robilliard JE et al 1979 Effects of the changes in maternal-fetal pH on the transplacental equilibrium of bupivacaine. Anesthesiology 51: 50–54

Kennedy RL, Miller RP, Bell JU et al 1986 Uptake and distribution of bupivacaine in fetal lambs. Anesthesiology 65: 247–253

Kennedy RL, Bell JU, Miller RP et al 1990 Uptake and distribution of lidocaine in fetal lambs. Anesthesiology 72: 483–489

Kihara S, Miyabe M, Kakiuchi Y et al 1999 Plasma concentrations of lidocaine and its principal metabolites during continuous epidural infusion of lidocaine with or without epinephrine. Regional Anesthesia and Pain Medicine 24: 529–533

Klein JA 1990 Tumescent technique for regional anesthesia permits lidocaine doses of 35 mg/kg for liposuction. Journal of Dermatology and Surgical Oncology 16: 248–263

Knudsen K, Beckman-Suurküla SM, Blomberg S, Sjövall J, Edvardsson N 1997 Central nervous and cardiovascular effects of i.v. infusions of ropivacaine, bupivacaine and placebo in volunteers. British Journal of Anaesthesia 78: 507–514

Kuhnert BR, Knapp DR, Kuhnert PM et al 1979 Maternal, fetal and neonatal metabolites of lidocaine. Clinical Pharmacology and Therapeutics 26: 213–220

Kuhnert PM, Kuhnert BR, Stitts JM et al 1981 The use of selected ion monitoring technique to study the disposition of bupivacaine in mother, fetus, and neonate following epidural anesthesia for Cesarean section. Anesthesiology 55: 611–617

Lofström B 1978 Tissue distribution of local anesthetics with special reference to the lung. International Anesthesiology Clinics 16: 53–58

Lönnqvist PA, Westrin P, Larsson BA et al 2000 Ropivacaine pharmacokinetics after caudal block in 1–8 year old children. British Journal of Anaesthesia 85: 506–511

Maclean D, Chambers WA, Tucker GT, Wildsmith JAW 1988 Plasma prilocaine concentrations after three techniques of brachial plexus blockade. British Journal of Anaesthesia 60: 136–139

Mazoit JX, Denson DD, Samii K 1988 Pharmacokinetics of bupivacaine following caudal anesthesia in infants. Anesthesiology 68: 387–389

McLean S, Starmer GA, Thomas J 1969 Methaemoglobin formation by aromatic amines. Journal of Pharmaceutics and Pharmacology 21: 441–450

Miyabe M, Kakiuchi Y, Kihara S et al 1998 The plasma concentration of lidocaine's principal metabolite increases during continuous epidural anesthesia in infants and children. Anesthesia and Analgesia 87: 1056–1057

Moore DC, Mather LE, Bridenbaugh PO et al 1976a Arterial and venous plasma levels of bupivacaine following peripheral nerve blocks. Anesthesia and Analgesia 55: 763–768

Moore DC, Mather LE, Bridenbaugh LD et al 1976b Arterial and venous plasma levels of bupivacaine (Marcaine) following epidural and intercostals nerve blocks. Anesthesiology 4: 39–45

Morikawa K-I, Bonica JJ, Tucker GT et al 1974 Effect of acute hypovolaemia on lignocaine absorption and cardiovascular response following epidural block in dogs. British Journal of Anaesthesia 46: 631–635

Nancarrow C, Runciman WB, Mather LE et al 1987 The influence of acidosis on the distribution of lidocaine and bupivacaine into the myocardium and brain of the sheep. Anesthesia and Analgesia 66: 925–935

Nation RL, Triggs EJ, Selig M 1977 Lignocaine kinetics in cardiac patients and aged subjects. British Journal of Clinical Pharmacology 4: 439–448

Palazzo MGA, Kalso EA, Argiras E, Madgwick R, Sear J 1991 First-pass lung uptake of bupivacaine: effect of acidosis in an intact rabbit lung model. British Journal of Anaesthesia 67: 759–763

Peeyush M, Ravishankar M, Adithan C et al 1992 Altered pharmacokinetics of lignocaine after epidural injection in Type II diabetics. European Journal of Clinical Pharmacology 43: 269–271

Pihlajamaki KK 1991 Inverse correlation between the peak venous serum concentration of bupivacaine and the weight of the patient during interscalene brachial plexus block. British Journal of Anaesthesia 67: 621–622

Pihlajamäki KK, Kanto J, Lindberg R, Karanko M, Kiilholma P 1990 Extradural administration of bupivacaine: pharmacokinetics and metabolism in pregnant and non-pregnant women. British Journal of Anaesthesia 64: 556–570

Post C, Eriksdotter-Behm K 1982 Dependence of lung uptake of lidocaine in vivo on blood pH. Acta Pharmacologica et Toxicologica 51: 136–140

Post C, Andersson RGG, Ryrfeldt A et al 1979 Physicochemical modification of lidocaine uptake in rat lung tissue. Acta Pharmacologica et Toxicologica 44: 103–109

Ramanathan J, Bottorf M, Jeter JN et al 1986 The pharmacokinetics and maternal and neonatal effects of epidural lidocaine in preeclampsia. Anesthesia and Analgesia 65: 120–126

Rice ASC, Pither CE, Tucker GT 1991 Plasma concentrations of bupivacaine after supraclavicular brachial plexus blockade in patients with chronic renal failure. Anaesthesia 46: 354–357

Rosenberg PH, Pere P, Hekali R, Tuominen M 1991 Plasma concentrations of bupivacaine and two of its metabolites during continuous interscalene brachial plexus block. British Journal of Anaesthesia 66: 25–30

Rothstein P, Arthur GR, Feldman H et al 1986 Bupivacaine for intercostal nerve blocks in children: blood concentrations and pharmacokinetics. Anesthesia and Analgesia 65: 625–632

Rothstein P, Cole JS, Pitt BR 1987 Pulmonary extraction of ($^3$H) bupivacaine: modification by dose, propranolol and interaction with ($^{14}$C) 5-hydroxytryptamine. Journal of Pharmacology and Experimental Therapeutics 240: 410–414

Routledge PA, Stargel WW, Barchowsky A et al 1982 Control of lidocaine therapy: new perspectives. Therapeutic Drug Monitoring 4: 265–270

Safran D, Kuhlman G, Orhant EE et al 1990 Continuous intercostal blockade with lidocaine after thoracic surgery. Clinical and pharmacokinetic study. Anesthesia and Analgesia 70: 345–349

Scott DB, Jebson PJR, Braid DP et al 1972 Factors affecting plasma levels of lignocaine and prilocaine. British Journal of Anaesthesia 44: 1040–1049

Scott DB, Lee A, Fagan D et al 1989 Acute toxicity of ropivacaine compared with that of bupivacaine. Anesthesia and Analgesia 69: 563–569

Scott DA, Emanuelsson B-M, Mooney PH et al 1997 Pharmacokinetics and efficacy of long-term epidural ropivacaine infusion for postoperative analgesia. Anesthesia and Analgesia 85: 1322–1330

Sharrock NE, Mather LE, Go G et al 1998 Arterial and pulmonary arterial concentrations of the enantiomers of bupivacaine after epidural injection in elderly patients. Anesthesia and Analgesia 86: 812–817

Simon RP, Benowitz NL, Culala S 1984 Motor paralysis increases brain uptake of lidocaine during status epilepticus. Neurology 34: 384–387

Takasaki M 1984 Blood concentrations of lidocaine, mepivacaine, and bupivacaine during caudal analgesia in children. Acta Anaesthesiologica Scandinavica 28: 211–214

Thomson P, Melmon KL, Richardson JA et al 1973 Lidocaine pharmacokinetics in advanced heart failure, liver disease, and renal failure in humans. Annals of Internal Medicine 78: 499–508

Tucker GT 1986 Pharmacokinetics of local anaesthetics. British Journal of Anaesthesia 58: 717–731

Tucker GT 1994 Safety in 'numbers' The role of pharmacokinetics in local anesthetic toxicity. Regional Anesthesia 19: 155–163

Tucker GT, Boas RA 1971 Pharmacokinetic aspects of intravenous regional anesthesia. Anesthesiology 34: 538–549

Tucker GT, Mather LE 1975 Pharmacokinetics of local anaesthetic agent. British Journal of Anaesthesia 47: 213–224

Tucker GT, Mather LE 1979 Clinical pharmacokinetics of local anaesthetic agents. Clinical Pharmacokinetics 4: 241–278

Tucker GT, Mather LE 1988 Physicochemical properties, absorption and disposition of local anaesthetic agents. In: Cousins MJ, Bridenbaugh PO (eds) Neural blockade in clinical anesthesia and management of pain, 2nd edn, pp. 47–110. JB Lippincott, Philadelphia

Tucker GT, Mather LE 1998 Properties, absorption, and disposition of local anaesthetic agents. In: Cousins MJ, Bridenbaugh PO (eds) Neural blockade in clinical anesthesia and management of pain, 3rd edn, pp. 55–95. Lippincott-Raven, Philadelphia

Tucker GT, Boyes RN, Bridenbaugh PO et al 1970 Binding of anilide-type local anesthetics in human plasma. II: Implications in vivo with special reference to transplacental distribution. Anesthesiology 33: 304–314

Tucker GT, Cooper S, Littlewood D et al 1977 Observed and predicted accumulation of local anaesthetic agents during continuous extradural analgesia. British Journal of Anaesthesia 49: 237–242

Van der Meer AD, Burm AGL, Stienstra R et al 1999 Pharmacokinetics of prilocaine after intravenous administration in volunteers. Anesthesiology 90: 988–992

Van Kleef JW, Burm AGL, Vletter AA 1990 Single dose interpleural versus intercostals blockade: nerve block characteristics and plasma concentration profiles after administration of 0.5% bupivacaine with epinephrine. Anesthesia and Analgesia 70: 484–488

Veering BT, Burm AGL, Van Kleef JW et al 1987 Epidural anesthesia with bupivacaine: Effects of age on neural blockade and pharmacokinetics. Anesthesia and Analgesia 66: 589–593

Veering BT, Burm AGL, Vletter AA et al 1991 The effect of age on systemic absorption and systemic disposition of bupivacaine after subarachnoid administration. Anesthesiology 74: 250–257

Veering BT, Burm AGL, Vletter AA et al 1992 The effect of age on the systemic absorption, disposition and pharmaco-dynamics of bupivacaine after epidural administration. Clinical Pharmacokinetics 22: 75–84

Vester-Andersen T, Christiansen C, Hansen A et al 1981 Interscalene brachial plexus block: Area of analgesia, complications and blood concentrations of local anesthetics. Acta Anaesthesiologica Scandinavica 25: 81–84

Wang J-S, Backman JT, Wen X et al 1999 Fluvoxamine is a more potent inhibitor of lidocaine metabolism than ketoconazole and erythromycin in vitro. Pharmacology and Toxicology 85: 201–205

Wang J-S, Backman JT, Taavitsainen P et al 2000 Involvement of CYP1A2 and CYP3A4 in lidocaine N-deethylation and 3-hydroxylation in humans. Drug Metabolism and Disposition 28: 959–965

Weidemann D, Mühlnickel B, Staroske E, Neumann W, Röse W 2000 Ropivacaine plasma concentrations during 120-hour epidural infusion. British Journal of Anaesthesia 85: 830–835

Wildsmith JAW, Tucker GT, Cooper S et al 1977 Plasma concentrations of local anaesthetics after interscalene brachial plexus block. British Journal of Anaesthesia 49: 461–466

Williams R, Blaschke TF, Meffin PJ et al 1976 Influence of viral hepatitis on the disposition of two compounds with high hepatic clearance: Lidocaine and indocyanine green. Clinical Pharmacology and Therapeutics 20: 290–299

Wing LMH, Miners JP, Birkett DJ et al 1984 Lidocaine disposition – sex differences and effects of cimetidine. Clinical Pharmacology and Therapeutics 35: 695–701

Yokoyama M, Mizobuchi S, Nagano O et al 2001 The effect of epidural insertion site and surgical procedure on plasma lidocaine concentration. Anesthesia and Analgesia 92: 470–475

# 6. Clinical use of local anaesthetic drugs

## J A W Wildsmith

The previous two chapters have described the dynamic and kinetic aspects of the pharmacology of the local anaesthetic drugs. The aim here is to draw on that detailed information and direct attention to the particular aspects which govern the safe, effective clinical use of this class of drugs. They have exactly the same membrane-stabilising effect on the cells of the heart and brain as they have on peripheral nerve fibres, but the systemic consequences of this are rare. This is not because there are large differences in the sensitivity of these three types of cell, but because injection of the drugs at, or close to, their sites of intended action usually ensures that the concentrations found in the systemic circulation are below those which produce overt toxic effects. This chapter will consider the prevention and treatment of such systemic toxicity, and other aspects of the clinical pharmacology of the local anaesthetics.

## SYSTEMIC TOXICITY

The most severe reactions result from accidental intravascular injection, but systemic toxicity may also follow repeated administration during prolonged pain control or simple overdosage.

### Clinical features

As concentrations of local anaesthetics in the blood/plasma increase, there is progressive depression of both central nervous and cardiovascular systems, with the neurological features predominating in most circumstances. The early features are all subjective, and patients may note numbness of the tongue or circumoral structures (due to a direct effect of drug in an area with a high blood supply), light-headedness or tinnitus. They may then become acutely anxious, with the more objective features including slurring of speech and muscle twitching. Drowsiness is an indication that the systemic concentration is close to that associated with severe toxicity which involves loss of consciousness, convulsions and, almost certainly, apnoea. Without immediate resuscitation, hypoxaemia and acidosis will develop rapidly, due not only to the apnoea, but also to the high oxygen consumption in the muscles of a convulsing patient.

The cardiovascular system has long been thought to be less sensitive to the effects of local anaesthetic drugs than the central nervous system. As a result, circulatory collapse during a toxic reaction was considered to be more likely to be a consequence of hypoxaemia and acidosis (which will increase the proportion of ionised, active drug present intracellularly) than a primary cardiac effect. In fact, the local anaesthetic drugs do have a primary depressant action on the myocardium which is proportional to their local anaesthetic potency, but the effect is of little significance at the systemic concentrations produced during uneventful regional anaesthesia or in the therapy of arrhythmias (Covino & Vassallo 1976).

Low concentrations of most of the drugs tend to produce slight vasoconstriction, but vasodilation occurs at higher concentrations. These peripheral and myocardial effects are modified by central actions which result in an increase in sympathetic nerve activity (Bonica 1971), so that the intravenous injection of 1–2 mg kg$^{-1}$ of lidocaine will produce measurable increases in blood pressure, heart rate and cardiac output. However, the epidural injection of about 400 mg of plain lidocaine will cause the expected decrease in these parameters (even though the systemic concentrations of drug are similar) because of the effects of sympathetic nerve block.

This relatively simple view of systemic toxicity was challenged by Albright (1979) who reported seven cases of primary cardiac toxicity produced after administration of one of the longer acting agents. There was some initial scepticism that agents belonging to a class of drugs with an anti-arrhythmic action could actually cause problems such as ventricular fibrillation, but that was soon recognised to be the case. Under certain circumstances, racemic bupivacaine, in particular, was identified as a potent cause of severe ventricular arrhythmias which are very difficult to treat (Davis & de Jong 1982, Mallampati et al 1984). Most such cases seem to have been associated with the rapid, accidental intravenous injection of a relatively large dose of bupivacaine, but as little as 50 mg (10 ml of 5 mg ml$^{-1}$ solution) has been known to produce ventricular fibrillation (Whiteside & Wildsmith 2001). Every user of local anaesthetics must be aware that rapid intravenous injection of even a relatively modest dose will almost certainly produce frank convulsions and, possibly, cardiorespiratory collapse without any of the more minor manifestations of systemic toxicity being apparent.

## Factors affecting toxicity

Systemic toxicity is related to the amount of drug in the blood supplying the brain and the heart. Several factors are relevant (Ch. 5), but a few are of crucial clinical importance.

### Dosage

The dose of drug administered for any procedure is the product of the volume injected and the concentration of the solution. However, neither the volume nor the concentration used has any direct effect on the systemic concentrations which result. It is the *mass* of drug injected which is important, that is, 20 ml of 2% lidocaine will produce virtually the same systemic concentrations as 40 ml of 1% solution.

It has become common for 'safe' maximum dose recommendations, particularly those related to the patient's weight, to be sought and proposed. Neither unqualified absolute, or weight-related, maximum doses have any great scientific validity in adults. For example, the epidural administration of a fixed dose of lidocaine to adult patients with a considerable range in weight produced no correlation with maximum plasma concentrations (Scott & Cousins 1980). The anaesthetist should be aware of all the factors which affect systemic concentrations of local anaesthetics and relate these to the *particular block, patient and drug* under consideration. Local anaesthetic drug requirements may be smaller in the pregnant patient and obviously extremes in size are important. It should be said that although dosage information for young children is somewhat limited, weight-related doses are a useful guide in this age group.

### Rate of absorption

Clearly the most rapid rate of entry of drug into the circulation will be produced by direct intravascular administration. Absorption of a correctly placed dose from the site of injection depends on the blood flow – the higher the blood flow the more rapid will be the rise in, and the greater will be the peak, systemic drug concentration. There is also much circumstantial evidence that the rate of rise in plasma concentration is as important as the absolute figure for the production of toxic symptoms (Scott 1975), although this is difficult to quantify.

Basal blood flow is quite different among the various sites of local anaesthetic administration, so that the rate of absorption is greatest after intercostal and interpleural administration, followed by epidural, brachial plexus and lower limb blocks. It is slowest after subcutaneous infiltration, but high concentrations may follow topical application to the upper respiratory and gastrointestinal tracts. Absorption may be reduced by the addition of a vasoconstrictor to the injected solution, and this will, in most cases, allow the safe dose to be increased by 50–100%, but use of a vasoconstrictor may not always be appropriate.

Intravenous regional anaesthesia (Bier's block) is a special case. Premature tourniquet release will result in the rapid entry of a large dose of local anaesthetic into the circulation. However, when the tourniquet has been applied for a minimum of 20 minutes, much of the drug will have diffused into the tissues of the limb. Tourniquet release then results in slower increases in systemic concentrations than after brachial plexus block.

The overall state of the circulation will also affect the systemic concentration achieved. For example, 400 mg of drug injected intravenously over 1 minute into a patient with a cardiac output of 4 l min$^{-1}$ will result (theoretically) in a peak concentration of 100 µg ml$^{-1}$. The resultant peak systemic concentration will increase directly with rate of injection, and inversely with cardiac output.

### Distribution and metabolism

Although the clinician can control the factors which affect the rate of entry of drug into the circulation, there is not the same ability to influence the distribution and metabolism of drug once it has been injected. Nevertheless, an understanding of these processes is essential to the decision making which underpins safe clinical practice.

Distribution throughout the body buffers the rise in systemic concentration as drug is absorbed. Before blood containing local anaesthetic reaches the systemic circulation it will pass through the right side of the heart, where it will have no effect, and then through the lungs, which are capable of temporarily sequestering, and possibly metabolising, large amounts of local anaesthetic. The percentage taken up by the lungs decreases as the dose increases, so their buffering capacity will be less able to prevent a toxic reaction should an intravenous injection be made rapidly.

After passage through the lungs, local anaesthetics are distributed to the organs of the body in proportion to their 'share' of cardiac output. The organs with a high blood supply (brain, heart, liver and spleen) also have a high affinity for the drugs, and tissue concentrations will increase rapidly. Fat and muscle, having low blood supplies, equilibrate slowly, but the high affinity of fat for local anaesthetic drugs means that large amounts may be absorbed there temporarily during continuous infusion, prior to release back to the circulation before metabolism.

Generally, the *ester* drugs are metabolised by plasma cholinesterase so rapidly that it is very difficult to measure their concentrations in blood after a regional block. Because of this rapid metabolism systemic toxicity is very rare. Theoretically, an abnormal cholinesterase level could result in an increased risk of toxicity (cf. suxamethonium), but enzyme activity must be reduced dramatically to impair significantly the rate of hydrolysis of the ester drugs.

The *amide* local anaesthetics are metabolised in the liver, although it is probable that prilocaine may undergo some extrahepatic metabolism as well. Hepatocellular damage has to be severe before the rate of breakdown is affected, but because some amides (*not* bupivacaine) have relatively high hepatic extraction ratios, their rate of metabolism is more dependent on hepatic blood flow. This has practical relevance to the use of lidocaine as an anti-arrhythmic agent in cardiogenic shock, where liver blood flow will be reduced.

### Protein binding

Like many other drugs, local anaesthetics bind to plasma proteins, primarily $\alpha_1$-acid glycoprotein and albumin,

**Table 6.1** Approximate percentages of amide local anaesthetics that are protein-bound at two different serum concentrations

| Drug | Serum concentration ($\mu$g ml$^{-1}$) | |
| --- | --- | --- |
| | 1 | 50 |
| Bupivacaine | 95 | 60 |
| Etidocaine | 95 | 60 |
| Ropivacaine | 94 | 63 |
| Mepivacaine | 75 | 30 |
| Lidocaine | 70 | 35 |
| Prilocaine | 40 | 30 |

to varying degrees. The former binds the drugs avidly, but has a limited capacity for them, whereas albumin has a low affinity, but a large capacity. As a result, the greater proportion of a low concentration is bound, but once the binding sites on $\alpha_1$-acid glycoprotein are occupied the proportion that is bound decreases as the concentration increases (Table 6.1). The measurement of protein binding was originally undertaken to provide a physicochemical property which related to duration of action in the laboratory assessment of new compounds. It is often assumed that drugs with greater affinity for protein are less toxic because only a small part of the total amount present in plasma is 'available' to diffuse into the tissues and produce toxic effects, but the analysis in Chapter 5 clearly refutes this argument. Finally, it is noteworthy that prilocaine, the least protein-bound of all the amides, is the least toxic. Figures for protein binding do not correlate with acute systemic toxicity.

## Prevention and treatment of toxicity

The single most important factor in the prevention of toxicity is the avoidance of accidental intravenous injection. Careful aspiration tests are vital and should be repeated each time the needle is moved. However, a negative test is not an absolute guarantee of extravascular placement, especially when a catheter technique is used. The initial injection of 2–3 ml of solution containing epinephrine (1:200 000) has been advocated – an increase in heart rate during the next 1–2 minutes indicating an intravascular injection. However, the heart rate may vary considerably while a block is being established (particularly during labour) and epinephrine is not the safest of drugs. In addition, no test dose can guarantee against subsequent migration of the catheter or needle into a vein.

An alternative to the test dose is to repeat the aspiration test after each 5 ml of solution, and to inject slowly while watching the patient carefully for any early signs of systemic effect. A very distinct pause in injection should be allowed after the first 5 ml increment to allow such features to appear. In the elderly, a period of at least a minute should elapse in case a slow circulation time delays the onset of symptoms such as tinnitus or circumoral numbness. Finally, particular care should be taken with head and neck blocks because the injection of only a small dose of drug into a carotid or vertebral artery will produce a major cerebral reaction.

Systemic toxicity from absorption of a correctly placed but excessive dose of drug is very rare and may be avoided by taking into account the known behaviour of the individual drug when injected at that particular site. Each chapter in the second part of this book indicates the appropriate drugs and doses for the various blocks considered. The pharmacokinetic basis for these figures lends little support to the principle of the 'maximum recommended dose', whether this is related to patient weight or not. Scott (1989) has argued cogently the case against adherence to such maximum doses because it can result in the use of an inadequate amount of drug for the procedure. A better concept is to keep in mind the 'median' dose required for a specific block and to modify this, *up or down*, in the light of the patient's physique and state of health.

Other aspects of the prevention of toxic reactions, and also their treatment, are discussed in Chapter 8.

## OTHER SIDE-EFFECTS

Local anaesthetics are relatively free from other side-effects. Complications of specific drugs will be discussed later, but four general features are worth mentioning here.

## Allergic reactions

Allergy to the ester class of local anaesthetics is relatively common, particularly with procaine, because *p*-aminobenzoic acid is produced when this agent is hydrolysed. Most reactions are dermal in personnel handling the drugs, but fatal anaphylaxis has been recorded in patients. Allergy to the amide drugs is extremely rare, and most 'reactions' are due to systemic toxicity, the effects of added vasoconstrictors, or are manifestations of anxiety (e.g. fainting). Allergic reactions do occur occasionally in association with administration of a local anaesthetic, but are usually due to a preservative in the local anaesthetic solution, or to some other substance to which the patient is exposed at or about the same time (e.g. latex). However, true drug allergy has been reported (Brown et al 1981).

Although true allergy to amide local anaesthetics is rare, it is not uncommon to meet a patient who claims to be allergic to such drugs, or who has been so-diagnosed by a medical or dental attendant. Such patients merit close investigation because the diagnosis is usually wrong. This can cause unnecessary difficulties in providing anaesthesia or analgesia in many clinical situations, and leaves the patient at risk of an even more major reaction on subsequent exposure if the original reaction was allergic in nature but attributed to the wrong precipitant. Very often the history will identify the correct nature of the problem, but considerable investigation of past medical and dental treatments may be necessary. A proportion of patients will need to undergo challenge testing, usually where the history is equivocal or the events described are somewhat bizarre, the latter often an indicator of a patient's attempt at needle or dentist 'avoidance'! Challenge testing, although considered inappropriate with most drugs, is useful with local anaesthetics to demonstrate to the patient that they can be administered safely. However, the testing must be performed in a structured manner with all resuscitation facilities to hand (Wildsmith et al 1998).

## Drug interactions

Interactions with other drugs, particularly of a pharmacokinetic nature (see Ch. 5), are possible, but rarely give rise to clinical problems. All local anaesthetics have a weak neuromuscular blocking action and, in theory at least, might potentiate the definitive drugs with that action or cause problems in myasthenic patients, but there is no clear evidence that this happens. Therapy with anticholinesterases for myasthenia, or the concomitant administration of other drugs hydrolysed by plasma cholinesterase, could slow the metabolism of ester drugs. The amide local anaesthetics are potent inhibitors of plasma cholinesterase (Zsigmond et al 1978) and the administration of an ester to a patient who has recently received an amide might have unexpectedly toxic effects.

The benzodiazepines can mask the early signs of systemic toxicity and may be used deliberately for that effect. Large doses given as premedication may even prevent convulsions, but cardiorespiratory collapse could then be the first sign of a toxic reaction. The dose of any anticonvulsant used to treat toxicity must be adjusted with care since it may exacerbate cardiorespiratory depression. Finally, the depressant action of drugs used in the treatment of cardiovascular disease might combine with the systemic effects of a local anaesthetic to precipitate cardiac failure.

## Tissue toxicity

The local anaesthetic drugs in clinical use rarely produce nerve damage. Any neuropathy developing after surgery is more likely to be due to other factors such as faulty patient positioning or trauma from the needle, the catheter or the operative procedure itself (Aitkenhead 1994). However, some years ago there were several reports in the American literature of neurological damage after the use of chloroprocaine. It would seem that this was caused by sodium bisulphite added to the solution as an antioxidant (Covino 1984). In the epidural space, the nerve sheath probably protected the nerve from the effects of this preservative, but when accidental intrathecal injection occurred – a feature common to most of the reported cases – the bisulphite had free access to the nerve tissue. This emphasises the particular care which must be taken with intrathecal injection.

Subsequently, renewed interest in continuous spinal anaesthesia was checked by the publication of several reports of cauda equina syndrome (Rigler et al 1991). The common factor seems to have been the repeated injection of local anaesthetic (usually, but not always, lidocaine with glucose) in unsuccessful attempts to extend an initially restricted block. The solution would seem to have accumulated in the sacral section of the theca and exposed the unsheathed nerve roots to unusually high concentrations of drug. The proper response to the limited block would have been careful consideration of the position of the intrathecal catheter and the way in which this was influencing drug spread, not simply repeating a failed injection (Denny & Selander 1998).

The most recent concern about tissue toxicity of local anaesthetics has been associated again, but not uniformly, with the intrathecal injection of lidocaine.

Reports of discomfort lasting 24–36 hours in the buttocks and thighs of patients who had received spinal anaesthesia, often as day cases in the lithotomy position, were labelled as 'Transient Radicular Irritation' or 'Transient Neurological Symptoms'. However, neither term is appropriate because it seems that the actual cause is overstretching of spinal ligaments by adoption of extremes of posture while the anaesthetic is effective (Selander 1999).

## Antiplatelet activity

One side-effect of local anaesthetic drugs may be looked upon as a benefit rather than a complication. Regional techniques can result in a reduction in the risk of the thromboembolic complications of surgery (Ch. 2). One of the mechanisms explaining this is a direct pharmacological effect of this group of drugs in decreasing both platelet aggregation and blood viscosity (Borg & Modig 1985, Henny et al 1986). The relative importance of this and the indirect effect of sympathetic block on lower limb blood flow in reducing stasis has yet to be established.

## PHARMACOLOGY OF INDIVIDUAL DRUGS

The available local anaesthetic drugs vary somewhat in their stability, potency, duration and toxicity. Differences in these features may be related to variations in physicochemical properties, and these in turn to the underlying chemical structures as has been discussed in Chapters 4 and 5.

## Clinical factors affecting drug profile

Before making direct comparisons between the various local anaesthetic drugs, it is important to emphasise that several clinical factors affect rate of onset, potency, duration of action and toxicity. Onset time will be decreased, and duration increased, by the use of a larger dose. Dose may be increased by increasing either volume or concentration, but given the same total dose, a large volume of a dilute solution will produce a better block than a small volume of a concentrated one. There are marked differences in onset time between the different types of block. Onset is almost immediate after infiltration and is progressively longer for spinal, peripheral nerve, epidural and brachial plexus blocks. This order correlates with variations in diffusion barriers, both around and within the nerve trunks, at the different sites. In the cerebrospinal fluid the nerve rootlets are bare, but they acquire a sheath after piercing the dura mater. Further coverings are acquired as the nerves leave the intervertebral foramina, but these become progressively thinner as the nerves spread distally and become smaller. The dose of drug required for the different blocks and the likely duration of action also increases in much the same order as onset time.

## Individual drug features

Because of the above factors, comparisons between different agents should be made using only data collected for the same block. It is at least questionable whether there are any significant differences in onset time between agents if *equipotent* concentrations are used. However, there are real differences in potency, duration and toxicity, and much of our understanding of the safe clinical use of local anaesthetics has come from studies of their pharmacokinetics as outlined in Chapter 5. The clinical features of the individual drugs are discussed below, but the definitive quantitative data on the more commonly used of these agents are to be found earlier in the book, in Tables 4.1, 5.1, 5.2, 5.3 and 5.4.

### The esters
**Cocaine** Because of its systemic toxicity, central nervous stimulant and addictive properties, and tendency to produce allergic reactions, cocaine has little if any place in modern anaesthesia. It is still used in ear, nose and throat practice for its vasoconstrictor action, but is becoming very difficult to obtain legitimately at a reasonable price. In animals the main site of metabolism is thought to be the liver, but there is evidence that plasma esterases are more important in man (Van Dyke et al 1976).

**Benzocaine** This ester does not contain the amine group common to all the other clinically useful agents. As a result it does not ionise and this has implications for our understanding of how local anaesthetic drugs act (see Ch. 4). Of more practical relevance, an inability to ionise means that benzocaine will not form water-soluble salts so it can only be applied topically, a use for which it is very effective. Benzocaine is hydrolysed very rapidly to p-aminobenzoic acid, and so it is of low toxicity, but may produce allergic reactions.

**Procaine and chloroprocaine** The short shelf-life, brief duration of action, incidence of allergic reactions and the introduction of better agents have all combined to limit the use of procaine. As its name suggests, chloroprocaine is structurally very similar. The simple addition of a chloride atom to the aromatic ring produces a drug which is hydrolysed even faster than procaine and is probably slightly more potent. Its metabolic product is 2-chloro-4-aminobenzoic acid which, from the lack of published reports, seems to be less likely to produce allergic reactions than *p*-aminobenzoic acid. The obvious advantages of this compound, which is used very widely in the USA, were offset by reports of permanent neurological damage, probably due to the bisulphite included in the solution to prevent spontaneous hydrolysis (see above).

**Tetracaine** This is the most potent and longest acting of the ester drugs in clinical use. It is hydrolysed by plasma cholinesterase, but relatively slowly, so it is quite toxic. In small doses it can be used safely and it has long been the standard drug for spinal anaesthesia in the USA.

### The amides
**Lidocaine** Lidocaine is today the standard agent against which all other local anaesthetics are compared. All the general features of the amides apply to it and it has no unusual properties. It has been used safely for all types of local anesthesia and is also a standard anti-arrhythmic agent.

**Mepivacaine** Although chemically somewhat different from lidocaine, mepivacaine is very similar clinically. It seems to have no particular advantage or disadvantage although it may be slightly less toxic.

**Prilocaine** Of all the amide drugs prilocaine has the lowest systemic toxicity. This is because it differs from lidocaine in several minor, but significant respects. It does not produce any vasodilatation, is sequestered (or perhaps metabolised) by the lungs (Akerman et al 1966a) in greater amounts, is distributed to the other tissues at a faster rate, and requires higher systemic concentrations to produce convulsions. As a result the safe dose of this agent is twice that of lidocaine. Because it is equipotent with lidocaine and probably has a slightly longer duration of action, it is surprising that it is not more widely used.

The reason for its lack of popularity is related to the fact that there is only one methyl group on the aromatic ring. This means that the first stage of its metabolism is hydrolysis to *o*-toluidine, the hydroxylated products of which have the ability to reduce haemoglobin (Akerman et al 1966b). It is anxiety about producing methaemoglobinaemia that seems to restrict the use of prilocaine, even though more than 600 mg must be used before the theoretical risk becomes real. This is far in excess of the amount which would be used for a single administration and *prilocaine is the agent of choice whenever the risk of systemic toxicity is high.*

It should not be used during labour, partly because 'top-up' injections may exceed the dose which will produce methaemoglobinaemia, but mainly because fetal haemoglobin is more sensitive to this transformation. It would seem wise to try and avoid using it in anaemic patients, although it is important to stress that when methaemoglobinaemia becomes clinically apparent as cyanosis, only 1.5 g 100 ml$^{-1}$ haemoglobin is reduced and the intravenous injection of 1 mg kg$^{-1}$ of methylene blue will rapidly reverse this. Smaller, titrated doses may also be effective.

*Bupivacaine* The introduction of bupivacaine was an important event because it is a long-acting agent, the acute toxicity of which is, relative to potency, much the same as that of lidocaine. Its duration allows single-shot local blocks to be used for more prolonged surgery, but more importantly, the risk of toxicity is less during catheter techniques because the intervals between injections are longer. The other advantage of bupivacaine for catheter techniques is that effective analgesia can be provided with less motor block than the agents previously available.

Unfortunately, bupivacaine was implicated in a series of very severe toxic reactions, some of which were fatal. In many of these instances the supervision of the patient left much to be desired, but evidence accumulated to suggest that the agent may occasionally produce cardiotoxicity before neurotoxicity, with primary ventricular fibrillation being described in both man and animals (see above, and Ch. 4 & 5). In some of the cases high concentrations were used for intravenous regional anaesthesia – a procedure for which this agent, in any concentration, is most unsuitable. Many of the other reactions were associated with the use of the 0.75% solution and it would seem that, should the needle or catheter be placed accidentally in a vein, this concentrated formulation allows the very rapid injection of a large dose into the circulation. Peak systemic concentrations are thus likely to be higher than if the same dose were injected as a more dilute solution.

Obviously, such serious reactions can be prevented if the drug is administered correctly. However, concern about the problem led to renewed interest in finding alternative agents with a similar clinical profile to bupivacaine, but less cardiotoxicity. Ropivacaine has been available for some time now, and levobupivacaine more recently.

*Ropivacaine* Chemically, this agent is intermediate in structure between mepivacaine and bupivacaine (Table 4.1), but unlike those two drugs it is presented as a pure solution of a single 'S' isomer (see Ch. 4). In man, the pharmacokinetic properties of ropivacaine compare well with bupivacaine (Lee et al 1989) and its cardiotoxicity is less (Scott et al 1989). Early clinical studies suggested that it performs very similarly to bupivacaine (Reynolds 1991), but that it produces an even greater degree of 'separation' of motor and sensory block (Brockway et al 1991). It is also more water soluble than bupivacaine so that higher concentrations can be made available for clinical use.

Subsequent clinical studies have confirmed the early promise (see McClure 1996 for a review). Continuous epidural infusions have been shown to produce less lower limb motor block than bupivacaine (Zaric et al 1996), but to provide effective analgesia for up to 3 days after major surgery (Scott et al 1999). A meta-analysis of obstetric epidural analgesia studies showed that the lower degree of motor block may translate into a reduced need for operative deliveries (Writer et al 1998). Finally, the higher concentrations may provide more effective block of major nerve trunks, such as in the brachial plexus (Casati et al 1999). However, the overall benefits of ropivacaine have been questioned on the grounds of both relative potency (Gautier et al 1999, McDonald et al 1999) and cost-effectiveness (D'Angelo 2000), although both claims have been refuted (Wildsmith 2000, 2001).

*Levobupivacaine* This agent is the single 'S' isomer derivative of bupivacaine (Ch. 4). It has become commercially available only recently (see McLeod & Burke 2001 for review). Its clinical performance seems to be identical to that of bupivacaine, although it should theoretically be less cardiotoxic. However, this benefit may not be achieved unless the consequences of changes in the regulations on labelling of new drugs are appreciated. As mentioned in Chapter 4, the older drugs (including ropivacaine) are presented in terms of the weight per unit volume of the hydrochloride salt, but for levobupivacaine it is *base* drug which is measured. This has a lower molecular weight so a solution of levobupivacaine '5 mg ml$^{-1}$' has 11% *more* drug in it than does bupivacaine '5 mg ml$^{-1}$'.

The whole issue of the differences, or otherwise, between racemic bupivacaine, ropivacaine and bupivacaine, both pharmacological and economic, is somewhat controversial at present and requires more comparative studies, particularly of ropivacaine with levobupivacaine, to establish the true position.

**Etidocaine** This is a long-acting derivative of lidocaine, which has not become anything like so widely used or available as bupivacaine. It seems to have the ability to produce a more profound effect on motor nerves than sensory ones and this may be related to its very high lipid solubility and low p$K_a$.

## ADDITIVES

In addition to the active agent, local anaesthetic solutions may contain several substances added to adjust factors such as pH, tonicity and baricity. Solutions in multidose bottles, and those with epinephrine in single-use ampoules, will also contain a preservative, which can be the cause of allergic phenomena. Manufacturers usually recommend that solutions containing preservative should not be used for spinal and epidural injection because of the risk of nerve damage. Other additions may be made to the solution for pharmacological rather than pharmaceutical reasons.

## Vasoconstrictors

Addition of a vasoconstrictor will reduce the toxicity, prolong the duration and probably improve the quality of block resulting from the injection of a local anaesthetic. Commendable though each of these features is, vasoconstrictors are not used universally. They are absolutely contraindicated for ring blocks and intravenous regional anaesthesia because they may produce tissue ischaemia. The most commonly used agent, epinephrine, has its own systemic effects and should be used with particular care, if at all, in patients with cardiac disease. Concentrations greater than 1:200 000 should not be used and the total dose should be limited. Doses greater

than 200 mg have been shown to cause cardiovascular disturbances during brachial plexus block (Kennedy et al 1966). Interactions with other sympathomimetic drugs, such as tricyclic antidepressants, may occur, especially when vasoconstrictors are used systemically to treat hypotension. Felypressin has less systemic effect, but it may be a coronary vasoconstrictor and is usually only available for dental use.

Finally, there is the question as to whether vasoconstrictors increase the risk of permanent neurological damage by making nerves ischaemic. Their widespread use in the USA suggests that this is not a matter for practical concern, but many anaesthetists feel that they should only be used if there is no alternative method of reducing toxicity or prolonging duration. As with chloroprocaine, it might be the preservative which has been responsible for nerve damage. Most commercial solutions containing epinephrine also contain sodium metabisulphite as an antioxidant. There is an argument, on safety grounds, for the addition of epinephrine to the local anaesthetic just before use to avoid administration of the antioxidant, but this needs to be done with great care to ensure that the correct concentration is produced.

## Other adjuvants

At various times solutions of local anaesthetics have been introduced containing substances which, it is claimed, may improve the block in some way. Some drugs have been prepared as the *carbonated* salt instead of the standard hydrochloride in an effort to speed the onset of block. Laboratory studies have consistently shown that this is effective due to a combination of direct axon depression by carbon dioxide, enhanced diffusion of the local anaesthetic and a decrease in intracellular pH, favouring formation of the ionised form of the drug (Catchlove 1972). Clinical studies are less consistent in their results, but the evidence suggests that carbonated solutions produce some improvement in blocks of slower onset (McClure & Scott 1981).

The *alkalinisation* of standard solutions of local anaesthetics by the addition of sodium bicarbonate has also been employed in an attempt to speed the onset of block. The theory is that an increase in the pH of the solution will increase the proportion of the drug in the non-ionised, membrane-permeant form and thus speed nerve penetration. The results of clinical studies have not been entirely consistent, and, even where a positive effect has been demonstrated, doubt has been expressed about its clinical usefulness (Swann et al 1991). There is always the risk that the pH change will cause the drug to precipitate before injection and the method has little to commend it.

A much older strategy for speeding onset is the addition of the tissue enzyme *hyaluronidase*. There is little objective evidence (Keeler et al 1992) to support its use except in ophthalmology (Nicoll et al 1986), where it continues to be popular.

Local anaesthetics have also been injected with *high molecular weight dextran* with the intention of prolonging their duration of action. Again the clinical results are inconclusive, but dextrans of very high molecular weight may be effective, especially in combination with epinephrine (Simpson et al 1982).

A number of substances have been added to local anaesthetic preparations to try and improve their rate of penetration through intact skin. For many years these attempts were not very successful, but a significant development was the *eutectic mixture of local anaesthetics* (EMLA). This is an oil-in-water emulsion of equal amounts of the base forms of lidocaine and prilocaine. When crystals of these bases are mixed together at room temperature they assume a 'liquid' form, because this eutectic mixture has a lower melting point than either constituent. This allows the drugs to be prepared in a formulation suitable for topical application. The cream has to be applied to the skin for about an hour, but sufficient base does penetrate to allow relatively painless venepuncture. In some patients it may even allow the cutting of skin grafts.

The addition of *opioids* to local anaesthetics for spinal and epidural use is now very standard practice in both postoperative (Ch. 11) and obstetric (Ch. 18) pain control. Other substances with analgesic actions at spinal cord level, such $\alpha_2$-adrenergic agonists (e.g. clonidine) and benzodiazepines (e.g. midazolam), are being used also. Great care must be taken when making any such addition that the correct concentration is produced, and that the substance is safe for administration into the vertebral canal. None of these substances has a product licence for these applications, and there are few, if any, relevant safety data for many of them. Such additions should be made only when it is clear that there is benefit, and in line with agreed hospital policies.

## CHOICE OF LOCAL ANAESTHETIC AGENT

One of the most important decisions to be made when using a local technique is how much of which drug is to be injected. First, the solution has to be of adequate strength. For lidocaine (the relative potencies of the

**Table 6.2 The clinical features of individual local anaesthetic drugs**

| Drug | Potency[a] | Duration[a] | Toxicity | Main use in UK |
|------|---------|----------|----------|----------------|
| **The esters** | | | | |
| Cocaine | 1 | $\frac{1}{2}$ | Very high | Nil |
| Benzocaine | NA | 2 | Low | Topical |
| Procaine | 2 | $\frac{3}{4}$ | Low | Nil |
| Chloroprocaine | 1 | $\frac{3}{4}$ | Low | Not available |
| Tetracaine | $\frac{1}{4}$ | 2 | High | Topical |
| **The amides** | | | | |
| Lidocaine | 1 | 1 | Medium | Infiltration, nerve block, epidural |
| Mepivacaine | 1 | 1 | Medium | Not available |
| Prilocaine | 1 | $1\frac{1}{2}$ | Low | Infiltration, nerve block, IVRA[b] |
| Ropivacaine | $\frac{1}{4}$ | 2–4 | Medium | Infiltration, nerve block, epidural |
| Bupivacaine | $\frac{1}{4}$ | 2–4 | Medium | Extradural, spinal, nerve block |
| Levobupivacaine | $\frac{1}{4}$ | 2–4 | Medium | Extradural, spinal, nerve block |
| Etidocaine | $\frac{1}{2}$ | 2–4 | Medium | Not available |

[a]Relative to lidocaine. [b]IVRA = intravenous regional anaesthesia.

other agents are in Table 6.2) the concentrations which are adequate to produce analgesia for skin incision are:

| | | |
|---|---|---|
| infiltration | } | 0.5% |
| intravenous regional | | |
| minor nerve block | } | 1.0% |
| brachial plexus | } | 1.0–1.5% |
| sciatic/femoral | | |
| epidural | } | 1.5–2.0% |
| spinal | } | 2.0–5.0% |

Greater concentrations than these may be used to produce more profound blocks of faster onset and longer duration. The volume to be injected will depend on the particular technique and, once the required concentration and volume are known, an appropriate drug should be selected on the basis of the likely rate of absorption and expected duration of surgery at that site.

Some workers employ mixtures of drugs, usually in an attempt to overcome the somewhat slower onset of the longer acting agents by adding a short-acting drug with a rapid onset. The evidence that this actually works is at best conflicting and it may be that pharmaceutical interactions between solutions are responsible for the failure of the technique to work (Covino 1986). In most situations it is simpler to insert a catheter and make sequential injections.

Further consideration of drug selection for particular blocks is given in the appropriate chapter later in this book. It is important to remember that availability of particular agents may be limited by commercial factors. However, it is often possible to arrange for a hospital pharmacy in Britain to import a supply of an otherwise unavailable drug from a country where it is on sale.

## Further Reading

Smith G, Scott DB (eds) 1986 A symposium on local anaesthesia. British Journal of Anaesthesia 58: 691–746

## References

Aitkenhead AR 1994 The pattern of litigation against anaesthetists. British Journal of Anaesthesia 73: 10–21

Akerman B, Astrom A, Ross S, Telc A 1966a Studies on the absorption, cv distribution and metabolism of labelled prilocaine and lidocaine in some animal species. Acta Pharmacologica et Toxicologica 24: 389–403

Akerman B, Peterson S A, Wistrand P 1966b Methemoglobin forming metabolites of prilocaine. Third International Pharmacological Congress (Abstracts), Sao Paolo, Brazil, p. 237

Albright GA 1979 Cardiac arrest following regional anesthesia with etidocaine or bupivacaine. Anesthesiology 51: 285–287

Bonica JJ 1971 Regional anesthesia: recent advances and current status, pp. 69–70. Blackwell, Oxford

Borg T, Modig J 1985 Potential antithrombotic effects of local anaesthetics due to their inhibition of platelet function. Acta Anaesthesiologica Scandinavica 29: 739–742

Brockway MS, Bannister J, McClure JH, McKeown D, Wildsmith JAW 1991 Comparison of extradural ropivacaine and bupivacaine. British Journal of Anaesthesia 66: 31–37

Brown DT, Beamish D, Wildsmith JAW 1981 Allergic reaction to an amide local anaesthetic. British Journal of Anaesthesia 53: 435–437

Casati A, Fanelli G, Aldegheri G et al 1999 Interscalene brachial plexus anaesthesia with 0.5%, 0.75% or 1% ropivacaine: a double-blind comparison with 2% mepivacaine. British Journal of Anaesthesia 83: 872–875

Catchlove RFH 1972 The influence of $CO_2$ and pH on local anesthetic action. Journal of Pharmacology and Experimental Therapeutics 181: 298–309

Covino BG 1984 Current controversies in local anaesthetics. In: Scott DB, McClure JH, Wildsmith JAW (eds) Regional anaesthesia 1884–1984, pp 74–81. ICM, Sodertalje

Covino BG 1986 Pharmacology of local anaesthetic agents. British Journal of Anaesthesia 58: 701–716

Covino BG, Vassallo HG 1976 Local anesthetics: mechanisms of action and clinical use, pp 131–140. Grune and Stratton, New York

D'Angelo R 2000 Are the new local anaesthetics worth their cost? Acta Anaesthesiologica Scandinavica 44: 639–641

Davis NL, de Jong RH 1982 Successful resuscitation following massive bupivacaine overdose. Anesthesia and Analgesia 61: 62–64

Denny NM, Selander DE 1998 Continuous spinal anaesthesia. British Journal of Anaesthesia 81: 590–597

Gautier PE, De Kock M, Van Steenberge A et al 1999 Intrathecal ropivacaine for ambulatory surgery: a comparison between intrathecal bupivacaine and intrathecal ropivacaine for knee arthroscopy. Anesthesiology 91: 1239–1245

Henny CP, Odoom JA, ten Cate H et al 1986 Effects of extradural bupivacaine on the haemostatic system. British Journal of Anaesthesia 58: 301–305

Keeler JF, Simpson KH, Ellis FR, Kay SP 1992 Effect of addition of hyaluronidase to bupivacaine during axillary brachial plexus block. British Journal of Anaesthesia 68: 68–71

Kennedy WF, Bonica JJ, Ward RJ, Tolas AG, Martin WE, Grinstein A 1966 Cardiovascular effects of epinephrine when used in regional anesthesia. Acta Anaesthesiologica Scandinavica 23: 320–333

Lee A, Fagan D, Lamont M, Tucker GT, Halldin M, Scott DB 1989 Disposition kinetics of ropivacaine in humans. Anesthesia and Analgesia 69: 736–738

Mallampati SR, Liu PL, Knapp RM 1984 Convulsions and ventricular tachycardia from bupivacaine with epinephrine: successful resuscitation. Anesthesia and Analgesia 63: 856–859

McClure JH 1996 Ropivacaine: a review. British Journal of Anaesthesia 76:300–307

McClure JH, Scott DB 1981 Comparison of bupivacaine hydrochloride and carbonated bupivacaine in brachial plexus block by the interscalene technique. British Journal of Anaesthesia 53: 523–526

McDonald SB, Liu SS, Kopacz DJ, Stephenson CA 1999 Hyperbaric spinal ropivacaine: a comparison to bupivacaine in volunteers. Anesthesiology 90: 971–977

McLeod GA, Burke D 2001 Levobupivacaine. Anaesthesia 56: 331–341

Nicoll JMV, Trueren B, Acharya PA, Ahlen K, James M 1986 Retrobulbar anesthesia: the role of hyaluronidase. Anesthesia and Analgesia 65: 1324–1328

Reynolds F 1991 Editorial: ropivacaine. Anaesthesia 46: 339–340

Rigler M L, Drasner K, Krejcie T C et al 1991 Cauda equina syndrome after continuous spinal anesthesia. Anesthesia and Analgesia 72: 275–281

Scott DA, Blake D, Buckland M et al 1999 A comparison of epidural ropivacaine infusion alone and in combination with 1, 2, and 4 microg/mL fentanyl for seventy-two hours of postoperative analgesia after major abdominal surgery. Anesthesia and Analgesia. 88: 857–864

Scott DB 1975 Evaluation of the clinical tolerance of local anaesthetic agents. British Journal of Anaesthesia 47: 328–331

Scott DB 1989 Editorial: 'maximum recommended doses ' of local anaesthetic drugs. British Journal of Anaesthesia 63: 373–374

Scott DB, Cousins MJ 1980 Clinical pharmacology of local anesthetic drugs. In: Cousins MJ, Bridenbaugh D (eds) Neural blockade in clinical anesthesia and management of pain, pp 86–127. Lippincott, Philadelphia

Scott DB, Lee A, Fagan D, Bowler GMR, Bloomfield P, Lundh R 1989 Acute toxicity of ropivacaine compared with that of bupivacaine. Anesthesia and Analgesia 69: 663–669

Selander DE 1999 Transient lumbar pain (TLP) after lidocaine spinal anaesthesia is not neurotoxic. In: Van Zundert A (ed.) Highlights in regional anaesthesia and pain therapy VIII, pp. 315–321. Hadjigeorgiou, Limassol.

Simpson PJ, Hughes DR, Long DH 1982 Prolonged local analgesia for inguinal herniorrhaphy with bupivacaine and dextran. Annals of the Royal College of Surgeons of England 64: 243–246

Swann DG, Armstrong PJ, Douglas E, Brockway M, Bowler GMR 1991 The alkalinisation of bupivacaine for intercostal nerve blockade. Anaesthesia 46: 174–176

Van Dyke C, Barash B G, Jatlow P, Byck R 1976 Cocaine: plasma concentrations after intranasal application in man. Science 191: 859–861

Whiteside J, Wildsmith JAW 2001 Developments in local anaesthetic drugs. British Journal of Anaesthesia 87: 27–35

Wildsmith JAW 2000 Correspondence: Relative potencies of ropivacaine and bupivacaine. Anesthesiology 92: 283

Wildsmith JAW 2001 Letters: New local anaesthetics – how much is improved safety worth? Acta Anaesthesiologica Scandinavica 45: 652–653

Wildsmith JAW, Mason A, McKinnon RP, Rae SM 1998 Alleged allergy to local anaesthetic drugs. British Dental Journal 184: 507–510

Writer WDR, Stienstra R, Eddleston JM et al 1998 Neonatal outcome and mode of delivery after epidural analgesia for labour with ropivacaine and bupivacaine: a prospective meta-analysis. British Journal of Anaesthesia 81: 713–717

Zaric D, Nydahl P, Philipson L, Samuelsson L, Heierson A, Axelsson K 1996 The effect of continuous lumbar epidural infusion of ropivacaine (0.1%, 0.2% and 0.3%) and 0.25% bupivacaine on sensory and motor blockade in volunteers: a double-blind study. Regional Anesthesia 21: 14–25

Zsigmond EK, Kothary SP, Flynn KB 1978 In vitro inhibitory effect of amide-type local analgesics on normal and atypical human plasma cholinesterases. Regional Anesthesia 3/4: 7–9

# 7. Preoperative considerations

## M R Checketts and J A W Wildsmith

Regional anaesthesia, when skilfully administered, is a hugely satisfying experience for the patient, anaesthetist and surgeon. It provides comfort for the patient, both during and after surgery, with little or no systemic upset, professional satisfaction for the anaesthetist and, very often, better operating conditions for the surgeon. However, success depends crucially upon the skill and knowledge of the anaesthetist. Meticulous attention to detail is essential, and the patient, the operation and the surgeon must all be taken into consideration when planning every phase of care. Many factors have to be considered, including the patient's general health, the nature, site and duration of the intended surgery, and the availability of appropriate equipment and facilities.

### PREOPERATIVE ASSESSMENT

Preoperative patient assessment is as important as, and identical to, that routinely carried out before general anaesthesia. A full history must be taken, a complete physical examination should have been performed, and the results of appropriate investigations must be available. The patient's case record will often contain relevant details of the past medical history, and records of previous anaesthetics should be consulted in particular, because they may record useful information such as the degree of difficulty in performing an earlier regional block. If additional investigation or specialist consultation is necessary, this should be arranged well before embarking on the planned operative procedure. All of the patient's details should be confirmed at a preoperative visit when the anaesthetist should also discuss and explain the planned technique, and ensure that the patient knows what to expect. Patients are becoming much better informed and clinicians must be prepared for, and respond to, their questions or worries. Finally, it is important to identify, and thus plan to deal with, potential technical difficulties such as anatomical abnormality at the block site at this early stage rather than in the anaesthetic room just before surgery.

### Pre-existing disease

Most medical conditions have at least some implication for the practice of regional anaesthesia, and the significance of this must be appreciated if blocks are to be used safely and effectively.

#### Cardiovascular system

Regional anaesthesia for patients with ischaemic or valvular heart disease is challenging, and a careful risk–benefit analysis should be performed on each patient. There may be potential benefits in avoiding the generalised cardiovascular depressive effects of general anaesthesia, but there are potential pitfalls with regional anaesthesia which cannot be ignored. However, expertly managed regional anaesthesia may contribute much to the management of even the highest risk patients undergoing very complex surgical procedures.

Surgery on patients with *ischaemic heart disease* carries a higher risk than usual and this risk is increased markedly if there is any episode of prolonged hypotension (Mauney et al 1970). In patients who had suffered a previous myocardial infarction, Steen and colleagues (1978) found a five-fold increase in re-infarction rate if the systolic pressure decreased by 30% or more for 10 minutes or longer, presumably because of a reduction in myocardial perfusion. Any situation which produces an imbalance between oxygen delivery and cardiac work leading to increased myocardial oxygen demand is to be avoided, so hypoxaemia, tachycardia, hypertension and hypotension are particularly likely to cause problems in the cardiac patient.

There is good evidence that regional anaesthesia can have a beneficial effect on the critical balance between myocardial oxygen supply and demand. Using the model of a dog with reduced coronary flow, Klassen and colleagues (1980) found that sympathetic block from an epidural caused a beneficial redistribution of coronary flow to the endocardium, probably due to alterations in the tone of transmural resistance vessels. Further, Davis and colleagues (1986), also working with dogs, found that thoracic epidural block reduced myocardial infarction size after coronary arterial occlusion. Human studies have shown that localised high thoracic epidural block ($T_1$ to $T_5$) causes a decrease in systolic arterial pressure, heart rate and pulmonary arterial and wedge pressures, without significant changes in coronary perfusion pressure, cardiac output, stroke volume or systemic and pulmonary vascular resistances in patients with unstable angina (Blomberg et al 1989). Thus, thoracic epidural block may reduce myocardial oxygen demand without jeopardising coronary arterial supply.

Reiz (1989) has reviewed current understanding of the circulatory changes induced by epidural anaesthesia in cardiac patients. A high thoracic epidural block ($T_1$ to $T_5$) improved left ventricular function during stress testing in patients with severe coronary artery disease (Kock et al 1990), but myocardial ischaemic events are more likely to occur in such patients if there is more extensive block ($T_1$ to $T_{12}$) (Reiz et al 1980). However, thoracic epidural block has been found to be effective in patients with severe angina refractory to conventional medical therapy (Blomberg et al 1989, Toft & Jorgensen 1989), and has been used successfully on a long-term (greater than 3 years) domiciliary basis in similar patients deemed unsuitable for coronary revascularisation (Blomberg 1994).

Despite these encouraging findings, at the present time only a handful of studies demonstrate a clear beneficial effect of regional anaesthesia on cardiac outcome in surgical patients (Liu et al 1995), although the evidence is stronger for high-risk patients (Yeager et al 1987, Tuman et al 1991). However, it may be that the most promising therapeutic intervention for these patients is perioperative β-adrenergic block, the Perioperative Ischemia Research Group arguing forcefully that this can reduce both mortality and cardiovascular complications in patients with ischaemic heart disease undergoing non-cardiac surgery (Mangano et al 1996). The American College of Physicians reviewed the whole issue of perioperative myocardial ischaemia and recommended a protocol for at-risk patients (American College of Physicians 1997, Palda & Detsky 1997). Thus, there is an alternative strategy to regional anaesthesia, although it must be remembered that it will not provide any of the other benefits of regional anaesthesia such as high-quality pain control.

Central nerve block in patients with *valvular heart disease* is also controversial because such patients often have a reduced ability to increase cardiac output and, hence, to respond to physiological insults. As a result the vasodilatation produced by sympathetic paralysis during spinal or epidural block may result in an exaggerated degree of hypotension. In the presence of aortic stenosis the effect on coronary artery blood flow can be catastrophic because systemic hypotension is not associated with a decrease in left ventricular pressure because of the pressure gradient across the narrowed aortic orifice.

Controlling the extent of sympathetic block will limit these problems, and a catheter technique will allow a central nerve block to be induced slowly and progressively. Any cardiovascular change will be similarly progressive and can be controlled with increments of appropriately chosen sympathomimetic agents, perhaps more readily than during the acute changes produced by induction of general anaesthesia. There are now several reports of uneventful spinal or epidural anaesthesia in patients with valvular disease (Collard et al 1995, Pittard & Vucevic 1998), but the report of the death of a pre-eclamptic parturient with aortic incompetence serves as a reminder that the block has to be very carefully controlled in such patients (Alderson 1987). Careful contemplation of the risks and benefits of the planned technique, as well as significant experience of managing both cardiac patients and regional block are obviously essential.

## Respiratory system

Patients with severe respiratory disease are among the most willing to accept regional anaesthesia for their operations. They are keenly aware of the limitations which their disease places upon their activity and of how local anaesthesia may be of benefit to them. For peripheral or lower abdominal surgery, neural block avoids the complications of both general anaesthesia and neuromuscular blocking agents, and enables patients to look after their airways and lung ventilation.

However, a supplementary general anaesthetic is usually necessary during upper abdominal and thoracic surgery, and block of at least some of the nerves supplying the respiratory muscles is inevitable (Freund et al 1967). This may lead to a decrease in vital capacity, maximum breathing capacity and the ability to cough and clear secretions.

The most important alteration in pulmonary function in patients undergoing surgery is an almost inevitable reduction in functional residual capacity which may result in atelectasis, ventilation perfusion mismatch, hypoxaemia and pneumonia. Unfortunately, there is no evidence that any form of preoperative respiratory function testing can predict which patients may become compromised, but well-known risk factors are obesity, advanced age, pre-existing pulmonary disease, thoracic or abdominal incisions and severe pain. The major advantage of regional anaesthetic techniques in upper abdominal and thoracic surgery is in the provision of postoperative analgesia. Published studies comparing the pulmonary sequelae of regional and systemic opioid analgesic techniques are conflicting. It seems that the benefits of epidural analgesia on pulmonary complications are only apparent in high-risk patients and only when epidural block is maintained well into the postoperative period (Liu et al 1995).

### Nervous system

Pre-existing disease of the nervous system presents the anaesthetist with a most contentious problem. Bromage (1978) has reviewed possible causes of neurological damage during the performance of regional anaesthesia, especially near the spinal cord. These include direct trauma, haematoma, infection, vasoconstriction and accidental injection of a neurotoxin. It is almost inevitable that, if a patient's neurological condition degenerates after a regional anaesthetic, the block will be blamed to the exclusion of all other possible causes. However, Bromage has elegantly shown that many peripheral nerve lesions occurring after extradural analgesia are not directly related to the technique itself. Marinacci and Courville (1958) carried out electromyography on 482 patients with neurological complications after subarachnoid anaesthesia and only in four cases were the complications considered to be due to the block.

Unfortunately, most of the literature relating to regional anaesthesia in patients with neurological disease is anecdotal. It is therefore difficult to define specific guidelines, but analysis of the few published series is helpful. There are several reports of permanent neurological deterioration after regional anaesthesia in patients with pre-existing problems (Chaudhari et al 1978, Hirlekar 1980, Ballin 1981), but there are protagonists of regional anaesthesia who believe that it exerts no influence upon the clinical course of a wide range of neurological conditions (Crawford et al 1981). Pre- and postoperative clinical evaluation and documentation are important regardless of the anaesthetic used, because changes in neurological status are common after surgery anyway. Accurate documentation is vital for medicolegal purposes also.

Patients with neurological conditions may be at risk from a number of complications which must be appreciated by the anaesthetist. A deterioration may not be due to the block itself, but a failure to recognise the implications of the existing condition. Respiratory compromise may occur secondary to musculoskeletal abnormalities or abnormal medullary control of ventilation. Autonomic hyperreflexia is common and can result in unwelcome rapid and dramatic changes in haemodynamic status, or even in cardiac arrest. A state of relative hypovolaemia is well recognised after spinal-cord injury and in patients with multiple sclerosis. The combination of this pre-existing problem with the sympathectomy caused by a central nerve block may result in profound hypotension.

*Multiple sclerosis (MS)* Stress, fatigue, infection and hyperthermia are well documented as factors that can exacerbate MS. These factors are common in the perioperative period so it is usually impossible to specify the cause of a relapse after surgery. There are no published data describing a large number of MS patients receiving regional anaesthetic techniques, but there are several small retrospective reports mainly concerning obstetric patients. Typically, MS goes into remission during pregnancy, but may then relapse in the early postpartum period (Abramsky 1994). There are conflicting reports on whether central nerve block is associated with such a relapse; Samford and colleagues (1978) suggest that it is, but others refute this (Crawford et al 1981, Bader et al 1988, Capdeville & Hoyt 1994). It is important to consider carefully the risks and benefits of regional anaesthesia in patients with MS, and to discuss the issues, particularly the risk of relapse, with the patient.

*Spinal cord injury* The spinal cord redevelops reflex activity about 1 month after transection. Autonomic hyperreflexia can be provoked by a skin incision or visceral stimulation such as a full bladder. These reflex responses may result in profound hypertension and bradycardia, and may be life threatening, especially if the transection level is above $T_6$. Procedures such as cystoscopy are particularly likely to provoke these reflexes and spinal anaesthesia can be employed with great benefit with the sole intention of blocking the reflex pathways (Schonwald et al 1981, Lambert et al 1982). However, there has been at least one report of such a mass reflex developing in the presence of an apparently adequate block (Lambert et al 1982), but subarachnoid baclofen may further attenuate these reflexes (Muller et al 1990) and central nerve block is probably the anaesthetic technique of choice in patients at risk of autonomic hyperreflexia.

**Peripheral neuropathy** The risks and benefits of regional techniques have to be considered carefully in patients with peripheral neuropathy, particularly if there is the possibility of co-existent autonomic neuropathy because it may be associated with greater cardiovascular morbidity (Page & Watkins 1978, Burgos et al 1989). However, regional anaesthesia will offer clear advantages in many patients with this combination of problems, particularly diabetics (see below).

**Other neuropathology** Regional anaesthesia also has potential advantages in patients with other types of neurological disease. A clear example is the avoidance of neuromuscular blocking drugs in patients with myotonic dystrophy and myasthenia gravis so that the respiratory morbidity, to which they are particularly susceptible, is reduced.

An individual approach to the patient, the intercurrent disease and the proposed surgery is necessary in order to decide on the most appropriate form of anaesthetic management.

### Renal system

Bromage and Gertel (1972) alleged that patients with chronic renal failure are more susceptible than healthy patients to toxicity from local anaesthetic agents. These authors suggested that this might stem from a difference in drug binding due to the hypoproteinaemia associated with renal failure. They also noted that anaemia may cause a high output circulation and thus lead to rapid systemic absorption. On the other hand, the sympathetic block caused by regional anaesthesia may improve circulation and perfusion to the site of operation, whether this is the kidney itself, or a limb

during the fashioning of an arteriovenous fistula. However, brachial plexus block, particularly by the axillary route, should be undertaken with great care in a patient with such a fistula because the associated venous distension will make accidental intravascular injection much more likely.

### Obesity

There may be significant technical problems with the performance of regional anaesthesia in the obese patient. Fisher and colleagues (1975) have suggested that difficulty in positioning, identifying landmarks and needle location all combine to make regional anaesthesia extremely difficult. Conversely, the benefits of combining light general anaesthesia with regional anaesthesia for upper abdominal surgery in the morbidly obese have been well documented by Buckley and colleagues (1983). Many of their patients also had cardiovascular and respiratory disease, and postoperative complications were less than in a similar group given general anaesthesia alone. However, the two groups and techniques employed were not matched or randomised, and the findings should be assessed in that light.

### Diabetes

Diabetic patients have an increased incidence of atherosclerosis and its attendant complications. They are particularly prone to episodes of painless myocardial ischaemia and the cardiovascular system should be the focus of unremitting vigilance. In addition, diabetes is associated with microangiopathy, peripheral neuropathy, autonomic dysfunction and infection. However, these problems are more than offset by the many occasions when regional anaesthesia allows surgery to be performed with minimal disruption of the diabetic patient's carbohydrate intake and insulin regime, and with minimal activation of the 'stress' hormones, all of which act to increase blood sugar and destabilise its control.

### Infection

Infection at or close to the site of injection is a major contraindication to the use of local anaesthetic techniques. Not only may it spread the infection, but the block is likely to be ineffective (Bieter 1936) because pH changes in the infected tissue will impair local anaesthetic action. It may be possible to block a nerve distant from the focus of infection, but this is not always effective, as many dental patients can confirm.

More distant foci of infection present more complicated challenges. Major infections such as meningitis, arachnoiditis or epidural abscess are rare after spinal or epidural anaesthesia and there is good epidemiological evidence that the incidence of meningitis after lumbar puncture is no higher than in the general population, even in bacteraemic patients (Eng & Seligman 1981). However, Carp and Bailey (1992) found that 12 out of 40 bacteraemic rats developed meningitis after cisternal puncture, although none of the comparative group, which had been given gentamicin, developed meningitis. This led Chestnut (1992) to recommend proceeding with central nerve block in bacteraemic patients *provided* that appropriate antibiotics have been given *and* that there is some evidence of clinical improvement (e.g. reduced pyrexia).

Leaving an epidural catheter *in situ* in a patient with systemic infection, even if this is being treated, is more controversial because, like any other foreign body, it may act as a focus for local infection so patients must be selected and monitored carefully (Carson & Wildsmith 1996). The belief that the caudal approach presents a greater risk than any other is unfounded as long as antiseptic precautions are adequate (Abouleish et al 1980).

## Muscle disease

Malignant hyperthermia is probably the best known example of a muscle disease with anaesthetic significance. Regional anaesthesia avoids the use of volatile agents and muscle relaxants, but may still be associated with increased temperature in susceptible individuals (Katz & Krich 1976, Wadhwa 1977). Amide agents such as lidocaine can release calcium from the sarcoplasmic reticulum and this would imply that they should be avoided, although prilocaine is used for muscle biopsy in the investigation of suspected patients (Hopkins 2000). Esters are probably safer (Gronert 1980), but there has been one report of a reaction in a susceptible individual (Katz & Krich 1976).

## Sickle cell disease

Regional techniques are the methods of choice in sickle cell disease (Howells et al 1972), although the usual precautions must still be taken to ensure good perfusion, maintain oxygenation and avoid tourniquets. On theoretical grounds, prilocaine should not be used in these patients.

## Allergy

Many patients claim to be 'allergic' to local anaesthetics, but the history usually reveals that a previous reaction was due to systemic toxicity, the effect of an added vasoconstrictor or a psychological reaction. Most patients have only been exposed to local anaesthesia in the dental chair where fear and anxiety are relatively common, epinephrine is used in high concentration and injections are made into vascular tissues. Allergy to local anaesthetics is rare, but each suspected case should be investigated (Wildsmith et al 1998). Failure to do so may force the anaesthetist to avoid regional anaesthesia unnecessarily in the future and, if the reaction was truly allergic in nature, may result in subsequent administration of the real cause of the reaction again.

Intradermal injection is the usual method of testing for local anaesthetic sensitivity, but false positive responses are not infrequent (Fisher 1984). Full resuscitation facilities should be available and the initial injection should be 0.1 ml of solution. Complete investigation should include progressive injection of increasing doses of the local anaesthetic drug (Weiss et al 1989). Cross-sensitivity is common between the ester drugs, but not between the amides, although the possibility that a reaction was due to a preservative should be kept in mind.

## Psychological problems

Regional anaesthesia is not contraindicated by psychological illness, but its use must be assessed in the context of the patient's ability to understand and consent to the intended procedure. The patient must be able to co-operate fully with the block procedure, and it may be that the nature of the illness makes this impossible. Moore (1976) states that hysteria and malingering are both relative contraindications to the use of regional anaesthesia.

## Coagulation considerations

Abnormalities of the coagulation process present particular problems for the regional anaesthetist. Even in the normal patient, there is the possibility of haematoma formation after regional anaesthesia where the nerve is so deeply placed that pressure cannot be used to control bleeding after needle insertion. The risk is obviously greater in cases where coagulation is deficient, and it has been argued that intercostal nerve block should be avoided in such patients (Nielsen 1989).

81

Disorders of coagulation may occasionally result from intercurrent disease, and the ideal solution is restoration of normal coagulation prior to the block, something which will usually require the help of a haematologist. If restoration of normal coagulation is not possible, clinical decisions should be based on the degree of disorder, and guidelines on a similar degree of drug induced abnormality followed. Many surgical patients are at high risk of thromboembolism, and drug therapy is used commonly to reduce the risk. Regional anaesthesia in this situation is a complex issue which requires careful consideration. The 'simple' approach is to avoid regional block in any patient receiving pharmacological thromboprophylaxis, but this will deny many patients the benefits of a regional technique, often quite unnecessarily.

### Vertebral canal haematoma

The extreme manifestation of this issue is vertebral canal haematoma formation after central nerve block. This is a potentially catastrophic complication because permanent paraplegia will ensue unless the haematoma is both diagnosed and evacuated rapidly, perhaps within as little as 8 hours. Anxiety about this happening can mean that the patient is denied *either* the benefits of the regional anaesthetic technique *or* appropriate deep vein thrombosis (DVT) prophylaxis, even though vertebral canal haematoma is a very rare complication with an estimated incidence of 1 in 220 000 associated with spinals and 1 in 150 000 with epidurals (Tryba 1993). It is thus crucial that the concern does not lead to suboptimal management which may well have greater *total* risks for the patient. Appropriate advice on the use of spinal and epidural block in patients receiving pharmacological prophylaxis for thromboembolism was published some years ago (Wildsmith & McClure 1991), but the concerns have been renewed recently by events in the USA (Lumpkin 1998). The advice has now been updated and the situation may be summarised as follows.

Most vertebral canal haematomas occur spontaneously, with an incidence estimated at one per million population per year (Holtas et al 1996). Many are associated with *disordered coagulation* (Groen & Ponssen 1990), which has also been identified as one of the major factors in the cases reported after spinal and epidural block (Vandermeulen et al 1994). *Technical difficulty* during instrumentation of the vertebral canal is another factor, with epidural block (especially with catheter insertion) carrying a greater risk than spinal.

*Catheter removal* is an important time of further risk. To put the subject into perspective, it should be noted that the review highlighting these points was able to identify only 61 case reports published between 1906 and 1994 (Vandermeulen et al 1994), but this was before the widespread use of low-molecular-weight heparin.

In 1998, a report appeared in the USA documenting over 40 cases of vertebral canal haematoma occurring in less than 5 years in patients receiving the low-molecular-weight heparin, enoxaparin (Lumpkin 1998). Most followed spinal or epidural block, although a few related to diagnostic lumbar puncture, and the report confirmed the other risk factors mentioned above as well as noting an association with enoxaparin. This American series is in direct contrast to experience in Europe, where enoxaparin has been available for much longer, but where only two cases of vertebral canal haematoma have been reported. Its incidence after spinal or epidural block in patients receiving enoxaparin has been estimated at 1 in 2 250 000 in Europe, but at 1 in 14 000 in the USA (Tryba & Wedel 1997), a difference which has to be explained.

Although there were other issues (Checketts & Wildsmith 1999), the major contributory factor seems to have been a difference in recommended dose of enoxaparin. In Europe the dose is 20–40 mg once daily, starting 12 hours before surgery, so that the peak effect of the drug (4–6 hours after administration) will be well past at the time of block administration and any risk will be minimal. In the USA, the recommended dose was 30 mg twice daily, starting 1 hour after surgery. Thus, there would be no effect at the time of institution of a block, but the long half-life of enoxaparin (10–12 hours) could lead to cumulation, particularly at the higher dose. The drug might well then produce an overt effect on coagulation and cause bleeding at the time of catheter removal. Even if dose were the major factor, other aspects provide lessons which will help to minimise the risk of this dreadful complication. The primary lesson is that surgeons and anaesthetists must communicate properly regarding policies for use of central nerve block and DVT prophylaxis. An overview of the more general points is that:

- Vertebral canal haematoma is a rare complication, but its serious nature requires that some precaution is taken to minimise the incidence
- The risk seems to be related to the degree of coagulation disturbance, and interactions between drugs may be particularly important (Wysowski et al 1998)

- Technical difficulty during block performance was reported in many cases, so technical skill and experience may be very relevant
- Coagulation status at the time of catheter removal needs as much attention as at its insertion

Against this background, specific aspects of the various pharmacological agents used in thromboprophylaxis can be considered.

*Warfarin* Frank anticoagulation is the ultimate contraindication to spinal or epidural block, and most authorities recommend that the INR should be 1.5 or lower for institution of a block or removal of a catheter (Horlocker et al 1994, Odoom & Sih 1983, Wu & Perkins 1996). However, warfarin is used infrequently for perioperative thromboprophylaxis in the UK and most patients presenting for anaesthesia are receiving the drug for other indications. Prior to elective surgery, such patients will have their coagulation managed actively in order to achieve an appropriate balance between the risks of bleeding and thrombus formation. In principle, this involves stopping the warfarin and replacing it with a method of pharmacological thromboprophylaxis with a shorter duration of effect once the INR is less than 1.7. Special provisions apply in ophthalmic surgery (see Ch. 17).

*Unfractionated heparin* Thromboprophylaxis with low-dose (5000 units), subcutaneous heparin given two to three times daily does not usually prolong the APTT and large numbers of such patients have received spinal or epidural block without sequelae (Schwander & Bachmann 1991). However, the numbers of patients involved in these studies are small relative to the risk of vertebral canal haematoma and a transient elevation of the APTT may occur (Cooke et al 1976). Thus, some anaesthetists prefer not to institute spinal or epidural block within 4–6 hours of a dose of heparin, and they delay the next dose until after the block has been performed (Wildsmith & McClure 1991). Similar considerations would apply to catheter removal. Because of the risk of thrombocytopaenia, the platelet count should be checked before the block is performed, or the catheter removed, if the patient has been receiving any heparin preparation for more than a few days.

*Low-molecular-weight heparin (LMWH)* LMWHs act by inhibiting factor Xa and have relatively little anti-IIa (thrombin) activity. They have a higher bioavailability and longer duration of action than unfractionated heparin. Peak anti-Xa activity occurs about 3–4 hours after subcutaneous injection, but even at 12 hours the anti-Xa effect has only reduced by 50%. The effects of LMWHs are predictable and dose related, and their pharmacokinetics and dynamics have to be appreciated by the regional anaesthetist. The evidence suggests that the standard European dose regimen (e.g. enoxaparin 20–40 mg, once daily) is not associated with any increased risk as long as the block is instituted, or the catheter removed, 10–12 hours after drug administration. There seems to be no definite reason why a first dose should not be given immediately after block administration or catheter removal, although the current American view is more cautious (American Society of Regional Anesthesia 1998). This recommends that 24 hours elapse before the next dose is given even after uneventful spinal or epidural block and only if there is adequate haemostasis.

*Antiplatelet agents* Much concern has been expressed about the potential for the anti-platelet effect of aspirin and similar drugs to increase the risk of vertebral canal haematoma in patients receiving spinal or epidural block. However, there is little or no evidence to support this concern, although interactions with other agents such as low molecular weight heparin may occur (Horlocker et al 1995, Wysowski et al 1998).

*Platelet abnormalities* Patients with disorders of platelet function or low platelet levels may present an increased risk of vertebral canal haematoma if they receive an epidural or spinal block. The risk is presumed to be high if there is clinical evidence of platelet dysfunction, that is, petechiae or spontaneous and easy bruising of the skin. Specialist advice may be useful if central neural block is considered appropriate because platelet therapy may be indicated before the patient undergoes surgery (Thomas 1997).

*Quantifying the risk* It is not unnatural to seek some numerical indicator of the actual risk in an individual patient. With warfarin and unfractionated heparin this is readily available in the clinical situation in the form of INR- and APTT-testing respectively. Unfortunately, testing for the activity of LMWH against factor Xa is not readily available so it is necessary to rely on knowledge of the time course of the agents. In platelet abnormalities a count may be of some use, but provides no information on the activity and effectiveness of those platelets. These difficulties have led to suggestions that the bleeding time can determine which patients are at risk, but this is a subjective screening test and not one on which to base clinical decisions. Thromboelastography (Sharma et al 1999, Whitten & Greilich 2000) may be more objective, but as with bleeding time (Thomas 1997) there is no epidemiological evidence on what is, or is not, a 'safe' or 'dangerous' result. It may be that taking a careful bleeding history from the patient is the simplest and most cost-effective way of identifying the risk (Colon-Otero et al 1991).

*An overview* Definitive recommendations should be based on the results of randomised, double-blind studies, but none are available and, given the incidence of vertebral canal haematoma, it is unlikely that such evidence will appear. A common-sense approach, based on the evidence reviewed briefly above, is needed for practice within a framework of agreed local policies. It is particularly difficult to lay down guidelines for the patient in labour, or presenting for emergency surgery, who has already received a thromboprophylactic drug. The agent used, the dose, and the time interval since its last administration should be noted. Any decision should be based on the balance of risks and benefits, which will often require discussion with the patient as well as with the surgeon. These discussions should be documented fully. Trainees must understand the issues and seek advice from consultants if they are in any doubt.

Because many of the reported cases were associated with 'difficult' or 'traumatic' procedures, as well as with disordered coagulation *the need for a cautious, gentle technique is self-evident.* When there is difficulty or bleeding during the block procedure (or any other unusual risk factor) it is essential that this is recorded and greater vigilance maintained during the postoperative period. It may also be advisable to omit or delay the next dose of thromboprophylactic agent. In the face of difficulty occurring during a block it may even be appropriate to review the situation and switch to an alternative anaesthetic method. Finally, although this discussion of vertebral canal haematoma has dealt with the factors likely to predispose to the condition, it should be appreciated that a haematoma will only produce symptoms if it can exert pressure on the cord or cauda equina, and this will depend on the local anatomy of the epidural space at the point where the bleeding occurs. A small, loculated haematoma may therefore produce symptoms whereas one which can spread unimpeded may not.

Combinations of thromboprophylactic agents may cause greater disturbance of coagulation and require more caution. The commonest situation is the patient who is already on aspirin and who is to undergo an operation for which the local protocol requires administration of heparin. However, there is new evidence that aspirin is an effective DVT prophylactic (Sors & Meyer 2000), so there may be no need to give another agent preoperatively, particularly since central block has been shown to prevent thromboembolism. Profound epidural block maintained for 24 hours will reduce the incidence of asymptomatic DVT after lower limb joint replacement surgery to about 25% (Modig et al 1983), a figure which compares well with the effect of low molecular weight heparin (Bergqvist et al 1996), and the combination of epidural block with aspirin therapy (with or without sequential calf compression) has been shown to produce very low DVT rates (Lieberman et al 1994).

## THE SURGICAL PROCEDURE

Regional anaesthesia is not suitable for all types of surgery. In some cases, the appropriate block may be technically difficult with a high failure rate, or the operation may be so extensive that more than one block is required, and the problem of drug toxicity may arise. In many other cases though, regional anaesthesia can provide effective postoperative analgesia even if sedative or general anaesthetic supplementation is required for the operation itself. One of the chief advantages of regional anaesthesia in obstetrics is that the mother can be fully conscious and unsedated at the time of delivery.

## Site and nature of the operation

Obviously, the chosen regional technique should provide anaesthesia over the area of the skin incision, but it must also be extensive enough to block stimuli arising from deeper structures manipulated during surgery. For example, a block limited to $T_{11}$ and $T_{12}$, although adequate for an inguinal herniorrhaphy incision, will be inadequate when the surgeon handles the spermatic cord and hernial sac. Similarly, perineal anaesthesia alone will be inadequate for a vaginal hysterectomy. When a spinal or epidural block is used, particular care should be taken to ensure that the segmental block provided gives adequate anaesthesia for the surgical procedure.

Even if it is technically possible to supply complete anaesthesia for all stages of an operation, it is not always desirable that the patient should be fully aware throughout. Many patients prefer to be lightly sedated during surgery and the availability of short-acting intravenous drugs such as midazolam and propofol makes this possible with minimal postoperative after-effects. A controlled infusion of propofol allows the depth of sedation to be very carefully controlled with rapid wake up and virtually no 'hangover' effect.

## Duration of surgery

This will have a major bearing on selection of the local anaesthetic drug and regional technique used. Insertion of a catheter allows increments of local anaesthetic to be given during surgery and should be used whenever there is the slightest risk that the operation may outlast the effect of a single dose. Single-injection techniques should be reserved for operations which are certain to be finished before a single dose has worn off, and do not require local analgesia for postoperative pain control.

The duration of the operation may also influence decisions regarding the choice of sedation or general anaesthesia. Operating tables are not designed for the comfort of the conscious patient, and lying on a firm surface for a long period can become an ordeal for even the most resilient and co-operative patient.

## Anaesthetist and surgeon

The extent to which regional anaesthesia is deemed suitable in various cases depends on the attitude of both anaesthetist and surgeon. The main source of surgical prejudice against regional anaesthesia is the concern that the smooth running of the operating list will be impaired, but there is evidence that, in experienced hands, regional anaesthetic techniques take very little longer to perform than a general anaesthetic (Dexter 1998). The co-operation and enthusiasm of surgeons should be cultivated at all times and it is common courtesy to inform them in advance when regional anaesthesia is planned. When the clear benefits of regional anaesthesia are apparent in terms of a rapid and pain-free recovery, surgeons encourage rather than resist it.

Another area of surgical concern is the possibility that the operation might be compromised by inadequate anaesthesia or muscle relaxation. The surgeon expects the best possible operating conditions, and the anaesthetist requires skill, experience and patience to

provide these consistently. If a regional anaesthesia 'culture' is established in an institution in which surgeons, nurses and patients are well informed about the many advantages, life becomes much easier for the anaesthetist. The atmosphere in the operating theatre should be relaxed and free of stress. There is wide variation among surgeons as to what constitutes an 'ideal' environment. Some enjoy the technical challenge and social contact provided by the conscious patient, whereas others value freedom of speech and prefer sedation or general anaesthesia. Many senior surgeons feel that surgical trainees should gain experience in operating on conscious patients. They point out that this refines surgical technique and tightens operating theatre discipline.

There is a similar variation in attitude towards regional anaesthesia among anaesthetists. Modern training requirements ensure that all trainee anaesthetists have some experience from an early stage, but not everyone is temperamentally suited to cope with the special challenges which regional anaesthesia presents. Such anaesthetists should aim to master one or two widely applicable blocks so that their repertoire is not restricted to general anaesthetic techniques, and their patients are not entirely denied the benefits of regional anaesthesia. At the other end of the scale, the enthusiast must make sure that his main concern is the patient's overall welfare, and not his own enthusiasm for regional block.

It is also crucial to accept readily failure of a regional technique should it occur and develop strategies to address such a failure, for example additional peripheral regional block or general anaesthesia. There are no guarantees in regional anaesthesia and anaesthetists should not promise 100% success to the patient or presume they can achieve it themselves.

## AVAILABLE FACILITIES

Before proceeding further it is necessary to consider the equipment and drugs required for the safe and effective performance of the chosen technique.

## Resuscitation

Intravenous access and fluids, a tipping trolley, an oxygen supply and resuscitation drugs and equipment *must* be available. The equipment must include an anaesthetic machine as a source of oxygen and means of lung ventilation, laryngoscopes, oropharyngeal airways, cuffed tracheal tubes, a stilette and efficient suction. The full range of anaesthetic and resuscitation drugs should be immediately available. A defibrillator must also be easily accessible and it is the anaesthetist's duty to be familiar with its function and to know the current guidelines on advanced cardiac life support.

## Local anaesthetic drugs

The pharmacology of local anaesthetic drugs has been described in Chapters 4, 5 and 6. Obviously the appropriate drug for the planned procedure should be used. *Every care should be taken to avoid injection errors and ensure that the intended local anaesthetic solution is injected.*

The contents of single-use glass or plastic ampoules from a reputable drug company are guaranteed sterile and should be used for all central blocks. The ampoules themselves may be double wrapped and autoclaved for use within a sterile field. Multidose vials contain additional bacteriostatic agents and are certainly not suitable for spinal or epidural anaesthesia. It has been suggested that they should not be used for any regional technique (Henderson & Macrae 1983) because pathogens may have been introduced during previous use. These objections can be overcome by using a multidose vial once only and then discarding it. Generic local anaesthetics should be regarded with suspicion unless the exact contents are known.

All solutions should be drawn up through a micropore filter needle, to exclude problems due to particulate matter from ampoules (Somerville & Gibson 1973) and from disposable regional anaesthetic trays (Seltzer et al 1977).

## THE PREOPERATIVE VISIT
## Explanation to the patient

It cannot be over-emphasised that the preoperative preparation of the patient is one of the keys to success with regional anaesthesia. It establishes rapport with the patient, ensures co-operation and makes technical performance of the block easier. Patients with pre-existing medical conditions, such as chronic obstructive airway disease, are often keen to have regional anaesthesia, but may be encouraged if they are not. Healthier patients can be offered a choice of regional anaesthesia, general anaesthesia or a mixture of both. Many patients prefer

to be asleep and their wishes should always be taken into account. It may be necessary occasionally to 'sell' the advantages of regional anaesthesia, but there should be no attempt at coercion.

An adequate explanation of what the patient can expect should be given in terms which are readily understood. Specific mention should be made of paraesthesiae if they are to be elicited or involuntary muscular twitching when a nerve stimulator is to be used. If the patient is to remain conscious during surgery, it is prudent to mention that some sensation may be preserved, and that feelings of pressure, movement, warmth or cold may be experienced; otherwise any stimulus may be interpreted as pain and this may result in unnecessary action being taken by the anaesthetist, although any truly painful sensation must be attended to immediately. Music can be a useful distraction during the procedure and patients can be encouraged to bring a favourite tape or disk to theatre if they wish.

It is good practice to point out the advantages associated with the chosen technique – early recovery, lack of postoperative pain, reduced amount of nausea and vomiting, etc. – and to follow this with an explanation of what the patient will experience before, during and after the block. An assurance that the patient will not see the operation is often required and the patient should be warned that motor block may outlast the sensory block postoperatively.

## Preparation of the patient

Patients for major blocks should be treated in the same way as patients receiving general anaesthesia and standard protocols regarding fasting should be followed, remembering that there is evidence that these protocols do not need to be as stringent as they used to be (Strunin 1993). The urinary bladder should be empty preoperatively because a full bladder in a patient with a peripheral block can be both uncomfortable and disruptive, and over-distention increases significantly the need for catheterisation after spinal or epidural block.

## Premedication

Some patients require no more premedication than a preoperative visit and adequate explanation of the intended procedure by the anaesthetist. However, drug premedication is often desirable, and its aim should be the relief of pain and anxiety.

## Opioids

Pain relief may be necessary in patients with fractures or other painful conditions. This will allow the patient to be transported to the operating theatre and positioned for the block with the minimum of distress. In these circumstances, opioid analgesics are appropriate, although they possess many properties which are undesirable in patients having regional anaesthesia, including nausea, vomiting, respiratory depression, sedation and delayed gastric emptying. However, opioid premedication prior to regional anaesthesia does have the advantage of further reducing postoperative analgesic requirements (McQuay et al 1988), although Grant and colleagues (1981) have suggested intramuscular ketamine (0.5 mg kg$^{-1}$) as an alternative.

## Benzodiazepines

Anxiolytic drugs such as diazepam, lorazepam and temazepam are useful premedicants for patients about to undergo surgery under regional anaesthesia. Oral temazepam (10–30 mg, 1–2 hours before surgery) is widely prescribed and is relatively short acting with minimal residual 'hangover' effect (Beechey et al 1981). However, it does not produce amnesia and one of the other benzodiazepines, such as lorazepam (2–4 mg, 2 hours before surgery), should be used if this is required. Lorazepam has a slow onset and long duration of action, but these properties make it useful for night sedation or premedication of anxious patients who are towards the end of the operating list. Oral midazolam (0.5 mg kg$^{-1}$) has become popular for calming the very anxious or agitated child before anaesthesia, but its short duration means that it has to be administered approximately 30 minutes before the patient comes to theatre.

## Other drugs

With the possible exception of trimeprazine in children, phenothiazines are rarely used for premedication now. There is no place for the butyrophenones such as droperidol because they may produce an apparently relaxed and co-operative patient who is, in reality, extremely apprehensive. Anticholinergic and antiemetic drugs are not usually required before regional anaesthesia although they may be used in special circumstances.

Before long operations, it can be useful to administer a long-acting *non-steroidal anti-inflammatory drug* (NSAID), not only as an analgesic adjunct, but also to minimise the discomfort caused by prolonged immobility. Even if a light general anaesthetic is to be administered, oral diclofenac 100 mg given the night before surgery, or ibuprofen 400 mg, 2–4 hours pre-operatively, can be helpful. However, NSAIDs are contraindicated in patients with active peptic ulceration, renal impairment (including prerenal problems) or brittle asthma, and a small dose of an opioid may serve the same purpose.

## The elderly patient

Heavy premedication should be avoided in older patients, and even the benzodiazepines may cause profound sedation, confusion and restlessness. Many elderly patients present for fracture surgery, and premedication may be better provided with an analgesic. Hyoscine should be avoided because it may cause confusion in older patients (Checketts & Coventry 1992).

# References

Abramsky C 1994 Pregnancy and multiple sclerosis. Annals of Neurology 36(suppl): S38–41

Abouleish E, Orig T, Amortegui AJ 1980 Bacteriologic comparison between epidural and caudal techniques. Anesthesiology 53: 511–514

Alderson JD 1987 Cardiovascular collapse following epidural anaesthesia for Caesarean section in a patient with aortic incompetence. Anaesthesia 42: 643–645

American College of Physicians 1997 Clinical guideline, Part I: guidelines for assessing and managing the perioperative risk from coronary artery disease associated with noncardiac surgery. Annals of Internal Medicine 127: 309–312

American Society of Regional Anesthesia 1998 Consensus statements on central nerve block and anticoagulation. Regional Anesthesia and Pain Medicine: 23(S2)

Ballin NC 1981 Paraplegia following epidural analgesia. Anaesthesia 36: 952–953

Bader AM, Hunt CO, Datta S 1988 Anesthesia for the obstetric patient with multiple sclerosis. Journal of Clinical Anesthesiology 1: 21

Beechey APG, Eltringham RJ, Studd C 1981 Temazepam as premedication in day surgery. Anaesthesia 36: 10–16

Bergqvist D, Benoni G, Bjorgell O et al 1996. Low molecular weight heparin (enoxaparin) as prophylaxis against venous thromboembolism after total hip replacement. New England Journal of Medicine 335: 696–700

Bieter RN 1936 Applied pharmacology of local anaesthetics. American Journal of Surgery 34: 500–510

Blomberg S, Emanuelsson H, Ricksten S-E 1989 Thoracic epidural anesthesia and central hemodynamics in patients with unstable angina pectoris. Anesthesia and Analgesia 69: 558–562

Blomberg S 1994 Long term home self treatment with high thoracic epidural anesthesia in patients with severe coronary artery disease. Anesthesia and Analgesia 79: 413–421

Bromage PR 1978 Epidural analgesia. WB Saunders, Philadelphia

Bromage PR, Gertel M 1972 Brachial plexus anesthesia in chronic renal failure. Anesthesiology 36: 488–493

Buckley FP, Robinson NB, Simonowitz DA, Dellinger EP 1983 Anaesthesia in the morbidly obese. A comparison of anaesthetic and analgesic regimens for upper abdominal surgery. Anaesthesia 38: 840–851

Burgos LG, Ebert TJ, Assiddao C et al 1989 Increased intra-operative cardiovascular morbidity in diabetics with autonomic neuropathy. Anesthesiology 70: 591–598

Capdeville M, Hoyt MR 1994 Anesthesia and analgesia in the obstetric population with multiple sclerosis: A retrospective review. Anesthesiology 81: 1173–1177

Carp H, Bailey S 1992 The association between meningitis and dural puncture in bacteraemic rats. Anesthesiology 76: 739–742

Carson D, Wildsmith JAW 1996 The risk of extradural abscess. British Journal of Anaesthesia 75: 520–521

Chaudhari LS, Kop BR, Dhruva AJ 1978 Paraplegia and epidural analgesia. Anaesthesia 33: 722–725

Checketts MR, Coventry DM. 1992 Transdermal hyoscine and confusion in the elderly. Anaesthesia 47(12): 1097

Checketts MR, Wildsmith JAW 1999. Central nerve block and thromboprophylaxis – is there a problem? British Journal of Anaesthesia 82: 164–167

Chestnut DH 1992 Editorial view: Spinal anesthesia in the febrile patient. Anesthesiology 76: 667–669

Collard CD, Eappen S, Lynch EP, Concepcion M 1995 Continuous spinal anesthesia with invasive hemodynamic monitoring for surgical repair of the hip in two patients with severe aortic stenosis. Anesthesia and Analgesia 81: 195–198

Colon-Otero G, Cockerill KJ, Bowie EJW 1991 How to diagnose bleeding disorders. Postgraduate Medicine 90: 145–150

Cooke ED, Lloyd MJ, Bowcock SA, Pilcher MF 1976. Monitoring during low-dose heparin prophylaxis. New England Journal of Medicine; 294: 1066–1067

Crawford JS, James FM, Nolte H, Van Steenberge A, Shah JL 1981 Regional anaesthesia for patients with chronic neurological disease and similar conditions. Anaesthesia 36: 821

Davis RF, DeBoer LWV, Maroko PR 1986 Thoracic epidural anaesthesia reduces myocardial infarct size after coronary artery occlusion in dogs. Anesthesia Analgesia 65: 711–717

Dexter F 1998 Regional anaesthesia does not significantly change surgical time versus general anaesthesia – a meta-analysis of randomized studies. Regional Anesthesia and Pain Medicine 23: 439–443

Eng RHK, Seligman SJ 1981 Lumbar puncture induced meningitis. Journal of the American Medical Association 245: 1456–1459

Fisher A, Waterhouse TD, Adams AP 1975 Obesity: its relation to anaesthesia. Anaesthesia 24: 208–216

Fisher MM 1984 Intradermal testing to anaesthetic drugs: practical aspects of performance and interpretation. Anaesthesia and Intensive Care 12: 115–120

Freund FG, Bonica JJ, Ward RJ, Akamatsu TJ, Kennedy WF 1967 Ventilatory reserve and level of motor block during high spinal and epidural anesthesia. Anesthesiology 28: 834–837

Grant IS, Nimmo WS, Clements JA 1981 Pharmacokinetics and analgesic effect of i.m. and oral ketamine. British Journal of Anaesthesia 53: 805–809

Groen RJ, Ponssen H 1990 The spontaneous spinal epidural hematoma. A study of the etiology (review). Journal of Neurological Science 98: 121–138

Gronert GA 1980 Malignant hyperthermia. Anesthesiology 53: 395–423

Henderson JJ, Macrae WA 1983 Complications. In: Henderson JJ, Nimmo WS (eds) Practical regional anaesthesia. 101 Blackwell, Oxford

Hirlekar G 1980 Paraplegia after epidural analgesia associated with an extradural spinal tumour. Anaesthesia 35: 363–364

Holtas S, Heiling M, Lonntoft M 1996 Spontaneous spinal epidural haematoma: findings at MR imaging and clinical correlation. Radiology 199(2):409–413

Hopkins PM 2000 Malignant hyperthermia: advances in clinical management and diagnosis. British Journal of Anaesthesia 85: 118–128

Horlocker TT, Wedel DJ, Schlichting JL 1994 Postoperative epidural analgesia and oral anticoagulant therapy. Anesthesia and Analgesia 79: 89–93

Horlocker TT, Wedel DJ, Schroeder DR et al 1995 Pre-operative antiplatelet therapy does not increase the risk of spinal hematoma associated with regional anesthesia. Anesthesia and Analgesia 80: 303–309

Howells TH, Huntsman RG, Boys JE, Mahmood A 1972 Anaesthesia and sickle-cell haemoglobin, with a case report. British Journal of Anaesthesia 44: 975–987

Katz JD, Krich LB 1976 Acute febrile reaction complicating spinal anaesthesia in a survivor of malignant hyperthermia. Canadian Anaesthetists' Society Journal 23: 285–289

Klassen GA, Bramwell RS, Bromage PR, Zborowska-Sluis DT 1980 Effect of acute sympathectomy by epidural anesthesia on the canine coronary circulation. Anesthesiology 52: 8–15

Kock M, Blomberg S, Emanuelsson H, Lomsky M, Stromblad S-O, Ricksten S-E 1990 Thoracic epidural anesthesia improves global and regional ventricular function during stress-induced myocardial ischemia in patients with coronary artery disease. Anesthesia and Analgesia 71: 625–630

Lambert DH, Deane RS, Mazuzan JE 1982 Anesthesia and the control of blood pressure in patients with spinal cord injury. Anesthesia and Analgesia 61: 344–348

Lieberman J, Huo M, Hanway J 1994 The prevalence of deep venous thrombosis after total hip arthroplasty with hypotensive epidural anaesthesia. Journal of Bone and Joint Surgery 76A: 341–348

Liu S, Carpenter RL, Neal JM 1995 Epidural anesthesia and analgesia. Their role in postoperative outcome. Anesthesiology 82: 1474–1506

Lumpkin MM. 1998 FDA Public Health Advisory: Reports of epidural or spinal hematomas with the concurrent use of low molecular weight heparin and with spinal/epidural anesthesia or spinal puncture. Anesthesiology 88(2): 27A–28A

McQuay HJ, Carroll D, Moore RA 1988 Postoperative orthopaedic pain – the effect of opiate premedication and local anaesthetic blocks. Pain 33: 291–295

Mangano DT, Layug EL, Wallace A, Tateo I 1996 Effect of atenolol on mortality and cardiovascular morbidity after noncardiac surgery. New England Journal of Medicine 335: 1713–1720

Marinacci AA, Courville CB 1958 Electromyogram in evaluation of neurological complications of spinal anaesthesia. Journal of the American Medical Association 168: 1337–1345

Mauney FM, Ebert PA, Sabiston DC 1970 Postoperative myocardial infarction. A study of predisposing factors, diagnosis and mortality rate in a high risk group of surgical patients. Annals of Surgery 172: 497–502

Modig J, Borg T, Bagge L, Saldeen T 1983. Role of extradural and of general anaesthesia in fibrinolysis and coagulation after total hip replacement. British Journal of Anaesthesia 55: 625–629

Moore D C 1976 Regional block, 4th edn. CC Thomas, Springfield

Muller H, Sarges R, Jouaux J, Runte W, Lampante L 1990 Intraoperative suppression of spasticity by intrathecal baclofen. Anaesthetist 39: 22–29

Nielsen CH 1989 Bleeding after intercostal nerve block in a patient anticoagulated with heparin. Anesthesiology 71: 162–164

Odoom JA, Sih IL 1983. Epidural analgesia and anticoagulant therapy. Experience with one thousand cases of continuous epidurals. Anaesthesia 38: 254–259

Page MM, Watkins PJ 1978 Cardiorespiratory arrest and diabetic autonomic neuropathy. The Lancet i: 14–16

Palda VA, Detsky AS 1997 Clinical guideline, Part II: perioperative assessment and management of risk from coronary artery disease. Annals of Internal Medicine 127: 313–328

Pittard A, Vucevic M 1998 Regional anaesthesia with subarachnoid microcatheter for Caesarean section in a parturient with aortic stenosis. Anaesthesia 53:169–173

Reiz S 1989 Circulatory effects of epidural anesthesia in patients with cardiac disease. Acta Anaesthesiologica Belgica 30: 21–27

Reiz S, Nath S, Rais O 1980 Effects of thoracic epidural block and prenalterol on coronary vascular resistance and myocardial metabolism in patients with coronary artery disease. Acta Anaesthesiologica Scandinavica 24: 11–16

Samford C, Sibley W, Laguna J 1978 Anesthesia in multiple sclerosis. Canadian Journal of Neurological Science 5: 41–48

Schonwald G, Fish KJ, Perkash I 1981 Cardiovascular complications during anesthesia in chronic spinal cord injured patients. Anesthesiology 55: 550–558

Schwander D, Bachmann F 1991. Heparin and spinal or epidural anesthesia. Decision analysis [review]. Annales Françaises d'Anesthesie Reanimation 10: 284–296

Seltzer JL, Porretta JC, Jackson BG 1977 Plastic particulate contaminants in the medicine cups of disposable non-spinal regional anesthesia sets. Anesthesiology 47: 378–379

Sharma SK, Philip J, Whitter CW, Udaya BP 1999 Assessment of changes in coagulation in parturients with preeclampsia using thromboelastography. Anesthesiology 90: 385–390

Somerville TG, Gibson M 1973 Particulate contamination in ampoules: a comparative study. Pharmaceutical Journal 211: 128–131

Sors H, Meyer G 2000 Commentary: Place of aspirin in prophylaxis of venous thromboembolism. Lancet 355: 1288–1289

Steen PA, Tinker JH, Tarhan S 1978 Myocardial infarction after anesthesia and surgery. Journal of the American Medical Association 239: 2566–2570

Strunin L 1993 Editorial: How long should patients fast before surgery? Time for new guidelines. British Journal of Anaesthesia 70: 1–3

Thomas DP 1997 Does low molecular weight heparin cause less bleeding? Thrombosis and Haemostasis; 78: 1422–1425

Toft P, Jorgensen A 1989 Continuous thoracic epidural analgesia for the control of pain in myocardial infarction. Intensive Care Medicine 13: 388–389

Tryba M 1993 Epidural anesthesia and low molecular weight heparin: Pro Anasth Intensivmed Notfallmed Schmerzther 28:179–181

Tryba M, Wedel DJ 1997 Central neuraxial block and low molecular weight heparin (enoxaparine): lessons learned from different dosage regimens in two continents. Acta Anaesthesiologica Scandinavica; 41: 100–103

Tuman KJ, McCarthy RJ, March RJ, DeLaria GA, Patel RV, Ivanovich AD 1991 The effects of epidural anesthesia and analgesia on coagulation and outcome after major vascular surgery. Anesthesia and Analgesia 73: 696–704

Vandermeulen EP, Van Aken H, Vermylen J 1994 Anticoagulants and spinal-epidural anaesthesia. Anesthesia and Analgesia 79: 1165–1177

Wadhwa RK 1977 Obstetric anesthesia for a patient with malignant hyperthermia susceptibility. Anesthesiology 46: 63–64

Weiss MG, Adkinson NF, Hirshman CA 1989 Evaluation of allergic drug reactions in the peri-operative period. Anesthesiology 71: 483–486

Whitten CW, Greilich PE 2000 Thromboelastography: Past, present and future. Anesthesiology 92: 1223–1225

Wildsmith JAW, Mason A, McKinnon RP, Rae SM 1998 Allergy to local anaesthetic drugs is rare but does occur. British Dental Journal 184: 507–510

Wildsmith JAW, McClure JH 1991 Editorial: anticoagulant drugs and central nerve blockade. Anaesthesia 46: 613–614

Wu CL, Perkins FM 1996. Oral anticoagulant prophylaxis and epidural catheter removal. Regional Anesthesia 21: 517–524

Wysowski DK, Talarico L, Bacsanyi J, Botstein P 1998 Spinal and epidural hematoma and low-molecular-weight-heparin. New England Journal of Medicine; 338: 1774–1775

Yeager MP, Glass DD, Neff RK, Brinck-Johnson T 1987 Epidural anaesthesia and analgesia in high risk surgical patients. Anesthesiology 66: 729–736

# 8. Managing the block

## J E Charlton

Attention to detail is always important in the practice of medicine, but it is absolutely vital for successful regional anaesthesia. The need for care in assessing and preparing the patient, and selecting the most appropriate block for the particular situation, has been emphasised in the previous chapter, but just as much attention is required during the performance of the block and its subsequent management.

## THE BASICS

Sufficient help must be available to ensure that transport of the patient from the ward to the induction room is achieved without discomfort, especially if the patient is in pain. It is a matter of personal choice whether the block is carried out with the patient on a tipping trolley or the operating table, but the trolley is usually marginally more comfortable and it offers greater space for positioning. It is wise to ensure that all the necessary equipment, including a stool and pillows if the block is to be performed in the sitting position, is ready before the patient arrives. This reduces both patient anxiety and delay.

The optimum design of a local anaesthetic induction room has been described by Rosenblatt and Shal (1984); it must be well lit, at a comfortable temperature and have adequate storage accommodation. Trained assistance must be available and more than one person may be needed, especially if the block is to be performed out of the patient's sight. One person provides direct help to the anaesthetist, passing the equipment, solutions and drugs required during block performance, while the other reassures and monitors the patient. Unnecessary distractions must be avoided, the most common such being a vagrant surgeon looking for notes or asking when the block will be completed.

Such individuals should be granted an interview to discourage this behaviour and to remind them that the induction room is for anaesthetic purposes alone.

Vital signs, such as pulse and blood pressure, should be recorded, and intravenous access established, before the patient is positioned for the block. Intravenous fluids and supplementary oxygen may be started at this time if either is indicated for the particular block, patient or operation. The patient is then reminded what is about to happen and what he/she is likely to experience during the performance of the block. Patients find regional anaesthesia much more acceptable if the procedure has been explained carefully beforehand (Bondy et al 1999), but appropriate repetition at each stage is good practice and avoids unpleasant surprises for everyone.

The patient should be positioned by, or at least under the immediate supervision of, the person who will perform the block. After the proper position has been achieved, the relevant surface anatomy is identified. Landmarks may be marked with a skin pencil, either for teaching purposes or as an *aide memoire*, because the anatomy may be less clear after the patient has been prepared and draped. The raising of a skin wheal at an early stage gives the patient an indication of what is to come, and the anaesthetist an opportunity to assess the patient's response. At every stage the anaesthetist must aim to be as gentle as possible, remembering that there is someone else's nervous system on the 'sharp end' of the needle.

## BLOCK PERFORMANCE
### Awake or asleep?

Whether the patient is awake or asleep when the block is being performed is a matter of some controversy

(Fischer 1998, Wildsmith & Fischer 1999). Ultimately, the choice will depend upon the anaesthetist's personal preference, training requirements and experience, as well as the needs and preferences of the patient. The debate has centred on the potential for increased risk of complications during block performance in the unconscious patient (Bromage & Benumof 1998), but equally impassioned pleas have been made for the prior induction of general anaesthesia, especially in children (Krane et al 1998). There are arguments in favour of each approach. When the patient is un-conscious, the more relaxed atmosphere in the anaesthetic room provides ideal conditions for regional anaesthesia. As a result, the block is easier to perform and therefore, arguably, safer. On the other hand, warning symptoms or signs of complications may be missed in the unconscious or heavily sedated patient, and the possibility exists for further problems if the sedated patient becomes uncontrollable. A conscious patient is an excellent monitor of events. If it is felt necessary to induce general anaesthesia first, the patient's condition must be stable before the block is performed.

## Equipment

Standard 'Luer' fittings should be used throughout for all equipment, but it is still wise to check and assemble as much of the equipment (e.g. syringe, extension line, etc.) as possible before insertion.

### Block packs

It is vital to have somewhere to put the necessary equipment during block performance, and an adequately sized trolley represents the best choice. A 'Mayo' table is an alternative, but the work area should be big enough for the block pack to be opened out fully, and for additional items to be added as needed, without sterility being impaired. The choice of pack is a matter for individual and departmental choice. A number are commercially available, varying in design and content, but all provide a range of equipment with guaranteed sterility. However, these packs may contain swabs, needles and syringes which are surplus to most requirements and many anaesthetists use a basic hospital preparation pack and add whatever they need for each procedure.

Cost is a significant factor and if regional block is performed frequently, trays produced locally may offer a distinct advantage. Most contain basic items for skin

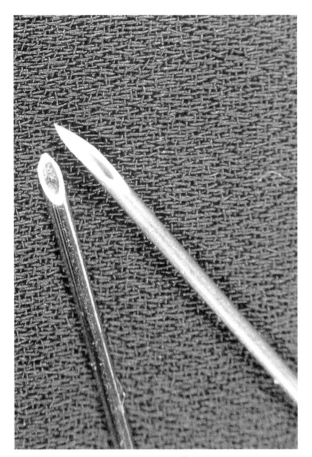

**Fig 8.1** Long- and short-bevel needle points

preparation and towelling, so that needles, syringes, filters, catheters, and drugs can be added aseptically as needed. This approach permits flexibility of use for both central and peripheral block. Care must be taken that sterility indicators are checked regularly, and this applies to drugs sterilised locally as well.

### Needles

A wide variety of specialised, sterile, disposable needles is available for all the major techniques, and they are discussed in the appropriate chapters, but it is possible to use needles designed for other purposes for many blocks. For example, paediatric spinal needles are excellent for minor peripheral and cranial nerve blocks, as well as trigger point injections. A translucent hub allows the early recognition of intravascular placement during a block and reduces the possibility of systemic toxicity by direct injection. It is argued that short bevel needles (Fig. 8.1) are less traumatic to the nerve when paraesthesiae are sought during block performance (Selander et al 1977). If a needle bends during the course of a block it should be discarded, *not* straightened, because of the risk of breakage. If a bony landmark is being used and firm osseous contact occurs, the needle should be inspected and replaced if there is any hint of damage. A 'bur' on the end of a needle after bony contact will tear tissue subsequently.

There is no place today for re-usable needles, except in the developing world where resources are limited. Where they are still used, a security bead near the hub is important, because repeated sterilisation and use may weaken the junction between the hub and shaft. This refinement is unnecessary for disposable needles.

### Catheters

Disposable catheters should be biochemically inert, easy to sterilise and have a low coefficient of friction with a high tensile strength. They should be reasonably rigid, should not kink easily and should be marked at intervals. Modern designs of catheter have modified tips so that they are less traumatic. Spinal and epidural catheters are considered further in Chapters 10 and 11. Special catheters are available for other blocks, but it is quite possible to use venous cannulae for plexus or caudal block, although they should, ideally, be radio-opaque and made of an inert material. They do offer the advantages of seeming to 'migrate' less and being easier to fix in place using proprietary dressings than epidural catheters.

### Syringes

Disposable plastic syringes are perfectly adequate for regional block, and glass syringes have fallen into disuse except in the developing world. When a glass syringe is used, preliminary aspiration of a small amount of local anaesthetic or saline will lubricate the barrel and make the plunger run smoothly. Although it may seem that the choice of syringe size will depend only upon the volume to be injected, it may be easier to control aspiration and injection with a small syringe. Thus it may be safer and more comfortable to use several small syringes than a single large one. An 'immobile needle' (see below) will reduce the possibility of needle movement when connections are being made and reduce the possibility of trauma to underlying tissues.

## Peripheral nerve location

The first requirement of a successful nerve block is accurate knowledge of the anatomy. This was highlighted in William Mayo's foreword to Gaston Labat's ground-breaking textbook 'Regional Anesthesia'. Mayo (1922) wrote:

> *The anesthetist must have an accurate knowledge of anatomy and a high degree of technical skill in order that the anesthesia be safe and satisfactory, and the operation not delayed.*

The importance of examining the patient and defining the anatomy has been highlighted quite recently by studies of factors which may predict technical difficulty with a block. Only physical characteristics (Sprung et al 1999) or age (Tessler et al 1999) had any predictive value. Interestingly, it is apparent that time to operation is not a factor when regional anaesthesia is compared to general anaesthesia, a recent meta-analysis showing that the difference is less than 2 minutes (Dexter 1998).

In the earliest days of regional anaesthesia the elicitation of paraesthesiae became the traditional method of confirming accurate needle placement, but the use of a nerve stimulator has become very wide-spread, both as a teaching aid and as part of normal practice (Franco & Vieira 2000). There are advantages and disadvantages to each method.

### Paraesthesiae

Paraesthesiae can be unpleasant for the patient and, if frankly painful, can produce sudden movement, which may move the needle and cause nerve damage (Selander et al 1979a). However, if there are paraesthesiae it indicates that the needle tip is very close to the nerve and that a successful block is more likely. It is good practice to explain fully what paraesthesiae feel like before the procedure starts and ask the patient to state clearly when these features occur. The distribution of the symptoms is identified and, if this is appropriate to the intended block, the injection is made. It is important to make sure the patient does not point to where the paraesthesiae have been felt, because this may move the needle tip and the whole process will have to start again.

Paraesthesiae are subjective feelings which may be misinterpreted even by alert and co-operative patients, especially if there has been difficulty in finding the exact location of the nerve (Raj et al 1980). Success rates in performing blocks using paraesthesiae may be poor if a patient gives inappropriate responses because of apprehension or inability to co-operate.

## Nerve stimulators

The *advantages* of using a nerve stimulator are:

- There is no need to produce paraesthesiae, although they may occur
- Patient co-operation is unnecessary and the technique can be used in patients who are sedated or anaesthetised
- Information about the optimal local anaesthetic injection point is provided as long as the unit displays current output
- Lack of a motor response from the target nerve indicates that the needle is not in the right place
- They are a useful teaching aid

The *disadvantages* are:

- It is possible to stimulate the nerve when the needle tip is still some distance away if the current used is too high
- It is not possible to stimulate sensory nerves in the same way as those with a motor component
- There is some cost associated with purchasing and maintaining a nerve stimulator, and the various disposable components required

However, a nerve stimulator should be available in all anaesthetising locations. If it has a dual function it can be used to test neuromuscular transmission as well as to locate nerves during regional anaesthesia, but for this it should have a visual display of the current and offer a range of stimulation frequencies. If too high a current is used, stimulation may cause a sudden, gross motor movement, which may be painful for the patient and surprise all parties. Some anaesthetists therefore argue that only stimulators with a specific low output should be used for nerve location. Even if the patient is sedated or anaesthetised, the initial current should be no greater than 1.5 mAmp, and a starting current of 1 mAmp is used by many practitioners. As the nerve is approached the current is progressively reduced, and it is generally accepted that a motor response in the target nerve distribution with a current of 0.5 mAmp or less indicates that the needle tip is close enough for injection to produce an adequate block. All the currents quoted are with the 'negative' (cathode) terminal of the stimulator attached to the needle.

**Insulated needles** Insulated needles and catheters of various designs are readily available for use with stimulators. The current field is located precisely at the tip and avoids the possibility that the shaft of the needle is close to the nerve when the tip is not. Thus, more accurate localisation of the nerve is possible. The extra expense of insulated needles and nerve stimulators can be justified easily because they produce greater accuracy in injection and thus higher success rates. They are particularly useful as teaching aids for beginners and make the performance of uncommon or unfamiliar blocks simpler. However, patient acceptance rates may be lower where multiple nerves are blocked using a stimulator (Fanelli et al 1999).

## Aseptic technique

Before any block procedure, the skin should be cleaned with an iodine-based bacteriocidal preparation, or with chlorhexidine, but it is important to establish first that the patient is not sensitive to the preparation. These solutions should be allowed to dry before towelling or before inserting needles because they are then most effective, and the risk of transferring what is a very neurolytic solution to the needle is minimised. Whether the skin preparation actually provides any protection against infection is uncertain, but it serves to focus the attention of the anaesthetist on the importance of maintaining a limited and relatively sterile area. The cleansing solution should be placed nearest to the patient on the block tray to avoid it dripping on to the equipment or the anaesthetist's gloves, and should be removed once cleaning is completed. Where it is necessary to shave the skin this should be done immediately before the block. Shaving any earlier may predispose to infection (Seropian & Reynolds 1971).

It is customary to wear sterile gloves for most regional procedures, and modern gloves give an excellent 'feel' to the skin and underlying tissues. Approaches to sterility have changed in the last few years and it is now rare to wear a gown as well as gloves for peripheral blocks. Conversely, central block procedures require a larger sterile area, if only because catheters are sometimes difficult to control, and some anaesthetists therefore wear a gown. In addition, it is prudent to wear a surgical mask while performing a central block. This will reduce contamination of the site (Philips et al 1992), a desirable aim because the consequences of infection are so serious, but the use of sterile *and* disposable equipment has probably done as much to reduce the possibility of infection as skin preparation and towelling.

## Needle insertion

All equipment should be checked and all solutions drawn up before the block procedure is started. If possible, anything used in connection with the block should be kept out of the patient's sight at all times. A local anaesthetic skin wheal is raised at the point of intended needle entry and, if a short-bevelled or pencil-point needle is to be used, it is useful to make a small 'nick' in the skin to ease insertion. If this is not done considerable force may be needed and this may cause the patient to become worried and tense. In addition, sudden skin penetration may cause the needle to pass to a greater depth than intended.

Every attempt should be made to avoid touching the shaft of the needle. This may prove quite difficult when long and flexible needles are used, but the shaft should be gripped as near to the hub as possible. The needle can be steadied by placing the back of the non-dominant hand against the patient, and using its thumb and index finger to grasp the needle hub. This will give excellent control while the needle and syringe are advanced by the dominant hand (see Fig. 11.10).

The needle should always be withdrawn somewhat before changes in direction are made. Withdrawing too little will result in virtually no change in direction of the needle if the tip is anchored in dense tissues. It also puts stresses upon the needle that may cause bending or even breakage. It is better to withdraw the needle until it lies in pliable tissue and can then be realigned appropriately.

*Intraneural injection* If paraesthesiae have been elicited, care must be taken that an intraneural injection does not occur, because it will cause considerable pain and may lead to permanent nerve damage (Lofstrom 1966, Selander et al 1979a). Anything more than very minor discomfort during the early part of the injection indicates the need for slight withdrawal of the needle and reassessment of the position of the tip.

## Special considerations

### Aids to success

A success rate of over 95% should be the aim in regional anaesthesia. Failure can be minimised by careful case selection and the rejection (especially by the beginner) of patients with abnormal or absent anatomical landmarks. Unsuccessful or inadequate block is usually due to failure to place the local anaesthetic close enough to the nerve, but it may also be due to the use of an inadequate volume or mass of drug. It has been argued for many years that the 'maximum' doses specified on data sheets represent very conservative safety margins for correctly administered nerve blocks (with the exception of the intercostal and interpleural techniques). The factors affecting systemic concentrations of local anaesthetic are the site of injection, the characteristics of the individual patient and the properties of the drug used. Adherence to fixed dose limits without considering these factors may contribute to high failure rates for the beginner and may inhibit even the most experienced anaesthetist. However, local anaesthetic drugs are being used with increasing frequency by non-anaesthetists. Lack of knowledge about the safe limits of local anaesthetic drugs when used in large volumes and injected over large areas (for the purposes of either pain relief or reduction in blood loss during cosmetic surgery) has led to problems.

Plenty of time must be allowed for the performance of any block, and just as much time allowed for it to work. The anaesthetist should never be rushed into abandoning a block: 'tincture of time' is often as effective as a supplement or a general anaesthetic. Every anaesthetist should become competent in one technique before learning another, and should never miss an opportunity to study the anatomy of any nerve block.

*The 'immobile needle'* Winnie (1983) advocated the use of a length of small bore, disposable intravenous extension tubing placed between the syringe and the needle (Fig. 8.2). This allows the anaesthetist to maintain the needle in the correct position without it being dislodged during an aspiration test or when the syringe is being changed by an assistant. This technique works well and should be standard practice when large volumes of drug are injected.

### Testing the block

Observing the onset of a block after injection of the solution has two purposes. It indicates that the distribution and quality of the block are adequate for the proposed surgery, but it also indicates whether spread has become excessive and complications such as hypotension are thus more likely to develop. For medicolegal as well as humanitarian reasons, formal testing of the block is mandatory before surgery is

95

vasodilatation in the area of the nerve or plexus block, heaviness of the arms or legs and some decrease in the blood pressure during central block.

The ability to manage patients confidently only comes with experience. The beginner should start with simple blocks and, when testing, use a non-invasive method (e.g. a blunt needle, a spirit soaked swab or gentle pinching with a clip). If there is doubt, the patient should be warned of movement and hot or cold sensations during preparation for the procedure, and be assured that no painful manoeuvres will be performed. In any circumstance it is good practice to ask the surgeon to test the operative site by squeezing the skin surreptitiously and progressively with a pair of forceps before any incision is made.

### Living with failure

Success in regional anaesthesia depends on many different factors, and may not always be achieved. The only true failure is a failure to learn something from the experience. A block may be slow in onset, inadequate in extent or a total failure. There may be time constraints and the reactions of the patients must be considered.

***Slow onset*** Time must be allowed for the block to develop, especially in the elderly. A spinal may be repeated if no effect is seen after 10 minutes, but it should not then be abandoned for at least 30 minutes after the first injection. An epidural may take as long as 45 minutes to develop. During this time, boluses of local anaesthetic and adjustments to the catheter position and the posture of the patient may be required, and extra time must be allowed for these changes to become effective. Peripheral nerve and plexus blocks with long-acting agents may also take up to 45 minutes to develop. When a block is only partially developed, or where the need for the list to proceed is becoming paramount, peripheral supplementation or local infiltration by the surgeon can be employed. This additional amount of local anaesthetic should be included in the total used, because much of the original dose will not have been metabolised at the time of the supplementary injections.

***Inadequate block*** The easiest way of coping with an inadequate block is to induce general anaesthesia, but this may be irritating for the patient who has been persuaded that regional anaesthesia is best for the planned procedure. Some patients prefer to remain awake despite some discomfort, and there are various

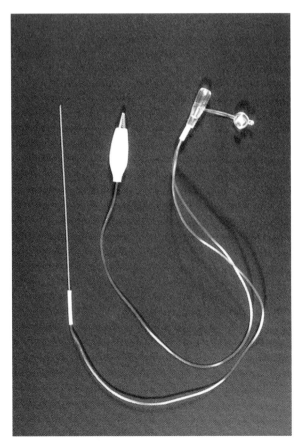

**Fig 8.2** An 'immobile' needle set. Note that this needle has an insulated sheath and that there is an integral attachment for a nerve stimulator

allowed to commence in the conscious patient, but total skin anaesthesia does not guarantee full anaesthesia of deeper tissues. Assessment of the intensity and spread of the block may be made by pinching the skin, movement of painful joints or observing motor or sympathetic block. Care should be taken to avoid trauma to the skin or underlying tissues during such assessment.

When patients are in pain (e.g. if they are in labour or have a fracture) the onset of analgesia is a perfect indication of block development. Surreptitious gentle movement of a painful limb will indicate whether or not it is ready for manipulation. For elective surgery, informal assessment is more difficult, but these are the patients who are more likely to be disturbed by excessive testing. The best defence against failure is to ensure that sufficient solution is injected in the correct place. It is customary to allow a latent period, appropriate to the block and the drug used, to elapse before looking for signs of the developing block. Useful signs are

methods of making the situation tolerable. Intravenous sedation (e.g. midazolam) may be sufficient to relieve minor discomfort, but this may simply disinhibit the patient and an analgesic may therefore be more appropriate. Small amounts of intravenous opioid (e.g. fentanyl) can be given, but inhalation of nitrous oxide (50% in oxygen from a facemask) is very useful in this situation and provides both sedation and analgesia. Whatever agent is used, 'conscious' sedation should be employed and verbal contact maintained with the patient. Large doses of parenteral sedatives and analgesics may lead to respiratory obstruction and depression, and will delay recovery. If this seems likely to happen, the induction of general anaesthesia is a better option.

**Complete failure** If the block does not work it can always be repeated, particularly if there are compelling reasons for avoiding general anaesthesia. Time must be allowed for some of the first dose of local anaesthetic to be metabolised, and there may be a need to modify both the technique and drug dose used for the second injection. In addition, rearrangement of the operating list will be necessary, and explanations should be offered to both the patient and one's colleagues.

The alternative to these options is general anaesthesia, but it is not uncommon to find, when the patient has woken after the operation, that a completely satisfactory block has developed – 'tincture of time' may have been the answer after all.

## PREOPERATIVE MANAGEMENT
### Systemic toxicity of local anaesthetic drugs

Local anaesthetic drugs possess the ability to stabilise all excitable membranes, an effect which is not confined to peripheral nerves. Given sufficient tissue concentration they will depress the function of both the central and cardiovascular systems. Properly performed regional anaesthesia should not result in blood concentrations of local anaesthetics sufficient to cause systemic effects, but because these are life threatening and usually of sudden onset (see Ch. 6), rapid action is necessary to counteract them.

### Prevention

A thorough understanding of pharmacokinetics, especially those factors influencing absorption, distribution and elimination, is essential. Knowledge of the blood concentration profile of the agent and the technique employed will help the anaesthetist to be most vigilant at the time of greatest risk. For this reason it is suggested that the inexperienced anaesthetist use a limited range of drugs and techniques until confidence in these is established.

The two main causes of toxicity are overdosage and accidental intravascular injection. Overdose can be avoided by paying attention to toxic limits appropriate to the solution used and the site of injection. Inadvertent intravascular injection can be minimised by careful technique and selection of the appropriate equipment. Sufficient time should be allowed for blood to become visible in the needle hub or catheter after aspiration. Aspiration should be carried out at frequent intervals (approximately each 5 ml injected) and should be done gently, otherwise the vessel wall may occlude the tip of the needle. A negative test should not be regarded as absolute proof of correct placement, and all injections should be made slowly.

Particular vigilance is required with injections into the head and neck, and with intravenous regional anaesthesia. In the former, accidental intra-arterial injection of a very small dose of local anaesthetic can cause convulsions and in the latter, faulty equipment, slipshod technique or early release of the tourniquet may result in the rapid entry into the circulation of large amounts of drug.

**Test doses** It is obvious that the needle or catheter has entered a vein or punctured the dura when blood or cerebrospinal fluid appears spontaneously or after aspiration. Unfortunately, intravenous, intra-arterial and subarachnoid injections can occur despite negative aspiration tests, and 'test doses' are commonly employed to help exclude these possibilities. The test solution will depend upon the hazards to be excluded, but three criteria must be satisfied:

1. The test solution must be capable of producing unequivocal and easily observable evidence of intravenous, intra-arterial or subarachnoid injection within a reasonably short time
2. The solution used for the test dose should be unlikely to produce any detectable effect if injected into the correct place
3. Sufficient time must be allowed for the test dose to produce an effect before the full dose is administered

The most common use of a test dose is during the institution of an epidural block and this is considered in Chapter 11. However, a test dose should be employed in other circumstances where a relatively large dose of local anaesthetic is used, and particularly in blocks of the head and neck. Intravascular injection into branches of the carotid and vertebral arteries will produce almost instantaneous cerebral signs, and quite small doses can produce major reactions. In this area, much smaller test volumes (0.5–1 ml) must be injected very slowly with close observation of the patient to avoid serious complications.

### Treatment

It is not usually necessary to treat the signs and symptoms of toxicity, with the exception of convulsions, provided that respiration and circulation are maintained. The most important aspect of managing local anaesthetic toxicity is the prevention of hypoxia. This requires scrupulous monitoring of oxygen saturation, the administration of oxygen and encouragement to breathe normally together with the mandatory constant verbal contact. Cardiovascular depression should be treated by elevation of the legs, intravenous fluids and the administration of a vasopressor such as ephedrine (5–30 mg). Major collapse requires full resuscitative measures.

If convulsions occur, the aim of treatment is to stop them as soon as possible and to treat any accompanying depression of the cardiovascular or respiratory systems before cerebral hypoxia and acidosis compound the situation. Convulsions may be treated in one of three ways. *Intravenous induction agents* will rapidly abort local anaesthetic-induced convulsions and have the advantages of being short acting, readily available and familiar to all anaesthetists. However, they may increase respiratory and cardiovascular depression and should be used in small, incremental doses. *Benzodiazepines* such as diazepam or midazolam have been shown to prevent and to abort local anaesthetic-induced seizures. Again, incremental dosage should be small. Convulsions induced by more potent, longer-acting agents such as bupivacaine appear to be more resistant to benzodiazepine treatment than those induced by drugs such as lidocaine (de Jong & De Rosa 1981). An alternative is a short-acting *neuromuscular blocking agent* such as suxamethonium or rocuronium. The argument for this approach is that it allows rapid control of the airway and lung ventilation to improve oxygenation, but their administration to a hypoxic patient carries the risk of cardiac arrest. Paralysis will stop the physical manifestations of convulsive activity,

but not the seizure activity within the brain, which will still need to be treated.

After successful treatment of a reaction to an intravascular injection of a local anaesthetic, it is wise to examine the patient to ascertain the extent of any block which has been produced. If a substantial area is affected it is reasonable to assume that only a small proportion of the solution was injected intravenously. If there is little or no evidence of anaesthesia it should be assumed that most, if not all, of the injection was intravascular. Subsequent management can be based upon this information.

## Other adverse drug reactions

### Treatment of allergy

True allergic reactions to local anaesthetic drugs are rare (see Ch. 6). If anaphylaxis occurs it is vital to follow the standard guidelines on the treatment of this life-threatening complication (Nimmo et al 1995). Administration of the drug(s) likely to have caused the reaction should be stopped, the airway maintained, 100% oxygen administered and 10–20 µg increments of epinephrine given intravenously over 1 minute. The total amount of epinephrine should be titrated to maintain blood pressure. Additional supportive measures include corticosteroids, other bronchodilators and the infusion of fluids, preferably colloid, to restore the blood volume. Antihistamines are only of value in milder reactions and may take some time to work.

### Epinephrine overdose

Treatment is symptomatic and will depend upon the patient's cardiovascular status. Oxygen and sublingual glyceryl trinitrate should be administered if angina develops. β-adrenoceptor blocking agents may be needed to control tachycardia, but they should be avoided when hypertension is the presenting clinical sign. In this circumstance a short-acting vasodilator such as sodium nitroprusside may be given, but great caution should be exercised because the initial hypertension can be followed by a rapid decrease in blood pressure.

### Methaemoglobinaemia

Some of the metabolites of prilocaine can cause the reduction of haemoglobin to methaemoglobin. Hjelm and Holmdahl (1965) showed that 600 mg of prilocaine will produce a methaemoglobin concentration of 5.3%. This dose is far greater than that usually used in clinical practice, but will lead to cyanosis which is just detectable clinically. In spite of this, almost theoretical, drawback, prilocaine remains the safest of the amide local anaesthetics and the cyanosis is of little significance in the healthy individual. Methaemoglobinaemia can be reversed within 30 minutes by the intravenous administration of methylene blue. A dose of $1–2$ mg kg$^{-1}$ is often quoted, but significantly less is usually needed so it would seem sensible to titrate the dose. Users of prilocaine should be aware that clinically indetectable and insignificant concentrations of methaemoglobin will reduce pulse oximetry readings.

## Hypotension and regional anaesthesia

The cardiovascular effects of central block have been known for many years, but much of the research has been performed on unpremedicated, healthy volunteers and patients. It may be inappropriate to rely upon such data when dealing with an elderly surgical patient who may be hypovolaemic and have cardiac disease, autonomic dysfunction or some other condition affecting the response. Cardiovascular depression can occur after both spinal and epidural block, and this is largely related to the level of sympathectomy, although there are some differences between the two types of block. Epidural anaesthesia usually develops more slowly than spinal anaesthesia, and there is time for compensation to occur, so that the initial decrease in blood pressure may be less dramatic. The cardiovascular response to epidural block may be modified by the systemic effects of both local anaesthetic and vasoconstrictor drugs.

Peripheral vasodilatation caused by sympathetic block decreases left ventricular afterload. Peripheral venous dilatation will decrease venous return and hence cardiac output, but only if the denervated veins are below the level of the right atrium. Mean arterial pressure will decrease in proportion to the change in cardiac output and, less importantly, to the reduction in peripheral vascular resistance. As the mean arterial pressure decreases, there is a reduction in coronary blood flow but, fortunately, this is accompanied by a similar decrease in myocardial oxygen requirement. The latter is reduced because of decreased left ventricular afterload and decreased preload and bradycardia (Hackel et al 1956).

The bradycardia may be due to the Bainbridge reflex, because right atrial pressure receptors respond to decreased venous return. It may also be due to block of the cardio-accelerator fibres from $T_1$ to $T_5$. Scott (1975) suggested that high sympathetic block may lead to an increase in parasympathetic activity and there is a possibility that severe bradycardia and hypotension are caused by vasovagal attacks in susceptible patients (Wetstone & Wong 1974).

Sympathetic block below $T_4$ causes dilatation of the splanchnic, pelvic and lower limb vessels. In healthy patients, various mechanisms come into play to compensate for this. Vasoconstriction above the level of the block occurs, mediated by unblocked sympathetic vasoconstrictor fibres ($T_1$ to $T_4$), and systemic release of catecholamines may be mediated by any unblocked fibres supplying the adrenal medulla. In addition, vascular tone below the level of the block may return because of the autoregulation of flow by precapillary sphincters (Granger & Guyton 1969). Unblocked cardiac sympathetic fibres mediate an increase in myocardial contractility and heart rate, and it has been suggested that low plasma concentrations of local anaesthetic drugs also cause cardiovascular stimulation (Bonica et al 1970).

Sympathetic block above $T_4$ reduces or abolishes compensatory vasoconstriction in the head, neck and upper limb, as well as the ability of the cardiac sympathetic fibres to stimulate the heart. However, cardiovascular changes seen with high thoracic blocks are relatively modest: a $15–20\%$ reduction in cardiac output and an increase in central venous pressure (Bonica et al 1971). There has been debate about the role of epidural block as part of the technique for anaesthesia in high-risk patients and the consensus view is that cardiac problems are reduced and regional anaesthesia improves matters rather than makes them worse (Kehlet 1998). Despite this, adverse change in cardiovascular parameters in a patient deprived of compensatory mechanisms requires prompt and efficient treatment from the anaesthetist.

### Hypovolaemia

Sympathetic block is particularly dangerous in the hypovolaemic patient. Massive cardiovascular changes were observed in volunteers who had been volume depleted by over $10\%$ (Kennedy et al 1968, Bonica et al 1972). There are important lessons to be learned from these studies, although it is unlikely that they could be repeated in today's ethical climate. The earlier study showed that spinal block to $T_5$ caused substantial decreases in mean arterial pressure, central venous pressure and peripheral resistance. Despite minimal changes in cardiac output and rate, two patients showed transient asystole accompanied by a marked decrease in blood pressure when the block level increased to $T_2$ to $T_3$. Similar effects were seen in the later study in which epidural injections of lidocaine were used to produce a block to $T_5$. In 5 out of 7 patients, vigorous resuscitation was required because of substantial hypotension. The hypovolaemia was much better tolerated when the local anaesthetic solution contained epinephrine. Lidocaine–epinephrine mixtures may cause an increase in cardiac output and heart rate with a decrease in peripheral resistance and mean arterial pressure. The increased heart rate may provide some protection against the increased vagal activity.

The practical lessons are vivid: spinal and epidural block should be avoided in any patient with uncorrected hypovolaemia; and any fluid lost during surgery must be replaced immediately.

### Concomitant general anaesthesia

Three studies have investigated the combination of epidural block with general anaesthesia and spontaneous ventilation (Stephen et al 1969, Scott et al 1977, Germann et al 1979). They suggest that light general anaesthesia combined with epidural block may cause slightly greater cardiovascular depression than an epidural alone. The sequence of performance of epidural block and general anaesthesia has not been shown to affect haemodynamic variables.

### Intermittent positive pressure ventilation (IPPV)

Very little information is available on the cardiovascular effects of the combination of spinal or epidural block with IPPV, but there are theoretical reasons to believe that it can cause marked cardiovascular depression (Lynn et al 1952). A decrease in blood pressure is likely because the sympathetic block associated with the regional technique prevents the vasoconstriction which normally compensates for reduced venous return and cardiac output seen with increased intrathoracic pressure. It may also be due to increased spread of solution in the epidural space when the patient is ventilated.

### Reduced venous return

Any condition which causes a reduction in venous return, such as a gravid uterus, an intra-abdominal mass, ascites, abdominal packs or the use of surgical retractors, may lead to marked hypotension. The response may be accentuated when these factors occur in conjunction with an epidural or spinal block.

### Autonomic dysfunction

Some degree of autonomic dysfunction may occur with diabetes, alcoholism, rheumatoid arthritis, Guillaine–Barré syndrome and in the elderly. In addition, there are the specific but extremely rare conditions with autonomic dysfunction such as the Riley–Day or Shy–Drager syndromes. Postural hypotension and high resting heart rates are common in all these conditions and the response of these patients to any form of anaesthesia is unpredictable (Page & Watkins 1978).

## Significance of hypotension

A decrease in blood pressure may be considered undesirable, or even dangerous. However, beneficial effects include decreased surgical blood loss, improved operating conditions and decreased myocardial work. Even in patients with ischaemic heart disease, modest degrees of hypotension are well tolerated. Hypotension during spinal and epidural anaesthesia can be regarded as a physiological effect rather than a complication, and Lund (1971) was one of the first to suggest that '*it may be a desirable phenomenon under certain circumstances*'.

The surest way to anticipate hypotension is to monitor the circulation. Measurement of pulse rate, blood pressure and oxygen saturation should be combined with direct observation of the peripheral circulation. The degree of block should be monitored carefully, especially after each injection during a continuous epidural, so that on the rare occasion when the catheter migrates into the cerebrospinal fluid the sudden development of a greater degree of block is noted before the hypotension becomes catastrophic.

## Prevention of excessive hypotension

The most obvious way of preventing hypotension is to limit the extent of sympathetic block. A block to $T_{10}$ results in very little sympathetic paralysis, yet a wide range of surgical procedures can be carried out. A more extensive block will result in a greater degree of sympathetic paralysis.

*Prophylactic fluid loading* is only logical in those situations where acute blood loss is anticipated, as in obstetrics. In such cases, expansion of the intravascular volume compensates for the dilated vascular bed caused by sympathetic block. The accompanying decrease in haematocrit may cause temporary improvement in blood flow and the delivery of oxygen to the tissues. However, routine preloading with fluid assumes that hypotension will always occur. In fact, this is not the case, even with blocks to the upper thoracic region, because many conscious patients are able to compensate without the need for volume expansion. Preloading can also lead to problems. Because most central blocks regress from above downwards, sympathetic tone returns before bladder sensation, and catheterisation is often necessary. In the elderly patient there is also the risk that the fluid may overload the pulmonary circulation.

*Prophylactic vasopressor therapy* is also unnecessary in most patients and has little to commend it (Smith & Corbascia 1970). Engberg & Wiklund (1978a) studied the effects of ephedrine 50 mg administered subcutaneously before high epidural block in middle-aged and elderly patients. They found that the haemodynamic effects of the block were minimised and cardiac work was unaltered from pre-induction levels, but arterial pressure and peripheral resistance increased. The addition of 1:20 000 phenylephrine to the local anaesthetic solution for epidural analgesia has been shown to maintain arterial pressure, but to reduce cardiac output slightly (Stanton-Hicks et al 1973).

Prophylactic fluid loading is wise for those patients in whom significant blood loss is anticipated, and prophylactic vasopressors may be indicated for patients in whom a sudden and dramatic decrease in blood pressure is likely, or for whom this is particularly undesirable. For example, carefully adjusted infusions of epinephrine may be used to maintain the circulation in the presence of a deliberately extensive epidural block for major orthopaedic surgery (Sharrock et al 1990).

## Treatment of excessive hypotension

Before performing spinal or epidural block it is important to decide what degree of hypotension is unacceptable. Treatment is rarely required in a healthy patient before mean arterial pressure decreases by more than 30% of the resting control figure, but in patients with one or more of the previously discussed risk factors, earlier intervention may be indicated.

**Oxygen** Additional oxygen is not essential for patients having regional analgesia, but it represents an additional safety factor and should certainly be administered to those at risk of developing hypotension. This will include the majority of patients over the age of 60 years. Supplementary oxygen should be given to all patients receiving sedation, and a pulse oximeter should be available (Smith & Crul 1989).

**Posture** A decrease in blood pressure during spinal anaesthesia is invariably due to a reduced cardiac output secondary to a decrease in venous return. The simplest and safest way to correct matters is to raise the legs. A steep head-down tilt has the same effect and, surprisingly, relatively little effect on cephalad spread of local anaesthetic (Sinclair et al 1982).

**Fluids** The rapid infusion of 500–1000 ml of balanced salt solution has been advocated as a safe way to restore arterial blood pressure to a satisfactory level. However, it is now apparent that it is relatively ineffective for the treatment or prophylaxis of hypotension induced by spinal anaesthesia in a patient with a normal circulating blood volume. Additional problems have been listed earlier and the mainstay of treating hypotension due to the block itself should be pharmacological.

**Vasopressors** The detailed pharmacology of vasopressors has been extensively reviewed by Smith and Corbascia (1970). Only a small proportion of healthy patients will require vasopressors, but they should never be withheld when rapid restoration of blood pressure is indicated. These drugs should be used sparingly and in minimal incremental dosage until the vasomotor tone, lost by sympathetic block, has been restored. The vasopressors most commonly used in the treatment of hypotension caused by spinal or epidural analgesia are ephedrine, methoxamine and phenylephrine.

*Ephedrine* is both a direct and an indirectly acting α- and β-adrenoceptor agonist. It increases heart rate, stroke volume, cardiac output and peripheral vascular resistance. The latter effect may increase cardiac work without excessive increases in blood pressure or heart rate (Engberg & Wicklund 1978b). It is probably the drug of choice in obstetric practice (Eng et al 1971) because its effect upon uterine blood flow appears to be less than that of other vasopressors (Ralston et al 1974). It is relatively short acting when given intravenously. Incremental doses of 3–5 mg are satisfactory, but larger doses may cause tachycardia or hypertension.

*Methoxamine* is a pure α-adrenoceptor agonist. It may be preferred to ephedrine when hypotension and tachycardia coexist, because it increases peripheral resistance and has little effect upon cardiac output (Li et al 1965). It does not increase (and usually slows) heart rate, causes few dysrhythmias and has been recommended as the drug of choice in patients with ischaemic heart disease (Gilbert et al 1958). However, its pure α-adrenoceptor action may result in pressure being maintained at the expense of flow. It is given slowly in increments of 1–2 mg intravenously.

*Phenylephrine* is also a pure α-adrenoceptor agonist and is a suitable alternative to methoxamine, but it has a much shorter duration of action. It may be given intravenously by infusion of a 20 µg ml$^{-1}$ concentration or in 20–40 µg boluses.

In some countries *dihydroergotamine* 0.5 mg is used to prevent and treat hypotension (McCrae & Wildsmith 1993). This drug acts mainly on venous capacitance vessels, but it may cause nausea and vomiting. It is contraindicated in antipartum obstetric patients.

**Vagolytics** Atropine is not a vasopressor and is not the drug of choice for hypotension due to sympathetic block. None the less, it has a role to play in the management of cardiovascular problems during regional anaesthesia. A heart rate of less than 60 beats per minute may be associated with an inadequate cardiac output. This is usually due to vagal overactivity combined with a high sympathetic block. Intravenous atropine, in increments of 0.3 mg, will correct bradycardia and, in the presence of a central block, is unlikely to cause tachycardia, but vagal overactivity may, in some situations, be treated as effectively by the cautious administration of intravenous sedatives (e.g. thiopental at 50 mg) (Burke & Wildsmith 2000).

## Respiratory effects

Regional techniques are not widely recognised as having any effect on respiratory function. This is true for very peripheral nerve blocks and central blocks below T$_{10}$, but some effects of other methods must be considered. Higher levels of epidural and spinal block may cause paralysis of respiratory muscles, and Freund and colleagues (1967) demonstrated marked decreases in expiratory reserve volume. This may make it difficult for the patient to cough effectively. In patients with pre-existing reduced respiratory reserve (those in whom regional anaesthesia may be most suitable) the effects of a high central block may be most unpleasant. The effects may be reduced by the concomitant use of other types of analgesics with a local anaesthetic agent which does not have a marked effect upon motor nerves at the concentration chosen.

Pneumothorax must always be considered where respiratory distress occurs when puncture of the pleura may have occurred, for example intercostal, paravertebral, interpleural, supraclavicular or stellate ganglion block. In addition, respiratory depression and arrest may be due to extensive sympathetic block, reduced cardiac output and cerebral hypoxaemia.

## Sedative and anaesthetic supplements

The advantages and disadvantages of having a patient awake during surgery have been discussed in Chapter 2. Decisions about supplementation should be made, where possible, at the preoperative visit because it is important that this issue should be considered before consent is obtained. The block may be used alone, with light sedation and preservation of consciousness, with sedation sufficient to produce sleep or with a full general anaesthetic. So-called 'deep sedation', where contact with the patient is lost, really equates to a general anaesthetic. Many factors influence the choice of supplement, including the preference of the patient, the presence of systemic disease or an airway problem, the type and duration of surgery, the facilities available (especially for recovery), the experience of all the staff involved, and training requirements.

### Light sedation

Most sedatives, anxiolytics and analgesics may be used to sedate patients undergoing regional anaesthesia. Unless the surgery is expected to be prolonged, long-acting agents, such as diazepam and morphine, may not be as appropriate as the shorter-acting, more controllable agents. Midazolam (1–2 mg increments i.v.), propofol (10–20 mg increments or as a slow infusion i.v.), fentanyl (25 mg increments i.v.) and the inhalation of nitrous oxide (25–50%) are all widely used.

During elective surgery these agents may be used singly or in combination to promote gentle sedation and the choice of drug will depend upon the patient's needs. The patient should be able to respond to question and command, although many will fall asleep once the block is effective.

### Deep sedation

The difference between 'deep sedation' and general anaesthesia is impossible to define. In the past, many anaesthetists premedicated the patient with a benzo-diazepine and then gave increments of intravenous agents such as methohexitone or thiopental. However, repeated administration of these agents may lead to cumulation and, in turn, to delayed recovery and pro-found cardiorespiratory depression. Deep sedation is difficult to control and, if the patient has an aversion to being awake, it may be better to give a formal general anaesthetic, either inhalational or intravenous with a short-acting drug such as propofol.

### General anaesthesia

It is sometimes argued that the administration of a general anaesthetic to a patient who has received regional anaesthesia is an unnecessary complication, but it has several advantages. No regional technique can be guaranteed to block all possible sources of discomfort in every patient undergoing surgery, and the conscious patient may interpret unblocked sensations from the operative field as pain. This is particularly true of abdominal surgery because the visceral supply may be by autonomic nerves from above the level of the somatic block. In addition, the discomfort of lying on an operating table for a long period of time may be intolerable despite the use of strategies to obviate it.

Hypotension due to sympathetic block is a feature of spinal and epidural anaesthesia. For many procedures it enhances the surgical field and may contribute to the success of the operation. However, the degree of hypo-tension required for this effect is below that which is well tolerated by the conscious patient, and the low pressure may trigger a vasovagal attack. General anaesthesia inhibits this reflex and allows the hypo-tensive effect of the block to become an advantage rather than a 'complication' requiring prevention or treatment.

Supplementary general anaesthesia also allows the patient to be positioned and prepared for surgery while the block is becoming effective. In the conscious patient, these preparations may have to be delayed while the block develops. Furthermore, the atmosphere in the operating theatre is more relaxed, allowing surgeon and anaesthetist to discuss any problems, and enabling trainee staff to be taught, without inhibition. General anaesthesia will also eliminate any overt toxic reactions to the local anaesthetic agent.

Early experience of the problems associated with the conscious patient often deters anaesthetists from persisting with regional anaesthesia. The planned administration of a light supplementary general anaesthetic ensures success in almost every case. Any of the standard agents is suitable for induction, and nitrous oxide, with a low concentration of a volatile agent, is suitable for maintenance, administered with oxygen from a face or laryngeal mask. This will usually suffice for superficial operations, but tracheal intubation is required for abdominal and thoracic procedures. Artifical ventilation may produce a quieter surgical field for operations near the diaphragm, but neuro-muscular block is often only needed at the time of intubation.

Apart from major surgery, perhaps the main reason for supplementing regional with general anaesthesia is to help the beginner learn how to use regional methods. As the necessary confidence is gained, regional anaesthetic techniques can be used without significant supplemen-tation. These methods are becoming more popular as their ability to improve postoperative recovery is recog-nised more widely. The most common reasons for delay in discharge after surgery are drowsiness, persistent pain, nausea and vomiting. Greater use of regional methods will help deal with these problems by producing better pain control and reducing the need for general anaesthetic and sedative drugs.

## Monitoring

Monitoring the patient undergoing a procedure under regional block should be exactly the same as that used for a general anaesthetic, and should include pulse, blood pressure, electrocardiograph and oxygen saturation. Baseline readings should be obtained before starting the block, and should be continued at regular intervals right through to the recovery area. Regular communi-cation with the patient is an important component of monitoring because there is no question that the patient is the most sensitive indicator for potential or actual problems. Observation of colour, pulse, respiratory pattern and the presence or absence of sweating will often give a quicker indication of problems than any machine. Knowledge of the likely time course of the block performed, and of the development of possible side-effects, will help in the intelligent anticipation and treatment of complications. During long operations repeated doses will be necessary and their effect should be monitored as closely as those of the original in-jection. As with general anaesthesia, temperature is not monitored frequently enough and significant hypothermia may go undetected and untreated during regional anaesthesia (Frank et al 1999).

*Block level* (see also 'Testing the block' p. 95)

The level of the block and anaesthesia of the surgical site should be monitored for as long as possible before surgery when a central block is used. With careful planning, it should be possible to establish a stable block before the patient is taken into theatre or is anaesthetised. This is not always possible, but further checks on the developing block can be made under the surgical drapes, which should be placed as soon as the patient is settled in position for surgery. Non-invasive methods such as a 'pressure palpator' are preferred (Fassoulaki et al 1999). The drapes should be kept away from the patient's face and a claustrophobic atmosphere can be avoided by use of a screen which allows clear access for, and conversation with, the anaesthetist.

The upper thoracic segments only are available for testing, but these are the most important because extension of the block to this level will forewarn the anaesthetist of possible problems. Testing at this level will not warn of missed segments so, as noted earlier, the surgeon should always be asked to check discreetly the adequacy of the block at the operative site before making the skin incision. The carefully timed inflation of the blood pressure cuff will serve to divert the patient's attention as the incision is made.

*Positioning*

Even greater attention than usual must be given to the position of the patient on the operating table when regional anaesthesia is employed. All anaesthetised areas should be padded and supported, and unanaesthetised parts of the body should be positioned carefully. A patient who is awake should be shown how much movement is allowed. Uncomfortable positions may be indications for supplementary general anaesthesia, but this may only become obvious after the operation has started.

## POSTOPERATIVE CARE

The quality of personnel and facilities required for postoperative care should be the same, whatever form of anaesthesia has been used. However, the emphasis will be different because of the particular features of regional anaesthesia. The patient recovering from regional anaesthesia supplemented with mild sedation or a light general anaesthetic will have few of the problems associated with recovery from full general anaesthesia such as severe pain, residual neuromuscular block, central depression of ventilation, respiratory obstruction and inadequate clearance of secretions. Patients who have had regional anaesthesia have a much lower risk of postoperative hypoxaemia than those who have received a general anaesthetic (Moller et al 1990).

The major hazard during recovery from regional anaesthesia is hypotension, particularly after spinal or epidural block. It is not uncommon for this to occur, due to redistribution of blood flow when the patient is moved from the operating table and transported to the recovery area. It is important that the administration of oxygen is continued at this critical time. Blood pressure limits should be set, beyond which the anaesthetist or other medical staff should be informed. Written instructions for continuation of oxygen and fluid therapy, and the action to be taken in the event of hypotension should be provided.

The frequency of recordings of vital signs will depend on the patient's condition, but particular attention must be directed to measurement of blood pressure until the block has obviously started to regress. These recordings may be required more frequently than after general anaesthesia. Severe hypotension has been reported up to 2 hours after the induction of spinal anaesthesia (Moore & Bridenbaugh 1966) and noted up to 90 minutes after the induction of epidural block (personal observation). Particular vigilance is required if vasopressors have been needed to maintain blood pressure perioperatively. The action of these agents is relatively short when given intravenously and hypotension may occur as the effects wear off. The recovery room staff must be told if vasopressors have been used and instructed to be particularly assiduous in measuring blood pressure. They should be given a clear indication of how long the action of the vasopressors is likely to be, and a realistic appraisal of the time during which problems may be anticipated.

Hypotension should be managed as described earlier, but it is particularly important that the staff looking after the patient should realise that the block is not the only reason why a patient may become hypotensive. The most likely cause is, of course, surgical bleeding, and this must be suspected when hypotension occurs suddenly in a patient in whom the block is regressing satisfactorily. Patients who have had spinal or epidural anaesthesia which extended to the thoracic segments may still have residual autonomic block for some time after the procedure. This may cause hypotension if the patient's posture is changed suddenly. These patients should be mobilised gradually as the block regresses, and care should be taken when the patient first sits and stands.

When an epidural or a spinal block has been used for day-care surgery, certain criteria have to be fulfilled before the patient is discharged (Pflug et al 1978). Ambulation can be allowed once these criteria have been met:

- Return of sensation in the perianal area ($S_4$ and $S_5$);
- Plantar flexion of the foot (while supine) at pre-anaesthetic strength;
- Return of proprioception in the big toe;
- Patient should not be hypovolaemic or sedated;
- Patient should have passed urine before discharge.

## Positioning and pressure areas

Positioning of the patient is just as important during recovery as it is in the operating theatre. It is quite possible for the anaesthetised lower limb to fall off the side of the bed and for the patient to be unaware of this (the 'dead leg'). Stretching or compression may then result in neural damage and similar problems have been seen in the upper limb (Lofstrom et al 1966). Sensory block prevents the patient from appreciating pressure over bony prominences, and it is possible that this may lead to skin necrosis. When analgesia is extended into the postoperative period by means of a catheter technique, pressure points must be checked and the patient's position changed regularly.

## Urinary retention

The bladder is innervated by the sacral autonomic fibres and these may be among the last to regain function after central block. Any patient who has received large volumes of fluid during surgery and who does not have a catheter in place should be regarded as being at risk of urinary retention. If the bladder is obviously distended, it should be catheterised, but there is no need to leave the catheter in place if prompt recovery of normal neural function is expected. If, on the other hand, the analgesia is to be continued into the postoperative period, an indwelling urinary catheter may be needed.

After spinal anaesthesia the incidence of retention requiring catheterisation is directly related to the length of action of the agent used. In one study, 6% of patients needed catheterisation after spinal anaesthesia with a short-acting agent, compared with 30% of those who received a long-acting agent (Ryan et al 1984).

## Regression of the block

Medical and nursing staff should be given an approximate indication of how long the block will last. The patient should be encouraged to report any subjective feelings. Failure to do this may mean that potentially serious side-effects of the block, such as epidural haematoma, may go unnoticed and early treatment may be delayed. Good rapport between the patient and staff aids both the detection of genuine complications and the tolerance of minor discomforts unconnected with the regional anaesthesia.

## Postoperative analgesia

The provision of excellent analgesia during the early postoperative period is a major benefit of regional anaesthesia. However, small doses of conventional parenteral analgesics may also be required to alleviate discomforts which lie outside the range of the block, and to encourage the sleep which all patients require after major surgery. In cases where the block is not to be continued into the postoperative period, parenteral analgesia should be given before the block wears off completely, rather than when the pain is fully established. A number of trials suggest that the use of regional anaesthesia reduces the requirement for postoperative analgesia, but it is still unclear what combination, dose and timing of administration of postoperative drugs offer the greatest clinical benefit (Kehlet & Dahl 1993).

## Complications

### Neurological sequelae

These can be caused by intraneural injection, incorrect use of tourniquets, and faulty positioning during or after surgery, as well as by direct damage by needles (Wooley & Vandam 1959, Lofstrom et al 1966, Kroll et al 1990). A note should always be made on the anaesthetic record whenever paraesthesiae are elicited because this may help an exact diagnosis to be made if there are persistent postoperative problems (Lim & Pereira 1984). There is some evidence that tourniquets can induce sensitivity to stimuli as well as producing direct damage to nerve. Abram (1999) suggests that tissue damage can be reduced by using the lowest possible tourniquet pressure, and by blocking nociceptive fibres with topical local anaesthetic, subcutaneous infiltration or regional block. The symptoms of neural damage can vary (Selander et al 1979b), and any such case should be reviewed and investigated to try to establish the cause. The possibility that some other substance, which may be neurolytic, may have been inadvertently injected instead of the local anaesthetic drug must never be forgotten.

Transient neurological symptoms or lumbar pain after the use of hyperbaric lidocaine was first described by Schneider and colleagues (1993). Since then such symptoms have been noted more frequently and appear to be dependent upon anaesthetic, surgical and probably undefined patient factors (Horlocker & Wedel 2000). Their significance has yet to be determined, but it is most important to differentiate between short-lived features and those which may be a manifestation of something more serious. This subject is considered further in Chapters 10 and 22.

### Backache

This is a common complaint in the postoperative period. Lund (1971) found an incidence varying between 2 and 25% after spinal anaesthesia, but there is no evidence for the commonly held belief that epidural block causes more backache because of the larger needles used. There is an increase in the amount of backache suffered by obstetric patients who have had an epidural when compared with those who have not (McArthur et al 1990). However, the most likely cause in this instance is postural and is related to relaxation of the back muscles, with loss of lumbar lordosis, due to the block. Patients who receive general anaesthesia supplemented by neuromuscular block also complain occasionally of backache. The use of non-steroidal anti-inflammatory drugs may be helpful.

### Headache

Most postoperative headaches occur in patients who have not had a dural puncture. These are often caused by stress and anxiety, and are usually ill-defined in site. They are not related to posture and are rarely incapacitating. Reassurance and symptomatic treatment are all that is required. However, anaesthetists must be aware of the characteristic features of post-lumbar puncture headache: it is postural, being noticed when the patient first sits or stands, and diminishing or disappearing when supine again; it is usually occipital with cervical radiation. Severe post-lumbar puncture headache may be accompanied by visual and auditory disturbances. Hearing loss is less when smaller needles are used (Fog et al 1990). Post-lumbar puncture headache can be relieved by dural blood patch (see Chapter 11) and must not be left untreated because intracranial haematoma can result.

### Pain at the injection site

There is sometimes pain and local tenderness at the site of injection. This is probably due to the mild trauma which inevitably occurs when a needle is inserted into tissues. It should settle down within a day or two, but if it fails to do so, other causes such as local infection, contamination with antiseptic, a neurolytic agent or nerve damage, should be considered.

### Haematoma

This can occur after any nerve block but, obviously, will be more common where nerves are closely related to blood vessels. At peripheral sites, it usually resolves in a couple of weeks and gives rise to few problems. This should be explained to the patient. Where puncture of a blood vessel is part of the technique, as in the transarterial approach to the axillary brachial plexus, a haematoma is more common and long-lasting paraesthesiae are frequent (Hartung & Rupprecht 1989). This sort of problem should be taken into account when the choice of technique is made.

A spinal or epidural haematoma may be followed by serious and permanent neurological sequelae if not diagnosed and treated immediately. Any patient with prolonged neural deficit and complaining of pain must be assessed urgently and immediate help should be sought from neurological, radiological and neurosurgical colleagues when there is even the slightest doubt. Imaging techniques are now so sophisticated that the rapid and accurate diagnosis of a haematoma pressing upon neural tissues can be made easily. The same applies to the diagnosis and treatment of isolated nerve palsies which occasionally occur.

### Nausea and vomiting

The commonest causes of postoperative nausea and vomiting are general anaesthesia, the use of opioid drugs and the ingestion of blood after ear, nose, throat and oral surgery. It is also related to the site of the surgery and is more common after eye, ear, breast and gynaecological surgery. The incidence is less after regional anaesthesia, but increases if the systolic blood pressure is below 80 mmHg. The administration of oxygen is helpful (Ratra et al 1972), as is the treatment of bradycardia if this accompanies the nausea and vomiting.

# References

Abram S 1999 Central hyperalgesic effects of noxious stimulation associated with the use of tourniquets. Regional Anesthesia and Pain Medicine 24: 99–101

Bondy LR, Sims N, Schroeder DR, Offord KP, Narr BJ 1999 The effect of anesthetic patient education on preoperative patient anxiety. Regional Anesthesia and Pain Medicine 24: 158–164

Bonica JJ, Berges PU, Morikawa K 1970 Circulatory effects of peridural block: I. Effects of level of analgesia and dose of lidocaine. Anesthesiology 33: 619–626

Bonica JJ, Akamatsu TJ, Berges PU, Morikawa K, Kennedy WF 1971 Circulatory effects of peridural block: II. Effects of epinephrine. Anesthesiology 34: 514–522

Bonica JJ, Kennedy WF, Akamatsu TJ, Gerbershagen HU 1972 Circulatory effects of peridural block: III. Effects of acute blood loss. Anesthesiology 36: 219–227

Bromage PR, Benumof JL 1998 Paraplegia following intracord injection during attempted epidural anesthesia under general anesthesia. Regional Anesthesia and Pain Medicine 23: 104–107

Burke D, Wildsmith JAW 2000 Correspondence: Severe vaso-vagal attack during regional anaesthesia for Caesarean section. British Journal of Anaesthesia 84: 823–824

de Jong RH, De Rosa RA 1981 Benzodiazepine treatment of seizures from supraconvulsant doses of local anesthetics. Regional Anesthesia 6: 51–54

Dexter F 1998 Regional anesthesia does not significantly change surgical time versus general anesthesia – a meta-analysis of randomized studies. Regional Anesthesia and Pain Medicine 23: 439–443

Eng M, Berges PU, Ueland K, Bonica JJ 1971 The effects of methoxamine and ephedrine in normotensive pregnant primates. Anesthesiology 35: 354–360

Engberg G, Wiklund L 1978a The use of ephedrine for the prevention of arterial hypotension during epidural blockade. A study of the central circulation after subcutaneous premedication. Acta Anaesthesiologica Scandinavica 66 (Supplement): 1–26

Engberg G, Wiklund L 1978b The circulatory effects of intra-venously administered ephedrine during epidural blockade. Acta Anaesthesiologica Scandinavica 66 (Supplement): 27–36

Fanelli G, Casati A, Garancini P, Torri G 1999 Nerve stimulator and multiple injection technique for upper and lower limb blockade: failure rate, patient acceptance, and neurologic complications. Anesthesia and Analgesia 88: 847–852

Fassoulaki A, Sarantopoulos C, Zotou M, Karabinis G 1999 Assessment of the level of sensory block after subarachnoid anesthesia using a pressure palpator. Anesthesia and Analgesia 88: 398–401

Fischer HBJ 1998 Editorial: Regional anaesthesia – before or after general anaesthesia? Anaesthesia 53: 727–729

Fog J, Wang LP, Sunberg A, Mucchiano C 1990 Hearing loss after spinal anesthesia is related to needle size. Anesthesia and Analgesia 70: 517–520

Franco CD, Vieira ZEG 2000 1,001 subclavian perivascular brachial plexus blocks: success with a nerve stimulator. Regional Anesthesia and Pain Medicine 25: 41–46

Frank SM, Nguyen JM, Garcia CM, Barnes RA 1999 Temperature monitoring practices during regional anesthesia. Anesthesia and Analgesia 88: 373–377

Freund FG, Bonica JJ, Ward RJ, Akamatsu TJ, Kennedy WF 1967 Ventilatory reserve and level of motor block during high spinal and epidural anesthesia. Anesthesiology 28: 834–837

Germann PAS, Roberts JG, Prys-Roberts C 1979 The combination of general anaesthesia and epidural block I. The effects of sequence of induction on haemodynamic variables and blood gas measurements in healthy patients. Anaesthesia and Intensive Care 7: 229–238

Gilbert JL, Lange G, Poleroy I, Brooks CM 1958 Effects of vasoconstrictor agents on cardiac irritability. Journal of Pharmacology and Experimental Therapeutics 123: 9–15

Granger HJ, Guyton AC 1969 Autoregulation of the total systemic circulation following destruction of the central nervous system in the dog. Circulation Research 25: 379–388

Hackel DB, Sancetta SM, Kleinerman J 1956 Effect of hypo-tension due to spinal anesthesia on coronary blood flow and myocardial metabolism in man. Circulation 13: 92–97

Hartung HJ, Rupprecht A 1989 Die axillare plexus brachialis-blockade. Eine studie an 178 patienten. Regional Anesthesie 12: 21–24

Hjelm M, Holmdahl MH 1965 Biochemical effects of aromatic amines. II Cyanosis, methaemoglobinaemia and Heinz-body formation induced by a local anaesthetic agent (prilocaine). Acta Anaesthesiologica Scandinavica 9: 99–120

Horlocker TT, Wedel DJ 2000 Neurologic complications of spinal and epidural anesthesia. Regional Anesthesia and Pain Medicine 25: 83–98

Kehlet H 1998 Modification of responses to surgery by neural blockade. In: Cousins M J, Bridenbaugh P O (eds) Neural blockade in clinical anesthesia and management of pain, 3rd edn, p. 160. Lippincott-Raven, Philadelphia

Kehlet H, Dahl JB 1993 The value of 'multimodal' or 'balanced analgesia' in postoperative pain treatment. Anesthesia and Analgesia 77: 1048–1053

Kennedy WF, Bonica JJ, Akamatsu TJ, Ward RJ, Martin WE, Grinstein A 1968 Cardiovascular and respiratory effects of subarachnoid block in the presence of acute blood loss. Anesthesiology 29: 29–35

Krane EJ, Dalens BJ, Murat I, Murrell D. 1998 The safety of epidurals placed during general anesthesia. Regional Anesthesia and Pain Medicine 23: 433–438

Kroll DA, Kaplan RA, Posner K, Ward RJ, Cheney FW 1990 Nerve injury associated with anesthesia. Anesthesiology 73: 202–207

Li T-H, Shimosato S, Etsten B 1965 Methoxamine and cardiac output in non-anesthetised man and during spinal anesthesia. Anesthesiology 26: 21–30

Lim EK, Pereira E 1984 Brachial plexus injury following brachial plexus block. Anaesthesia 39: 691–694

Lofstrom JB, Wennberg A, Widen L 1966 Late disturbance in nerve function after block with local anaesthetic agents. Acta Anaesthesiologica Scandinavica 10: 111–122

Lund PC 1971 Principles and practice of spinal anesthesia. CC Thomas, Springfield

Lynn RB, Sancetta SM, Simeone FA, Scott RW 1952 Observations on the circulation in high spinal anesthesia. Surgery 22: 195–213

Mayo W 1928 Foreword in Labat G 1928 Regional anesthesia – its technic and clinical application. WB Saunders: Philadelphia

McArthur C, Lewis M, Knox EG, Crawford JS 1990 Epidural anaesthesia and long term backache after childbirth. British Medical Journal 301: 9–12

McCrae AF, Wildsmith JAW 1993 Prevention and treatment of hypotension during central neural block. British Journal of Anaesthesia 70; 672–680

Moller JT, Wittrup M, Johansen SH 1990 Hypoxemia in the postanaesthetic care unit: An observer study. Anesthesiology 73: 890–895

Moore DC, Bridenbaugh LD 1966 Spinal (subarachnoid) block. A review of 11,574 cases. Journal of the American Medical Association 195: 907–912

Nimmo WS, Edwards AE, Aitkenhead AR 1995 Suspected anaphylactic reactions associated with anaesthesia, vol. 2, p. 14. Association of Anaesthetists, London

Page MM, Watkins PJ 1978 Cardiorespiratory arrest and diabetic autonomic neuropathy. Lancet i: 14–16

Pflug AE, Aasheim GM, Foster C 1978 Sequence of return of neurological function and criteria for safe ambulation following subarachnoid block. Canadian Anaesthetists' Society Journal 25: 133–139

Philips BJ, Ferguson S, Armstrong P, Anderson FM, Wildsmith JAW 1992 Surgical facemasks are effective in reducing bacterial contamination caused by dispersal from the upper airway. British Journal of Anaesthesia 69: 407–408

Raj PP, Rosenblatt RM, Montgomery SJ 1980 Use of the nerve stimulator for peripheral blocks. Regional Anesthesia 5: 14–21

Ralston DH, Shnider SM, De Lorimier AA 1974 Effects of equipotent ephedrine, metaraminol, mephentermine and methoxamine on uterine blood flow in the pregnant ewe. Anesthesiology 40: 354–370

Ratra CK, Badola RP, Bhargava KP 1972 A study of factors concerned in emesis during spinal anaesthesia. British Journal of Anaesthesia 44: 1208–1211

Rosenblatt RM, Shal R 1984 The design and function of a regional anesthesia block room. Regional Anaesthesia 9: 12–16

Ryan JA Jr, Adye BA, Jolly PC, Mulroy MF 1984 Outpatient inguinal herniorrhaphy with both regional and local anesthesia. American Journal of Surgery 148: 313–316

Schneider M, Ettlin T, Kaufmann M, Schumacher P, Urwyler A, Hampl K, von Hochstetter A 1993 Transient neurologic toxicity after hyperbaric subarachnoid anaesthesia with 5% lidocaine. Anesthesia and Analgesia 76: 1154–1157

Scott DB 1975 Management of extradural block during surgery. British Journal of Anaesthesia 47: 271–272

Scott DB, Littlewood DG, Drummond GB, Buckley FP, Covino BG 1977 Modification of the circulatory effects of extradural block combined with general anaesthesia by the addition of adrenaline to lignocaine solutions. British Journal of Anaesthesia 49: 917–925

Selander D, Dhuner K-G, Lundborg G 1977 Peripheral nerve injury due to injection needles used for regional anaesthesia. Acta Anaesthesiologica Scandinavica 21: 182–188

Selander D, Edshage S, Wolff S. 1979a Paresthesia or no paresthesia? Nerve lesions after axillary blocks. Acta Anaesthesiolgica Scandinavica 23: 27–33

Selander D, Brattsand R, Lundborg G, Nordborg C, Olsson Y 1979b Local anaesthetics: importance of mode of application, concentration and adrenaline for the appearance of nerve lesions. Acta Anaesthesiolgica Scandinavica 23: 127–136

Seropian R, Reynolds BM 1971 Wound infections after preoperative depilatory versus razor preparation. American Journal of Surgery 121: 251–254

Sharrock NE, Mineo R, Urquhart B 1990 Hemodynamic response to low-dose epinephrine infusion during hypotensive epidural anesthesia for total hip replacement. Regional Anesthesia 15: 295–299

Sinclair CJ, Scott DB, Edstrom HH 1982 Effect of the Trendelenberg position on spinal anaesthesia with hyperbaric bupivacaine. British Journal of Anaesthesia 54: 497–500

Smith DC, Crul JF 1989 Oxygen desaturation following sedation for regional anaesthesia. British Journal of Anaesthesia 62: 206–209

Smith NJ, Corbascia AN 1970 The use and misuse of pressor agents. Anesthesiology 33: 58–101

Sprung J, Bourke DL, Grass J, Hammel J, Mascha E, Thomas P, Tubin I 1999 Predicting the difficult neuraxial block: a prospective study. Anesthesia and Analgesia 89: 384–389

Stanton-Hicks M d'A, Berges PU, Bonica JJ 1973 Circulatory effects of peridural block IV: Comparison of the effects of epinephrine and phenylephrine. Anesthesiology 39: 308–314

Stephen GW, Lees MM, Scott DB 1969 Cardiovascular effects of epidural block combined with general anaesthesia. British Journal of Anaesthesia 41: 933–938

Tessler MJ, Kardash K, Wahba RM, Kleiman SJ, Trihas S, Rossignol M 1999 The performance of spinal anesthesia is marginally more difficult in the elderly. Regional Anesthesia and Pain Medicine 24: 126–130

Wetstone DL, Wong KC 1974 Sinus bradycardia and asystole during spinal anesthesia. Anesthesiology 41: 87–89

Wildsmith JAW, Fischer HBJ 1999 Correspondence: Regional anaesthesia – before or after general anaesthesia? Anaesthesia 54: 86

Winnie AP 1983 Plexus anesthesia, vol. 1, p. 211. Churchill Livingstone, Edinburgh

Wooley EJ, Vandam LJ 1959 Neurological sequelae of brachial plexus nerve block. Annals of Surgery 149: 53–60

# 9. Anatomy and physiology of the vertebral canal

## M Brockway and W A Chambers

## THE VERTEBRAL COLUMN

The vertebral column is a strong curved pillar, which extends from the base of the skull to the pelvis in the midline (Fig. 9.1). It is formed by a series of vertebrae, which contribute about three-quarters of its length, the remainder deriving from the intervening fibrocartilaginous discs. Only a small degree of movement occurs between any two adjacent vertebrae, but the cumulative effect results in a column of considerable flexibility that is strong and stable. The vertebral column has three major functions.

1. It is the means whereby the upper body weight is transmitted to the pelvis and then to the lower limbs and the ground.
2. It provides the sites of attachment of the muscles of posture and locomotion.
3. It forms a protective canal for the spinal cord and its covering meninges.

Typically, there are 24 'true' vertebrae, making up the cervical (7), thoracic (12) and lumbar (5) regions of the column. There are normally 9 'false' vertebrae, which constitute the sacrum and coccyx.

In the embryo, the spine is curved into a 'C' shape, concave forwards. This primary curvature persists throughout life in the thoracic and sacral regions, and may return to some extent in the lumbar and cervical region with ageing. Extension of the head when it is held up, and of the lower limbs when standing erect, produces secondary curvatures in the cervical and lumbar regions which are concave backwards (Fig. 9.1). All of these curves are produced predominantly by moulding of the intervertebral discs, with the 'high' points in the supine position being $C_4$ to $C_5$ and $L_2$ to $L_4$, and the 'low' points $T_5$ to $T_7$ and $S_2$. The lumbar curve is more marked in women, particularly during pregnancy, while the cervical curve usually includes the first two thoracic vertebrae. Most curvature occurs in the anterior/posterior plane, but minor lateral curves may also occur. In the thoracic region the column may deviate somewhat laterally, usually towards the right and be compensated for by curves above or below.

## The vertebra (Fig. 9.2)

### A typical vertebra

The general features of vertebrae change gradually between regions, but are similar enough to be considered together. Viewed from above, the 'typical' vertebra has an anterior body through which the weight of the person is transmitted. This body increases in size down the column to accommodate the increase in transmitted weight. The flat superior and inferior surfaces are the sites of attachment of the intervertebral discs, which separate adjacent vertebrae and act as shock absorbers to dissipate the forces placed on the column. The posterior surface of the body is flat, while the anterior and lateral faces are curved. Posteriorly, there is a vertebral or neural arch, which completes the boundaries of the vertebral foramen. Anteriorly, this arch is formed by two stout 'pedicles' and is completed posteriorly by two laminae which unite in the midline to form the base of the spinous process. The pedicles attach to the upper posterior surface of the vertebral body – a feature which allows confirmation of vertebral orientation. When viewed laterally, each pedicle carries two notches of uneven depth, the inferior notch usually being deeper than the superior. Articulation of two neighbouring vertebrae forms the intervertebral foramina, through which the roots of spinal nerves and the vascular structures supplying the spinal cord pass.

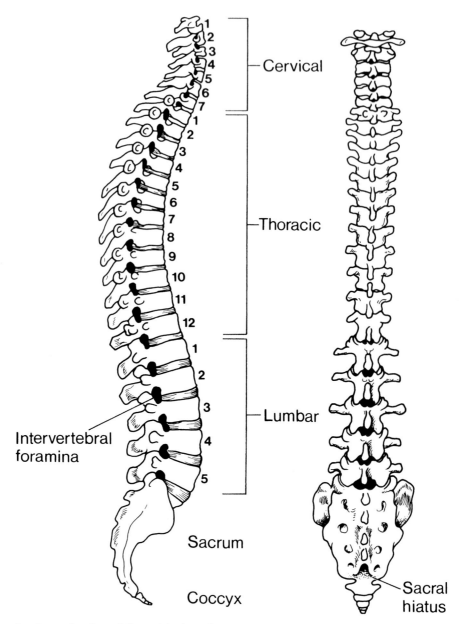

**Fig 9.1**  Lateral and posterior views of the vertebral canal

An articular pillar of paired superior and inferior articular processes lies behind the pedicles. The superior articular process of one vertebra articulates with the inferior articular process of the vertebra above through synovial 'facet' (or zagapophysial) joints. The spinous process projects posteriorly, and paired transverse processes project posterolaterally, from the neural arch. The laminae and spinous process together form a large surface area for muscle and ligament attachment.

*Cervical vertebrae*
The typical cervical vertebrae have relatively small bodies and are found in the middle of this region: the $C_1$ (atlas), $C_2$ (axis) and $C_7$ (vertebra prominens) are atypical. The transverse processes contain the foramen transversarium for the passage of the vertebral artery, the spinous processes are short and horizontal, and the laminae are flat, long and increase in depth from $C_3$ downwards.

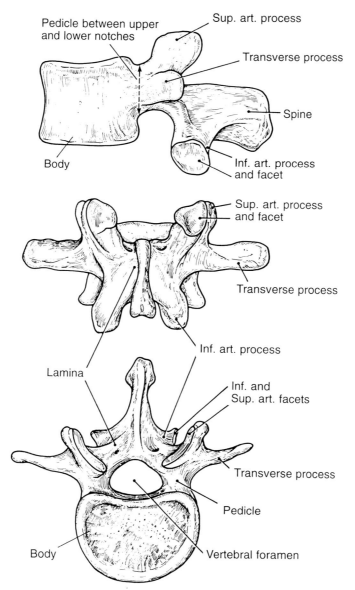

Pedicle between upper and lower notches

Sup. art. process

Transverse process

Spine

Inf. art. process and facet

Body

Sup. art. process and facet

Transverse process

Inf. art. process

Lamina

Inf. and Sup. art. facets

Transverse process

Pedicle

Vertebral foramen

Body

**Fig 9.2** Lateral, posterior and superior views of a 'typical' vertebra

The atlas ($C_1$) is essentially a ring of bone, there being no vertebral body. The axis ($C_2$) is the pivot, or axis, upon which the head turns, there being a projecting odontoid process or dens. The seventh cervical vertebra ($C_7$) is essentially transitional, having some of the characteristics of the cervical vertebrae above, and others of the thoracic vertebrae below.

### Thoracic vertebrae

The pedicles pass directly backwards, carrying deep inferior notches and virtually no superior notch ($T_1$ excepted). From $T_1$ to $T_8$ the pedicles bear superior and inferior articular surfaces, the upper articulating with the head of the corresponding rib and the lower with the head of the rib below. A similar surface on the large transverse process articulates with the rib tubercle. $T_1$ and the last two or three thoracic vertebrae have complete articular surfaces for the corresponding rib only. The vertebral foramina are large and triangular, freely accommodating the relatively thick spinal cord. The spinous processes are long and generally angled caudally to overlap the spine below.

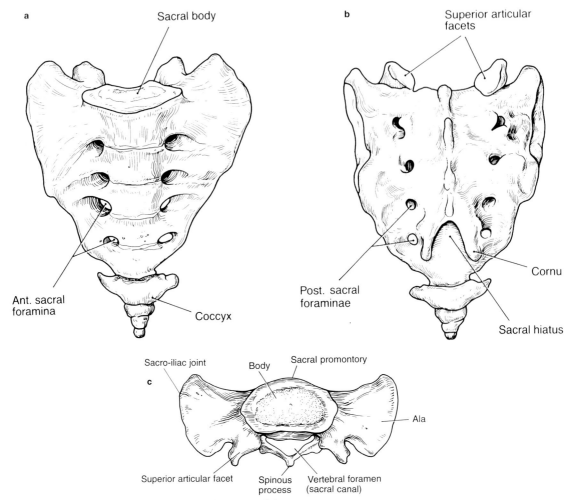

**Fig 9.3**  Anterior (a), posterior (b) and superior (c) views of the sacrum

The intervertebral discs are thin in comparison with other regions and this, together with the overlap of the spinous processes and the presence of the ribs, greatly restricts movement in the thoracic region.

### Lumbar vertebrae

In the lumbar region the vertebral bodies are large and kidney shaped, the pedicles are short and stout with shallow superior notches, and the transverse processes are generally slender except for $L_5$ where they are short, thick, strong and arise from the vertebral body as well as the neural arch. The laminae are deep and short and the spinous processes horizontal, thick and square. The body of $L_5$ is wedge shaped, being thicker anteriorly and forming the characteristic lumbosacral angle.

## The sacrum (Fig. 9.3a–c)

In the adult, the five (sometimes six) vertebrae below the lumbar segment fuse to form the sacrum, the central part of the pelvic girdle. It is a wedge-shaped bone, wider above than below, and concave anteriorly, both from above downwards and from side to side. The central part of the sacrum is formed by the fusion of the vertebral bodies, and there are four transverse ridges on the anterior surface representing the obliterated intervertebral discs. At the lateral ends of these ridges are the four anterior sacral foramina, the remnants of the anterior ends of the intervertebral foramina, through which pass the ventral rami of the sacral spinal nerves. The posterior surface of the sacrum is formed by the fusion of the neural arches. A midline crest derives from the laminae and has three or four tubercles on it, representing the fused spinous processes. Lateral to this is the intermediate crest (the fused articular process) and, directly opposite the anterior foramina, the four posterior foramina for the posterior rami of the sacral nerves. The lateral crest is the result of fusion of the transverse processes.

Inferiorly, the laminae of the last sacral arch, and occasionally those of the adjacent arch, fail to meet and leave a roughly triangular sacral hiatus, bounded by the cornua which are the remnants of the lowest articular process. The sacral hiatus shows considerable variation in both length and width, but can usually be found approximately 5 cm above the tip of the coccyx, directly above the uppermost limit of the natal cleft. The hiatus is traversed by the fifth sacral nerves.

## Vertebral anomalies

Variations in the bony anatomy of the spine are of more than passing interest because they may make the performance of spinal or epidural block difficult or impossible. Common anomalies include fusion of two or more vertebrae (particularly the fifth lumbar vertebra to the sacrum), separation of the first sacral segment, and absent or additional vertebrae. Grossly abnormal development can result in hemi-vertebra or even in spina bifida, caused by failure of fusion of two developmental centres in the neural arch. This is not usually associated with any neurological defect, although there may be an overlying dimple, lipoma or tuft of hair, but only rarely is there a gross defect of one or more arches with protrusion of the cord or its coverings. Variations in the structure of the sacrum are dealt with in Chapter 12.

## INTERVERTEBRAL JOINTS AND LIGAMENTS

The individual vertebrae articulate with each other through the column of bodies and intervertebral discs. Additionally, the neural arches articulate through the superior and inferior processes on each side at the facet joints. The vertebrae are linked to each other by a complicated system of ligaments, with only the pedicles not being connected directly to a ligament. There are four groups of ligaments. True ligaments connect:

 (i) The vertebral bodies to each other;
 (ii) The neural arches and other posterior structures; and
(iii) The vertebral column to other bony structures.

A fourth group of (false) ligaments protect or separate vertebral components, for example, the intertransverse and transforaminal ligaments.

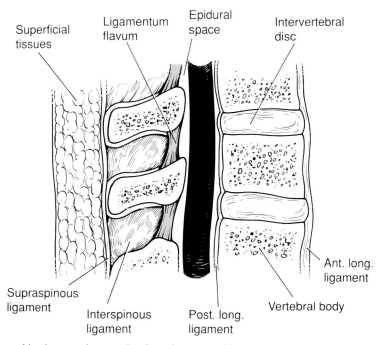

**Fig 9.4** Sagittal section of lumbar vertebrae to the show the principal ligaments

## Ligaments of the vertebral body (Fig. 9.4)

The anterior longitudinal ligament runs along the front of the vertebral bodies from $C_2$ to the sacrum, becoming wider as it descends. It is attached primarily to the anterior margins of the vertebral bodies and secondarily to the curved anterior surfaces. Over the intervertebral discs it is attached only loosely to the annuli fibrosi. Its deep fibres are unisegmental whereas the more superficial ones may cover four or five segments. The posterior longitudinal ligament runs over the posterior surfaces of the vertebral bodies and discs, being attached mainly to the annuli fibrosi, but also to the margins of the adjacent vertebral bodies. The shortest fibres of the posterior longitudinal ligament extend across two spinal segments, that is, from disc or superior margin of one vertebral body to the inferior margin or disc of the body two above. Longer more superficial fibres may extend over four or five segments.

The annuli fibrosi are structurally and functionally the principal ligaments of the vertebral bodies. They lie in the peripheral part of the intervertebral disc, the collagen fibres running from the disc of one vertebral body to the next in a series of concentric lamellae, which are often deficient posterolaterally. These fibres act to resist movement between the vertebrae.

## Posterior ligaments

The ligamentum flavum is a series of paired ligaments arising from the lower border and adjacent inner surface of one lamina and the inferior aspect of the pedicle (Fig. 9.4) and then dividing into medial and lateral components. The medial component attaches to the upper border and outer surface of the lamina below, while the lateral part attaches and contributes to the facet joint capsule. The thickness of the ligament varies considerably (2–10 mm), and increases from above downwards. It is 80% elastin in young adults, but its elasticity decreases with increasing age and it may calcify. The exact function of the ligamentum flavum is unknown, although its elasticity will serve to prevent buckling and encroachment on to other structures. Each pair of ligaments may meet in the midline at an attenuated junction, but fail to do so in approximately 50% of cervical and thoracic segments. Any deficiency is usually filled by the anterior surface of the interspinous ligament, although this too may be deficient in the cervicothoracic region (Westbrook et al 1993, Hogan

1996). It is theoretically possible therefore that a needle inserted in the midline could enter the epidural space without traversing the ligamentum flavum or interspinous ligament, and therefore without any loss of resistance.

The interspinous ligaments run between the shafts of adjacent spines, but they are thin and it is doubtful whether they are effective in limiting spinous separation. The supraspinous ligament is a powerful fibrous structure attaching to the posterior edges of the vertebral spines from $C_7$ downwards. It reaches $L_3$ in 20%, $L_4$ in 75%, and $L_5$ or the sacrum in 5% of individuals. Although called a ligament, this structure consists mainly of the tendinous attachments of the long back muscles, with only the most superficial (posterior) layers lacking any continuity with muscle. The supraspinous ligament offers little resistance to the separation of spinous processes and may become ossified in old age, so making penetration with a fine needle difficult or impossible. Above $C_7$ the supraspinous ligament is continuous with the ligamentum nuchae.

## The intervertebral discs

Whatever an individual's height, the vertebral column is about 70 cm in length in the male and 60 cm in the female, with the intervertebral discs accounting for 20–25% of this. With ageing, atrophy of the discs and osteoporosis of the vertebrae lead to kyphotic deformity and a decrease in height. The discs allow 'rocking' between adjacent vertebrae during flexion, extension and lateral bending, and some rotation (a ball and socket joint in this position would compromise weight bearing ability).

An intervertebral disc requires to be:

- Strong, in order to sustain body weight without collapsing;
- Deformable enough to allow the movements outlined above; and
- Resilient enough to avoid damage during those movements.

To achieve these properties the disc is formed in two parts. The ligamentous annulus fibrosus (see above) surrounds the nucleus pulposus, a semifluid, mucoid mass which will deform, but not compress, under pressure. These properties result in applied pressure being transmitted in all directions, as when a water-filled balloon is compressed. With ageing the nucleus gradually changes until it cannot be distinguished from the annulus fibrosus, the disc becoming thinner and less resilient.

## Movement of the spine

Extension is the freer movement and is greatest in the lumbar and least in the thoracic regions. Flexion, which is largely restrained by tension in the spinal extensor muscles, is most marked in the thoracic region and almost absent in the lumbar. It should be noted that natural forward bending is largely flexion at the hip joints and not flexion of the trunk. The ligamentum flavum stretches freely on flexion and its elastic recoil avoids the formation of folds which might be caught between bones on extension. Because of the ribs, lateral flexion is very limited in the thoracic region, but significant rotation is possible. Lateral flexion is greatest in the lumbar region, but only slight rotation is possible.

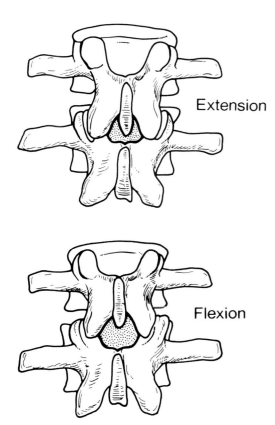

**Fig 9.5** Effect of flexion and extension on the interlaminar space in the lumbar region

If the vertebral column is viewed from behind, the laminae and spines can be seen to overlap each other so that the spinal canal is completely hidden except in the lower lumbar region. The gap between the lumbar spinous processes can be widened by flexion of the spine (Fig. 9.5), but this manoeuvre has a more limited effect in the thoracic region. Rotation may distort the bony structures, so that a direct approach to the vertebral canal is not possible from the midline. This is more likely to be a problem in the thoracic region where, as noted above, a greater degree of rotation is possible.

## THE VERTEBRAL CANAL

The vertebral canal extends from the foramen magnum to the sacral hiatus. It is formed by the neural arches, the posterior surfaces of the vertebral bodies and the ligaments and other structures that link them. The curves of the vertebral column are mirrored in the canal, which has a roughly triangular cross-sectional shape with the apex posteriorly. However, it is more oval in cross-section in the cervical and upper thoracic regions, with the surface area tending to increase from above downwards. The most notable openings of the canal are 29 pairs of intervertebral foramina, which are formed by the inferior and superior notches of the adjacent pedicles together with contributions from the vertebral bodies and discs anteriorly, and the laminae and facet joints posteriorly. Twenty-five of the foramina face laterally whereas four (sacral) face anteroposteriorly. The intervertebral foramina tend to increase in diameter from above downwards, except between $C_5$ to $T_1$ and $L_4$ to $S_1$, through which the larger spinal nerves (supplying the upper and lower limbs) pass. The vertebral canal communicates with the thoracic and abdominal cavities through these foramina, and with the cranial cavity through the foramen magnum. The sacrococcygeal ligament usually seals the sacral hiatus completely.

## The meninges and dural sac

The spinal cord has three covering membranes or meninges – the dura, arachnoid and pia maters – which divide the vertebral canal into three distinct compartments: the epidural, subdural and subarachnoid spaces. The epidural space lies between the dura mater and

117

the margins of the spinal canal, but the subdural compartment is a potential space only, the arachnoid mater being approximated to the inner surface of the dural sac and separated from it by only a thin film of serous fluid. The subarachnoid space contains cerebrospinal fluid (CSF), the spinal cord and the nerve roots. The dura mater is a continuation of the inner layer of cerebral dura and is composed of dense longitudinally orientated fibrous tissue. The outer, endosteal layer of cerebral dura is continued, often deficiently, as the periosteal lining of the vertebral canal.

Extensions of the dura mater and the applied arachnoid continue along each spinal nerve root as far as the ganglion on the dorsal root and sometimes further, progressively thinning to become continuous with the coverings of the peripheral nerves (see Fig. 4.1). These extensions of the subarachnoid space, known as dural 'cuffs', contain a pocket of CSF and are pierced by numerous veins, arteries and lymphatics as they pass between the subarachnoid and epidural spaces. Additionally, arachnoid granulations protrude through the dura to communicate with the epidural veins and lymphatics, thus facilitating drainage of CSF and the removal of foreign material. The pia mater, the innermost membrane, is a vascular sheath which closely invests the spinal cord and thereafter continues caudally, closely invested with dura, as the filum terminale to attach to periosteum on the posterior surface of the coccyx. The blood vessels supplying the spinal cord lie within the tissue of the pia mater (see below).

### Dural sac

The dural sac extends from the foramen magnum to the second, or occasionally third, sacral segment where it continues distally as a covering of the filum terminale. However, there is some variation. The termination of the sac is lower in children, and in some adults it may be as high as the fifth lumbar segment. The sac lies rather loosely within the vertebral canal, being attached to the edge of the foramen magnum above, the posterior longitudinal ligament anteriorly, the ligamentum flavum and laminae posteriorly, the pedicles laterally and the coccyx by the filum terminale inferiorly. These attachments, together with the continuation of dura laterally along each spinal nerve root (see above), stabilise both the dural sac and the spinal cord, and are responsible for the roughly triangular cross-sectional shape (apex posteriorly) of the sac.

## Subarachnoid space

The subarachnoid space lies deep to the arachnoid mater. It contains the spinal cord, dorsal and ventral nerve roots, and CSF. The spinal cord extends from the medulla oblongata, with which it is continuous, to end as the conus medullaris near the lower border of the first lumbar vertebra. The exact level is variable (Fig. 9.6). The pia mater continues caudally as a thread-like filum terminale, ultimately attaching to the coccyx. The adult cord has an average length of 45 cm and weight of 30 g in the adult male, is elliptical in cross-section (with a

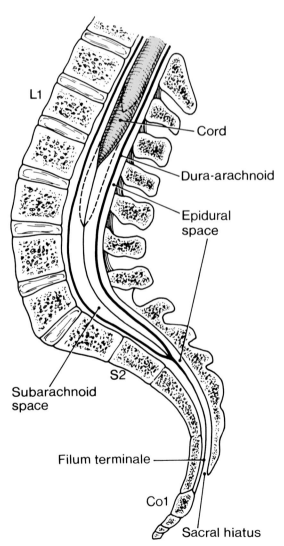

**Fig 9.6** Sagittal section of lumbar and sacral regions of the spine. The dotted lines indicate the range for the termination of the spinal cord

greater transverse diameter at all levels) and tapers caudally except for two distinct expansions. The first, and larger of these, is the cervicothoracic enlargement, which reaches maximum width at the level of $C_5$ and reflects the extensive upper limb innervation. The second, lumbosacral, enlargement innervates the lower limbs, and is situated between the ninth and twelfth thoracic vertebrae. There are 31 pairs of spinal nerves (8 cervical, 12 thoracic, 5 lumbar, 5 sacral and 1 coccygeal), each formed from a dorsal and a ventral root. These roots are formed from several smaller rootlets or fibrils, and every dorsal root has a ganglion where the cell bodies of the sensory nerves are situated.

Up to the third month of intrauterine life the cord extends the full length of the canal, but thereafter the vertebrae grow much more rapidly, and this results in the neonatal conus medullaris being at the third lumbar level. The differential growth means that, in the adult, there is increasing obliquity of the nerve roots from above downwards, so that the lumbar and sacral roots lie freely within CSF below the level of the conus medullaris to form the cauda equina. Numerous delicate trabeculations run between the arachnoid and pia maters, the pattern varying between individuals, with more to be found along the dorsal aspect of the cord than ventrally (Nauta et al 1983) (Figs. 9.7 & 9.8). A midline dorsal septum, the septum posticum (Di Chiro & Timins 1974, Nauta et al 1983) typically extends from the midcervical to lumbar regions. Generally, it is attached to the pia mater along the course of the dorsal

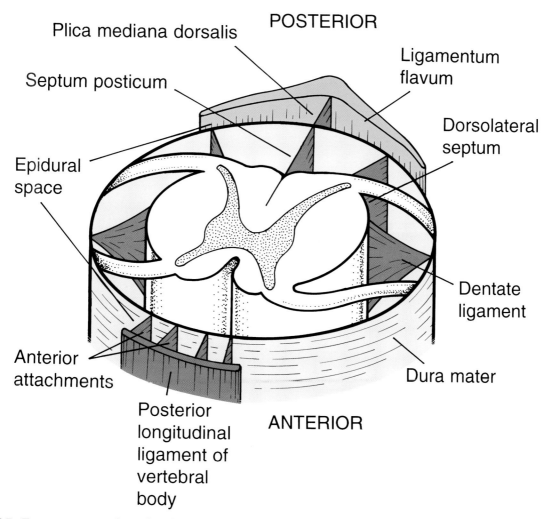

**Fig 9.7** Transverse section of spinal cord to show its attachments

vein of the spinal cord (Nauta et al 1983) and has irregular perforations, particularly towards its upper and lower ends. Lateral to the septum posticum, two other septa extend from the region of the dorsal rootlets and attach to the dorsolateral arachnoid mater. These dorsolateral septa tend to be more irregular, more densely fenestrated, to atrophy with age and to extend further rostrally and caudally than the septum posticum; they probably serve to tether the dorsal rootlets, keeping them clear of the lateral parts of the spinal cord (Nauta et al 1983). Substantial lateral projections from the pia mater, known as denticulate or dentate ligaments, attach to the dura mater and act to support the spinal cord. There are no attachments anterior to the dentate ligaments.

Spinal cord blood supply is provided by an anterior and two posterior spinal arteries (Fig. 9.8), all of which run within the pia mater. The anterior spinal artery is a single midline vessel, formed at the foramen magnum from a branch of each vertebral artery. It is the largest of the spinal vessels and supplies a substantial portion of the anterior cord. There is one posterior spinal artery (occasionally two) on each side, each derived from the posterior inferior cerebellar artery. Spinal branches of the vertebral, ascending cervical, posterior intercostal, lumbar and lateral sacral arteries pass through the intervertebral foramina to augment blood supply. Most of these are insignificant, but some contribute substantially, especially those at $T_4$ and $T_{11}$. The arterial supply to the cord is vulnerable to the consequences of occlusion, such as may follow trauma, hypotension or the use of vasoconstrictors. Blockage of a posterior vessel may have little effect, but occlusion of the anterior spinal artery usually leads to ischaemia of a large section of the spinal cord. Venous drainage is through a plexus of anterior and posterior veins which drain along the nerve roots into epidural and segmental veins.

## Epidural space

The epidural space is the compartment between the periosteal lining of the vertebral canal and the dural sac, which lies in the anterior part of the canal. Thus the epidural space has a small anterior compartment (roughly 10% of the total) and a much larger posterolateral compartment (90%). The distance from the posterior border of the vertebral canal to the dura varies according to spinal segment, being as little as

0.5 mm in the cervical region and up to 9 mm in the lumbar (Hirabayashi et al 1997). The space itself is largest in the sacral region because there is no dural sac, whereas in the cervical region the narrowness of the vertebral canal may obliterate the epidural space altogether, the two layers of dura being opposed. At the foramen magnum the two dural layers fuse.

The nerve roots on either side cross the posterolateral part of the epidural space to the two intervertebral foramina present at each segmental level. Inferiorly, their course is increasingly oblique, and they may lie in channels, known as radicular canals, leading to the foramina. At the foramina the nerves, together with fat and blood vessels, are tethered to the canal walls by connective tissue structures known as Charpy's ligaments. With increasing age the foramina tend to occlude (Reynolds 1984, Atkinson et al 1987), although this is not the case with the anterior sacral foramina (Luyendijk 1963, Luyendijk & Van Voorthuisen 1966).

Epidural fat, inconsistently filling the rest of the space, is very vascular and has a semifluid consistency. With age the nature of the fat changes so that it offers progressively more resistance to injection (Cousins & Bromage 1988), although the amount present may decrease (Igarashi et al 1997). More fat is found in the lumbar than the thoracic region, and this may be one of the reasons for enhanced spread of local anaesthetic at the thoracic level (Hogan 1996, Igarashi et al 1998). Magnetic resonance imaging (MRI) has shown that there is virtually no fat in the cervical region (Hirabayashi et al 1997). Interestingly, the fat is discontinuous in the lumbar region, being present only at the levels of the intervertebral discs, whereas it is continuous in the thoracic region, even though there is less of it (Hogan 1996, Hirabayashi et al 1997).

The epidural veins, known as the plexus of Batson, are large, valveless vessels which lie in the anterolateral part of the space and run vertically in four principal trunks. These communicate freely, through a venous ring at each vertebral level, with the sacral (and hence iliac and uterine) venous plexus, and the abdominal and thoracic veins. Thus pressure changes within the body's cavities are reflected in the epidural veins, most notably in pregnancy when the veins are distended and the effective volume of the epidural space is decreased. Lymphatics and arteries, which are relatively small, lie mainly in the lateral part of the space, pass through the intervertebral foramina to supply adjacent vertebrae and ligaments, and contribute to the supply of the spinal cord (see above). Cryomicrotomy has revealed that a vein often enters the posterior epidural space, in the midline between the pair of ligamenta flava. Less commonly, this vein is found more laterally, actually piercing the ligament (Hogan 1996).

Computerised axial tomography (CAT) has shown that the dorsal part of the epidural space, in sagittal section, has a 'sawtooth' outline because of the attachment, position and bulk of the ligamentum flavum. MRI and cryomicrotomy have revealed that the widest section is that nearest the cephalad lamina (Hogan 1996, Igarashi et al 1998). MRI scanning also shows that the dorsal epidural compartment is triangular in cross-section in the lumbar region, but more crescent shaped in the thoracic region (Hirabayashi et al 1997). The ventral epidural space varies in depth, being larger behind the vertebral body and smaller behind the protruding intervertebral disc (Luyendijk 1963). The posterior longitudinal ligament has numerous connections to the anterior dural sac and the two are often fused in the lumbar region. The close attachment, or even opposition, of the dural sac to the anterior canal wall may serve to separate completely the ventral epidural compartment (Harrison et al 1985, Savolaine et al 1988).

Periduroscopy has demonstrated the existence of dorsal midline strands connecting the dura mater to the ligamentum flavum, a finding confirmed later by epiduroscopy (Blomberg 1986, Savolaine et al 1988). These strands have been described as producing a fold in the dura mater termed the plica mediana dorsalis (Luyendijk 1976), which narrows the epidural space in the midline to its point of attachment to the ligamentum flavum, although others have suggested that the folding is an artefact (Hogan 1996). The strands are particularly well developed in the region of the vertebral arches and, in some cases, may alter epidural catheter direction, especially as the amount of catheter in the space increases. On occasion the strands form a complete membrane capable of preventing a catheter crossing from one side to the other (Blomberg 1986).

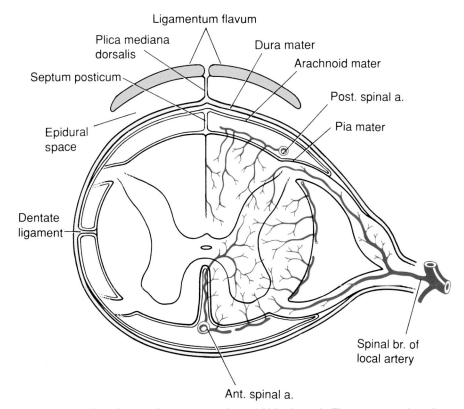

**Fig 9.8** Transverse section to show the spinal meninges and arterial blood supply. The nerve roots have been omitted on the left for clarity

CAT and MRI studies have confirmed this midline division of the posterior epidural space (Savolaine et al 1988, Hirabayashi et al 1997).

Other connective tissue bands have been described, originating from the plica mediana dorsalis and extending laterally, subdividing further the posterolateral compartment of the epidural space into lateral and posterior sections (Savolaine et al 1988) (Fig. 9.8). However, it has been argued that these strands represent simple distortions of the septa responsible for loculating fat in the lateral compartment (Hogan 1991). The posterolateral space is split into posterior and lateral compartments at the level of each neural arch by the opposition of the dura with the laminae. The posterior and lateral compartments themselves are generally discontinuous longitudinally, being separated by intervening laminae and pedicles, though this is less marked in the thoracic region (Westbrook et al 1993).

## PHYSIOLOGY OF THE VERTEBRAL CANAL

### Cerebrospinal fluid

The CSF is normally clear and colourless with a specific gravity of approximately 1.005 at 37 °C, though this may be increased slightly in conditions such as old age, uraemia, hyperglycaemia and hypothermia, but decreased during pregnancy (Richardson & Wissler 1996). It fills all the cavities in, and spaces around, the central nervous system and its function is to support and protect it. CSF is isotonic with plasma (280–290 mOsmol l$^{-1}$) and has similar constituents except that it contains only traces of protein (Table 9.1). Small numbers of blood cells are present in healthy CSF. It is produced in the choroid plexuses (small tufts of capillaries in direct contact with the ventricular lining) of the lateral ventricles, and also by plexuses in the third and fourth ventricles and on the surface of the brain. The differences between CSF and plasma imply that it is actively secreted rather than an ultrafiltrate. This is confirmed by the effects of drugs that influence sodium transport (such as acetazolamide) on CSF composition and rate of formation. The total volume is approximately 130 ml in the adult, with a daily production of approximately 150 ml, although this may decrease when the pressure is high, and increase up to threefold should the volume be low. Spinal CSF accounts for about 35 ml of the total, the majority being in the area of the cauda equina. CSF formation varies linearly with serum osmolality, decreasing when this is increased.

After secretion the fluid passes from the lateral ventricles into the third and then fourth ventricles through the interventricular foramen of Munro and the aqueduct of Sylvius respectively. It reaches the cisterna magna and cerebral subarachnoid space through the foramina of Luschka and Magendie (Fig. 9.9). Most flows upwards over the brain to be reabsorbed through the arachnoid villi (herniations of arachnoid mater through the dura that come to lie in contact with the vascular endothelium) into the superior sagittal and transverse sinuses and other sinuses to a lesser extent. There is very little active CSF flow within the vertebral canal, the character of the fluid being maintained by a combination of diffusion and the bulk

**Table 9.1** Constituents of cerebrospinal fluid (CSF) and plasma

| Constituent | CSF | Plasma |
|---|---|---|
| H$^+$ mmol l$^{-1}$ | 32–36 | 36–44 |
| Na$^+$ mmol l$^{-1}$ | 140 | 142 |
| Cl$^-$ mmol l$^{-1}$ | 115 | 98 |
| K$^+$ mmol l$^{-1}$ | 2.9 | 4.5 |
| Urea mmol l$^{-1}$ | 5.0 | 5.0 |
| Glucose mmol l$^{-1}$ | 4.5 | 5.0 |
| HCO$_3^-$ mmol l$^{-1}$ | 22 | 25 |
| Ca$^{2+}$ mmol l$^{-1}$ | 1.2 | 2.3 |
| Mg$^{2+}$ mmol l$^{-1}$ | 1.0 | 0.8 |
| Protein mg ml$^{-1}$ | 20–40 | 6000–8000 |

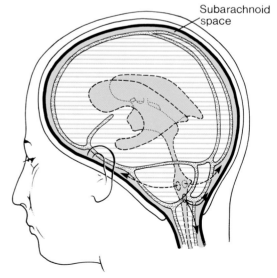

**Fig 9.9** Circulation of CSF. The arrows show the movement of CSF through the foramina of Lushka and Magendie

flow produced by alterations in posture. Most of the spinal CSF returns to the cranial cavity, but some is absorbed by the arachnoid granulations in the dural cuffs (see above). Normal pressure in the lumbar region is 60–100 mmH$_2$O in the lateral position and 200–250 mmH$_2$O when sitting, and it oscillates in time with both arterial pulsation and respiration. Respiration can cause pressure changes of up to 30 mmH$_2$O (a decrease with inspiration, an increase with expiration), while the arterial waves may have an amplitude of 2–15 mmH$_2$O (Usubiaga et al 1967a). These pressure variations are consistent throughout the CSF, unlike the situation in the epidural space (see below).

## Epidural pressure

The presence of a subatmospheric pressure in the epidural space was first reported in 1926 (Janzen 1926), and the 'hanging drop' sign as a method of utilising this pressure to identify the space, in 1932 (Gutierrez 1933). Pressure as low as −10 cm H$_2$O on deep inspiration (Bryce-Smith 1950, Usubiaga et al 1967b) has been recorded in the upper and middle thoracic regions where it is due largely to transmission of the negative intrathoracic pressure through the intervertebral foramina. Pressure increases with distance from the thorax so that it is least negative (if negative at all) in the lumbar and sacral regions (Usubiaga et al 1967a, b). The negative pressure in the thoracic and cervical regions is enhanced when sitting and when the spine is flexed (Usubiaga et al 1967a) whereas in chronic obstructive airways disease it may cease to be negative. Coughing and the Valsalva manoeuvre have been shown to increase the epidural pressure in all regions (Usubiaga et al 1967a, b)

Cyclical variations in epidural pressure have been demonstrated. Small pressure waves, synchronous with arterial pulsation, are found in the thoracic and cervical regions, but less consistently in lumbar pressure traces and never in sacral recordings. Larger amplitude pressure variations, synchronous with respiration, also occur. In the cervical and thoracic regions, pressure decreases with inspiration and increases with expiration, whereas in the lumbar region the reverse is found. This is unlike the pattern of pressure changes in CSF discussed above. These respiratory patterns are also found in the superior and inferior venae cavae respectively (Usubiaga et al 1967a). When the pressure in each venous system is elevated independently, for example by the Queckenstedt manoeuvre or abdominal compression, epidural pressure changes are largely confined to the adjoining space. A Valsalva manoeuvre or cough results in increased epidural pressure except in the sacral region. These observations led to the conclusion that the epidural space has three functional compartments: (a) cervicothoracic, which is the largest, and is influenced by pressure changes in the superior vena cava; (b) the lumbar, which is influenced by intra-abdominal pressure; and (c) the sacral canal, which has no negative pressure, no pressure oscillations and does not respond to abdominal compression. It is thought (Usubiaga et al 1967a) that the lipid tissues of the epidural space serve to isolate the regions (Hogan 1996, Hirabayashi et al 1997), allowing them to reflect the pressure changes in the cavities with which they communicate most directly.

During pregnancy there is an increase in intra-abdominal pressure, and consequent venous engorgement of the epidural space results in an increase in baseline epidural pressure, especially during uterine contractions, such that a negative pressure in the epidural space can no longer be demonstrated (Usubiaga et al 1967b). This pressure increase is more marked when the patient is supine during the second stage of labour (Galbert & Marx 1974).

## References

Atkinson RS, Rushman GB, Lee JA 1987 Spinal analgesia: intradural; epidural. A synopsis of anaesthesia, 10th edn, pp 662–721. John Wright, Bristol

Blomberg R 1986 The dorsomedian connective tissue band in the lumbar epidural space of humans: an anatomical study using epiduroscopy in autopsy cases. Anesthesia and Analgesia 65: 747–752

Bryce-Smith R 1950 Pressures in the extra-dural space. Anaesthesia 5: 213–216

Cousins MJ, Bromage PR 1988 Epidural neural blockade. In: Cousins MJ, Bridenbaugh PO. Neural blockade in clinical anesthesia and management of pain, 2nd edn, pp 253–360. Lippincott, Philadelphia

Di Chiro G, Timins EL 1974 Spinal myelography and the septum posticum. Radiology 111: 319–327

Galbert MW, Marx GF 1974 Extradural pressures in the parturient patient. Anesthesiology 40: 499–502

Gutierrez A 1933 Valor de la aspiracion liquida en el espacio peridural en la anestesia peridural. Revue Circulation, Buenos Aires 12: 225

Harrison GR, Parkin IG, Shah JL 1985 Resin injection of the lumbar extradural space. British Journal of Anaesthesia 57: 333–336

Hirabayashi Y, Saitoh K, Fukuda H, Igarashi T, Shimizu R, Seo N 1997 Magnetic resonance imaging of the extradural space of the thoracic spine. British Journal of Anaesthesia 79: 563–566

Hogan QH 1991 Lumbar epidural anatomy. A new look by cryomicrotome section. Anesthesiology 75: 767–775

Hogan QH 1996 Epidural anatomy examined by cryomicrotome section. Regional Anesthesia 21: 395–406

Janzen E 1926 Der negative vorschlag bei lumbalpunktion. Deutsche Z Nerven Heilk 94: 280–292

Igarashi T, Hirabayashi Y, Shimizu R, Saitoh K, Fukuda H, Mitsuhata H 1997 The lumbar extradural structure changes with increasing age. British Journal of Anaesthesia 78: 149–152

Igarashi T, Hirabayashi Y, Shimizu R, Saitoh K, Fukuda H 1998 Thoracic and lumbar extradural structure examined by extraduroscope. British Journal of Anaesthesia 81: 121–125

Luyendijk W.1963 Canalography. Journal Belge de Radiologie 46: 236–254

Luyendijk W 1976 The plica mediana dorsalis of the dura mater and its relation to lumbar peridurography. Neuroradiology 11: 147–149

Luyendijk W, Van Voorthuisen AE 1966 Contrast examination of the spinal epidural space. Acta Scandinavica Radiologica 5:105–166

Nauta HJE, Dolan E, Yasargil MG 1983 Microsurgical anatomy of the spinal subarachnoid space. Surgical Neurology 19: 431–437

Richardson MG, Wissler RN 1996 Density of lumbar cerebrospinal fluid in pregnant and nonpregnant humans. Anesthesiology 85: 326–330

Savolaine ER, Pandaya JB, Greenblatt SH, Conover SR 1988 Anatomy of the human lumbar epidural space: new insights using CT-Epidurography. Anesthesiology 68: 217–220

Usubiaga JE, Moya F, Usubiaga LE 1967a Effect of thoracic and abdominal pressure changes on the epidural space pressure. British Journal of Anaesthesia 39: 612–618

Usubiaga JE, Wikinski JA, Usubiaga LE 1967b Epidural pressure and its relation to spread of anesthetic solutions in the epidural space. Anesthesia and Analgesia 46: 440–446

Westbrook JL, Renowden SA, Carrie LES 1993 A study of the anatomy of the extradural region using magnetic resonance imaging. British Journal of Anaesthesia 71: 495–498

# 10. Spinal anaesthesia

## A P Rubin

Spinal anaesthesia is induced by the injection of local anaesthetic into the subarachnoid space. This route is also used for the co-administration of other drugs, such as opioids, to produce more prolonged pain control. It has the particular advantages that it is a very simple method and that only very small doses of drugs produce profound effects. Thus systemic toxicity is very unlikely to be a problem.

The popularity of the technique has waxed and waned since its introduction by August Bier in 1898. Widespread use in the 1930s and 1940s was followed by a decline in the 1950s and 1960s, coinciding with improvements in general anaesthetic techniques (notably the introduction of the neuromuscular blocking drugs) and the adverse publicity regarding neurological sequelae in the Woolley and Roe case (Cope 1954, Hutter 1990). Over the last two decades, the technique has regained a significant place in anaesthetic practice, so that it may be used in all age groups from premature neonates to the most elderly, and in a wide range of clinical situations.

Lumbar puncture should be performed below the termination of the spinal cord, which is at or about $L_1$ in the adult, the subarachnoid space ending at the level of the second sacral vertebra (Ch. 9). The tough dura mater and flimsy arachnoid are closely applied to each other, but there remains a potential (subdural) space between them. If the whole bevel of the spinal needle is not within the subarachnoid space, some of the solution may be deposited within the subdural space and this can account for some failures. The posterior subarachnoid space contains several membranous structures (see Fig. 9.7) and, in the lumbar region particularly, the septicum posticum may be well developed. These structures can lead to maldistribution of solutions, and account not only for failure to achieve adequate block, but also for neurotoxicity and the development of the cauda equina syndrome.

The site of action is primarily the nerve roots, but the dorsal root ganglia and the superficial parts of the cord may be affected also (Greene & Brull 1993). Differential effects may result in wide differences in the rostral levels of different types of block: up to seven segments between sympathetic and sensory block (Chamberlain & Chamberlain 1986), and 2.5 segments between sensory and motor block (Freund et al 1967).

## INDICATIONS AND CONTRAINDICATIONS

Spinal anaesthesia is restricted largely to operations performed below the level of the umbilicus. The likely duration of surgery is important, because spinal anaesthesia will not regularly produce surgical anaesthesia for longer than 2–3 hours unless a continuous method is used. It is particularly indicated for older and some poor-risk patients, such as those suffering from chronic respiratory, diffuse hepatic and renal disease, diabetes mellitus and some forms of cardiovascular disease. The higher the sensory block, the more extensive will be the sympathetic block and the greater the degree of vasodilatation produced. Sympathetic block, with reduced afterload and cardiac work, may be beneficial in patients with congestive cardiac failure or ischaemic heart disease, but reduced perfusion pressure could be disastrous in a patient with a fixed cardiac output (Ch. 7).

The advantages and disadvantages to the individual patient must be balanced, and only when the risks outweigh the benefits is the technique contraindicated. Many of the contraindications to spinal anaesthesia apply equally to other forms of regional block (Ch. 2 & 7). These include anticoagulant therapy and other coagulation disorders, refusal by the patient, disease or

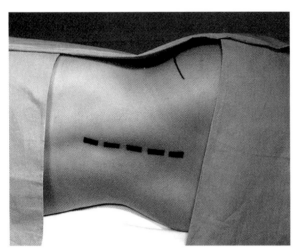

**Fig 10.1** Position for lumbar puncture in the lateral horizontal position. The hips and shoulders are vertical to eliminate rotation. A sandbag has been placed beneath the patient's loin to prevent lateral curvature of the spine

in day-care surgery, particularly the discharge criteria, are considered in Chapter 22.

## TECHNIQUE OF LUMBAR PUNCTURE

The patient should be on a firm surface on a tilting table or trolley. Intravenous access must be established, and oxygen saturation, blood pressure and ECG monitored. Resuscitation equipment must be available and checked. An understanding of the anatomy of the spine and a scrupulous aseptic technique are essential.

## Position

In choosing the position for lumbar puncture, various factors should be considered, notably the patient's general condition, level of sedation, girth, spinal anatomy and the baricity of the solution to be used.

### Lateral horizontal position (Fig. 10.1)

This is the usual position because it is easily adopted and maintained, and is easier in less co-operative or sedated patients. The patient is placed in the lateral position, with the back vertical and level with the edge of the trolley. It is very important to avoid rotation of the spine by ensuring that both hips and shoulders remain vertical. Maximum flexion of the lumbar spine, produced by flexing the legs acutely at the hips and knees, is essential to open the spaces between the spines and laminae in order to facilitate the passage of the needle through the ligaments and into the vertebral canal. The needle entering in the midline will continue in the midline if it is kept at right angles to the back and parallel to the top of the trolley.

### Sitting position (Fig. 10.2)

This position is helpful in the obese patient and in others in whom the spines are difficult to palpate, because it may be easier to identify the midline and assess the angles. However, it may be more dangerous in the sedated or anxious patient because vasovagal effects or pooling of blood in the lower limbs may precipitate a sudden bradycardia with marked hypotension.

The patient is placed with the buttocks near to the edge of the trolley, and the legs over the opposite side with feet supported on a stool. The patient rests the elbows on the thighs, or folds the arms forwards over pillows, to flex the spine. An assistant should support

severe deformity of the spinal column, active neurological disease, localised or systemic infection, severe hypovolaemia and other forms of shock. Lumbar puncture is contraindicated in the presence of raised intracranial pressure because it may lead to escape of CSF and coning of the brain stem. A history of headache does not contraindicate spinal anaesthesia, but may give rise to diagnostic difficulty in the postoperative period.

For many years, day-care surgery was thought to be a contraindication to spinal anaesthesia because of the risks of postdural puncture headache (PDPH). However, a wider range of day-care surgery is now performed on patients who are increasingly elderly, and the balance of risk has changed. The use of fine gauge, pencil point needles has reduced the incidence of PDPH to an acceptable level (Halpern & Preston 1994), and techniques with lidocaine, prilocaine or low dose bupivacaine have been advocated (Mulroy & Wills 1995). They provide rapid onset, reliable effects and similar discharge rates as general anaesthesia, but without residual sedation or the higher incidence of nausea and vomiting. There may be some uncertainty about the adequacy of duration of effect with both the short-acting agents and low-dose bupivacaine/ropivacaine (Mulroy & Wills 1995, Tarkkila et al 1997, Liam et al 1998, Gautier et al 1999). Therefore some clinicians favour the combined spinal–epidural (CSE) technique (see below) to increase flexibility (Urmey et al 1995). The general aspects of regional anaesthesia

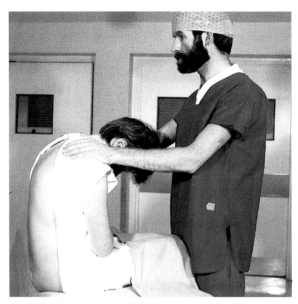

**Fig 10.2** Position for lumbar puncture in the sitting position

the patient from the front and ensure that the patient remains vertical when viewed in the sagittal plane.

## The midline approach (Fig. 10.3)

The midline approach is recommended because the angles are easier to identify, and the ligaments are less sensitive than the paraspinal muscles. A line drawn between the highest points of the iliac crests (Tuffier's line) will usually cross the spine at the level of the fourth lumbar spine, although this line may be as high as the third lumbar spine or as low as the $L_5/S_1$ interspace (Broadbent et al 2000, Reynolds 2000). Other vertebral levels may be identified from this line. Because the spinal cord ends at approximately the first lumbar interspace in the adult, the needle is usually inserted below this level. The widest appropriate interspace is usually selected, although the intended area of block may influence the choice because a higher level of injection will usually result in greater spread (Tuominen et al 1989).

The area is prepared carefully with antiseptic, which should be allowed to dry to allow time for it to be effective and to eliminate any risk of it being carried into the epidural or subarachnoid spaces. Sterile drapes are applied over a wide area to allow palpation of the relevant spines and iliac crests without compromising

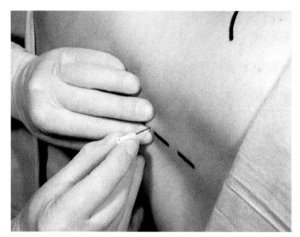

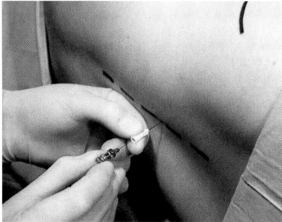

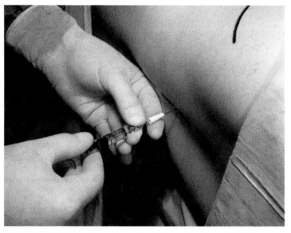

**Fig 10.3** Midline insertion of a 25 g spinal needle. The fingers of the left hand straddle the spine as an introducer needle is inserted into the supraspinous ligament with a very slight cephalad angulation. The guide needle is then held steady and the spinal needle passed through it. Once the dura has been punctured, the spinal needle assembly is immobilised between thumb and fingers and a syringe attached

the aseptic technique. Local anaesthetic for infiltration of the skin and subcutaneous tissues is drawn up into one syringe, and the exact volume of solution for the spinal injection drawn into a different size syringe to avoid confusion. It is essential that the preliminary infiltration includes the dermis as well as the subcutaneous tissues and the deeper ligaments. The index and middle fingers of the non-dominant hand are placed on either side of the midline so that only the spines, supraspinous ligament and interspace remain between the fingers to ensure that the infiltration is made in the midline. Sufficient local anaesthetic should be injected to allow painless insertion of the introducer and spinal needle, but not to obscure the bony landmarks of the interspace. Care should be taken to ensure that the spinal needle passes through the anaesthetised area by keeping the 'straddling' fingers in place throughout.

## Lateral and paramedian approaches

Both these approaches involve insertion of the needle about a centimetre from the midline. In the *lateral approach*, the needle is inserted lateral to the midpoint of the interspace, and is angled medially only. In the *paramedian approach*, the needle is inserted about 2 cm caudal and 1 cm lateral to the selected interspace, and the needle has cephalad as well as medial angulation. These approaches may be used if there is little space in the midline, the ligaments are calcified, or the anaesthetist prefers one of them. It is important to recognise that these approaches are only lateral or paramedian at the skin because the angulation of the needle ensures that it still enters the vertebral canal in the midline. Determining the precise angles required makes these approaches more difficult to understand and practise. The paramedian approach is considered further in Chapter 11.

## Spinal needles (Fig. 10.4)

Spinal needles are usually 9 cm long, and should have a close-fitting stilette, a smooth lining and a transparent hub, so that the flow of cerebrospinal fluid (CSF) is fast and can be identified quickly. The needle should produce minimal trauma and the smallest hole in the dura mater. The tip may be cutting (Quincke) or pencil point (Sprotte, Whitacre), but most practitioners now use a fine gauge pencil point needle to reduce the incidence of postdural puncture headache (Halpern &

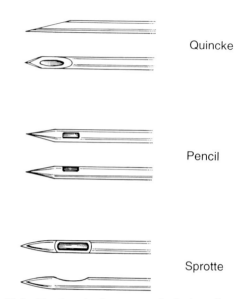

Quincke

Pencil

Sprotte

**Fig 10.4** The three basic patterns of spinal needles

Preston 1994, Hoskin 1998). Needles smaller than 27 g are difficult to use in practice, and may result in repeated attempts to identify CSF. The bevel or orifice of the spinal needle should be short to prevent partial injection into other spaces such as the subdural or epidural spaces (Crone & Vogel 1991).

### Needle insertion

A fine needle (24 g or finer) should be inserted through an 'introducer needle' to avoid bacterial contamination from the skin, implantation of skin into the deeper structures, and to act as a guide to keep the needle on the desired path. Most modern disposable sets include a suitable introducer, which should be short to avoid traversing the ligaments completely. The needle with stilette in place, and the bevel facing laterally if it has a Quincke tip, is inserted through the introducer needle. It is advanced at right angles to the back or in a slightly cephalad direction, because the interlaminar space may be at a slight cephalad angle to the interspinous space, especially in the older patient. If the needle leaves the midline, it enters the paraspinal muscles and will tend to drop rather than be gripped and held by the midline ligaments. Once this 'grip' is identified, the midline position and the degree of cephalad angulation should be confirmed, and the needle advanced further.

The tissues between the skin and the subarachnoid space offer different degrees of resistance to the passage of a needle, and the anaesthetist should use this feature to try to identify the different layers as the needle is inserted. The increasing resistance of the ligamentum flavum is usually recognised, as is a loss of resistance as the needle enters the epidural space. Insertion of the needle should be gentle and unhurried at all times, but especially so once the epidural space has been entered. At this point, the anaesthetist should ease the needle forward a millimetre at a time, rather than actively pushing it. It is almost a case of allowing the patient to 'breathe' him or herself on to the needle. After each small advance of the needle the stilette is removed so that CSF is identified as soon as the dura and arachnoid have been penetrated. A further loss of resistance, more often appreciated as a slight 'pop' or 'click', is usually noticed as the tip of the needle enters the subarachnoid space.

If bone is contacted, this is likely to be the lamina of the vertebra. The anaesthetist should check first that the spine is not rotated and remains fully flexed, and then that the needle direction is correct. If these checks do not produce success the needle should be withdrawn and reinserted, usually in a more cephalad direction.

### Use of 22 g needles

Many practitioners have now abandoned the use of the relatively large 22 g needle, but it has a place in the more difficult punctures, especially in the elderly. It is relatively rigid and an introducer is not required. However, a cutting needle should be used to puncture the skin first and care should be taken that the needle does not bend or deviate from the midline. The needle, if it has a Quincke tip, should pierce the dura with the bevel facing laterally to reduce the incidence of PDPH (Mihic 1985, Norris et al 1989). The advantage of the Quincke tip is that CSF is identified as soon as it enters the subarachnoid space and multi-compartment injection, paraesthesiae and neural trauma are less likely.

## Confirmation of dural puncture

The correct position of the needle is confirmed by free flow of CSF when the stilette is withdrawn. It will be slow with fine needles and occasionally slight rotation of the spinal needle may be required. If the fluid is blood stained, time must be allowed for it to clear before injecting the solution. If it does not clear quickly, another puncture should be made. Once there is a free flow of clear CSF, the syringe containing the spinal solution is carefully attached. The hub of the spinal needle should be firmly gripped to prevent displacement during the entire procedure. A small quantity of CSF is aspirated to ensure that the needle tip is still in the subarachnoid space and the solution injected at a rate of about 1 ml 5 s$^{-1}$. Some anaesthetists perform a further aspiration halfway through the injection, but care must be taken not to displace the needle tip. A final aspiration may be performed at the end, to confirm that all the solution has been deposited into the subarachnoid space. This final aspirate must be reinjected because it contains a high concentration of local anaesthetic. The needles are withdrawn carefully, an adhesive plaster or plastic spray is applied to the puncture site, and the patient placed in the desired position to ensure appropriate spread of solution.

## FACTORS AFFECTING THE SPREAD OF SPINAL ANAESTHESIA

Three groups of factors (the physical features of the solution, the technique of injection and the characteristics of the patient) influence intrathecal drug spread (Greene & Brull 1993). The most important factors, in order of clinical importance, are:

1. the relationship between patient posture and the baricity of the solution;
2. the level of injection;
3. the dose, volume and speed of injection.

Ideally, the spread of spinal anaesthesia should be predictable and controllable. However, there is considerable variation between patients in the spread achieved by a particular technique. Since the pioneering work of Barker (1907), it has been thought that the spread of solution in the subarachnoid space depends mainly on its baricity in relation to CSF, and the posture of the patient. There has been a firm belief that further spread could be achieved by increasing the volume injected, and that the curves of the spinal column might be used to limit spread. However, these concepts have been questioned and have been the subject of much recent clinical research and are reviewed below (Stienstra & Veering 1998).

### Posture and baricity

It is vital to use the correct definitions when considering spinal anaesthesia.

- *Density* of a liquid is its weight per unit volume.
- *Specific gravity* of a liquid is the ratio of its density relative to that of water. Both density and specific

gravity are temperature dependent, and the temperature at which the measurements are made should be quoted.

- *Baricity* of a liquid is the ratio of its density relative to that of CSF at 37 °C.

The specific gravity of CSF is 1.006–1.008, taking water as 1.000 at 25 °C. It decreases 0.001 for each 5° rise in temperature, so that at 37 °C it is usually 1.004–1.006. Any injected solution reaches body temperature within 60 seconds and it is the specific gravity at body temperature that determines baricity. Thus a solution of specific gravity greater than 1.010 at 37 °C is hyperbaric, and one less than 1.000 at 37 °C is hypobaric. Between these two values, solutions can be considered to be isobaric. Hyperbaric solutions are made by the addition of up to 10% glucose, giving a specific gravity of 1.020–1.030. Osmolality may be important and the osmolality of CSF at 37 °C is about 280 mOsm. The ideal spinal solution would be isotonic, but some are hypertonic. Any potential hazardous effect is decreased by the immediate dilution of the solution by the CSF.

A spinal anaesthetic solution may continue to spread under the influence of gravity for as long as 30 minutes after injection. This means that using posture to control spread is not a straightforward issue and anaesthetists should be aware of the relationship between posture and baricity with each solution used (Wildsmith et al 1981).

Glucose-free bupivacaine acts at body temperature as a hypobaric solution so that injections in the sitting position will spread two or three segments higher than when injected in the lateral position (Kalso et al 1982). Hyperbaric solutions produce blocks which are influenced by posture initially. Thus the block may be limited in spread while the patient is kept in the sitting or lateral position, but once the patient is placed supine, the block may spread upwards or to the other side.

Solutions are usually made hyperbaric by the addition of 5–8% glucose, but there is evidence that as little as 0.8% may be sufficient (Bannister et al 1990, Sanderson et al 1994). This concentration may be achieved by adding 1 ml of 0.5% bupivacaine with 8% glucose to 9 ml of the glucose-free solution and mixing well. The glucose may act in part by 'holding' the solution together, making it more viscous, so decreasing its tendency to diffuse into, and be diluted by, the CSF. Thus a more concentrated bolus of local anaesthetic moves through the CSF.

When equal volumes of solution are injected in supine patients, hyperbaric solutions spread higher than isobaric or hypobaric ones (Chambers et al 1981a). Plain (glucose-free) local anaesthetic solutions are less predictable and their use should be restricted to patients having surgery of the lower limb and perineum (Logan et al 1986).

## Level of injection

The level of injection plays some role in determining the height of block achieved by a given solution. The standard level of injection is $L_3/L_4$. Moving above or below this level will result in more extensive or restricted blocks respectively. With a higher level of injection there is greater bulk spread along the narrow channel between the spinal cord and dura. With a lower level injection the solution may be trapped below the apex of the lumbar curve, especially with a hyperbaric solution.

## Effect of dose, volume and speed of injection

Dose rather than volume or concentration seems to be the most important. Clearly there is a critical dose below which minimal block is achieved. Equally, the accidental subarachnoid injection of a 'full' epidural dose will produce a total spinal block. However, there is not a direct correlation between dose administered and final level of block. Within the range normally used for spinal anaesthesia the amount of drug injected has little effect on the spread of block. Increasing the dose has a more important effect on the quality and duration of block.

Slow injections (1 ml 10 s$^{-1}$ or less) tend to produce more predictable spread, while more rapid injections are like barbotage (repeated aspiration and injection of CSF with the local anaesthetic) and decrease predictability (McClure et al 1982).

## FACTORS AFFECTING THE DURATION OF SPINAL ANAESTHESIA

After injection the block produced ascends progressively to its maximal spread over 20 to 30 minutes. Regression then proceeds from above downwards and the rate of regression depends on:

- individual drug properties
- the dose injected
- the total spread achieved
- the use of adjuvants
  - vasoconstrictors
  - opioids
  - clonidine
- the general condition of the patient.

## Individual drug properties

Ideally, a range of drugs with different durations should be available, but commercial factors and licensing regulations limit choice. In the UK at present, only hyperbaric bupivacaine and plain levobupivacaine are licensed for intrathecal use, but the plain solutions of bupivacaine (0.5% and 0.75%) are used widely. The duration of surgical anaesthesia produced ranges from 1 to 3 hours, depending on other related factors (see below). A shorter duration of action may be achieved using lidocaine in either plain or hyperbaric solution. In other countries, mepivacaine (intermediate duration) and tetracaine (long duration) are also used. The density of the solution also influences duration (Concepcion 1989). At low segmental levels the longest duration follows the use of glucose-free bupivacaine (Cummings et al 1984).

Ropivacaine is undergoing preliminary evaluation as a spinal anaesthetic and produces a shorter duration of action than bupivacaine (Gautier et al 1999, McDonald et al 1999).

## Dose

Larger doses will increase the duration of action – an effect which is useful for long operations. Increasing the dose by 50% will extend the duration at $T_{12}$ by about 50% (Wildsmith & Rocco 1985).

## Spread

The greater the spread achieved with a given dose of drug, the shorter will be the duration of action. A drug limited to a small segmental area will last longer because the concentration in each of the nerves which it has reached will be higher.

## Adjuvants

### Vasoconstrictors

Both epinephrine (0.1–0.2 mg ≡ 0.1–0.2 ml of 1 in 1000 solution) and phenylephrine (1 mg) constrict dural

and spinal cord blood vessels, and inhibit nociception (Concepcion et al 1984). These actions may increase duration, but the effects are neither consistent nor reliable (Chambers et al 1981b, 1982). Manipulation of dose is a more reliable way of influencing duration.

### Opioids

Opioids inhibit pain transmission in the dorsal horn. A small dose of fentanyl (12.5–25 µg), sufentanil (2.5–5 µg) or morphine (0.2 mg) added to local anaesthetic exerts a synergistic action and prolongs duration of analgesia (Kalso 1983, Dahlgren et al 1997). There may also be more rapid onset and more profound block with the addition of an opioid, but their use introduces the risk of respiratory depression in the postoperative period.

### Clonidine

Clonidine is a selective $\alpha_2$-adrenergic agonist which acts on receptors in the dorsal horn and also affects neural transmission. Doses of 75–150 µg will prolong the block (Racle et al 1987, Fogarty et al 1993).

## General physical condition

It is likely that spread will be greater and duration of action prolonged in patients in poor physical condition. In addition, the cardiovascular effects may be greater. Neither the age of the patient (Pitkanen et al 1984) nor the pH of the CSF (Park et al 1975) seems to affect spread.

## ACHIEVING THE DESIRED BLOCK (Fig. 10.5)

'*The anaesthetist should never forget the capricious nature of spinal analgesia*' (Lee 1984).

Although the factors which affect spread and duration of spinal block have been identified in studies of groups of patients, there is still considerable variation of the effect obtained among individual patients. Thus, the minimum and maximum effects are more important than the mean effect when choosing a particular technique. The minimum effect will determine the clinical utility of the technique, while the maximum effect will determine the risk of complications, especially hypotension. Therefore a technique should be chosen to give the best chance of achieving adequate block for the proposed surgery, without the risk of unnecessary spread to the upper thoracic sympathetic outflow.

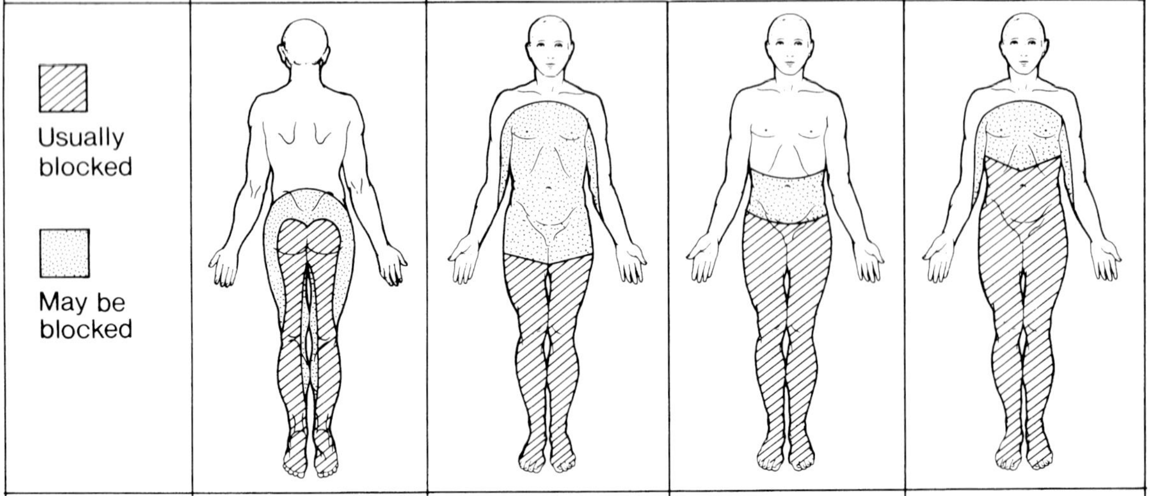

| | Saddle block | Upper lumbar blocks | | Mid-thoracic block |
|---|---|---|---|---|
| [hatched square] Usually blocked [dotted square] May be blocked | | | | |
| SOLUTION | Any hyperbaric | Plain bupivacaine | Plain amethocaine | Any hyperbaric |
| VOLUME (ml) | 1 | 3 | 2 | 2-3 |
| POSTURE | Sitting for 5 min | Patient placed supine after injection | | |

**Fig 10.5** Techniques of spinal anaesthesia

## Mid-thoracic block

For all lower abdominal surgery, including herniorrhaphy, a block to the mid-thoracic level is desirable, and a hyperbaric solution is preferred. Hyperbaric bupivacaine (2.5–3 ml) may be injected in the lateral position and the patient turned supine immediately afterwards. Very often this solution results in a high thoracic block which is more extensive than is needed. This reflects the effect of the high concentration of glucose on the movement of drug within CSF. The use of lower concentrations of glucose (0.8–1%) will result in blocks which are adequate for lower abdominal surgery, but do not have the same risk of spreading to the upper thoracic sympathetic outflow (Bannister et al 1990, Sanderson et al 1994).

## Upper lumbar block

For blocks up to $L_1$, 3–4 ml of glucose-free solution is usually sufficient whichever posture is used. This is particularly advantageous if patients have a painful condition such as fractured neck of femur, because they do not have to lie on the painful side during administration of the spinal. However, glucose-free solutions are unpredictable, and on occasion the block may not reach $L_1$. Injection at $L_2/L_3$ will reduce this risk, but will increase the possibility of spread to the cervical region (Logan et al 1986). A truly isobaric solution is not associated with these risks (Fig. 10.5).

## Saddle (perineal) block

When the maximum height of block required is $S_1$, 1–2 ml of hyperbaric solution may be injected in the sitting position, which should be maintained for at least 5 minutes. A risk of the sitting position is venous pooling with decreases in venous return, cardiac output and blood pressure. In addition, the hip joint will not be blocked and this may lead to discomfort if the patient is placed in the lithotomy position. Alternatively, 2–3 ml of plain solution may be administered to the supine patient, but this can produce a much higher level of block than is required for perineal surgery.

## Unilateral block

True unilateral spinal anaesthesia is probably impossible to achieve, owing to the proximity of the spinal roots of both sides within the theca. However, with careful manipulation of both posture and the baricity of the injected solution, together with a slow injection through a pencil point needle with a lateral orifice, it is possible to achieve a block predominantly on one side of the lower half of the body. This results in greater haemo-dynamic stability, and the duration of anaesthesia on one side greatly exceeds that on the other.

The technique essentially involves using a low dose of local anaesthetic (e.g. 1.6 ml of 0.5% hyperbaric bupivacaine) given over 30 seconds through a pencil point needle with the lateral orifice pointing towards the dependant side. The patient must remain on the dependant side for 30 minutes (Pittoni et al 1995), and the delay may not be worth the minimal advantage, especially because the low dose injected will limit total duration.

With all these techniques, a proportion of patients will develop hypotension. Measures for its prevention, recognition and treatment must always be available (Ch. 8). A contingency plan of management in the event of the rare partial or total failure should also be made. In essence, the options are to repeat the spinal anaesthetic (probably at an adjacent space in case some local factor has limited spread), or to give a general anaesthetic instead. The choice will depend very much on the circumstances of the case.

## SPECIAL TECHNIQUES
## Continuous spinal anaesthesia

The problems of variability in extent and duration of block make catheter-based spinal anaesthesia an attractive concept (Denny & Selander 1998). It allows the repeated injection of small doses of local anaesthetic to be titrated to the desired effect, but use of the method has been inhibited by fears of a high incidence of paraesthesiae, neurological complications and PDPH.

Interest was rekindled in the 1980s with the advent of 28 and 32 g microcatheters (Hurley & Lambert 1990), but reports of cauda equina syndrome (CES) (Rigler et al 1991), possibly associated with pooling of highly concentrated, hyperbaric local anaesthetic in the sacral segments, inhibited the initial enthusiasm. These microcatheters are technically difficult to use, and the

direction the catheter takes in the subarachnoid space is unpredictable. The inevitable slow injection prevents turbulence and decreases mixing of the local anaesthetic with CSF. All of these factors make for a very variable extent of block.

Larger catheters, such as 20–24 g, continue to be used by some enthusiasts, especially for elderly and poor-risk patients in whom slow titration of local anaesthetic is desirable. The reported failure rates average 2.5%. A 'catheter-over-needle' design system is available (in two sizes: 22 g over 27 g, and 24 g over 29 g). A thin wire is attached to the stilette, and it protrudes from the injection end of the catheter so that the stilette can be withdrawn once CSF is identified in the catheter. It has the advantage that the hole in the dura is the same size as the catheter (De Andres 1997, Denny & Selander 1998).

Continuous spinal anaesthesia is very much a technique for the experienced practitioner. Its safety and efficacy may be enhanced by using the larger sized systems, using a paramedian approach to ensure cephalad direction for the catheter, only inserting the minimum necessary length of catheter, and using plain solutions of local anaesthetic in the first instance. The headache rate may be less than 1% in very experienced hands (Denny et al 1987, Mahisekar et al 1991).

## Combined spinal epidural block

Recognition of the potential advantages of continuous spinal anaesthesia, but with concerns about its efficacy and safety confirmed, led to the development of systems for combining spinal and epidural block. A spinal needle may be inserted through a Tuohy needle until it enters the CSF, an appropriate subarachnoid dose of local anaesthetic injected, the spinal needle removed, and then a catheter passed into the epidural space. The technique is said to have the advantages inherent in spinal anaesthesia, that is, rapid onset and high quality anaesthesia, together with the flexibility of use of an epidural catheter. This gives the anaesthetist the ability to titrate accurately the subsequent block level and to continue the analgesia into the postoperative period. The method is most used in obstetric practice at present (see Ch. 18).

## SIDE-EFFECTS

The technique of spinal anaesthesia is so simple that it might lead to complacency. A complete understanding of the relevant physiology and complete clinical training are essential to ensure safe management.

## Cardiovascular system

Sympathetic block results in both arteriolar dilatation and venous pooling. The sympathetic outflow extends from $T_1$ to $L_2$, and therefore the height of block determines the extent of sympathetic block, and the likely degree of hypotension. However, when venous return or the sympathetic stimulation to the heart decreases, unopposed parasympathetic overactivity may lead to sudden bradycardia, hypotension, a decrease in cardiac output, and even asystole. This can occur with relatively restricted blocks and is more likely in patients who are awake, or those who are hypovolaemic, have aortocaval compression, or are excessively sedated (Caplan et al 1988). Unlike epidural block, the mass of local anaesthetic or vasoconstrictor absorbed is too small to modify the cardiovascular changes. The prevention and treatment of hypotension have been discussed in Chapter 8, but the benefits of maintaining venous return by keeping the patient in a slight head-down tilt should not be forgotten. This does not result in a significant extension of block height.

## Respiratory system

Spinal anaesthesia is unlikely to affect resting ventilation or produce changes in blood gases. However, if the block is very high, there may be a 20% decrease in inspiratory capacity, and a marked reduction in expiratory reserve volume. Cough strength may also be impaired (Egbert et al 1961, Freund 1969). The patient may have difficulty in taking a deep breath and may even feel dyspnoeic. Apnoea, in the absence of opioids, is rare and is usually secondary to hypotension and brainstem ischaemia, but if the block reaches the upper cervical level, it may be caused by bilateral phrenic nerve root involvement. Management of the total spinal is discussed in Chapter 11.

## Gastrointestinal and genitourinary systems

The intestine becomes contracted, peristalsis continues and the sphincters relax. Upper abdominal and intra-peritoneal visceral stimuli, probably transmitted by un-blocked vagal afferent fibres, may be perceived as pain, and provoke nausea and vomiting (Ratra et al 1972).

Nausea and vomiting may also be an early sign of hypotension. Hepatic and renal blood flow seem to be blood pressure dependent.

Urinary retention may be a problem in males because sacral autonomic fibre function, and thus detrusor muscle contraction, are among the last functions to recover (Axellson et al 1974). It is difficult to micturate while lying supine, and the patient must stay in bed until the risk of postural hypotension has passed. Fluid preload is a potential cause of overdistension of the bladder and should be avoided unless a urinary catheter is to be inserted.

## Other effects

Blood loss is reduced and the stress response, while often incompletely blocked, may be delayed (Webster et al 1991). It is likely that the incidence of deep venous thrombosis is also reduced, and early morbidity and mortality decreased as compared to general anaesthesia (Rodgers et al 2000).

## COMPLICATIONS
## Post-dural puncture headache

Headache is a very common symptom and it must not be assumed that all headaches following spinal anaesthesia are PDPH. Aseptic and bacterial meningitis should be considered in the differential diagnosis, and a condition known as spontaneous intracranial hypotension, with similar symptoms and signs to PDPH, has been described (Weitz & Drasner 1996).

PDPH is probably due to CSF leak from the subarachnoid to the epidural space. Low CSF pressure allows descent of the brain and this stretches the dura, tentorium, venous sinuses, and dural and cerebral blood vessels, and thus the nerve endings they contain. PDPH is occipito-frontal, appears within a few days of the event, and severely incapacitates the patient. It should be mild or absent in the supine position and be aggravated by sitting up. It may be accompanied by photophobia, nausea and vomiting, neck stiffness or cranial nerve palsies.

The incidence may be reduced to less than 1%, even in the obstetric population, by using fine, pencil point needles (Halpern & Preston 1994) and avoiding multiple dural punctures (Seeberger et al 1996). The bevel should be aligned longitudinally rather than transversely to separate rather than cut dural fibres (Mihic 1985,

Norris et al 1989). It has been suggested that extreme flexion of the spine tenses the dura and increases the size of the puncture hole. Extension of the head on the neck may lessen this tension.

Age decreases the incidence of PDPH possibly because decreased elasticity of the tissues allows less stretching of intracranial structures. Dehydration from any cause results in low CSF pressure, which increases the severity of the headache. The headache usually resolves spontaneously within a few days, but may persist for long periods. It may be dangerous because rupture of a bridging vein as the brain moves away from the dura may lead to a subdural haematoma (Newrick & Read 1982). Thus effective treatment for the established case is essential.

### Management of dural puncture

All patients who have had a spinal anaesthetic must be kept well hydrated and should avoid straining. Maintenance of the supine position after lumbar puncture does not decrease the incidence although it reduces the symptoms (Kang et al 1992), and may prevent complications. Patients should be encouraged to drink freely and to use mild, non-opioid analgesics. Manoeuvres such as tight abdominal binders and assuming the prone position have been used to raise the epidural pressure, and may help to reverse the gradient and reduce the CSF leak. However, they are largely historical. Caffeine 300–500 mg, given intravenously or as several cups of coffee, may relieve the symptoms (Camann et al 1990).

If the headache does not resolve within one or two days, or is very incapacitating, a dural blood patch must be considered (see Ch. 11).

## Backache

This is a common symptom and may be due to stretching of anaesthetised ligaments and joints during surgery. It is more common when the patient has been placed in the lithotomy position. The patient should be positioned carefully, and extreme postures should not be allowed while the block is effective because the protective effect of pain will have been removed.

## Neurological complications

### Local neurotoxicity
Neurological complications are extremely rare (Dripps & Vandam 1954). However, drugs which are innocuous when administered intravenously or epidurally may be neurotoxic in the subarachnoid space. It is thus essential that all drugs injected into the subarachnoid space have been shown to be safe in formal studies.

All neurological complications should be identified and investigated early by a competent neurologist with knowledge of the specific subject. The vast majority will be found to be incidental to the technique (Marinacci 1960), but they may result from the injection of inappropriate chemicals, preservatives or drugs, or from the introduction of infection. This may result in adhesive or proliferative arachnoiditis, or transverse myelitis, usually affecting the cauda equina first (CES), but often spreading higher. There may be low back pain, sphincter disturbances, sacral analgesia and perhaps some numbness and weakness of the legs. The onset is variable, and the clinical course is unpredictable with recovery uncertain.

Although the signs of damage to nerve roots are almost always due to incorrect posture, pressure or trauma during surgery, direct needle trauma may occur. Recently, Reynolds (2000, 2001) has drawn attention to a series of patients in whom the conus medullaris has been damaged by insertion at a vertebral level higher than the clinicians had assumed. She has emphasised the importance of careful identification of vertebral level, but it should be noted that all these cases involved the use of a 'pencil' point needle. Because the orifice of this needle is laterally placed, the first millimetre or two of the shaft must enter the subarachnoid space before any evidence of CSF is obtained. Also, the blunter nature of the 'pencil' point needle may lead to more precipitant entry into the subarachnoid space. Both these factors may contribute to an increased risk of cord puncture if insertion is at a level above $L_2/L_3$. Given the difficulty of identifying vertebral level with certainty in the clinical situation, these reports emphasise the need for the cautious, gentle and controlled needle insertion described earlier.

### Space-occupying lesions
If neurological features produce any suspicion of a space-occupying lesion such as a haematoma, abscess or tumour mass, a neurological opinion must be sought urgently because surgical decompression must be performed within hours. (The use of central neural block in the presence of anticoagulant therapy is discussed in Ch. 8.) Epidural abscesses are more often due to haematogenous spread than to the local introduction of infection.

### Anterior spinal artery syndrome

Interference with the vascular supply to nerves or the spinal cord may be devastating in its consequences. The classical condition is the 'anterior spinal artery syndrome', which manifests itself as a painless paralysis of the legs and sphincters due to infarction of the anterior segments of the spinal cord. The syndrome may follow periods of hypotension especially in older patients, but may also be associated with surgical interruption of the blood supply to the cord.

### Cerebral damage

Brain damage can occur due to cardiac arrest or a prolonged period of hypotension. While this is more likely with a total spinal following an intended epidural, it can occur with deliberate spinal anaesthesia (Caplan et al 1988). Careful monitoring and appropriate treat-ment of the cardiovascular and respiratory effects should prevent it.

### Transient neurological symptoms

The syndrome known as transient neurological symptoms (TNS) (formerly called transient radicular irritation) is a relatively recent concern. It seems to occur after day-care surgery particularly (Corbey & Bach 1998), and is thought to reflect musculoskeletal strain rather than neurotoxicity. TNS comprise radicular pain or dysaesthesia, which radiates to the buttocks and legs, and resolves spontaneously in a few days (Hampl et al 1995). These effects are not dependent on dose, concentration or osmolality, and seem to occur primarily after 5% hyper-baric lidocaine. However, they may, like most cases of backache after spinal anaesthesia, reflect extremes of posture more than anything else.

## References

Axellson KH, Mollefors K, Ollson JO, Lingardh G, Widman B 1974 Bladder function in spinal anaesthesia. Linkoping University Medical Dissertation, 184: v3–v21

Bannister J, McClure JH, Wildsmith JAW 1990 Effect of glucose concentration on the intrathecal spread of 0.5% bupivacaine. British Journal of Anaesthesia 64: 232–234

Barker AE 1907 A report on clinical experiences with spinal analgesia in 100 cases. British Medical Journal I: 665–674

Broadbent CR, Maxwell WB, Ferrie R, Wilson DJ, Gawne-Cain M, Russell R 2000 Ability of anaesthetists to identify a marked lumbar interspace. Anaesthesia 55: 1122–1126

Camann WR, Murray RS, Mushlin PS, Lambert DH 1990 Effects of oral caffeine on postdural puncture headache. A double-blind, placebo-controlled trial. Anesthesia and Analgesia 70: 181–184

Caplan RA, Ward RJ, Posner K, Cheney FW 1988 Unexpected cardiac arrest during spinal anesthesia: a closed claims analysis of predisposing factors. Anesthesiology 68: 5–11

Chamberlain DP, Chamberlain BD 1986 Changes in the skin temperature of the trunk and their relationship to sympathetic blockade during spinal anesthesia. Anesthesiology 65: 139–143

Chambers WA, Edstrom HH, Scott DB 1981a Effect of baricity on spinal anaesthesia with bupivacaine. British Journal of Anaesthesia 53: 279–282

Chambers WA, Littlewood DG, Logan MR, Scott DB 1981b Effect of added epinephrine on spinal anesthesia with lidocaine. Anesthesia and Analgesia 60: 417–420

Chambers WA, Littlewood DG, Scott DB 1982 Spinal anesthesia with hyperbaric bupivacaine: effect of added vasoconstrictors. Anesthesia and Analgesia 61: 49–52

Concepcion MA 1989 Spinal anesthetic agents. International Anesthesiology Clinics 27: 21–25

Concepcion MA, Maddi R, Francis D, Rocco A, Murray E, Covino BG 1984 Vasoconstrictors in spinal anesthesia with tetracaine – a comparison of epinephrine and phenylephrine. Anesthesia and Analgesia 63: 134–138

Cope RW 1954 The Woolley and Roe case: Woolley and Roe versus Ministry of Health and others. Anaesthesia 9: 249–270

Corbey MP, Bach AB 1998 Transient radicular irritation (TRI) after spinal anaesthesia in day-care surgery. Acta Anaesthesiologica Scandinavica 42: 425–429

Crone LL, Vogel W 1991 Failed spinal anaesthesia with the Sprotte needle. Anesthesiology 75: 717–718

Cummings GC, Bamber DB, Edstrom HH, Rubin AP 1984 Subarachnoid blockade with bupivacaine. A comparison with cinchocaine. British Journal of Anaesthesia 56: 573–579

Dahlgren G, Hulstrand C, Jakobsson J, Norman M, Eriksson EW, Martin H 1997 Intrathecal sufentanil, fentanyl, or placebo added to bupivacaine for cesarean section. Anesthesia and Analgesia 85: 1288–1293

De Andres J 1997 Continuous spinal anaesthesia. Current Opinion in Anaesthesiology 10: 341–344

Denny NM, Selander DE 1998 Continuous spinal anaesthesia. British Journal of Anaesthesia 81: 590–597

Denny N, Masters R, Pearson D, Read J, Sihota M, Selander D 1987 Postdural puncture headache after continuous spinal anesthesia. Anesthesia and Analgesia 66: 791–794

Dripps RD, Vandam LD 1954 Longterm follow-up of patients who received 10,098 spinal anesthetics. I: failure to discover major neurological sequelae. Journal of the American Medical Association 156: 1486–1491

Egbert LD, Tamersoy K, Deas TC 1961 Pulmonary function during spinal anesthesia: the mechanism of cough depression. Anesthesiology 22: 882–885

Fogarty DJ, Carabine UA, Milligan KR 1993 Comparison of the analgesic effects of intrathecal clonidine and intrathecal morphine after spinal anaesthesia in patients undergoing total hip replacement. British Journal of Anaesthesia 71: 661–664

Freund FG 1969 Respiratory effects of subarachnoid and epidural block. In: Bonica JJ (ed) Clinical anesthesia 2 Regional anesthesia: recent advances and current status, pp 98–107. FA Davis, Philadelphia

Freund FG, Bonica JJ, Ward RJ, Akamatsu TJ, Kennedy WF Jr 1967 Ventilatory reserve and level of motor block during high spinal and epidural anesthesia. Anesthesiology 28: 834–837

Gautier PE, De Kock M, Van Steenberge A et al 1999 Intrathecal ropivacaine for ambulatory surgery. Anesthesiology 91: 1239–1245

Greene NM, Brull SJ 1993 Physiology of spinal anesthesia, 4th edn. Williams and Wilkins, Baltimore

Halpern S, Preston R 1994 Postdural puncture headache and spinal needle design. Metaanalyses. Anesthesiology 81: 1376–1383

Hampl KF, Schneider MC, Ummenhofer W, Drewe J 1995 Transient neurologic symptoms after spinal anesthesia. Anesthesia and Analgesia 81: 1148–1153

Hoskin MF 1998 Spinal anaesthesia – the current trends towards narrow gauge atraumatic (pencil point) needles. Case reports and review. Anaesthesia and Intensive Care 26: 96–106

Hurley RJ, Lambert DH 1990 Continuous spinal anesthesia with a microcatheter technique: preliminary experience. Anesthesia and Analgesia 70: 97–102

Hutter CDD 1990 The Woolley and Roe case. A reassessment. Anaesthesia 45: 859–864

Kalso E 1983 Effects of intrathecal morphine, injected with bupivacaine, on pain after orthopaedic surgery. British Journal of Anaesthesia 55: 415–422

Kalso E, Tuominen M, Rosenberg PH 1982 Effect of posture and some c.s.f. characteristics on spinal anaesthesia with isobaric 0.5% bupivacaine. British Journal of Anaesthesia 54: 1179–1184

Kang SB, Goodnough DE, Lee YK et al 1992 Comparison of 26- and 27-g needles for spinal anesthesia for ambulatory surgery patients. Anesthesiology 76: 734–738

Lee JA 1984 Personal communication

Liam BL, Yim CF, Chong JL 1998 Dose response study of lidocaine 1% for spinal anaesthesia for lower limb and perineal surgery. Canadian Journal of Anaesthesia 45: 45–50

Logan ML, McClure JH, Wildsmith JAW 1986 Plain bupivacaine – an unpredictable agent. British Journal of Anaesthesia 58: 292–296

McClure JH, Brown DT, Wildsmith JAW 1982 Effect of injected volume and speed of injection on the spread of spinal anaesthesia with isobaric amethocaine. British Journal of Anaesthesia 54: 917–920

McDonald SB, Liu SS, Kopacz DJ, Stephenson CA 1999 Hyperbaric spinal ropivacaine: a comparison to bupivacaine in volunteers. Anesthesiology 90: 971–77

Mahisekar UL, Winnie AP, Vasireddy AR, Masters RW 1991 Continuous spinal anesthesia and post dural puncture headache. A retrospective study. Regional Anesthesia 16: 107–111

Marinacci AA 1960 Neurological aspects of complications of spinal anesthesia with medicolegal implications. Bulletin of the Los Angeles Neurological Society 24: 170–192

Mihic DN 1985 Postspinal headache and relationship of needle bevel to longitudinal dural fibres. Regional Anesthesia 10: 76–81

Mulroy MF, Wills RP 1995 Spinal anesthesia for outpatients: Appropriate agents and techniques. Journal of Clinical Anesthesia 7: 622–627

Newrick P, Read D 1982 Subdural haematoma as a complication of spinal anaesthetic. British Medical Journal 285: 341–342

Norris MC, Leighton BL, DeSimone CA 1989 Needle bevel direction and headache after inadvertent dural puncture. Anesthesiology 70: 729–731

Park WY, Balingit PE, Macnamara T E 1975 Effects of patient age, pH of cerebrospinal fluid and vasopressors on onset and duration of spinal anesthesia. Anesthesia and Analgesia 54: 455–463

Pitkanen M, Haapaniemi L, Tuominen M, Rosenberg PH 1984 Influence of age on spinal anaesthesia with isobaric 0.5% bupivacaine. British Journal of Anaesthesia 56: 279–284

Pittoni G, Toffoletto F, Cacarella G, Zanette G, Giron GP 1995 Spinal anesthesia in outpatient knee surgery: 22-gauge versus 25-gauge Sprotte needle. Anesthesia and Analgesia 81: 73–79

Racle JP, Benkhadra A, Poy JY, Gleizal B 1987 Prolongation of isobaric bupivacaine spinal anesthesia with epinephrine and clonidine for hip surgery in the elderly. Anesthesia and Analgesia 66: 442–446

Ratra CK, Badola RP, Bhargrave KP 1972 A study of factors concerned in emesis during spinal anaesthesia. British Journal of Anaesthesia 44: 1208–1211

Reynolds F 2000 Logic in the safe practice of spinal anaesthesia. Anaesthesia 55: 1045–1046

Reynolds F 2001 Damage to the conus medullaris following spinal anaesthesia. Anaesthesia 56: 238–249

Rigler ML, Drasner K, Krejcie TC et al 1991 Cauda equina syndrome after continuous spinal anesthesia. Anesthesia and Analgesia 72: 275–281

Rodgers A, Walker N, Schug S et al 2000 Reduction of post-operative mortality and morbidity with epidural or spinal anaesthesia: results from overview of randomised trials. British Medical Journal 321: 1493–1497.

Sanderson P, Read J, Littlewood DG, McKeown D, Wildsmith JAW 1994 Interaction between baricity (glucose concentration) and other factors influencing intrathecal drug spread.

British Journal of Anaesthesia 73: 744–746

Seeberger MD, Kaufmann M, Staender S, Schneider M, Scheidegger D 1996 Repeated dural punctures increase the incidence of post dural puncture headache. Anesthesia and Analgesia 82: 302–305

Stienstra R, Veering B 1998 Intrathecal drug spread: Is it controllable? Regional Anesthesia and Pain Medicine 23: 347–351

Tarkkila P, Huhtala J, Tuominen M 1997 Home-readiness after spinal anaesthesia with small doses of hyperbaric 0.5% bupivacaine. Anaesthesia 52: 1157–1160

Tuominen M, Taivainen T, Rosenberg PT 1989 Spread of spinal anaesthesia with plain 0.5% bupivacaine: Influence of vertebral interspace used for injection. British Journal of Anaesthesia 62: 358–361

Urmey WF, Stanton J, Peterson M, Sharrock NE 1995 Combined spinal–epidural anesthesia for outpatient surgery: dose–response characteristics of intrathecal isobaric lidocaine using a 27-gauge Whitacre spinal needle. Anesthesiology 83: 528–534

Webster J, Barnard M, Carli F 1991 Metabolic response to colonic surgery: extradural vs. continuous spinal. British Journal of Anaesthesia 67: 467–469

Weitz SR, Drasner K 1996 Spontaneous intracranial hypotension: a series. Anesthesiology 85: 923–925

Wildsmith JAW, Brown D 1998 (eds) Centennial spinal section issue. Regional Anesthesia and Pain Medicine 23: 333–387

Wildsmith JAW, Rocco AG 1985 Current concepts in spinal anesthesia. Regional Anesthesia 10: 117–121

Wildsmith JAW, McClure JH, Brown DT, Scott DB 1981 Effects of posture on the spread of isobaric and hyperbaric amethocaine. British Journal of Anaesthesia 53: 273–278

# 11. Lumbar and thoracic epidural block

## E N Armitage

The first epidural block was performed in the UK over 50 years ago, but only in recent years has the technique become firmly established as a substitute for, or an adjunct to, general anaesthesia for operative surgery, and for the effective control of pain in the postoperative period. Several factors have contributed to this increase in popularity.

1. Research into the physiological effects of central neural block, notably by workers in Seattle, Boston and Edinburgh, has provided a rational basis for the optimal management of epidural block and for the treatment of side-effects.
2. The long duration of action of bupivacaine has made epidural block much more practical clinically, and its recently introduced *n*-propyl homologue, ropivacaine, has the advantages of an improved safety profile and, for a given degree of sensory block, less motor impairment.
3. Appropriately sited epidural blocks can provide anaesthesia and analgesia of almost any distribution and may be used for a wide range of major surgery.
4. Placement of a catheter in the epidural space is a straightforward procedure and allows the benefits of the block to be extended into the postoperative period, provided that the anaesthetist has a sound technique based on the correct application of the basic sciences.
5. Acute pain teams are now active in all units where major surgery is performed, and their involvement in the management of postoperative epidural analgesia has improved the efficacy of the technique and facilitated the early detection and treatment of side-effects.

There are, however, disadvantages.

1. Visceral sensation remains intact, and although it is possible to block autonomic plexuses as surgery proceeds, general anaesthesia is the more practical alternative as a supplement to epidural block for major surgery of the thorax and abdomen.
2. A dermatomal 'mismatch', where the area of analgesia does not correspond to the area of surgery, may result in ineffective analgesia and unwanted side-effects.
3. To be successful for abdominal and thoracic surgery, the epidural should affect thoracic dermatomes. This, in turn, requires that the tip of the epidural catheter should lie in the thoracic region. Some anaesthetists are concerned that damage to the spinal cord may occur if the needle is inserted at this level.
4. Performance of a regional block adds to anaesthesia time, and while surgeons quickly come to appreciate the advantages of a smoothly performed and effective epidural, they are less understanding if blocks regularly disrupt the operating list, have to be abandoned, or are not fully effective.
5. Pre-existing neurological conditions, coagulation disorders and certain types of pharmacological thromboprophylaxis are weightier contraindications to epidural block than to other regional techniques because bleeding into the epidural space is not always immediately apparent. Furthermore, it cannot be controlled directly and may only be revealed when it causes symptoms (see Ch. 7).

## Equipment

The basic requirements for a regional block have been described in Chapter 8. More equipment (much of it specially designed) is needed for an epidural block than for most others and anaesthetists vary in their preference for these items.

### Needles

All epidural needles are now disposable and can be obtained from several manufacturers (e.g. Portex,

Steriseal, Becton Dickinson, Vygon and Abbott). They are of consistent high quality and are provided in sterile packs. The standard shaft is 8 cm long, although other lengths are available (Vygon, 9 cm), but it is recommended that each department standardises on one manufacturer for routine use in order to avoid confusion. (Shah et al 1999, Devine & Romer 2000). A needle with an 11 cm shaft (Portex) is available for use in the morbidly obese.

The *Tuohy* needle (Fig. 11.1) is widely used throughout the world. The shaft is graduated in centimetres and available in 16 g, 17 g and 18 g diameters, the former being most commonly used in adults. The needle wall is thin so that the lumen will admit a catheter of reasonable size. A stilette prevents coring of the superficial tissues and, when made of metal, increases the rigidity of the needle. The needle point is relatively blunt and is contoured so that a catheter emerges at an angle of about 20° (the Huber tip), but this design does have the important disadvantage that the catheter cannot be withdrawn through the needle without the risk of it being transected (Fig. 11.2). If it is necessary to withdraw the catheter, the needle must be withdrawn

simultaneously. Versions of the Tuohy needle are available with both fixed or detachable 'wings' at the hub.

The *Crawford* needle (Fig. 11.3) has a short bevel of conventional design. A catheter therefore emerges straight from the tip without any deflection so it can be withdrawn from the needle with less risk of transection. However, it will impinge on the dura if introduced at right angles to the skin by the conventional midline route. Therefore, the Crawford needle, and others of similar design, are better suited to the paramedian approach, which permits greater cephalad angulation than can be obtained from the midline. Furthermore, when cephalad angulation is used, the needle can be introduced with the bevel facing anteriorly (i.e. away from the anaesthetist), so that the bevel plane lies parallel to the long axis of the epidural space (see Fig. 11.15 p. 148). This has the advantage that the chances of dural puncture are reduced. The availability of these needles is a reminder that a Tuohy needle, although almost universally used for the performance of an epidural, is not essential for it.

### Syringes

If the epidural space is to be located by the loss of resistance method, it is essential that the syringe plunger runs smoothly along the entire length of the barrel. Although ordinary disposable syringes are perfectly satisfactory, most commercially prepared epidural packs contain a specifically designed 10 ml plastic, loss of resistance (LOR) device. Traditionally, reusable glass syringes have been used and, if scrupulously maintained, are excellent. Unfortunately, it is very difficult to obtain

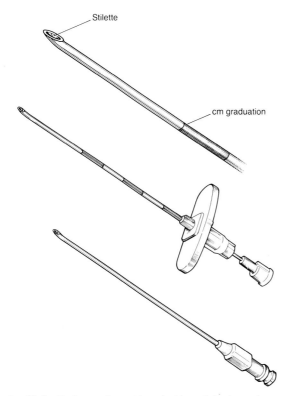

**Fig 11.1** Tuohy needles, with and without 'wing' attachment

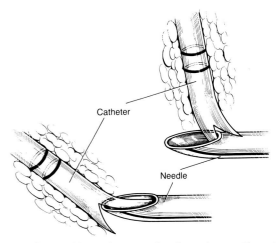

**Fig 11.2** Possible mechanisms of catheter damage if one is withdrawn through a Tuohy needle

'jet' of liquid produced as the space is entered is likely to push the dura away from the needle point. Some anaesthetists feel that this liquid also facilitates the subsequent passage of the epidural catheter by 'lubricating' the space, and there is evidence from work in obstetric patients that it also reduces the risk of blood vessel puncture (Verniquet 1980).

## Insertion of the catheter

When the catheter has passed through the full length of the needle, there is almost always some resistance to its emergence from the tip into the epidural space. This can usually be overcome by gripping centimetre-lengths of catheter close to the needle hub and inserting the catheter a little at a time. If a catheter refuses to pass, the probable reason is that the proximal part of the needle bevel still lies in the ligamentum flavum (Fig. 11.11). Obviously, a catheter will not pass until all the bevel is clear of the ligament, so the needle must be carefully advanced a further millimetre. A second injection of 5 ml of saline may also help a catheter to pass by 'opening up' the epidural space.

Although this description of the midline approach has stressed the importance of keeping the needle at right angles to the skin in both planes, this can be modified if there is difficulty in advancing the catheter. Unless the vertebral spines are very close together, it is usually possible to re-introduce the needle with some cephalad angulation and this, together with the manoeuvres described above, generally results in the catheter passing easily. If it does not, another interspace should be selected.

The epidural space is vascular, and blood occasionally tracks back along the catheter. If this happens, the catheter should be withdrawn until the flow stops and then flushed with saline to prevent it becoming occluded with blood clot. Clear fluid tracking along the catheter may be either CSF or injected saline. CSF usually flows briskly and can be aspirated easily. A catheter which has punctured the dura or which, despite slow withdrawal, remains in a vein should be removed and inserted at the same or an adjacent interspace.

When the catheter has been suitably positioned, a small amount of saline or local anaesthetic should be injected to ensure that it is still patent and has not kinked in the epidural space. The catheter must be fixed firmly so that it cannot be accidentally dislodged on the operating table or during nursing procedures on the ward. However, if it is applied too closely to the skin at its entry point, it may kink. This can be avoided by leading the catheter in a gentle curve over a small swab. Some catheter packs contain a special device designed to fulfil the same function (Fig.11.12). The whole area should then be covered with a waterproof adhesive dressing (Fig. 11.13). Increasingly, many anaesthetists feel that this dressing should be transparent so that any signs of skin infection at the puncture site and dislodgement of the catheter can be detected early. The remaining length of catheter is led up the back to the shoulder under a *narrow* strip of adhesive tape.

Once the patient has been turned supine again, the patency of the catheter should be tested once more to make sure that the change of position has not occluded it. A catheter inserted with the patient in the flexed position occasionally becomes kinked at its point of entry into the supraspinous ligament when the back is straightened. Asking the patient to straighten out prior to final catheter fixation can help prevent this. Catheters can also become occluded if they are nipped between the bony prominences of the vertebrae or kinked in the skin folds of the very obese.

## The test dose

The object of a test dose is to exclude intrathecal or intravascular placement of a catheter. The general principles have been discussed in Chapter 8, but it is worth re-emphasising here that:

- The test drug must be capable of exerting the desired 'test' effect;
- The dose must be large enough to produce it;

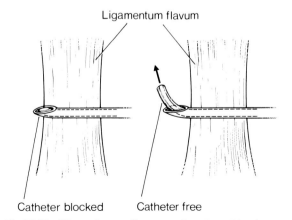

Ligamentum flavum

Catheter blocked    Catheter free

**Fig 11.11** The catheter will not pass into the epidural space unless the entire bevel is through the ligamentum flavum

145

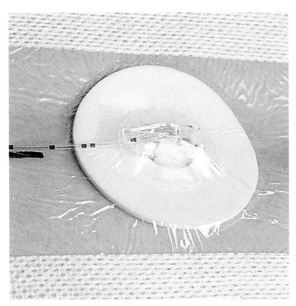

**Fig 11.12**  Epidural catheter fixation device in position

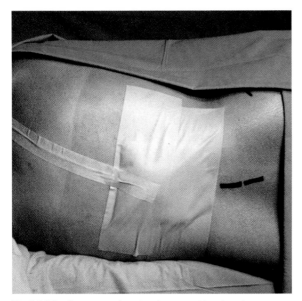

**Fig 11.13**  Protective dressing for an epidural catheter

- The drug and the dose must be *incapable* of producing the 'test' effect when injected into the correct place;
- The 'test' effect must be allowed sufficient time to develop;
- The 'test' effect should be easily observable.

There is disagreement about the value of test doses. Scott (1983) has argued that they are a ritual rather than a practical exercise. Certainly, they will be of no help, and may actually be misleading, if the above criteria are not applied. For example, a test dose may fail to provide definite evidence of an intrathecal injection if the patient is under general anaesthesia because it is impossible to obtain adequate neurological information. Blood appearing in a catheter indicates that an epidural vessel has been damaged, and it should not be assumed that intravascular injection cannot occur just because the catheter has been withdrawn and blood no longer flows. Local anaesthetic solutions containing epinephrine (20 µg) may give a more objective warning of an intravascular injection, but the effect of epinephrine may be minimal if the patient is being treated with β-sympathomimetic blockers and any effect may be difficult to interpret in a mother in painful labour.

If the patient is conscious and is to undergo major surgery with an epidural block unsupplemented by general anaesthesia, concentrated solutions of local anaesthetic will be required. In that situation, a small volume will contain sufficient drug to cause cerebral symptoms if it is given inadvertently by intravascular injection. Numbness or tingling of the tongue, light-headedness or tinnitus are indications that this has occurred. In order that these symptoms are detected early, injections should be given slowly (10 ml min⁻¹) with frequent aspiration tests. Continuous verbal contact with the patient must be maintained (Scott 1983) and if signs or symptoms of toxicity appear, the injection should be stopped before a dose likely to cause major systemic toxicity has been given.

## Alternative methods

### Loss of resistance to air

Advocates of this method point out that if clear fluid appears from the epidural needle it must be CSF and therefore dural puncture has definitely occurred. They claim that the issue may be in doubt if loss of resistance to saline has been used. The disadvantage of using loss of resistance to air is that air, unlike saline, is compressible and, because it is possible to 'spring' the plunger in the barrel even when the needle tip is in the ligamentum flavum, the loss of resistance sign may be inconclusive. Furthermore, those who use air tend to 'spring' the plunger intermittently so that the advance of the needle–syringe assembly is not a smooth, steady movement. Consequently, those who routinely use liquid find the end-point much more definite than with air. Moreover, detection of dural puncture after the use of liquid is not a problem in practice. It is usually very apparent that it has occurred.

It has been known for some time that loss of resistance to air is more likely to be associated with unblocked segments, at least in obstetric patients (Valentine et al 1991), but evidence is accumulating that the injection of air may also be responsible for more serious complications, such as cord and nerve root compression, subcutaneous emphysema, air embolism and paraesthesia (Saberski et al 1997). On balance, therefore, it seems prudent to choose liquid, which gives the most clear-cut indication of entry to the epidural space (an essential requirement every time an epidural is performed), rather than air, the features of which may be helpful only in the occasional case.

### The 'Doughty' technique (Fig. 11.14)

This method is important because it was successfully taught by Doughty for several years and has been widely used and taught by anaesthetists who were trained by him.

The stance differs from that described above in that the anaesthetist stands sideways on to the patient and faces caudad. There are three components to the technique. First, the thumb and first and second fingers of the right hand grip the rim of the syringe barrel and are responsible for advancing the needle–syringe assembly through the ligamentum flavum towards the epidural space. Second, the thumb and first finger of the left hand grip the hub of the needle to control its forward progress. The stability necessary for this important function is obtained by pressing the hand and the whole length of the forearm against the patient's back. Third, loss of resistance is detected by pressure exerted on the syringe plunger by the base of the right index finger or by the palm of the right hand. This pressure is separate from that applied by the thumb and fingers of the right hand and it does not contribute to the advance of the needle.

The amount of liquid in the syringe must be such that the plunger 'fits' the anaesthetist's hand and is in comfortable contact with the base of the index finger or the palm of the hand. The optimal volume of liquid therefore depends on the size of the anaesthetist's hand. The Doughty method, didactically taught and carefully supervised, results in inadvertent dural puncture in only about 1 in 200 cases (A Doughty, personal communication).

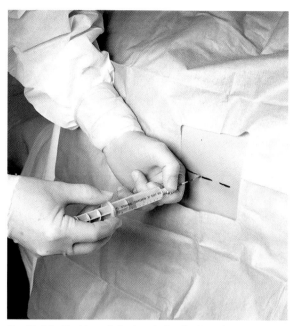

**Fig 11.14**  Position of the hands for the Doughty method

### Subatmospheric pressure

In the spontaneously breathing patient, some negative pressure from the intrapleural space is transmitted through the intervertebral foramina to the epidural space, the negative pressure being slightly greater in the thoracic than the lumbar region. Two techniques were described in the early days of epidural anaesthesia to take advantage of this.

In the *hanging drop* method (Soresi 1932), a drop of liquid is applied to the hub of the epidural needle when its tip is embedded in the ligamentum flavum. As the tip enters the epidural space, the liquid is sucked in. In the *balloon* method (Macintosh 1950), a small balloon is attached to the needle and is inflated through a side port. As the needle enters the space, the balloon deflates.

Unfortunately, a negative pressure in the epidural space is only observed in 80–90% of patients, and it may be absent in those with chronic obstructive airways disease and, of course, during artificial ventilation. The techniques are therefore unreliable and are mentioned here only for their historical interest.

## Paramedian approach with cephalad angulation

### Advantages

Because the 'paramedian' needle passes between the laminae of adjacent vertebrae, the interspinous ligaments,

**147**

which are often calcified in the elderly, are avoided. The needle is therefore less likely to be diverted from its course and less force is required to insert it. Also, the track of the needle need not be dictated by the amount of space between adjacent vertebral spines. This allows the needle to be inserted at a cephalad angle which is independent of the position or angle of the vertebral spines and which can therefore be selected by the anaesthetist. Another advantage of the method is that the deliberate location of a bony landmark provides direct evidence of the position of the needle *before* it enters the ligamentum flavum and the epidural space.

*Cephalad angulation* conveys several advantages which improve the safety and effectiveness of epidural anaesthesia.

1. The needle is less likely to puncture the dura because it crosses the epidural space obliquely, so the distance from the needle's point of emergence from the ligamentum flavum to the dura is greater

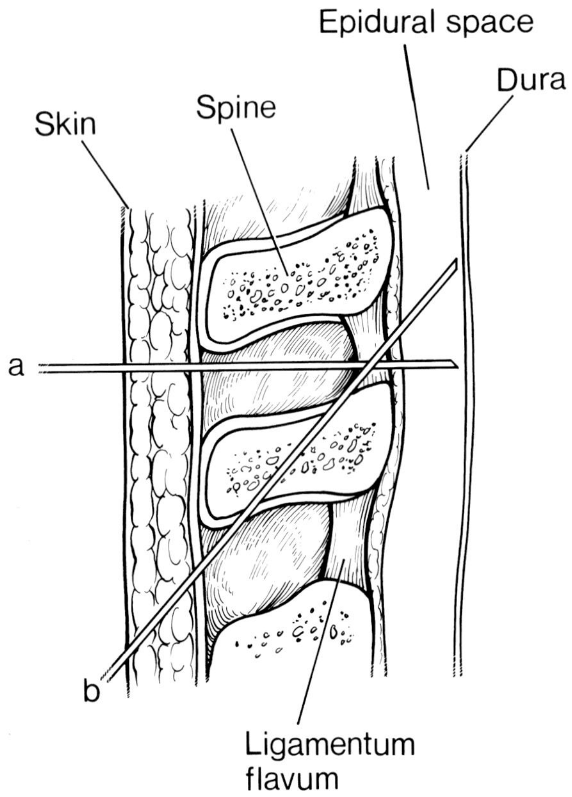

**Fig 11.15** Needle angles for the midline (a) and paramedian (b) approaches. Note that the distance from the ligamentum flavum to the dura with the paramedian approach is almost twice that of the midline.

than with the midline approach. The chances of dural puncture can be further reduced if a Crawford needle is used and inserted with its bevel facing anteriorly (Fig. 11.15).

2. Insertion of the catheter is usually very easy because the cephalad angle of the needle directs the catheter along the long axis of the epidural space. The small deflection of the catheter from the tip of a Tuohy needle further assists this process. Blomberg (1988), using epiduroscopy in cadavers, found that all catheters introduced by the paramedian approach followed a straight cephalad path. In the clinical situation, the final position of the catheter tip cannot be precisely known unless it is verified radio-graphically, but the catheter is obviously less likely to impinge on the dura, kink, or form loops and knots. As a result, it is feasible and safe to introduce as much catheter as is required to position the tip at a specific dermatomal level.

3. The catheter is less likely to be accidentally pulled out if several centimetres have been inserted.

4. With the paramedian approach, the vertebral lamina is deliberately located and the needle 'walked' off it superiorly into the ligamentum flavum. This bony landmark is very reassuring in the obese and, once found, allows the needle to be re-angled and further advanced with confidence. When the midline approach is used, it is unnerving for an anaesthetist to preside over the steady disappearance of a needle into the back of an obese patient with no sign of loss of resistance and no information as to where the tip is in relation to the epidural space.

*Technique*

The approach to the epidural space by the paramedian route differs from the midline approach in that neither of the two final angles of insertion is a right angle. The following description again assumes that the patient is lying on the left side and that the anaesthetist is right handed. The skin over the chosen vertebral spine is immobilised with the second and third fingers of the left hand, but the skin is pierced about 1 cm from the midline and level with a spine (Fig. 11.16). The needle is then inserted perpendicular to the skin until it strikes the vertebral lamina and the depth at which this occurs is noted from the centimetre graduations. It is now necessary to redirect the needle in both cephalad and medial directions (Fig. 11.17) and each angulation will be described separately.

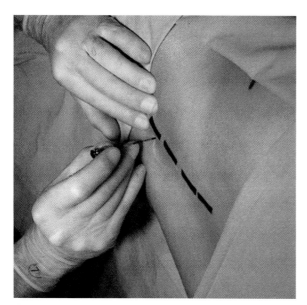

**Fig 11.16** Initial needle position for the paramedian approach. The tip is about 1 cm from the midline

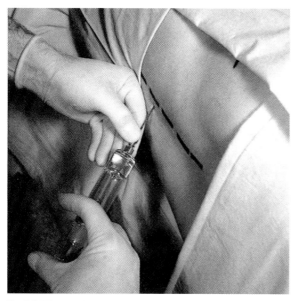

**Fig 11.17** Final needle angulation for the paramedian approach. Note that it is directed cephalad

*Cephalad angulation* The needle tip must be 'walked' along the lamina in a cephalad direction until it eventually clears it and enters the ligamentum flavum between the chosen lamina and the one above it. When performing this manoeuvre, two important points of technique must be born in mind. First, it is essential that the needle is withdrawn about 1 cm before each

cephalad probe of the lamina. Attempts to realign the needle without withdrawal will cause it to bend and this will increase the force required to advance it through the tissues. Second, the change of angle between each probing must not be more than about 15°. A larger angle may result in the needle tip passing from the superior edge of the chosen lamina to the inferior edge of the one above, and missing the ligament between them.

It will be apparent that the more caudad the initial insertion of the needle, the greater will be the cephalad angulation when it clears the lamina and the smaller will be the acute angle between needle and skin. However, establishment of this important cephalad angle does not alter the paramedian position of the needle tip which is still approximately 1 cm from the midline. If the needle were now to be advanced without being directed medially, it would enter the lateral part of the epidural space (often rich in blood vessels), or miss it altogether.

*Medial angulation* The second objective must therefore be to redirect the needle so that its tip passes 1 cm medially and enters the epidural space in the midline. Experience is required to judge this angle correctly. It will be greatest in lean patients in whom the distance between the skin and epidural space is short, and in cases where the anaesthetist inserts the needle some distance from the midline. The angle will be smallest in obese patients in whom the 1 cm correction is made over a large distance, and in cases in which a narrow paramedian approach is selected and the needle is inserted close to the midline.

Although the beginner will find it helpful to concentrate on these angles one at a time, it is possible, as experience and confidence increase, to create them simultaneously and to minimise probing of the lamina. In straightforward cases, the experienced anaesthetist can correctly angle the needle into the ligamentum flavum immediately after the initial perpendicular location of the lamina.

## THORACIC EPIDURAL ANAESTHESIA

Because the chest and abdominal walls are innervated by thoracic dermatomes (see Fig. 3.3 p. 24), epidural anaesthesia for all types of thoracic and abdominal surgery must block the appropriate thoracic nerves. In the thoracic region it is important that this is achieved with the minimum dose of local anaesthetic in order that extensive sympathetic block is avoided. Minimal dosage will only be effective if the dermatomal extent of the block precisely matches the dermatomal extent of the surgery, and the most important factor in determining this is the level at which local anaesthetic drug enters the epidural space. *It is therefore essential that a technique be used which allows accurate placement of the catheter tip.*

The paramedian approach with cephalad angulation (see above) is the method of choice because its advantages are particularly applicable to thoracic epidural anaesthesia. Although the midline approach can be used below the eighth thoracic vertebra where the spines are less acutely angled, a mismatch in which the upper dermatomes involved in the surgery are not anaesthetised is more likely to occur above this level because it is difficult to ensure that the catheter is placed at the appropriate level. Attempts to remedy this situation by injecting large volumes of local anaesthetic and hoping for cephalad spread are usually unsuccessful and result instead in extensive sympathetic block with its attendant cardio-vascular disturbances. Holmdahl and colleagues (1972) have shown that hypotension is more marked with a thoracolumbar block than with a block centred upon the mid-thoracic dermatomes. In addition, the patient may suffer from 'dead' legs, an insensitive bladder and loss of sphincter control. The side-effects and compli-cations then heavily outweigh any benefits and when this happens it is not surprising if surgeons, nurses and patients feel hostile towards epidural anaesthesia. In summary, abdominal surgery under epidural anaesthesia requires a thoracic block, and a dermatomal match is essential. However, thoracic epidural anaesthesia should not be attempted until the anaesthetist has first mastered the lumbar route and become experienced in the anaesthetic management of major surgery.

## FACTORS AFFECTING SPREAD OF SOLUTIONS

It is obviously important to identify the factors which may influence spread of a local anaesthetic in the epidural space, and to define their effects, where possible. Anatomical differences and physiological effects within the epidural space, the age, height, weight and posture of the patient, the rate of injection, the direction of the needle bevel at the time of injection, and the mass of drug injected have all been studied. However, in the

individual patient these factors interact, so that it is difficult to predict accurately the effect of a given dose of local anaesthetic.

## Epidural anatomy

The detailed anatomy of the epidural space is considered in Chapter 9. Only points of special relevance to epidural anaesthesia are considered below. Modern imaging techniques have shown that it is not a simple, uniform tube surrounding a cylindrical theca. The plica mediana dorsalis and other fibrous strands have been implicated in impeding the passage of a catheter and preventing the even spread of local anaesthetic solution, resulting in 'missed' segments and, in extreme cases, unilateral block. In view of these potential obstacles, it is perhaps surprising that epidural anaesthesia is as effective as it is.

In the cervical region, the dura is more closely applied to the ligamentum flavum than elsewhere, and it is even adherent to the periosteum in places. Consequently, the cervical epidural space is very narrow and in some cases may be little more than a potential space. This may account for the clinical observation that, even when the thoracic segments are profoundly blocked, the cervical segments are rarely affected (Grundy et al 1978a).

The 'periosteum' on the anterior surface of the ligamentum flavum and the vertebral laminae forms the posterior boundary to the epidural space. Although the ligamentum flavum is referred to as a single structure, it is in fact bilateral. The two components usually meet in the midline and provide the resistance to an advancing needle that is lost when the space is entered. However, gaps do occur in the midline between the right and left sides of the ligament, so it is possible for a needle intro-duced in the midline to enter the epidural space without encountering any resistance. This is obviously less likely to happen if the needle is inserted by the paramedian route.

## Epidural physiology

Negative pressure in the epidural space is due to transmission of negative intrathoracic pressure through the intervertebral foramina. It is greatest in the upper and middle thoracic regions and least in the lumbar and sacral regions as distance from the thorax increases. Greater negative epidural pressure is produced in the sitting position than in the supine, and in the flexed spinal position than in the extended. It has been suggested that negative pressure can be produced by 'tenting' the dura with the point of the needle (Aitkenhead et al 1979). On the other hand, there may be no negative pressure in conditions such as chronic obstructive airway disease in which intrathoracic pressure is abnormal, and in patients with raised intra-abdominal pressure.

## Patient factors

### Age

Bromage (1969) introduced the concept of the *segmental dose requirement*, which he defined as the mass of drug required to block one segment. He showed that this was greatest at about 19 years of age, when 1.5 ml per segment of 2% lidocaine was required, and found that the dose requirement declined linearly as age increased. However, Sharrock (1978), using 0.75% bupivacaine with epinephrine, found that the segmental dose requirement was virtually constant at about 1.3 ml per segment in patients between the ages of 20 and 40 years, but in patients over 60 years, the spread of anaesthesia did not correlate with the dose. Indeed, in some cases in this age group, 10 ml or less, injected at $L_2$–$L_3$, produced blocks up to $T_4$ and higher, and the segmental dose requirement varied between 0.35 and 1.2 ml.

This difference between the young and the old may be due to the fact that the intervertebral foramina tend to become occluded with age. Radiopaque dye injected epidurally can be seen tracking laterally into the paravertebral region in young patients, and it is at least possible that a local anaesthetic exerts some of its action there. No such tracking is seen in the elderly so solution is confined to the epidural space and spread within it is therefore likely to be more extensive. Also, more drug is available to diffuse through the dura into the CSF and this may explain why a comparatively small epidural dose sometimes results in an extensive block (Sharrock 1978).

### Height

Although tall patients tend to require large doses of drug for block of a given number of segments, the correlation between dose and height is poor. Indeed, it has been calculated that if two patients 30 cm different in height are given the same dose, the resulting block will only be one segment higher in the short patient (Grundy et al 1978a).

### Weight

Obese patients carry most of their excess fat subcutaneously, but they also have increased deposits in all areas where fat normally occurs. Any such increase in fat in the epidural space might be expected to affect the spread of drugs. The spread of 20 ml of 0.75% bupivacaine was studied in patients about to undergo Caesarean section, some of whom were lean and some grossly obese. The drug was injected with patients in either the horizontal or the sitting position. It was found that although posture made no difference to the eventual height of the block in the lean group, the sitting position resulted in lower blocks in the obese (Hodgkinson & Husain 1981).

### Posture

Posture and gravity are of limited value in controlling the spread of local anaesthetic in the epidural space. In patients who were given 2% lidocaine with epinephrine and maintained in the lateral position, the block developed earlier on the dependent side and lasted about 20 minutes longer, but it extended only one or two segments further than on the upper side (Apostolou et al 1981). Another study using 0.75% lidocaine produced similar findings (Grundy et al 1978b). Nevertheless, the effect of posture is sufficient to be of some clinical use. For example, it occasionally happens that an area of skin, usually in the groin region, remains sensitive when areas above and below are analgesic. If the patient is turned so that this 'missed' segment is dependent, and a further injection is given, anaesthesia often results. Posture can also be used to obtain perineal analgesia during lumbar epidural block.

## Injection factors

### Rate of injection

This exerts very little influence on the spread of local anaesthetic in the epidural space. A three-fold increase in the rate of injection of 0.75% plain bupivacaine produced a mean block less than one segment higher (Grundy et al 1978a).

### Direction of needle bevel

In patients under the age of 40 years, the segmental spread of an epidural block is the same whether the needle bevel faces cephalad or caudad. In patients over 40 years, there is a tendency towards more cephalad spread when the bevel faces cephalad, but the difference is slight and never more than two segments (Park et al 1982b).

### Mass of drug

The extent of sensory block produced by a particular agent is in general determined by the mass of drug injected rather than by the volume. However, this principle does not hold for extremes of concentration and volume, nor does it apply to the degree of motor block, as this is very closely related to drug concentration. The characteristics of individual local anaesthetics are considered below.

## CLINICAL PROFILE OF BLOCK

The onset, duration and quality of a block are determined by the intrinsic properties of the individual local anaesthetic agent, the concentration in which it is used and the effect of any adjuvants. There is wide variation between agents regarding speed of onset, duration of action and density of motor block. Increase in the concentration of a drug or the addition of epinephrine usually speeds the rate of onset of a block, prolongs its duration, and improves its quality.

## Methods of clinical assessment

Much of the work designed to define and compare the characteristics of local anaesthetics has given inconclusive and sometimes conflicting results because different criteria have been used for assessment. However, the most important clinical features of a local anaesthetic may be established if the typical pattern of onset and regression of an epidural block is understood (Fig. 11.18).

### Onset time

Any thorough assessment should take into account not only the time for the onset of analgesia (defined as inability to appreciate pinprick), but also anaesthesia (defined as inability to appreciate touch). These times, charted bilaterally for each spinal segment affected, give the *mean segmental latency profile* for a particular drug.

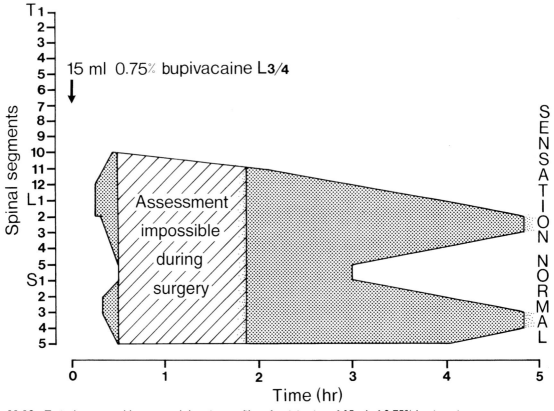

**Fig 11.18**  Typical segmental latency and duration profiles after injection of 15 ml of 0.75% bupivacaine

## Duration of block

Determination of the time at which bilateral analgesia and anaesthesia were last detectable for each affected segment provides a *mean segmental duration profile*. A simpler assessment of duration can be made by measuring the *two-segment regression time*. This is done by noting the maximum spread of the block and measuring the interval from the time of injection to the time at which the block has regressed two segments from this maximum. The method is valid when applied to patients who have been conscious throughout the procedure. However, if they have received a general anaesthetic in addition to the epidural, and have undergone major surgery, two-segment regression may have occurred before the end of the procedure or before the patient is sufficiently conscious to co-operate in the assessment. In such cases, four- or six-segment regression times may be used.

A wholly clinical approach to the assessment of duration of block is to note the interval from the time of injection to the time at which the patient first complains of pain. Comparison between agents with this method is only valid if surgical factors, such as type of incision and operation, are standardised, and the method lacks the quantitative precision of the duration profile and the segment regression assessments. However, it does provide the clinical anaesthetist with the most valuable information of all – the time by which an epidural infusion should be running or a top-up injection given, or some alternative form of analgesia commenced.

## Density of motor block

This is usually assessed clinically on the *Bromage scale*. The original scale ranged from 1 to 4, the lower numbers representing increasing motor block. The scale in current use has been modified and reversed, and is graded from 0 to 3: 0 = no motor block; 1 = inability to raise the extended leg; 2 = additional inability to flex the knee, and 3 = the additional inability to flex the ankle. This last sign is taken to indicate total paralysis of the affected muscles. A further modification, with grades from 1 to 6, has been developed for use in ambulant obstetric patients (Breen et al 1993). It permits finer discrimination and may be of value when early ambulation after major surgery becomes the norm. Confusingly, this scale has reverted to Bromage's original format: 1 represents complete block; 2 – ability to move the feet only; 3 – ability to move the knees; 4 – detectable weakness in the hip flexors; 5 – no detectable weakness in the hip flexors; 6 – ability to perform partial knee bending when the patient is upright.

The Bromage scales give useful clinical information and are quick and easy to apply. They do not, however, supply the quantitative information required when the motor effects of two local anaesthetic agents are being compared. Two methods, essentially research tools, have been devised for this. Average Rectified Electromyography (AREMG) measures electromyographic signals generated by the rectus abdominis muscle when the patient attempts to sit up. The signals are detected by skin electrodes placed at different dermatomal levels (Nydahl et al 1988). Mechanical Measurement of Isometric Muscle Force (MMIMF) uses mechanotransducers to measure the isometric force developed by muscles of the lower limb with the patient in the lithotomy position (Axelsson et al 1985).

## Local anaesthetics in the epidural space

### Lidocaine

A 2% solution is required to produce the muscle relaxation required for major abdominal and lower limb surgery. The onset time is short, and analgesia is detectable after about 6 minutes in dermatomes close to the site of injection. The duration of action is also short, although it can be prolonged by about 50% by the addition of epinephrine 1:200 000, but two-segment regression still takes place between $1\frac{1}{2}$ and 2 hours after injection.

The 1% solution produces analgesia, but it is inadequate for major surgery unless a large mass of drug is used.

### Prilocaine

Prilocaine is the least toxic of the amide local anaesthetics and this is its main advantage. The 2% solution provides conditions suitable for major surgery, but the onset time is somewhat slower than 2% lidocaine, a block being detectable after about 9 minutes and complete within 20 minutes. The duration exceeds that of lidocaine and the 6-segment regression time is between $2\frac{1}{2}$ and 3 hours.

### Bupivacaine

This long-acting agent is commercially available in the UK as 0.25, 0.5 and 0.75% solutions. The 0.25 and 0.5% solutions can also be obtained containing epinephrine at 1:200 000. The stronger solutions produce excellent analgesia, anaesthesia and muscle relaxation. The 0.75% solution is ideal for major surgery in the conscious patient because it provides profound and prolonged sensory and motor block (Fig. 11.18).

Plain bupivacaine is comparatively slow to act, and since this is the only disadvantage of an otherwise excellent agent, attempts have been made to overcome it. The addition of epinephrine to the 0.75% solution significantly decreases the onset time, and analgesia can be detected within 5 minutes (Sinclair & Scott 1984). Plain bupivacaine in 0.75% solution will provide 4–6 hours of analgesia and this pain-free period is increased to between 6.5 and 8 hours if epinephrine is added.

### Ropivacaine

With the exception of etidocaine (1972), ropivacaine, introduced into clinical practice in 1996, was the first significant local anaesthetic to be developed since 1963 when bupivacaine became available. It was developed in response to the need for a drug that was less cardiotoxic than bupivacaine. It is available in 0.2, 0.75 and 1% solutions

For *surgical procedures* requiring muscle relaxation, 0.75 or 1% solutions are required. Katz and colleagues (1990) compared 0.75% ropivacaine with 0.5% bupivacaine and found no major differences in onset or recovery time for either sensory or motor block. Comparison of 1% ropivacaine and 0.75% bupivacaine produced similar results, though the duration of sensory block was longer with ropivacaine (Wood & Rubin 1993). Similarly, there was no difference in the onset, spread and duration of sensory block when equal concentrations (0.5 and 0.75%) of the two drugs were compared. However, the motor block produced by ropivacaine was less intense, its onset slower and its duration of action shorter (Brockway et al 1991).

For *postoperative pain control* the separation of sensory and motor effects seen with ropivacaine should be an advantage where early ambulation is required. Schug and colleagues (1996) compared 0.1, 0.2 and 0.3% ropivacaine infused at a rate of 10 ml h$^{-1}$ after upper abdominal surgery. They found that the 0.3% infusion gave the lowest scores for pain on coughing and the highest scores for patient satisfaction. However, the only patient to develop a Bromage grade 3 block (see above) was in the 0.3% group. Although most studies have demonstrated minimal motor block with ropivacaine, a clear-cut advantage over bupivacaine has not always emerged. Jørgensen and colleagues (2000) compared

0.2% ropivacaine to 0.2% bupivacaine, both given at a rate of 8 ml h$^{-1}$ after abdominal hysterectomy, and found no difference in pain scores, motor block, the ability to walk, the time to discharge from hospital or the number of patients requesting supplementary ketorolac. Indeed, of the patients who did request ketorolac in the first 24 hours, those in the ropivacaine group needed significantly more. The consensus view seems to be that the 0.2% solution infused at 10 ml h$^{-1}$ gives the best balance between analgesia and preservation of motor function.

### Effects of epinephrine

In addition to its effects on the clinical profile of the local anaesthetic drug, epinephrine can also exert systemic effects in the amounts commonly used in epidural block. Twenty ml of a 1:200 000 solution contains 100 µg and will cause an increase in heart rate, systolic pressure, cardiac output and stroke volume, and a decrease in total peripheral resistance. These are the effects of β-adrenergic stimulation. The α-adrenergic effects of epinephrine are not seen, presumably because higher doses are required to produce them (Goodman & Gilman 1997).

If the local anaesthetic used for the epidural contains epinephrine, the simultaneous use of halothane is theoretically contraindicated due to the risk of cardiac arrhythmias. In practice, these do not seem to occur, probably because, in the presence of epidural block, minimal concentrations of inhalation agent are required. Sinclair & Scott (1984) used 0.5% halothane in a mixture of nitrous oxide and oxygen, and concluded that 100 µg of epinephrine was unlikely to cause harmful systemic effects. The risk of arrhythmias has diminished with the introduction of the ether-based inhalational agents and can be regarded as remote with desflurane and sevoflurane.

## MANAGEMENT OF EPIDURAL ANAESTHESIA

### The operative period

#### Epidural block in the conscious patient

If operations are to be performed on conscious patients, a profound degree of block is required. For short procedures, 2% lidocaine is suitable, but when a longer duration of effect is required the choice lies between appropriate doses of 0.75% bupivacaine and 1%

ropivacaine, and bolus injections of lidocaine given through a catheter. These are concentrated solutions and should be injected with the precautions previously described, that is, slowly ($10\,ml\,min^{-1}$) with frequent aspiration tests, while constant verbal contact is maintained with the patient. It should be emphasised, however, that the relative safety of ropivacaine makes it less satisfactory as a test drug for detecting accidental intravascular injection because symptoms do not appear until a significant dose has been given (Morton et al 1997). The drug should be injected at the appropriate vertebral level, so that the extent of anaesthesia 'matches' the operation. It is important that the anaesthetist takes into account not only the innervation of the skin incision, but also that of structures likely to be handled during surgery. For example, $10\,ml$ of solution injected at $L_1-L_2$ is adequate for inguinal herniorrhaphy, but for abdominal hysterectomy $15-20\,ml$ is required to ensure that perineal sensation is blocked.

Careful selection of patients and a knowledge of the principles, practice and limitations of epidural block are essential for satisfactory and consistent results, but supplementary sedation, systemic opioids and even light general anaesthesia may still be required at some stage in a patient's management. Their use, far from implying that the block has failed, acknowledges that there are sources of discomfort which an epidural is intrinsically incapable of relieving. For example, afferent stimuli from the coeliac plexus may cause distress, and supplementary analgesia in these cases enhances rather than devalues the effect of the block. The choice of appropriate agents has been discussed in Chapter 8.

### 'Balanced' epidural anaesthesia

Traditional fears that the superimposition of general anaesthesia on an extensive epidural block might cause profound hypotension do not appear to be justified. Significant decreases in mean arterial pressure do occur (see Ch. 8), but treatment with vasopressors is not generally required provided that the state of the circulation is constantly monitored and normovolaemia maintained.

For upper abdominal and thoracic procedures, control of ventilation is essential, so general anaesthesia and neuromuscular blocking agents are needed to produce muscle relaxation. In such cases, the object of the block is to provide analgesia only. Combining epidural block with general anaesthesia in this way has several advantages. First, the anaesthetist can be sure that the patient's airway is safe and pulmonary ventilation is adequate. Second, the fact that analgesia and muscle relaxation are obtained by different means results in versatility and refinement. Smaller amounts of local anaesthetic are required than if this one agent is expected to provide both effects, and because the epidural anaesthetises muscle spindle afferent fibres (see Ch. 4), the requirement for neuromuscular blocking drugs is also reduced. Reversal of the relaxant at the end of surgery is therefore rarely a problem, and is unnecessary in many cases. Third, the technique is suitable for patients in whom spontaneous ventilation may be undesirable because of obesity, severe respiratory disease, head-down tilt or the nature of the surgery.

For reasons given previously, the author prefers the paramedian approach to the epidural space with cephalad angulation of the needle for abdominal and thoracic surgery. The vertebral interspace chosen for needle insertion should correspond, in dermatomal terms, to the *lower* end of the anticipated surgical incision. When the epidural space has been located, $5\,ml$ of 0.25% bupivacaine or 0.2% ropivacaine is injected through the needle. The catheter is then passed until its tip is judged to have reached a level corresponding to the *upper* extent of the anticipated surgical incision – a dermatomal 'distance' of between five and seven segments if a vertical incision is to be used. In a typical patient, this usually results in the $15\,cm$ mark on the catheter being close to the skin entry point. Local anaesthetic ($5\,ml$) is then injected through the catheter. The patient has therefore received two $5\,ml$ increments ('dumb-bell' boluses) to cover the upper and lower ends of the incision. This ensures that, by the time the patient has been transferred to theatre, catheterised, 'prepped' and draped, an effective block has developed and the incision causes little or no cardiovascular response.

### Perioperative epidural infusion

The epidural infusion should be commenced as early as possible in the operation so that its effect can be observed while physiological measurements are still stable. The choice of drugs is considered later, but the regimen for major surgery usually consists of a low concentration of ropivacaine or bupivacaine with the addition of an opioid. The infusion is commenced at a rate of $20\,ml\,h^{-1}$ and continued until a steady trend

155

towards reduction in mean arterial pressure and heart rate is seen. This indicates that a block has developed which is sufficiently extensive to obtund virtually all afferent input. It is important to continue the initial infusion rate to this point. Failure to do so may result in bolus injections being required after surgery and, in addition, it may well be the reason why epidurals have only a small effect on reduction of the stress response after major abdominal and thoracic surgery (Kehlet 1994). The time for this effect to occur varies. In the small, elderly female it may be seen in about half an hour, but in the well-built, middle-aged male, it may take up to 2 hours. The infusion is then reduced to a maintenance rate which will depend on the patient's response to the initial infusion, but will usually be in the region of 5–10 ml h$^{-1}$. The advantage of this method of management is that the patient's individual response to the block, and evidence of its effectiveness, is established early. As a result, the patient is pain free when consciousness is regained, bolus doses of local anaesthetic are rarely necessary and the maintenance infusion rate is likely to be appropriate for the patient's needs in the postoperative period.

## The postoperative period

If the full potential of an epidural block is to be realised after major surgery, it should be continued into the postoperative period and be used, either alone or in conjunction with other analgesic methods, to prevent pain for as long as the individual patient needs it (Kehlet 1994). *There should be no arbitrary time after which all epidurals are routinely discontinued.*

It should be stressed that the object is to prevent pain rather than to relieve it. There is now good evidence that prevention or pretreatment is a more effective way of controlling a variety of acute pain states than treatment after the pain has occurred (Bach et al 1988, Woolf 1989). *No system of analgesia will yield its full potential unless it is targeted at prevention rather than relief.* The continued use of the term 'pain relief' is probably doing more than anything else to retard progress in this field (Armitage 1989).

### Personnel and organisation

After surgery, the patient is moved to an adjacent *recovery area* where the anaesthetist hands over to the recovery nurse. This involves a brief description of the type and course of the anaesthetic, a review of the record chart (with particular reference to the patient's response to the epidural infusion), the setting of limits for physiological variables beyond which corrective action must be taken, and any other suggestions for management.

When the patient is conscious, rational and stable, and has confirmed the effectiveness of the analgesia, he/she is ready for transfer to another area. When epidurals were first extended into the postoperative period, patients were nursed either on surgical wards or in intensive care units. Although there were, and still are, some notable instances of successful management of patients on wards, there were serious concerns that nurses lacked the experience or training to be familiar with the new technique. Furthermore, nurses themselves were limited in the responsibilities which they were allowed to undertake with regard to epidurals, and staffing levels were inadequate to provide the quality of care required. It therefore became usual for 'epidural' patients to be admitted to intensive care units where the nurse-to-patient ratio was high and anaesthetists were instantly available. However, bed availability seriously limited the number of patients who could benefit. Also, intensivists may now come from a medical, surgical or accident and emergency background, and a local culture and ethos is sometimes found in which postoperative pain control in a conscious, spontaneously breathing patient is neither properly understood nor highly prioritised.

The problem of how to control postoperative pain has been addressed in the USA by Ready and colleagues (1988). In the UK, interest has been stimulated by two Reports (1990, 1991). They recommended, firstly, the establishment of surgical *high dependency units* to provide a level of care intermediate between the intensive care unit and the ward, and orientated towards management of the surgical patient. Some hospitals have responded by upgrading the theatre recovery area to provide 24-hour cover; in others, the unit is run as an offshoot from the intensive care unit. The Reports further recommended the setting up of *acute pain teams* consisting of nurses and anaesthetists trained and experienced in all aspects of pain control. The teams are responsible for the patient's comfort and for providing continuity of care, and ideally they should have no other duties. In practice, the anaesthetist who has initiated the block and who therefore bears ultimate responsibility for it must liaise closely with the acute pain team. The teams have not only improved all aspects of pain control, but have also made it feasible for epidural infusions to be continued efficiently and safely beyond the confines of the high dependency unit, thus removing some of the objections to this form of management. For example, Coleman and Booker-Milburn (1996) found that the appointment of an Acute Pain Nurse contributed to patient care on surgical wards by improving the ward nurses' knowledge of pain management, increasing the efficacy of epidural infusions and reducing their side-effects.

## Principles of administration

The aim of a 'continuous' epidural is to produce a band of analgesia which encompasses the sensory nerves supplying the area of the wound. Four interacting factors must be considered when epidural analgesia is being planned. It is obviously essential that the anaesthetist knows the likely *dermatomal extent of the incision*. This is central to success and the surgeon must be consulted if there is doubt. A dermatomal 'mismatch' between the incision and the analgesia is the commonest cause not only of an ineffective epidural, but also of complications arising from efforts to correct it, such as high infusion rates and large bolus injections. The importance of the *position of the catheter tip* has already been emphasised and the tip should lie at the upper end of the required analgesia level because, firstly, the upper 'dumb-bell' bolus dose can be given at this point and, secondly, it is much easier to withdraw a catheter which is too high than to re-insert one which is too low. However, the optimal site will be determined by the mode of administration and the posture of the patient. Local anaesthetic solution may be administered by *bolus or infusion*. With a bolus, a relatively high pressure is generated as the solution enters the epidural space and this has an effect on its spread, rendering it independent of gravity. Burn and colleagues (1973) injected radiopaque solution by the lumbar route and showed that 20 ml spreads mostly cephalad, to the lower and mid-thoracic segments, and that this spread is not affected by the patient's posture at the time of injection. With a continuous infusion, on the other hand, the *patient's posture* can influence the effect of gravity on spread. For example, Dawkins (1966) showed in a classic paper that when local anaesthetic is infused into the epidural space of patients in the semi-upright position, gravity favours more caudad spread as the infusion progresses, an effect which tends to be more marked when comparatively low infusion rates are used. The same infusion in a horizontal patient spreads

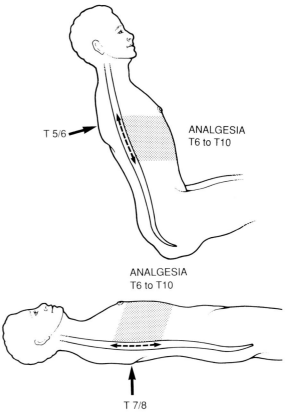

**Fig 11.19** Influence of posture on the distribution of analgesia during continuous epidural infusion in sitting and supine positions

cephalad as well as caudad (Fig. 11.19). The implications for the positioning of the catheter tip are obvious: if, as is usual, the epidural is to be given by infusion to a patient who will be in the semi-upright position, the catheter tip must be at the upper dermatomal level. Only if the epidural is to be given by intermittent bolus injections and/or the patient is to be nursed horizontal may a lower catheter position be satisfactory.

Modern pumps are accurate and reliable, but it is reassuring to have a burette in the delivery system so that the progress of an infusion can be checked visually. Also, if the contents of the burette are limited to, say, 50 ml, it is possible to prevent a serious overdose reaching the patient in the rare event of a pump malfunction. The burette reading should be charted hourly and compared with the 'volume infused' reading on the pump. The two figures should of course agree.

## Local anaesthetic regimens

**Bolus injections** Scott and colleagues (1982), using a pump capable of delivering bolus injections at variable time intervals, found that 8 ml of 0.5% plain bupivacaine, given 2-hourly, resulted in virtually complete analgesia, and more predictable analgesia than a continuous infusion. However, their regimen tended to cause some hypotension after the injections. They postulated that this might be avoided by giving smaller boluses more frequently. Schweitzer and Morgan (1987) confirmed this in a study in which they programmed a special automatic pump to give 3 ml boluses of 0.5% bupivacaine with epinephrine 1:200 000 every 60 minutes at a rate of 2.5 ml min$^{-1}$. More recently, Duncan and colleagues (1998) used an electromechanical pump to deliver 5 ml boluses of 0.375% bupivacaine at hourly intervals. Precise timing of injections is essential. Scott and colleagues (1982) found that when nursing staff were responsible for giving the boluses, analgesia was sometimes inadequate because it was not always possible for them to be given frequently enough.

**Infusions** Variable-rate infusion pumps are available for the administration of a steady flow of local anaesthetic solution. They must be accurate, reliable, quiet, and powerful enough to overcome the resistance of the 90 cm length of narrow epidural catheter. They are suitable for use with commercially prepared infusion packs of local anaesthetic. Syringe drivers are also available, but the syringe size is usually limited to 60 ml. They are therefore only practical for infusion of concentrated solutions at slow rates if frequent syringe changes are to be avoided.

Numerous infusion regimens have been used, ranging from small volume/high concentration to large volume/low concentration, the present trend being towards the latter. Mitchell and colleagues (1988) found that 6 out of 9 patients who received 0.125% bupivacaine at 15 ml h$^{-1}$ after major abdominal gynaecological surgery had adequate analgesia, but the study period lasted only 6 hours. Ross and colleagues (1980) infused 0.125% bupivacaine at a rate of 20 ml h$^{-1}$ for 2 days in patients who had undergone major abdominal and thoracic surgery. Plasma concentrations in the region of 3 µg ml$^{-1}$ were reached towards the end of the study period, but there were no clinical signs of toxicity.

Bupivacaine is now available in packs of 500 ml in concentrations of 0.1%, 0.125% and 0.25%. Ropivacaine is marketed in a concentration of 0.2% in rather less convenient 100 ml packs.

*Regression of a block* usually indicates that the infusion rate is too low. This should be corrected by first giving a bolus dose of the infusion solution via the pump to re-establish the extent of the block, and then re-setting the pump at a higher rate. Simply resetting the pump at a higher rate does not usually re-establish a regressing block, and if any effect is produced, it takes too long to become apparent.

The move towards early mobilisation after major surgery and the consequent need to leave motor function unimpaired has led to a trend towards the use of very low concentrations of local anaesthetic. However, *although early ambulation is undeniably an important advance in postoperative management, it must be accompanied by good pain control.*

## Opioid regimens

The discovery of opioid receptors in the spinal cord opened up an entirely new avenue for the treatment of postoperative pain (see Ch. 3). Unfortunately, the early promise of the technique was not confirmed: the transition from animal studies to widespread clinical use was far too rapid and anecdotal reports greatly outnumbered properly controlled trials. Morphine was the first agent to be used epidurally, and its relatively poor lipid solubility is probably responsible for both its long duration of action – the feature which, more than any other, has marked out epidural opioids as a major clinical advance – and its rostral spread, which can result in its more serious side-effects: delayed and unpredictable respiratory and central nervous system depression. Although initial reports claimed that 2 mg gave excellent analgesia, 10 mg in 10 ml was soon being used, but it requires 30 minutes to act and does not always produce adequate pain control. Pruritis is a side-effect of most epidural opioids, but is commonest with morphine and occurs even when preservative-free solutions are used (Weddell & Ritter 1980). Retention of urine is dose-dependent, with an incidence as high as 90% in one series (Bromage 1981). Where the quality of pain control provided by epidural morphine *or* bupivacaine has been compared, the latter has proved superior (Torda & Pybus 1984).

Highly lipid-soluble drugs such as diamorphine, fentanyl and sufentanil are only effective in doses approaching those used parenterally, but they produce a more distinct segmental block and there is less risk of rostral spread and respiratory depression. They need to be injected at a level close to the intended site of action. They have short onset times; diamorphine produces its effect within 15 minutes and a dose of 0.1 mg kg$^{-1}$ gives analgesia very similar in quality to the same dose given intramuscularly, though it lasts considerably longer (Jacobson et al 1983). Diamorphine, 5 mg in 10 ml saline, has been shown to reduce the stress response to surgery as measured by plasma glucose and cortisol concentrations, an effect which could not have been due to plasma diamorphine concentrations and must therefore have been spinally mediated (Cowen et al 1982). In a study investigating the effects of different concentrations of fentanyl, Welchew (1983) concluded that 100 µg in 10 ml of saline was the optimal dose.

### Combination regimens

As the concept of multimodal treatment of postoperative pain has gained ground, the epidural administration of drug combinations has become increasingly popular. Lee and colleagues (1988) studied the epidural infusion of 0.125% bupivacaine, diamorphine 0.5 mg h$^{-1}$, and a mixture of the two and found the mixture to be significantly more effective. Dahl and colleagues (1990) found that the use of combinations allowed reduction in the dose of both opioid and local anaesthetic as well as producing better analgesia. They used a mixture of 0.25% bupivacaine and morphine at 0.05 mg ml$^{-1}$ which many still consider to be the gold standard. As the preservation of motor function for early postoperative ambulation has become more important, lower concentrations have been used, such as 0.15% bupivacaine with diamorphine at 0.05 mg ml$^{-1}$, and 0.0625% bupivacaine with fentanyl at 0.125 mg ml$^{-1}$, at infusion rates between 4 and 15 ml h$^{-1}$.

### α$_2$-adrenergic agonists

An adrenergic pain modulating system, independent of the opioids, was described by Yaksh and Reddy (1981). It is thought to work by mimicking norepinephrine, which activates descending inhibitory pathways and reduces the release of substance P from Aδ and C afferent fibres in the dorsal horn. Clonidine, which also has some α$_1$ activity, is the agonist most commonly used. As the sole agent, in a dose of 150 µg, it produces significant analgesia, but hypotension, sedation and the relatively short duration of action limit its usefulness.

However, it enhances and prolongs epidural analgesia provided by local anaesthetics and opioids (Rostaing et al 1991, Carabine et al 1992).

### Supplementary medication

This is sometimes needed to treat symptoms which are beyond the scope of the epidural block. These include anxiety about the operation, sleeplessness, and discomfort from sites other than the wound, such as shoulder tip pain due to pneumoperitoneum, and the presence of a nasogastric tube. These are problems which are dealt with 'automatically' in patients receiving opioid analgesics in conventional doses. In patients receiving only epidural local anaesthetic, small doses of *systemically administered opioid* may be given safely and effectively. However, in patients receiving combinations of epidural local anaesthetic and opioid, there is an increased risk of respiratory depression if additional systemic opioids are given. In practice, problems are more likely to arise when the opioids are given to augment an inadequate block rather than to treat symptoms beyond its scope. In the former circumstance, epidural boluses and high infusion rates will have been tried already, and systemic opioids, even in modest doses, may then produce signs of depression. This emphasises further the importance of planning and precision when an epidural is being performed.

Non-steroidal anti-inflammatory drugs (NSAIDs) have been used both for a pre-emptive analgesic effect and as a third component in multimodal pain control. However, although the results of animal studies suggested that pre-injury treatment with NSAIDs reduced subsequent analgesia requirements, Murphy and Medley (1993) were unable to demonstrate a pre-emptive effect in surgical patients. Furthermore, NSAIDs do not improve the pain control at the wound site obtained with epidural opioid–local anaesthetic regimens, though they can relieve other causes of discomfort and are therefore a useful alternative to systemic opioids. NSAIDs are potentially toxic agents. They are contraindicated in elderly patients and in those with impaired renal function – groups which form a sizeable proportion of the surgical population – and should be used with discretion in view of the limited benefits they confer as supplements to epidural analgesia.

Once the operation is over and pain is controlled, anxiety decreases in most patients. Nevertheless, some patients may benefit from a small dose of an *anxiolytic agent*, though it must be appreciated that this may contribute to cardiorespiratory depression and will have no analgesic action.

## Aspects of management

**Protocols** Acute pain teams have greatly improved the management of postoperative pain and have helped to make pain prevention, as opposed to pain relief, a reality. However, because it is the ward nurse who is likely to be the first to observe an adverse event or the need for an adjustment, clear management protocols should be drawn up and readily available so that prompt and appropriate action can be taken in an emergency. There is much to be said for having them in written form at each patient's bedside. Nurses should be familiar with the operation of the pump, the significance of its alarms and the most common causes of malfunction.

**Hypotension** In general, the circulation is more stable than many anaesthetists believe, but both nursing and surgical staff must be aware that it is normal for the arterial blood pressure of epidural patients to be lower than those receiving conventional analgesia – inexperienced staff tend to give unnecessary treatment to 'hypotensive' epidural patients. A 'hypotensive' patient who is comfortable, rational, well perfused, producing urine and able to move the lower limbs is unlikely to be in immediate danger. However, it is vitally important that hypovolaemia is not allowed to occur because it is not tolerated in patients with a sympathetic block. Arbitrary blood pressure readings at which treatment should be given are inappropriate, and when the lowest acceptable limit is being determined, or when treatment is being considered, due regard should be given to the preoperative reading. The treatment of hypotension is considered later in this chapter and in Chapter 8.

Fears that the relative hypotension and complete analgesia may mask abdominal signs, thus causing *delay in the diagnosis of surgical complications*, are groundless. Patients suffering from haemorrhage or an anastomotic leak look and feel unwell, in marked contrast to those running a normal postoperative course with an epidural. However, when haemorrhage is suspected, it is important to appreciate that continued bleeding can lead to significant hypotension *without* tachycardia.

**Motor weakness** When an epidural is used as the sole anaesthetic agent, significant motor block of the lower limbs may extend into the early postoperative period, the duration depending on the agent used and the time of the last dose. With the low concentrations now used for infusions, any motor block should regress, but if it does not – and especially if, having regressed, it returns – it must be assumed that the catheter has migrated intrathecally.

**The patient in pain** One of the more difficult aspects of management is to decide whether a patient who is in pain requires supplementary medication or an increase in epidural dosage. If the pain is unilateral or associated with pinprick evidence of regression, it is likely that the epidural needs reinforcing. The dose of the bolus injection (which can be given via the infusion pump, set at a high rate) must take into account the fact that there is still a significant amount of drug in the epidural space, even though the block is inadequate, and 5 ml of solution is usually sufficient. Although gravity does not have a profound effect on spread, the patient with unilateral pain should lie on the unblocked side when the bolus is given and for at least 15 minutes afterwards.

**Colic** As a result of the sympathetic block induced by the epidural, the return of bowel motility is rapid and paralytic ileus is virtually unknown. However, excessive motility, which may occur if opioids are avoided, occasionally produces distressing colic which is quite distinct from wound pain. It responds to hyoscine butylbromide (Buscopan) 20 mg intravenously.

**Systemic toxicity** Concern about the toxicity of bupivacaine was one of the reasons for the development of ropivacaine, and infusions of the latter are less likely to cause refractory cardiac symptoms if the epidural catheter should accidentally migrate intravascularly. With bupivacaine, the total plasma concentrations reached during the 2-day course of an uncomplicated epidural infusion are relatively high (Ross et al 1980). However, it is the plasma concentration of free bupivacaine that determines the risk of toxicity, and this quotient remains constant after surgery because there is a concurrent rise in the level of $\alpha_1$-acid glycoprotein, which binds bupivacaine in the plasma. However, the appearance of symptoms does not depend solely on the plasma concentration. Scott (1975) administered intravenous bupivacaine at different rates to conscious volunteers and found that symptoms appeared at low plasma concentrations when the infusion rate was high. When dilute bupivacaine is given by epidural infusion, the rate of increase in plasma concentration tends to be very slow, and this may explain why Ross and colleagues

(1980) observed no toxic symptoms in their patients. One advantage of an infusion technique is that, if a catheter does migrate into an epidural vein, there will not be a sudden increase in plasma concentration, as will happen when a bolus is given.

*Discontinuing the epidural* In general, the more radical the surgery, the longer will the epidural be needed. For example, after thoraco-abdominal procedures, epidural analgesia should be continued for as long as intensive chest physiotherapy is required and, preferably, until after the chest drains have been removed. Most patients who have undergone major surgery require effective analgesia for at least 48 hours so it makes no sense to discontinue the infusion before this. Similarly, the practice of removing an epidural catheter immediately after surgery, when a patient's future analgesia requirements are unknown, has nothing to commend it. Indeed it is questionable whether it is justifiable to perform an epidural at all unless the anaesthetist intends to use it to maximum effect in the postoperative period.

The nature of the operation influences both the type of analgesia most suited to take over from the epidural and the timing of its introduction. For example, oral analgesia can be introduced sooner after orthopaedic procedures than after major bowel surgery, and paracetamol will not be absorbed until gastric motility has recommenced.

In theory, gradual reduction in the epidural infusion rate over a period of days – *weaning* – is illogical because a certain minimum rate is required to provide the necessary dermatomal spread and rates less than this result in an inadequate block. Some anaesthetists therefore maintain the infusion at a constant rate until alternative analgesia can be introduced and then discontinue the epidural. However, a block is not an all-or-nothing phenomenon in the postoperative period. Analgesia requirements diminish with the passage of time (though not at a steady rate) and it is not uncommon to find that on, say, the third postoperative day, a patient is pain free on an infusion rate two-thirds of that required immediately after surgery. Furthermore, sudden withdrawal of such a highly effective method of pain control can cause the patient much anxiety. The infusion rate should therefore be reduced gradually while alternative analgesia is being introduced, and the patient encouraged to decide when the epidural is no longer necessary. When the infusion is eventually stopped, the catheter must be left *in situ* until normal sensation has returned so that, in the rare case where pain is unexpectedly severe, the epidural can be re-activated.

## COMPLICATIONS OF EPIDURAL ANAESTHESIA

The side-effects of epidural anaesthesia, such as hypotension and shoulder tip pain, have already been mentioned and the general complications of regional anaesthesia have been dealt with in Chapter 8. There are, however, complications which arise specifically from epidurals.

### Dural puncture

The incidence varies with the skill and experience of the anaesthetist, but if the technique is taught according to sound anatomical principles and is carefully performed, dural puncture should not occur in more than 1% of cases. Dural puncture by the epidural needle is usually obvious because it results in a brisk flow of warm liquid. Puncture by the catheter may be harder to diagnose because flow of CSF down the catheter is comparatively slow and CSF may be mistaken for saline or local anaesthetic if these have been injected previously through the needle. A catheter accurately positioned in the epidural space does not necessarily remain there. It can migrate through the dura so that subsequent injections or infusions are intrathecal rather than epidural.

If dural puncture occurs, it is usual to withdraw the needle or catheter and to attempt epidural puncture and cannulation at an adjacent interspace. This occasionally results in a widespread block, presumably because local anaesthetic leaks through the hole in the dura and produces an intrathecal effect. An effective and carefully observed test dose is essential in these cases. Another approach, when accidental dural puncture occurs, is simply to insert the catheter to the subarachnoid space and convert to a continuous spinal technique (see Ch. 10).

*Total spinal* If dural puncture is not recognised and a full epidural dose is injected into the CSF, a profound and extensive block will develop for which full cardiorespiratory resuscitation may be required. Covino and colleagues (1980) recommend that a volume of CSF equal to the volume of solution injected should be withdrawn through the catheter as soon as the error is discovered. Some of the drug will hopefully be present in the aspirate, leaving a smaller intrathecal dose which will eventually be diluted as more CSF is formed.

Resuscitation should be continued until the effects of the block subside.

### Symptoms

Headache occurs commonly after dural puncture. The traditional explanation – and probably the right one – is that the leak of CSF into the epidural space causes reduction of CSF pressure in the theca, and the resulting tendency for the cord to descend puts increased tension on the pain-sensitive blood vessels of the supporting meninges. The headache classically comes on when the patient sits up or stands, disappears when he/she lies flat, and usually affects the occipital and nuchal areas. The incidence increases when large needles are used – a Tuohy needle produces symptoms in up to 40% of obstetric patients (Norris et al 1989).

### Treatment

The condition is self-limiting and will usually resolve within a week. Mild cases should be treated with analgesics, a high fluid intake, laxatives to minimise straining at stool and bedrest. More severe cases, as well as being intolerable for the patient, carry the risk of intracranial haemorrhage, and active steps should be taken to prevent CSF leakage.

A *dural blood patch* is the most effective method of sealing the dural puncture site. The patient's own blood is drawn under aseptic conditions and a sample sent for culture. Then 15–20 ml of blood is injected epidurally, ideally at the interspace at which the dural puncture occurred. An indwelling catheter should not be used for this because the catheter tip may be some distance from the dural hole and the blood clot may not extend far enough to cover it. The patient, after lying supine for 30 minutes, is allowed to be fully mobile, and Crawford (1980), reporting on 98 obstetric patients treated by this method, recorded only one whose headache was not relieved. Treatment with a blood patch does not appear to affect the success of subsequent epidural blocks and is certainly not a contraindication to them (Abouleish et al 1975).

An anaesthetist who has already punctured the dura and has, perhaps with difficulty, located the epidural space and passed a catheter at the second attempt, may be reluctant to perform a blood patch in case he/she punctures the dura yet again. In these circumstances, an *epidural infusion of 0.9% saline* may be given through the epidural catheter. A bacterial filter should be incorporated in the system, and the infusion continued at a rate of 60 ml h$^{-1}$ for 24 hours (Crawford 1972). The method results in a cure in over 70% of cases, but the patient must obviously remain in bed while the infusion is in progress.

Caffeine may be effective and if oral therapy is inappropriate, an intravenous infusion of 500 mg in 500 ml can be infused over 4 hours (Baumgarten 1987). The serotonin receptor agonist sumatriptan, 6 mg subcutaneously, has also been recommended (Carp et al 1994).

## Venous puncture

The insertion of a needle and catheter into the epidural space is a blind technique, so accidental venous puncture is a complication which all anaesthetists occasionally encounter. It is more likely to occur when the needle enters the epidural space a few millimetres from the midline because the venous plexuses occupy the lateral parts of the space. The appearance of blood from a needle which has entered the epidural space is rare, though it is sometimes seen before the space has been reached. Venous puncture with a catheter is more common, and occurs in up to 10% of obstetric cases. The injection of 10 ml of liquid before insertion of the catheter reduces the incidence to about 3% (Verniquet 1980). Venous puncture occasionally occurs as a result of migration of the catheter tip. If the epidural is being maintained with bolus injections, blood is discovered in the catheter when a top-up is about to be given. The catheter should be cleared with sterile 0.9% saline and withdrawn until blood can no longer be aspirated. A test dose of local anaesthetic containing epinephrine should then be given. Intravenous migration of the catheter should be suspected when a previously satisfactory infusion becomes ineffective.

### Epidural haematoma

Because any bleeding into the epidural space may not be revealed and is impossible to control directly, a haematoma may form and go undetected. Epidural block is therefore contraindicated in patients with coagulopathies and those receiving anticoagulants (see Ch. 7). The neurological symptoms and signs caused by a haematoma may be confused with those of epidural block and depend more on the location of the haematoma and the pressure it exerts than on its size. If sensory loss or lower limb weakness progress or outlast the expected duration of the block, neurological advice should be sought, and investigations commenced, at an early stage if permanent sequelae are to be avoided. If an unexpected neurological deficit or backache develop during an epidural infusion, the infusion must be stopped and the patient's neurological status assessed.

## Hypotension

The discussion in Chapters 2 and 8 on the physiology and significance of hypotension resulting from regional block provides a basis for deciding on the degree of hypotension acceptable in the individual case. Some decrease in systolic blood pressure, often accompanied by a reduction in heart rate, is usual after epidural block and indeed is a useful indication that the block is effective. Because this is associated with a low rate–pressure product and, hence, low myocardial oxygen demands, there is a beneficial effect on the normal myocardium, and flow becomes more important than pressure for ensuring tissue perfusion. In the patient with ischaemic heart disease though, perfusion pressure is more important than flow in forcing oxygenated blood past atheromatous obstructions, so systolic pressure (and heart rate) should be kept within 20% of normal, angina-free limits (Merin 1981).

If serious hypotension develops, the central venous pressure should be checked, the patient tilted head-down and 6 mg increments of ephedrine given intra-venously up to 30 mg. If this fails to restore and maintain blood pressure, other causes for the hypotension, such as undetected surgical haemorrhage, should be sought.

## Retention of urine

This is a recognised complication of epidural block. In many cases, such as major gynaecological, arterial, abdominal and thoracic surgery, a catheter will in any case be required for urinary output measurements. In others though, catheterisation may be necessary solely to deal with urinary retention resulting from the epidural, particularly when the block is continued into the postoperative period. Some orthopaedic surgeons believe that bladder catheterisation may increase the

risk of infection in newly inserted orthopaedic prostheses. However, when antibiotic prophylaxis is given before catheterisation, the infection rate in knee and hip prostheses is below the accepted mean for even the lowest risk categories (DJR Connolly 2000, personal communication; Semiannual Report of the US Department of Health and Human Resources Public Health Service 1999).

## Catheter problems

*Transections* and *kinking* of epidural catheters, and methods for avoiding these complications have been discussed earlier in this chapter. Studies in which radiopaque dye has been injected down epidural catheters have shown that a catheter inserted by the midline approach may loop if excessive length is introduced, and a *knot* may form when an attempt is made to remove it and the loop is drawn tight (Nash & Openshaw 1968). This complication may be avoided by inserting a short length of catheter, but although this may be adequate for the operation, it is likely to be displaced when the patient becomes mobile afterwards. The risk of knotting is reduced if the catheter is introduced through a needle inserted by the paramedian approach (see p. 147 above). A knotted catheter, or one which for any reason is *difficult to remove*, may be freed by flexing the patient to the position in which it was originally inserted and exerting traction. If this is ineffective, extension of the back may allow it to be withdrawn. If this also fails, or the catheter breaks, surgical removal may have to be considered, but it is worth bearing in mind that Dawkins (1969), faced with this problem, left the broken end *in situ* and no symptoms had occurred 2 years later when he reported the case.

## Infection

Not every case is reported, but infection of the epidural space is nevertheless very rare. When it does occur, it is generally secondary to sources in the skin, the respiratory or urinary tracts and most often occurs in patients with immunological compromise, for example, those on steroid therapy or with diabetes. A review of 39 cases of epidural abscess, collected over 27 years (Baker et al 1975), revealed only one case in which the infection could have been due to an epidural catheter, although this review extended over a period when epidural anaesthesia was not so widely practised as it is now. Saady (1976) reported an abscess attributable to epidural anaesthesia, the probable cause being the development of infection in the haematoma produced, presumably, when the catheter was inserted. Epidural abscess has also been described after a *single-shot* epidural injection in a diabetic patient (Goucke & Graziotti 1990) and after spinal anaesthesia (Loarie & Fairlie 1978, Beaudoin & Klein 1984). In the last 15 years, reports of infective sequelae appear to be increasing, perhaps due to better record keeping and audit, and concern about them should equal that regarding haematoma (Carson & Wildsmith 1995). There are certainly no grounds for complacency.

Two of the invariable signs of an epidural abscess – pyrexia and leukocytosis – first appear 3 or 4 days after the block. They may easily be attributed to surgical causes or respiratory infection, but local tenderness and back pain also are always present, CSF protein levels are raised and magnetic resonance imaging reveals narrowing or obstruction of the theca at the level of the abscess. Antibiotics, surgical decompression and drainage are required before irreversible neurological damage occurs. *Staphylococcus aureus* is usually the causative organism.

Neurological symptoms may take days or weeks to develop so the epidural may be overlooked as a possible cause. The situation is compounded in cases where the patient presents at a different hospital where clinical records of an admission elsewhere are unavailable (Bromage 1993). A high index of suspicion is therefore essential. Delay in making the diagnosis and in starting surgical treatment almost always result in a poor outcome.

# Neurological sequelae

Permanent neurological disability following an epidural attracts wide publicity, so it is not surprising that the occasional patient is unhappy about having a block. Such complications are very rare, but patients often expect the anaesthetist to know the incidence of complications. Unfortunately, the quotation of risk requires the collection of epidemiological data which includes an accurate record of the number of epidural blocks performed in large populations, and the incidence of complications within this population. Such information is not available at the moment though the increasing requirement for medical audit may yield it in the future (Wildsmith 1993).

However, studies do exist in which both the numerator and denominator are known. For example, Kane (1981) found that three out of a total of 50 000 patients had persistent paralysis of the lower limbs. More recently, Scott & Hibbard (1990) undertook a retrospective study of complications associated with epidural block in obstetric practice. The total number of epidurals given during the review period was over half a million, and 38 mothers suffered damage to a single spinal nerve or nerve root. In one case, the neuropathy appeared to be permanent but symptoms resolved within 3 months, in the other 37 patients. A further two patients developed irreversible lesions of the spinal cord, but the contribution, if any, of the epidural to their symptoms is uncertain. One developed thrombosis in a congenital cervical haemangioma 10 days after delivery, and the other probably developed anterior spinal artery syndrome 12 hours after delivery when she had apparently recovered from the effects of the epidural.

Permanent neurological damage has occurred when the treatment of complications such as hypotension, haematoma, abscess and accidental subarachnoid injection was inadequate or was commenced too late. It has also followed the accidental epidural injection of a highly irritant solution such as potassium chloride. However, direct needle trauma has almost certainly caused permanent damage in some cases, a point which emphasises the need for the highest standards of instruction, supervision and performance.

## Sequelae of uneventful blocks

Nerve damage has apparently followed the otherwise uncomplicated administration of a local anaesthetic solution. Preservatives, such as metabisulphite and methylparaben, and vasoconstrictors have been suspected of contributing to this. Metabisulphite added to chloroprocaine was almost certainly responsible for permanent paralysis after the accidental intrathecal injection of an epidural dose (Covino 1984). Solutions containing preservative should be avoided when epidural and spinal block is to be performed.

Many of the affected patients had received epinephrine, but this may simply reflect the frequency of its use. However, the dose given has often been unacceptably high and it is unwise to exceed the optimal concentration of 1:200 000. Commercial solutions which contain a vasoconstrictor are more acidic than those which do not, so it is better practice to add the epinephrine just before use.

## Latent neurological disease

Occasionally, some previously symptomless pathology may be unmasked by an epidural block. During epidural injection, pressure up to 60 cmH$_2$O may be generated, and although this dissipates rapidly, it could serve to hasten the onset of symptoms in a patient who was on the point of developing them. One patient who developed paraplegia after an epidural was cured when a laminectomy relieved her spinal stenosis (Chaudhari et al 1978), and the only case of permanent paralysis in Dawkins' personal series of 4000 patients was a man who was found to have secondary spinal deposits from a carcinoma of the prostate (Dawkins 1969).

# References

Abouleish E, Wadhwa RK, de la Vega S, Tan RN, Uy NTL 1975 Regional analgesia following epidural blood patch. Anesthesia and Analgesia (Current Researches) 54: 634–636

Aitkenhead AR, Hothersall AP, Gilmour DG, Ledingham I McA 1979 Dural dimpling in the dog. Anaesthesia 34: 14–19

Apostolou GA, Zarmakoupis PK, Mastrokostopoulos GT 1981 Spread of epidural anesthesia and the lateral position. Anesthesia and Analgesia (Current Researches) 60: 584–586

Armitage EN 1989 Postoperative pain – prevention or relief? British Journal of Anaesthesia 63: 136–137

Axelsson K, Hallgren S, Weidman B, Olstrin P-O. 1985 A new method for measuring motor block in the lower extremities. Acta Anaesthesiologica Scandinavica 29: 82–88

Bach S, Noreng MF, Tjellden NU 1988 Phantom limb pain in amputees during the first 12 months following limb amputation after preoperative lumbar epidural blockade. Pain 33: 297–301

Baker AS, Ojemann RG, Swartz MN, Richardson EP 1975 Spinal epidural abscess. New England Journal of Medicine 293: 463–468

Baumgarten RK 1987 Should caffeine become the first line treatment for postdural puncture headache? Anesthesia and Analgesia 66: 913–914

Beaudoin MG, Klein L 1984 Epidural abscess following multiple spinal anaesthetics. Anaesthesia and Intensive Care 12: 163–164

Blomberg RG 1988 Technical advantages of the paramedian approach for lumbar epidural puncture and catheter introduction. A study using epiduroscopy in autopsy subjects. Anaesthesia 43: 837–843

Breen TW, Shapiro T, Glass B, Foster-Payne D, Oriol NE 1993 Epidural anesthesia for labor in an ambulatory patient. Anesthesia and Analgesia 77: 919–924

Brockway MS, Bannister J, McClure JH, McKeown D, Wildsmith JAW 1991 Comparison of extradural ropivacaine and bupivacaine. British Journal of Anaesthesia 66: 31–37

Bromage PR 1969 Ageing and epidural dose requirements. Segmental spread and predictability of epidural analgesia in youth and extreme age. British Journal of Anaesthesia 41: 1016–1022

Bromage PR 1981 The price of intraspinal narcotic analgesia: basic constraints. Anesthesia and Analgesia (Current Researches) 60: 461–463

Bromage PR 1993 Spinal extradural abscess: pursuit of vigilance. British Journal of Anaesthesia 70: 471–473

Burn JM, Guyer PB, Langdon L 1973 The spread of solutions injected into the epidural space. A study using epidurograms in patients with the lumbosciatic syndrome. British Journal of Anaesthesia 45: 338–345

Carabine UA, Milligan KR, Moore J 1992 Extradural clonidine and bupivacaine for postoperative analgesia. British Journal of Anaesthesia 68: 132–135

Carp H, Singh PJ, Vadhera R, Jayaram A. 1994 Effects of the serotonin receptor agonist sumatriptan on the post dural puncture headache: report of six cases. Anesthesia and Analgesia 79: 180–182

Carson D, Wildsmith JAW 1995 The risk of extradural abscess. British Journal of Anaesthesia 75: 520–521

Chaudhari LS, Kop BR, Dhruva AJ 1978 Paraplegia and epidural analgesia. Anaesthesia 33: 722–725

Coleman SA, Booker-Milburn J 1996 Audit of postoperative pain control. Influence of a dedicated acute pain nurse. Anaesthesia 51: 1093–1096

Covino BG 1984 Current controversies in local anaesthetics. In: Scott DB, McClure JH, Wildsmith JAW (eds) Regional anaesthesia 1884–1984, pp 74–81. ICM, Sodertalje

Covino BG, Marx GF, Finster M, Zsigmond EK 1980 Prolonged sensory/motor deficits following inadvertent spinal anesthesia. Anesthesia and Analgesia (Current Researches) 59: 399–400

Cowen MJ, Bullingham RES, Paterson GMC et al 1982 A controlled comparison of the effects of extradural diamorphine and bupivacaine on plasma glucose and plasma cortisol in postoperative patients. Anesthesia and Analgesia (Current Researches) 61: 15–18

Crawford JS 1972 The prevention of headache consequent upon dural puncture. British Journal of Anaesthesia 44: 598–600

Crawford JS 1980 Experiences with epidural blood patch. Anaesthesia 35: 513–515

Dahl JB, Rosenberg J, Dirkes WE, Mogensen T, Kehlet H 1990 Prevention of postoperative pain by balanced analgesia. British Journal of Anaesthesia 64: 518–520

Dawkins CJM 1966 Postoperative pain relief by means of continuous epidural block. Acta Anaesthesiologica Scandinavica 23 (Supplement): 438–441

Dawkins CJM 1969 An analysis of the complications of extradural and caudal block. Anaesthesia 24: 554–563

Devine A, Romer H. 2000 The importance of confirming the length of a Tuohy needle. [Letter] Anaesthesia 55: 304

Duncan LA, Fried MJ, Lee A, Wildsmith JAW 1998 Comparison of continuous and intermittent administration of extradural bupivacaine for analgesia after lower abdominal surgery. British Journal of Anaesthesia 80: 7–10

Goodman LS, Gilman A 1997 The pharmacological basis of therapeutics, 9th edn, Macmillan, New York.

Goucke CR, Graziotti P 1990 Extradural abscess following local anesthetic and steroid injection for chronic low back pain. British Journal of Anaesthesia 65: 427–429

Grundy EM, Ramamurthy S, Patel KP, Mani M, Winnie AP 1978a Extradural re-visited. A statistical study. British Journal of Anaesthesia 50: 805–809

Grundy EM, Rao LN, Winnie AP 1978b Epidural anesthesia and the lateral position. Anesthesia and Analgesia (Current Researches) 57: 95–97

Hodgkinson R, Husain FJ 1981 Obesity, gravity and spread of epidural anesthesia. Anesthesia and Analgesia (Current Researches) 60: 421–424

Holmdahl MH, Sjogren S, Strom G, Wright B 1972 Clinical aspects of continuous epidural blockade for postoperative pain relief. Uppsala Journal of Medical Science 77: 47–56

Jacobson L, Phillips PD, Hull CJ, Conches ID 1983 Extradural versus intramuscular diamorphine. A controlled study of analgesic and adverse effects in the postoperative period. Anaesthesia 38: 10–18

Jørgensen H, Fomsgaard JS, Dirks J, Witterslev J, Dahl JB 2000 Effect of continuous epidural 0.2% ropivacaine vs 0.2% bupivacaine on postoperative pain, motor block and gastrointestinal function after abdominal hysterectomy. British Journal of Anaesthesia 84: 144–150

Kane RE 1981 Neurologic deficits following epidural and spinal anesthesia. Anesthesia and Analgesia (Current Researches) 60: 150–161

Katz JA, Knarr D, Bridenbaugh PO 1990 A double-blind comparison of 0.5% bupivacaine and 0.75% ropivacaine administered epidurally in humans. Regional Anaesthesia 15: 250–252

Kehlet H 1994 Postoperative pain relief. A look from the other side. Regional Anesthesia 19(6): 369–377

Lee A, Simpson D, Whitfield A, Scott DB 1988 Postoperative analgesia by continuous epidural infusion of bupivacaine and diamorphine. British Journal of Anaesthesia 60: 845–850

Loarie DS, Fairlie HB 1978 Epidural abscess following spinal anesthesia. Anesthesia and Analgesia 57: 351–353

Macintosh RR 1950 New inventions 2: extradural space indicator. Anaesthesia 5: 98

Merin RG 1981 Local and regional anesthetic techniques for the patient with ischemic heart disease. Cleveland Clinic Quarterly 48: 72–74

Michael S, Richmond NM, Birks RJS 1989 A comparison between open-ended (single hole) and closed-ended (three lateral holes) epidural catheters. Complications and quality of sensory blockade. Anaesthesia 44: 578–580

Mitchell RWD, Scott DB, Holmquist E, Lamont M 1988 Continuous extradural infusion of 0.125% bupivacaine for pain relief after lower abdominal surgery. British Journal of Anaesthesia 60: 851–853

Morton CPJ, Bloomfield S, Magnusson A, Jozwiak H, McClure JH 1997 Ropivacaine 0.75% for extradural anaesthesia in elective Caesarean section: an open clinical and pharmacokinetic study in mother and neonate. British Journal of Anaesthesia 79: 3–8

Murphy DF, Medley C 1993 Preoperative indomethacin for pain relief after thoracotomy: comparison with postoperative indomethacin. British Journal of Anaesthesia 70: 298–300

Nash TG, Openshaw DJ 1968 Unusual complication of epidural anaesthesia. British Medical Journal i: 700

Norris MC, Leighton BL, De Simone CA 1989 Needle bevel direction and headache after inadvertent dural puncture. Anesthesiology 70: 729–731

Nydahl P-A, Axelsson K, Hallgren S, Larsson P, Leissner P, Philipson L 1988 Evaluation of motor blockade by isometric force measurement and electromyographic recording during epidural anaesthesia: A methodological study. Acta Anaesthesiologica Scandinavica 32: 477–484

Park WY, Poon KC, Massengale MD, MacNamara TE 1982 Direction of needle bevel and epidural anesthetic spread. Anesthesiology 57: 327–328

Ready LB, Oden R, Chadwick HS et al 1988 Development of an anesthesiology-based postoperative pain management service. Anesthesiology 68: 100–106

Report 1990 Pain after Surgery. Commission on the provision of surgical services. The Royal College of Surgeons of England and The College of Anaesthetists, London

Report 1991 High dependency care – acute care in the future. Association of Anaesthetists of Great Britain and Ireland, London

Ross RA, Clarke JE Armitage EN 1980 Postoperative pain prevention by continuous epidural infusion. A study of the clinical effects and the plasma concentrations obtained. Anaesthesia 35: 663–668

Rostaing S, Bonnet F, Levron JC, Vodinh J, Pluskwa F, Saada M 1991 Effect of epidural clonidine on analgesia and pharmacokinetics of epidural fentanyl in postoperative patients. Anesthesiology 75: 420–425

Saady A 1976 Epidural abscess complicating thoracic epidural analgesia. Anesthesiology 45: 244–246

Saberski LR, Kondamuri S, Osinubi OYO 1997 Identification of the epidural space: is loss of resistance to air a safe technique? Regional Anesthesia 22: 3–15

Schug SA, Scott DA, Payne J, Mooney PH, Hägglöf B. 1996 Postoperative analgesia by continuous extradural infusion of ropivacaine after upper abdominal surgery. British Journal of Anaesthesia 76: 487–491

Schweitzer S, Morgan DJ 1987 Plasma bupivacaine concentrations during postoperative continuous analgesia. Anaesthesia and Intensive Care 15: 425–430

Scott DB 1975 Evaluation of the clinical tolerance of anaesthetic agents. British Journal of Anaesthesia 47: 328–331

Scott DB 1983 Abdominal and perineal surgery. In: Henderson JJ, Nimmo WS (eds) Practical regional anaesthesia pp. 215–237 Blackwell, Oxford.

Scott DB, Hibbard BM 1990 Serious non-fatal complications associated with extradural block in obstetric patients. British Journal of Anaesthesia 64: 537–541

Scott DB, Schweitzer S, Thorn J 1982 Epidural block in postoperative pain relief. Regional Anesthesia 7: 135–139

Semiannual Report of the US Department of Health and Human Resources Public Health Service 1999

Shah J, Mariappan M, Jeyapalan I 1999 A long 17-G Vygon needle. [Letter] Anaesthesia 54: 1022

Sharrock NE 1978 Epidural anesthetic dose responses in patients 20 to 80 years old. Anesthesiology 47: 425–428

Sinclair CJ, Scott DB 1984 Comparison of bupivacaine and etidocaine in extradural blockade. British Journal of Anaesthesia 56: 147–153

Soresi AL 1932 Peridural anesthesia: a preliminary report. Medical Record (New York) 35: 165–166

Torda TA, Pybus DA 1984 Extradural administration of morphine and bupivacaine. A controlled comparison. British Journal of Anaesthesia 56: 141–146

Valentine SJ, Jarvis AP Shutt LE 1991 Comparative study of the effects of air or saline to identify the extradural space. British Journal of Anaesthesia 66: 224–227

Verniquet AJW 1980 Vessel puncture with epidural catheters. Experience in obstetric patients. Anaesthesia 35: 660–662

Weddell SJ, Ritter RR 1980 Epidural morphine: serum levels and pain relief. Anesthesiology 53: 419

Welchew EA 1983 The optimum concentration for epidural fentanyl. A randomised double-blind comparison with and without 1:200 000 adrenaline. Anaesthesia 38: 1037–1041

Wildsmith JAW 1993 Extradural abscess after central neural block. British Journal of Anaesthesia 70: 387–388

Wood MB, Rubin AP 1993 A comparison of epidural 1% ropivacaine and 0.75% bupivacaine for lower abdominal gynecologic surgery. Anesthesia and Analgesia 76: 1274–1278

Woolf CJ 1989 Recent advances in the pathophysiology of acute pain. British Journal of Anaesthesia 63: 139–146

Yaksh TL, Reddy SVR 1981 Studies in the primate on the analgesic effects associated with intrathecal actions of opiates, alpha-adrenergic agonists and baclofen. Anesthesiology 54: 451–467

# 12. Sacral epidural (caudal) block

## L V H Martin and E Doyle

The sacral approach to the epidural space provides a more reliable and effective block of the sacral nerve roots than does the lumbar route, and is often preferred for operations which involve the sacral dermatomes. The technique of using a single injection of local anaesthetic via the caudal approach combines the advantages of simplicity with a high success rate and a low incidence of side-effects. It is applicable to many surgical procedures and can be combined with general anaesthesia to reduce the requirement for volatile agent and opioid, allowing rapid pain-free recovery with minimal postoperative vomiting and an early resumption of eating and drinking.

The technique of caudal block depends upon the accurate localisation of the sacral hiatus through which access to the sacral epidural space is gained. Unfortunately, there are considerable anatomical differences in the size and shape of the hiatus, which may make its identification difficult, and in some cases the insertion of a needle into the sacral canal may be impossible.

### Anatomical variations (Fig. 12.1)

Interest in the anatomy of the sacrum was aroused in the 1940s in the USA and was associated with the development of continuous caudal anaesthesia for the relief of pain in childbirth (Edwards & Hingson 1942, Hingson 1947a, b). Reviews of large collections of skeletons delineated the wide range of normal measurements and recorded the variations which may occur (Trotter & Letterman 1944, Trotter & Lanier 1945).

The adult sacrum is formed from five distinct semicartilagenous sacral vertebrae, which ossify and fuse but in differing degrees, so that many variations of 'normal' may occur. The important variations relate to the dorsal wall of the sacral canal (Trotter 1947). The sacral hiatus, which is roughly triangular in shape, results from failure of fusion of the laminae of the fifth sacral vertebra, and is covered by the sacrococcygeal ligament. Sometimes the fourth, and occasionally the third vertebrae, also fail to fuse, so that there is considerable variation in the position of the apex of the hiatus, and in its distance from a line joining the two sacral cornua. The 'classical' position of the apex is level with the lower third of the body of $S_4$, but this is found to be the case in only 35% of patients, being higher in 45% of them and lower in 20%. The mean distance between the apex and a line joining the cornua is 20 mm, but with a range of 0–66 mm. However, occasionally there may be complete failure of all the sacral arches or the hiatus can be completely obliterated by bone. Failure of fusion of the upper sacral vertebrae may also occur and result in separate defects through which solution may escape during injection. The base of the hiatus (the line joining the sacral cornua) is subject to some variation also, having a mean length of 16 mm and a range of 7–28 mm.

In Trotter's study the mean anteroposterior diameter of the sacral canal was 5.3 mm (range 0–16 mm), but it was less than 2 mm in 5.5% of cases. Complete obliteration of the canal was found in a very small proportion, caused either by a transverse fold in the posterior wall of the canal, with a corresponding projection from the anterior wall, or by the dorsal projection of a sacral body into the canal. Studies in cadavers (Lanier et al 1944) have shown similar variations in the position of the inferior extremity of the dura, which was found to have a mean position at the middle third of the body of $S_2$, being caudad to this in 46% of cases and cephalad in 38%. The mean distance from the dura to the apex of the sacral hiatus was 47 mm, with a range of 19–75 mm.

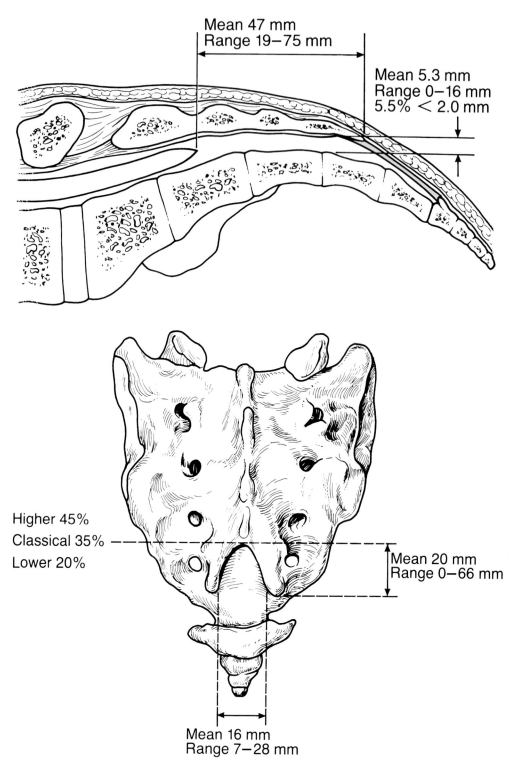

**Fig 12.1** Variations in sacral anatomy

Recently, magnetic resonance imaging (MRI) has been used to study the anatomy of the adult sacrum during life (Crighton et al 1997). Overall, there is reasonable congruence between these new measurements and the older studies, although some differences emerge. The median and modal position of the apex of the sacral hiatus was found to be lower, that is, at the level of the upper third of the body of $S_5$. The mean length of the sacrococcygeal ligament was similar at 22.6 mm, but with a smaller range (upper limit 36 mm). The anteroposterior dimensions of the canal were similar also, and it was noted that the maximum diameter of the canal was adjacent to the upper third of the sacrococcygeal ligament. The position of the inferior extremity of the dura was confirmed at the middle third of $S_2$, but the mean distance from the dura to the apex of the hiatus was greater at 60.5 mm (range 34–80 mm) no doubt reflecting the smaller variability of the sacral hiatus in this series.

## Technique of sacral epidural block

Explanation of the procedure, including the likelihood of some postoperative lower limb motor block, and consent from the patient are required preoperatively. Some patients are concerned at the thought of an epidural technique being performed for what they may regard as minor surgery and a simple explanation of the procedure and its benefits is often reassuring.

### Indications and contraindications
Caudal epidural block has a defined place in surgery on the anus, rectum, penis, prostate, urethra, vagina and cervix. Local infection and bleeding disorders may contraindicate use of this method and require careful consideration (Ch. 7). Anatomical abnormalities of the sacrum or overlying skin, which may lead to difficulty in identifying the sacral hiatus, and neurological abnormalities are relative contraindications.

### Position of patient
Caudal injections are usually carried out either with the patient prone or in the lateral position. The *prone position* is easier for the operator, but is less comfortable for the patient, particularly if there is any respiratory embarrassment. The patient's head and shoulders should be supported by a suitable pillow or padding, and another pillow should be placed under the pelvis to tilt it and bring the sacral hiatus into greater prominence. The ankles should also be supported on a pillow with the lower limbs slightly abducted and the feet internally rotated. This prevents tightening of the gluteal muscles, which can make identification of the landmarks more difficult.

In *the lateral position* the patient should arch the back and draw up the knees in front of the abdomen, and the sacral region should be brought to the edge of the table to allow the operator greater freedom of movement. The anaesthetist should sit or crouch and, if right handed, should place the patient in the left lateral position so that the natural movement of the wrist facilitates the insertion of the needle. In this position the patient's buttock may fall over the sacral region and obscure the region of the hiatus.

Caudal injection with the patient in the lithotomy position has been described (Berstock 1979).

### Location of sacral hiatus
The approximate position of the sacral hiatus can be identified in two ways. First, an equilateral triangle with its base on the line joining the two posterior superior iliac spines will have its apex over the sacral hiatus (Fig. 12.2). Second, if the anaesthetist's index finger is laid in the natal cleft with the distal end at the tip of the coccyx, the sacral hiatus will be level with the proximal interphalangeal joint (Fig. 12.3). When the approximate position has been indicated, the sacral spines are palpated with a gradual movement in a caudal direction until a depression is felt. Identification of the sacral cornua laterally will then confirm the exact location.

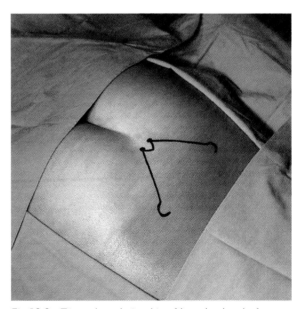

**Fig 12.2** Triangular relationship of bony landmarks for caudal block

171

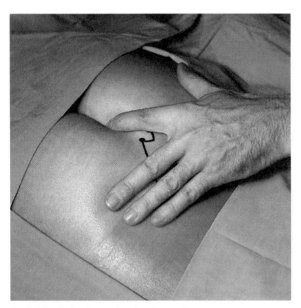

**Fig 12.3**   Index finger level with tip of coccyx

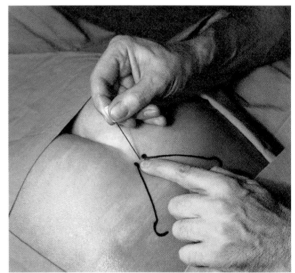

**Fig 12.4**   Needle alignment for initial insertion

## Choice of needle

Ordinary disposable hypodermic needles may be used for injection, but their length may be inadequate, particularly in obese patients, and breakage is always a possibility. It is more satisfactory to use a longer, more substantial needle, preferably with a trocar *in situ*, because this prevents the possibility of introducing a core of skin into the epidural space. Spinal needles of 18 or 19 g can be used, as can epidural needles with a straight point. Huber pointed needles, although recommended by some, are less satisfactory and are more difficult to insert through the sacrococcygeal ligament. A short bevelled needle will also reveal an appreciable loss of resistance, or 'click', as the sacrococcygeal ligament is pierced.

## Needle insertion

During preparation of the skin, care should be taken to avoid antiseptic solutions irritating the perineum. A skin wheal should be raised over the hiatus and the subcutaneous tissue infiltrated with a small quantity of local anaesthetic. The sacrococcygeal ligament and the adjacent periosteum should also be infiltrated, but large amounts of anaesthetic should be avoided because the landmarks, which may already be difficult to palpate, are easily obscured.

The caudal needle should then be inserted (Fig. 12.4) through the skin wheal, close to the apex of the sacral hiatus, and at right angles to the sacrococcygeal ligament. It is advanced through the ligament until the bone of the underlying sacral body is reached. The needle should be withdrawn slightly to disengage the tip from the periosteum, and the hub 'depressed' through 55–60° to bring the shaft into alignment with the sacral canal (Fig. 12.5). The needle is then advanced along the canal. There is often a sensation of a 'give' at this stage and the needle is then firmly held by bone and ligament. It should be kept in the midline and sufficient length inserted to establish its position, but without risk of penetration of the dura. The measurements and variations detailed earlier must be borne in mind throughout.

## Incorrect insertion

It is easy to place the needle incorrectly and a number of possibilities exist. The needle may be inserted superficial to the canal (Fig. 12.6A), so that the injection is made into the subcutaneous tissue. It is usually possible to see or palpate a swelling if this occurs, but in cases of doubt the injection of a few millilitres of air will produce localised surgical emphysema which will confirm the misplacement. Alternatively, the needle may enter the canal, but become embedded in the periosteal lining. Attempts at injection will then meet with considerable resistance. It is also possible for the needle to enter the canal, but leave it through a superior defect so that the injection will again be subcutaneous.

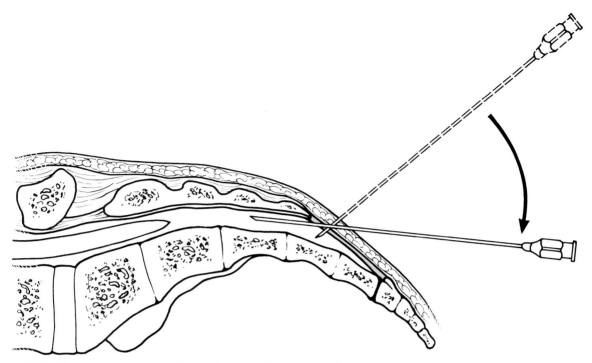

**Fig 12.5**  Change of alignment needed to advance needle along sacral canal

A more serious malposition may occur if the needle is inserted too vigorously and too far. It will then pass through the sacrococcygeal joint, or lateral to the coccyx, and into the pelvic cavity beyond (Fig. 12.6B). In this case both the rectum and birth canal may be entered and the needle will become contaminated. Subsequent withdrawal and re-insertion into the sacral canal will carry with it the danger of infection. If this malposition is suspected the procedure should be abandoned. Failure to recognise incorrect placement during labour has resulted in the injection of local anaesthetic into the fetal skull (Sinclair et al 1965). It is also possible to force the point of the needle into the marrow cavity of a sacral vertebra and any local anaesthetic injected will be absorbed rapidly (DiGiovanni 1971, McGown 1972).

Misplacement, as opposed to malposition, may occur if the needle enters an epidural vein, or is advanced too far and punctures the dura.

### Injection

When the needle is satisfactorily positioned it should be left 'open' for 10–20 seconds to help detect blood or cerebrospinal fluid in case of accidental venous or dural puncture. The syringe with local anaesthetic should then be attached and a gentle aspiration test performed. A dural 'tap' is, in fact, very rare, but should it occur it is wise to abandon the procedure and consider an alternative technique such a 'saddle block' spinal. A 'bloody tap' is more common and is usually due to bleeding into the sacral canal from veins damaged during needle insertion, rather than to intravenous placement of the needle tip. The needle should be withdrawn slightly and, if the aspiration test is now negative, a small quantity of local anaesthetic injected. The patient is questioned and observed for any sign of systemic effect and, if none appears, the full dose of anaesthetic is injected slowly, in small increments. It should be remembered that aspiration from small epidural veins may be negative and intravenous injection can still occur after a negative test. If the needle is correctly placed in the sacral canal there will be only slight resistance to injection, similar to that experienced with an epidural or venous injection. If any force is required, malposition should be suspected, but the needle should be rotated to see whether that helps before it is repositioned.

If there is doubt about the position of the needle tip, the anaesthetist may inject 2–5 ml of air through it while listening with a stethoscope placed over the lower lumbar vertebrae. If the needle is within the sacral

173

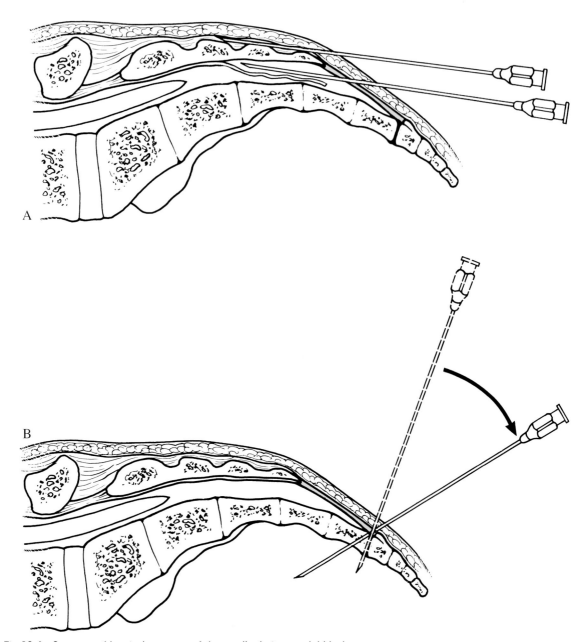

**Fig 12.6**  Some possible misplacements of the needle during caudal block

canal a loud bruit will be heard (Lee 1988, Lewis et al 1992). This procedure, sometimes referred to as the 'whoosh test', has been the subject of some controversy regarding both its usefulness (Atherton 1998, Eastwood et al 1998) and the advisibility of injecting air into the epidural space (Sethna & Berde 1993, Guinard & Borboen 1993). When a clear bruit is heard, it is a useful confirmatory sign of correct placement. When there is no bruit, or there is some doubt about it, the position of the needle should be reviewed.

## Volume of solution

The spread of solution in the sacral canal is dependent on the volume injected. The early anatomical studies suggested that the mean volume of the sacral canal in adults is slightly more than 30 ml (range 12–65 ml). However, this volume was measured in 'dry' bones, and the canal is filled with dura, nerves, blood vessels and connective tissue in life. Thus the MRI studies showed the mean volume of the canal to be 14.4 cm$^2$ (range 9.5–26.6 cm$^3$). In addition to the volume injected, cranial spread of solution is affected by the speed of injection, and by variable and unpredictable leakage through the sacral foramina (Burn et al 1973).

Cousins and Bromage (1971), using a standard dose (20 ml) of 2% lidocaine, found wide variations in the upper level of analgesia, there being no correlation with age, height or weight of the patient. However, 20 ml of solution can be relied upon to produce analgesia of the sacral nerves. Spread to the lower thoracic region may occur occasionally, but this seldom causes clinical problems and 20 ml is recommended as the standard volume for adults irrespective of the drug used.

## Suitable local anaesthetics

All local anaesthetic agents may be used to produce caudal anaesthesia. However, provision of postoperative analgesia is the usual reason for performing caudal epidural block, and bupivacaine, in a concentration of 0.25%, is the most commonly used agent. This concentration is occasionally associated with motor block, which may delay discharge in outpatients, so lidocaine or prilocaine (1%) is usually preferred in that situation. The less toxic long-acting local anaesthetic, ropivacaine, is now in clinical use and may produce less motor block than an equivalent dose of bupivacaine. Given that the consequences of the venous injection of bupivacaine are among the most serious complications of caudal epidural block, ropivacaine may offer an advantage.

An effective caudal block may be followed by severe pain when it wears off. This must be anticipated and sequential analgesia provided. Inpatients should have adequate systemic or oral analgesia prescribed for them, and day-patients should be discharged with a supply of appropriate analgesic drugs and instructions for home use. In either case, the first dose should be timed in advance of complete block regression.

## Additives

Epinephrine 1:200 000 will prolong the action of the local anaesthetic drug, but there is wide and unpredictable variation in its effect. This is particularly noticeable after haemorrhoidectomy when analgesia may last many hours and outlast recovery of other sensations. It may be that the prevention of the initial muscle spasm prevents the onset of a 'pain–spasm–pain' cycle.

The caudal route has been used for epidural opioid administration, with morphine being given alone and in combination with local anaesthetics. The results have been variable (Jensen et al 1982, Farad & Neguib 1985).

Clonidine and ketamine have been used as additives to improve caudal analgesia in children, but their use in adults has not been reported.

## Continuous caudal analgesia

When this was originally developed for use in obstetrics, catheters of suitable size were not available and the technique had to be performed using semi-rigid needles. With the development of epidural catheters it is now possible to insert a catheter in the sacral region. Because the size of the canal may limit the diameter of the needle, the smallest available catheter should be used. Provided that the needle tip is lying freely in the canal, no difficulty should be experienced in threading the catheter through it. About 5 cm should be advanced beyond the needle. After the needle is withdrawn, the catheter entry point in the skin should be dressed and secured with waterproof tape.

An alternative to an epidural catheter for a continuous caudal is an ordinary venous cannula. This is simpler to insert, but difficult to secure, and it may be uncomfortable for the patient when sitting or lying supine.

## References

Atherton AMJ 1998 Caudal epidurals: the 'whoosh test'. Anaesthesia 53: 927

Berstock DA 1979 Haemorrhoidectomy without tears. Annals of the Royal College of Surgeons of England 61: 51–54

Burn JM, Guyer PB, Langon L 1973 The spread of solutions injected into the epidural space. A study using epidurograms in patients with the lumbosciatic syndrome. British Journal of Anaesthesia 45: 338–344

Cousins MJ, Bromage PR 1971 A comparison of the hydrochloride and carbonated salts of lignocaine for caudal anaesthesia in out-patients. British Journal of Anaesthesia 43: 1149–1155

Crighton IM, Barry BP, Hobbs GJ 1997 A study of the anatomy of the caudal space using magnetic resonance imaging. British Journal of Anaesthesia 78: 391–395

DiGiovanni AJ 1971 Inadvertent interosseous injection – a hazard of caudal anesthesia. Anesthesiology 34: 92–94

Edwards WB, Hingson RA, 1942 Continuous caudal anesthesia in obstetrics. American Journal of Surgery 57: 459–464

Eastwood D, Williams C, Buchan I 1998 Caudal epidurals: the whoosh test. Anaesthesia 53: 305–307

Farad H, Naguib M 1985 Caudal morphine for pain relief following anal surgery. Annals of the Royal College of Surgeons of England 67: 257–258

Guinard J-P, Borboen M 1993 Probable venous air embolism during caudal anesthesia in a child. Anesthesia and Analgesia 76: 1134–1135

Hingson RA 1947a Continuous caudal analgesia in obstetrics, surgery and therapeutics. Current Researches in Anesthesia and Analgesia 26: 177–191

Hingson RA 1947b Continuous caudal analgesia in obstetrics, surgery and therapeutics – conclusion. Current Researches in Anesthesia and Analgesia 26: 238–247

Jensen PJ, Siem-Jorgensen P, Nielsen BN, Wichmand-Nielsen H, Wintherreich E 1982 Epidural morphine by the caudal route for postoperative pain relief. Acta Anaesthesiologica Scandinavica 26: 511–513

Lanier VA, McKnight HE, Trotter M 1944 Caudal analgesia: an experimental and anatomical study. American Journal of Obstetrics and Gynecology 47: 633–641

Lee MG 1988 Identification of the caudal epidural space. Anaesthesia 43: 705–706

Lewis MPN, Thomas P, Wilson LF, Mulholland RC 1992 The 'whoosh' test. Anaesthesia 47: 57–58

McGown RG 1972 Accidental marrow sampling during caudal anaesthesia. British Journal of Anaesthesia 44: 613–614

Sethna NF, Berde CB 1993 Venous air embolism during identification of the epidural space in children. Anesthesia and Analgesia 76: 925–927

Sinclair JC, Fox HA, Lenty JF, Fuld GL, Murphy J 1965 Intoxication of the fetus by a local anesthetic. New England Journal of Medicine 273: 1173–1177

Trotter M 1947 Variations of the sacral canal: their significance in the administration of caudal analgesia. Current Researches in Anesthesia and Analgesia 26: 192–202

Trotter M, Lanier PF 1945 Hiatus canalis sacralis in American whites and negroes. Human Biology 17: 368–381

Trotter M, Letterman GS 1944 Variations of the female sacrum. Surgery, Gynecology and Obstetrics 78: 419–424

# 13. Regional anaesthesia of the trunk

## A Lee

## INNERVATION OF THE TRUNK

### The somatic supply

The thoracic and first lumbar spinal cord segments supply the major part of the innervation of the trunk (see Fig. 3.3). The course, branches and relations of the first 11 thoracic nerves are sufficiently similar to allow them to be described as 'typical' segmental nerves (Fig. 13.1). Each has a ventral and a dorsal ramus, the latter passing posteriorly to supply the muscles and skin of the paravertebral region. Close to its origin the ventral ramus communicates with the associated sympathetic ganglion through the white and grey rami communicantes. It then continues as the intercostal nerve which has three main branches:

1. *The lateral cutaneous branch* arises approximately in the mid-axillary line and pierces the internal and external intercostal muscles obliquely before dividing into anterior and posterior branches. The anterior branch runs forward to supply skin over the pectoral region ($T_1$–$T_6$) or that of the anterior abdominal wall ($T_7$–$T_{12}$). The posterior supplies skin over the scapula and latissimus dorsi.
2. *The anterior cutaneous branch* pierces the external intercostal and pectoralis major muscles to supply the skin of the anterior part of the thorax near the midline ($T_1$–$T_6$) or pierces the posterior rectus sheath to supply the rectus muscle and the overlying skin ($T_7$–$T_{12}$).
3. *A collateral branch* arises from most nerves in the posterior intercostal space and runs forward in the inferior part of the space. It lies parallel to the main nerve and may rejoin it anteriorly or end as a separate anterior cutaneous nerve.

Other branches exist, but are less easily defined. Numerous slender filaments supply the intercostal muscles and parietal pleura and these branches may cross to adjoining intercostal spaces.

Exceptions to this typical pattern occur at either end of the thoracic outflow. Most of the fibres from $T_1$ join those from $C_8$ to form the inferior trunk of the brachial plexus. Some fibres from $T_2$ and $T_3$ join to form the intercostobrachial nerve which supplies the medial aspect of the upper arm. The nerve from $T_{12}$ is subcostal and most of its ventral ramus joins that of $L_1$ to form the iliohypogastric, ilio-inguinal and genitofemoral nerves (Fig. 13.2).

The course and relations of an intercostal nerve (Fig. 13.1) must be understood if safe, effective blocks are to be produced. In its most posterior course, medial to the angle of the rib, the nerve lies deep to the posterior intercostal membrane with very little tissue separating it from the pleura. At the angle of the rib it comes to lie in the subcostal groove, inferior to the intercostal artery and between the subcostal and internal intercostal muscles. The nerve continues in the subcostal groove until it reaches the anterior end of the space. It is apparent that any solution placed in the same tissue plane as the nerve may track centrally and gain access to the paravertebral space, the sympathetic ganglion and even the epidural space. Posteriorly, there are communications with the adjacent spaces.

These nerves may be blocked at several 'central' sites, that is, in the subarachnoid, epidural and paravertebral spaces. More peripherally, the intercostal nerves and even their cutaneous branches may be blocked.

### The autonomic supply (Fig. 13.3)

The 12 thoracic, together with the first and occasionally the second lumbar, segments give rise to the entire sympathetic innervation of the trunk.

177

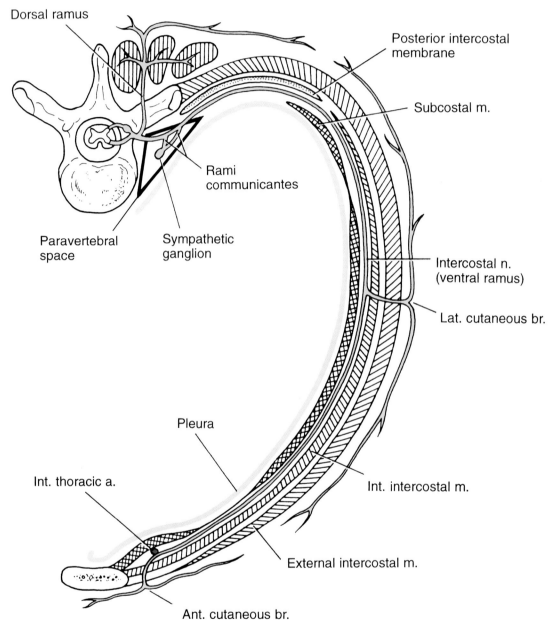

**Fig 13.1** Anatomy of a typical intercostal nerve, showing also the boundaries of the paravertebral space. The recurrent and smaller branches have been omitted for clarity.

The parasympathetic supply is primarily through the vagus, which runs a completely separate anatomical course. The pelvic viscera receive their parasympathetic supply through the second to fourth sacral nerves. Preganglionic sympathetic fibres from each segment run forward from the intervertebral foramen in white rami communicantes to the paravertebral sympathetic ganglia where they either synapse diffusely or pass uninterrupted to peripheral sites such as the coeliac plexus and adrenal glands. In the thoracic region the sympathetic chain and ganglia are located immediately anterior to the heads or necks of the ribs and, from there, postsynaptic fibres travel to segmental nerves in the grey rami communicantes (Fig. 13.3).

The sympathetic outflow from $T_1$ to $T_3$ forms the stellate ganglion which lies in the thoracic inlet,

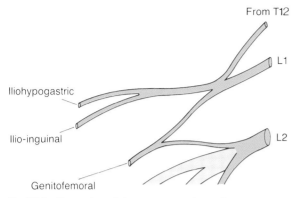

**Fig 13.2** Formation of the nerves supplying the inguinal region

anterior to the neck of the first rib in close proximity to the vertebral artery and the pleura (see Fig. 21.1). The sympathetic rami from $T_3$ to $T_5$ form a diffuse network of cardiac sympathetic nerves. From $T_5$ to $T_{12}$ the rami are more discrete, running caudally and somewhat anteriorly as the great, lesser and least splanchnic nerves. At first these are closely applied to the vertebral bodies of $T_{11}$ and $T_{12}$ but, after piercing the crus of the diaphragm, they coalesce to form the diffuse coeliac

plexus overlying the aorta and the coeliac axis at the level of the first lumbar vertebral body (see Fig. 21.3). From there sympathetic fibres accompany blood vessels to supply the abdominal viscera. The sympathetic supply to the pelvis and urogenital tract is derived from $T_{10}$ to $L_1$ and runs in the lumbar sympathetic chain and the ill-defined hypogastric plexus.

The sympathetic and somatic innervation are thus closely related near the neuraxis, but become separated peripherally. It follows that spinal or paravertebral block will cause significant sympathetic block, which may result in major cardiovascular changes and other physiological effects. Conversely, peripheral nerve blocks only affect somatic innervation and leave sympathetic efferents intact. It is also apparent that, if complete denervation of the viscera is required, vagal afferents have to be obtunded by a separate procedure such as coeliac plexus block.

## INTERCOSTAL NERVE BLOCK

The intercostal nerve may be blocked at any point in its course, but for the best analgesia and muscle relaxation the injection should be made proximal to the origin of

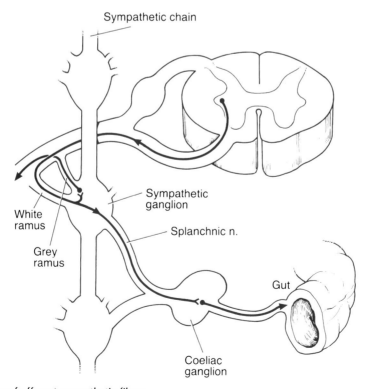

**Fig 13.3** Synaptic sites of efferent sympathetic fibres

the lateral branch (i.e. posterior to the mid-axillary line).

## Positioning and preparation

In the premedicated patient the prone or lateral decubitus position is recommended, whereas the ambulant patient can be seated leaning forwards over the edge of the bed or operating table, head on hands (Fig. 13.4). A pillow should be placed under the chest of the prone patient. In either position the shoulders should be abducted and the arms forward so that the scapulae move laterally and allow access to the posterior rib angles where the rib is usually easily palpated. At this point the intercostal space is relatively deep and the nerve is separated from the pleura by the subcostal muscle. In very obese or muscular individuals, the ribs and spaces may be more easily defined in the posterior axillary line, anterior to latissimus dorsi.

Surface markings can greatly help accurate needle placement. A line is drawn along the edge of the paraspinous muscles, approximately 8–10 cm from the midline, and the point at which it crosses the lower border of each rib is marked.

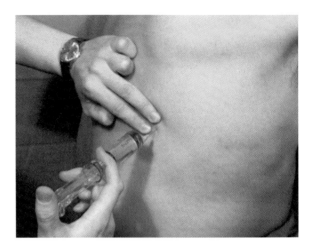

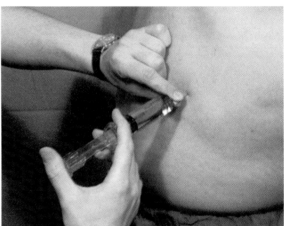

**Fig 13.5** Technique of intercostal nerve block. (A) The fingers of the left hand have pushed the skin that normally lies over the rib headwards. The needle tip has been advanced down to the rib. (B) The left hand then grips the needle hub and the needle is 'walked' down until it slides under the rib

## Injection technique (Fig. 13.5)

The skin is drawn cephalad with the 'palpating hand' and a 23 or 25 g short-bevelled needle is introduced over the rib and advanced perpendicular to the skin until bony contact is made. A small quantity of local anaesthetic may be injected on to the periosteum as this is the most painful part of the procedure. The 'palpating hand' then holds the hub of the needle firmly between thumb and index finger with the hypothenar eminence pressed firmly on to the patient's back. The 'injecting hand' then gently walks the needle caudally while the skin is allowed to move back over the rib until the tip just passes under its lower edge.

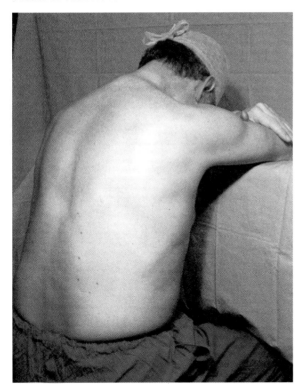

**Fig 13.4** Position for intercostal block in ambulant patient

Occasionally, a slight 'pop' is felt as the needle is advanced through the external intercostal muscle and the posterior intercostal membrane. The patient is asked to hold his breath as the needle is passed under the rib and while the injection is made. This minimises lung movement over the needle point so that if it has accidentally penetrated the pleura the risk of pneumothorax is decreased. If a careful aspiration test is negative for air and blood, up to 5 ml of local anaesthetic solution is injected.

For upper abdominal midline surgery, 12 nerves have to be blocked ($T_6$–$T_{11}$ bilaterally) and up to 60 ml of solution may be required. Systemic absorption of local anaesthetic is very rapid due to the vascularity of the area and this technique may produce high blood concentrations (Scott et al 1972, Moore et al 1976), particularly after liver transplantation (Bodenham & Park 1990). The concentrations produced are surpassed only by those which may follow inadvertent intravascular injection or endotracheal instillation (Braid & Scott 1965). These factors mean that the drug and its concentration have to be chosen with care. From the point of view of toxicity prilocaine would have much to offer, but if the block is to be of real benefit to the patient, a longer acting agent is needed. Bupivacaine 0.25% with 1:200 000 epinephrine is recommended. The addition of epinephrine decreases the rate of absorption and the peak blood concentration, but there is little evidence that it significantly prolongs the duration of this block. A significant dose of epinephrine may be administered, so it is important to bear in mind the contraindications to this drug and to use solutions without vasoconstrictor when indicated. Ropivacaine may be a preferable alternative to bupivacaine, but the optimum dose for comparable block to bupivacaine has yet to be determined. Intercostal blocks are by no means painless and they involve multiple injections, so additional systemic analgesia or sedation may be needed.

The anatomical distribution of solution deposited in the intercostal space is of relevance to both the resultant analgesia and the likely complications, but remains subject to debate. A claim that it is anatomically possible for a single large-volume injection to spread to several adjacent spaces (Nunn & Slavin, 1980) resulted in further studies suggesting that medial spread to the paravertebral space might be responsible for this effect (Moore 1985, Mowbray et al 1987, Crossley 1988). Moore (1985) suggested that the posterior intercostal membrane has to be pierced before solution will spread to adjacent

spaces, and this requires that the needle be placed posteriorly and close to the pleura, with concomitant risk of pneumothorax. It is debatable (Moore 1981) whether this is useful in practice, with further evidence suggesting that multiple injections are more effective and reliable than the single-injection technique (Renck et al 1984, Mowbray & Wong 1988). However, repeat injection through an indwelling catheter has been used to extend the duration of analgesia by eliminating the need for further painful injections and the increased risk of pneumothorax (Ablondi et al 1966, Murphy 1983, Kolvenbach et al 1989).

## Indications

For unilateral thoracic procedures, intercostal block produces rather better postoperative analgesia than conventional opioid therapy. It may be performed by the anaesthetist before or immediately after surgery, or by the surgeon from inside the chest. When the chest is open, the intercostal nerves can be injected under direct vision, a catheter inserted (Sabanathan et al 1988, 1990) or a cryoprobe used to freeze the nerves (Glynn et al 1980). Intercostal block has no effect on visceral structures so by itself it is inadequate for conventional surgery, although the introduction of minimally invasive techniques has increased the use of intercostal block, and video-assisted talc pleurodesis may be safely performed under intercostal blocks and sedation alone (Danby et al 1998). The duration of analgesic effect is 4–8 hours with bupivacaine and some analgesia may be demonstrable by pinprick for up to 18 hours.

Unilateral intercostal block ($T_6$–$T_{11}$) provides good somatic analgesia for a subcostal incision, but muscle relaxation is usually inadequate for the surgical procedure and neuromuscular blocking drugs are required. Better relaxation is produced by bilateral block, but again this may not be sufficient for upper abdominal surgery.

Body surface surgery may be performed under intercostal blocks alone.

## Complications

The *physiological effects* of intercostal block are usually slight. Minimal cardiovascular changes are seen unless either large quantities of epinephrine have been used or the injected solution has tracked posteriorly to involve the sympathetic chain. As well as upper limb sympathetic block (Purcell-Jones et al 1987), dramatic hypotension

(Benumof & Semenza 1975, Cottrell 1978, Brodsky 1979, Skretting 1981) and total spinal anaesthesia (Friesen & Robinson 1987) have been recorded, so the anaesthetist must be ready to deal with such rare, but potentially serious, complications. With regard to the respiratory system, intercostal block offers some slight advantages in the postoperative period when compared with conventional analgesia, but the results of different studies are not always comparable or conclusive. Intercostal block tends to reduce the impairment of respiratory function which occurs after thoracic and upper abdominal procedures. It improves the result of effort-dependent tests such as vital capacity, forced expiratory volume and peak expiratory flow rate and reduces to some extent the degree and duration of postoperative hypoxaemia (Engeberg 1975, Kaplan et al 1975). There is some evidence to suggest that postoperative chest infection is slightly less common than with opioid analgesia (Engeberg 1983).

The incidence of *pneumothorax* depends on the skill of the operator and the zeal with which this complication is sought. Published series quote an incidence of between 0.075 and 19% (Moore 1975, Cronin & Davies 1976). If a pneumothorax occurs, it is usually small and resolves spontaneously, but occasionally an intercostal drain is required, particularly if the patient is being artificially ventilated because tension pneumothorax is then a real danger. Significant haemorrhage may occur after intercostal nerve block if coagulation is impaired (Nielsen 1989); so, as with all regional techniques, the coagulation status of the patient must be taken into account.

## INTERPLEURAL BLOCK

Interpleural analgesia was first described by Kvalheim & Reiestad (1984). After initial scepticism, the analgesic action of interpleural injection of local anaesthetic was confirmed, but the duration of effect of a single injection is less than originally reported (VadeBoncouer et al 1989). The technique has proved useful after rib fractures and unilateral trunk operations (Reiestad & Stromskag 1986, Rocco et al 1987), but it does not appear that respiratory function is better maintained with this technique than with systemically administered opioids (Oxorn & Whatlet 1989, Scott et al 1989, Lee et al 1990b). The place of interpleural analgesia in anaesthetic practice is limited, particularly since the widespread adoption of laparoscopic cholecystectomy.

## Mechanism of block

Radiographic studies have demonstrated that 20 ml of solution spreads posteriorly in the pleural cavity from the diaphragm to the apex of the lung in the supine subject (Brismar et al 1987). It is probable that the local anaesthetic diffuses through the parietal pleura to produce multiple intercostal nerve block and this is supported by the finding of diminished sensitivity to cold in the same dermatomes (Lee et al 1990b). Both sympathetic and splanchnic nerve block may also be produced. Horner's syndrome and upper limb vasodilatation have been described in association with the technique (Parkinson et al 1989) and the sympathetic block may contribute to the analgesia. Splanchnic nerve block may alleviate visceral pain and account for the profound analgesia described after left-sided interpleural block in a patient with severe pancreatic pain.

## Technique

Local anaesthetic may be injected through a previously inserted chest drain which is then clamped for up to 30 minutes, or through a catheter placed in the pleural cavity at thoracotomy. More commonly, a catheter is inserted percutaneously into the closed chest. Great care must be taken to avoid producing a pneumothorax secondary to either lung puncture or accidental air entry during catheter insertion.

The catheter is inserted through an intercostal space using full aseptic precautions. The skin is first punctured with a sharp hypodermic needle and then a Tuohy epidural needle is advanced until a rib is contacted. The needle is then 'walked' superiorly off the rib into the intercostal space, where its passage through the external intercostal muscle is easily appreciated. Methods of insertion vary from this stage and may be described as 'open' or 'closed'.

### Open techniques
During open techniques the pleural space is in direct communication with the atmosphere at some stage.

1. In the original technique, the anaesthetist identifies subatmospheric pressure in the pleural cavity by attaching an air-filled syringe to the epidural needle and watching for movement of the plunger in the barrel of the syringe (Reiestad & Stromskag 1986). The syringe is then removed and the catheter threaded expeditiously through the needle.

2. A 'hanging drop' technique, similar to that used for epidural catheter insertion, may be employed (Squier et al 1989).

3. The catheter is placed in the epidural needle when its tip is in the intercostal muscles. One hand advances the needle and the other tries to thread the catheter. This becomes possible when the pleural space is reached (Gin et al 1990).

4. The pleural space may be identified using loss of resistance to the injection of air or saline (Seltzer et al 1987).

With the first two methods it is necessary to have the patient breathing spontaneously, but even with the latter two methods the patient should be disconnected from positive-pressure ventilation to minimise the risk of lung puncture.

### Closed techniques

Systems which allow the catheter to be fed through a silicone or rubber seal will prevent air entry during catheter insertion. The pleural space is identified by the collapse of a small balloon on a side arm or by the ability to run in saline rapidly from a bag attached to that side arm (Scott 1991).

The potential space immediately superficial to the parietal pleura has a subatmospheric pressure at times during the respiratory cycle and it is possible for the catheter to be mistakenly placed in this space. Analgesia may still be effective (Lee et al 1990b).

### Dosage

A 20 ml dose of 0.5% bupivacaine with 1:200 000 epinephrine will last 4–5 hours (VadeBoncouer et al 1989). Infusions of 0.2–0.25% bupivacaine at 10 ml h$^{-1}$ have been used effectively by the author in adults, and smaller volumes are effective in children (McIlvaine et al 1988).

### Indications

Interpleural analgesia may be useful after mastectomy, open cholecystectomy and nephrectomy (Lee et al 1990a, Reiestad & Stromskag 1986). Results after thoracotomy are more variable (Rosenberg et al 1987, McIlvaine et al 1988). Bilateral blocks for midline abdominal surgery carry the risk of bilateral pneumothoraces and require large doses of local anaesthetic (El-Naggar et al 1988).

Interpleural analgesia may have a role after chest trauma or in the management of some chronic pain states (Rocco et al 1987, Durrani et al 1988).

### Complications

Small pneumothoraces secondary to air entry through the needle are of little consequence and resolve spontaneously (Brismar et al 1987). Pneumothorax secondary to lung puncture is more serious and may require insertion of an underwater seal drain.

Local anaesthetic toxicity has followed injection of bupivacaine into an inflamed pleural cavity (Seltzer et al 1987). Peak plasma concentrations of bupivacaine after interpleural injection are reduced when epinephrine-containing solutions are used (Kambam et al 1989, Gin et al 1990).

Hemidiaphragmatic paralysis has been reported (Landesberg et al 1990, Lee et al 1990b). Sympathetic block of the upper extremity may occur (Parkinson et al 1989).

Contraindications are relative, but a past or present history of pleurisy, pneumonia, pulmonary embolus, severe chronic obstructive airways disease or other major lung or pleural pathology should probably rule out the use of this technique.

## PARAVERTEBRAL BLOCK

Paravertebral block was used extensively in the first half of the 20th century and has recently been used to provide analgesia after unilateral surgery or in some chronic pain states (Eason & Wyatt 1979, Richardson & Lonnqvist 1998). In concept, it is an attractive technique because it can produce relatively localised unilateral analgesia with a reduced incidence of hypotension and urinary retention compared to epidural block (Matthews & Govenden 1989). The block requires expertise to perform, the degree of spread is variable, and there remains the potential for hypotension, bilateral block, pneumothorax, or even a total spinal (Gilbert & Hultman 1989, Lonnqvist et al 1995). However, these risks must be placed in context with alternative techniques, and recent developments in catheter placement, such as image intensification, can reduce the risks in some circumstances. Indeed, in chronic pain practice the use of an image intensifier is mandatory if reliable diagnostic results from low volumes of local anaesthetic are to be obtained, or if neurolytic procedures are to be undertaken safely.

## Anatomy (Fig.13.1)

The paravertebral space is triangular and situated at the head and necks of the ribs. Medially it is bounded by the vertebrae, intervertebral foramina and intervertebral discs. Anteriorly is the parietal pleura, and the posterior boundary is formed by the superior costotransverse ligament and posterior intercostal membrane. Solution can spread superiorly and inferiorly to affect more than one intercostal nerve, as well as medially through the intervertebral foramen and laterally along the intercostal space. The sympathetic chain and rami communicantes are present within the paravertebral space and are invariably blocked. Anatomical studies, using radiopaque contrast media or computerised tomography (CT) scanning in patients, and injections of dyes or latex in cadavers, have shown considerable variation in the dimensions of the paravertebral space (Lonnqvist & Hildingsson 1992). Highly variable patterns of spread may be seen with injected solutions tracking over several segments in either cephalad or caudad directions, into the pleural space (which implies pleural puncture), and by no means infrequently, into the epidural space (Conacher & Kokri 1987, Conacher 1988, Purcell-Jones et al 1989).

## Technique

Paravertebral block may be carried out with the patient in the prone, lateral or sitting position, and at any appropriate level from high-thoracic to mid-lumbar regions (Moore 1979). Both single-injection and catheter techniques may be employed. The space is most commonly identified using a loss-of-resistance technique. A needle is inserted 2–3 cm lateral to the appropriate spinous process until the transverse process is contacted. The needle is then passed superior to the transverse process and may be felt to pass through the superior costotransverse ligament (see Fig. 13.6). Passage of the needle superior to the transverse process probably reduces the likelihood of spread through the adjacent intervertebral foramen. Paraesthesiae in the anterior ramus of the thoracic segmental spinal nerve indicates correct placement. Anatomical structures are less well defined than for epidural needle placement and this has led to the development of other methods of identifying the paravertebral space.

The pressure in the paravertebral space is subatmospheric on inspiration in contrast to the pressure in posterior spinal muscles in which the pressure is positive on inspiration. Pressure monitoring during needle insertion can identify the space by inversion of the pressure waveform on inspiration as the space is entered. During thoracotomy the position of a catheter placed percutaneously preoperatively can be verified by injection of methylene blue. Surgical placement of a catheter, introduced percutaneously through a Tuohy needle towards the end of thoracotomy, ensures reliable analgesia.

The bolus dose employed is commonly 20 ml of 0.25–0.5% bupivacaine in adults, and the addition of epinephrine may reduce peak plasma concentrations in some individuals (Snowden et al 1994). With a sub-

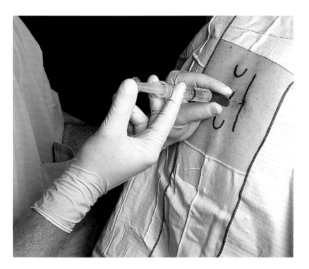

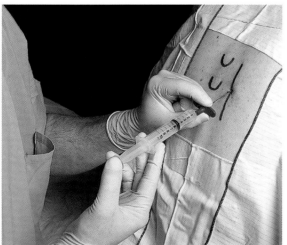

**Fig 13.6** (A) Needle insertion for location of transverse process. (B) Needle re-angled to pass cephalad to transverse process and pierce costotransverse ligament

sequent infusion, steady state plasma concentrations may not be reached for up to 4 days, but there are no reports of toxicity with this infusion technique. In chronic pain conditions, both local anaesthetics and neurolytic solutions may be injected.

## Indications

Paravertebral blocks may be used for postoperative pain control after thoracotomy, open cholecystectomy or nephrectomy. They have been used successfully as the sole anaesthetic for breast cancer surgery (Greengrass et al 1996, Coveney et al 1998) and inguinal hernia repair (Klein et al 1998), enabling these procedures to be performed on day-care patients. Paravertebral blocks not only provide excellent analgesia, but have been shown, in the case of unilateral procedures, to lead to better suppression of the stress response, better preservation of pulmonary function, reduced incidence of postoperative pulmonary complications, reduced hospital stay and reduced incidence of post-thoracotomy neuralgia than epidural or intrapleural block or systemic opioids (Matthews & Govenden 1989, Richardson et al 1995, Richardson et al 1999).

## PERIPHERAL BLOCKS

Due to the branching of segmental nerves, there is considerable overlap in their distribution. The more peripheral the block, the more widespread must be the infiltration of local anaesthetic drug. The use of such blocks for abdominal surgery necessitates multiple injections of large volumes of solution and brings with it the problems of overdosage. The requirement for infiltration of the skin incision, multiple injections into the rectus sheath on each side, infiltration of the parietal peritoneum and either coeliac plexus block or intra-peritoneal local anaesthetic lavage are impractical in everyday anaesthetic practice. Two important peripheral blocks are used.

## Field block for herniorrhaphy

This technique can be used alone for day-care surgery or poor-risk patients. When combined with light general anaesthesia, it gives good operating conditions and post-operative pain control. The musculocutaneous innervation of the inguinal region is through the ventral rami of $T_{11}$

and $T_{12}$ and two upper branches of the lumbar plexus, the iliohypogastric and ilio-inguinal nerves (see Fig. 13.2).

### Anatomy (Fig. 13.7)

The ventral ramus of the 12th thoracic or *subcostal nerve* is larger than the other thoracic roots and sends a large branch to join the first lumbar root. The anterior branch follows the lower border of the 12th rib, continues between the transversus and internal oblique muscles, becomes superficial at the lower end of the rectus sheath and supplies skin over the lower anterior abdominal wall.

The anterior cutaneous branch of the *iliohypogastric nerve* lies first between the internal oblique and transversus muscles. About 2 cm medial to the anterior iliac spine it passes through the internal oblique to lie between it and the external oblique. About 3 cm above the superficial ring it pierces the external oblique aponeurosis to supply the skin above the pubis and medial end of the inguinal ligament.

The *ilio-inguinal nerve* pierces the internal oblique muscle a little lower and further forward than does the iliohypogastric nerve. In the male it then enters the inguinal canal and lies below the spermatic cord. It accompanies the cord through the superficial ring and supplies skin over the root of the penis and scrotum. Throughout its course it supplies branches to the cord and cremaster muscle.

The genital branch of the *genitofemoral nerve* also runs in the inguinal canal and may supply skin in the medial part of the groin.

*Autonomic fibres* supply the spermatic cord throughout its length, originating from the lower thoracic segments and travelling with the testicular blood vessels and somatic nerves.

### Technique

Because the subcostal, iliohypogastric and ilio-inguinal nerves lie close together, anteromedial to the anterior superior iliac spine (Fig. 13.7) and between the abdominal muscle layers, they may be conveniently blocked here. With the patient supine, a point 2 cm anterior and inferior to the iliac spine is marked and infiltrated with local anaesthetic. A short-bevelled blocking needle is inserted at this point and directed posteriorly. Then 10–15 ml of local anaesthetic is infiltrated through the full thickness of the abdominal wall to ensure spread of solution between all muscle layers. From the same point, the needle is directed

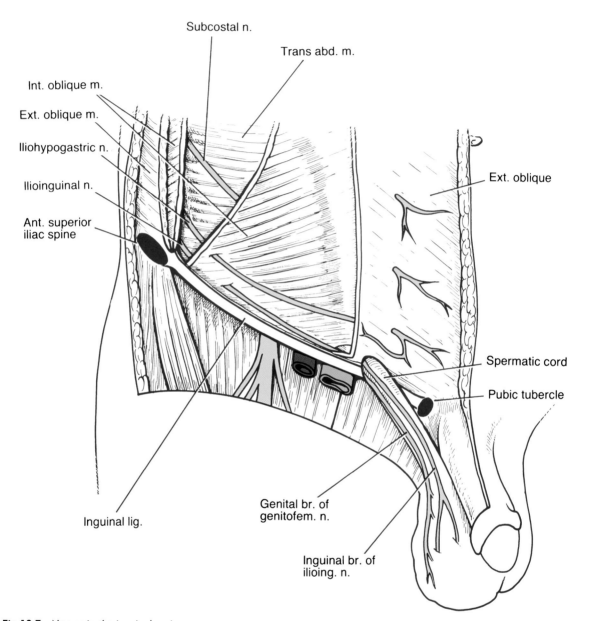

**Fig 13.7** Nerves in the inguinal region

inferomedially, parallel to the inguinal ligament, and more anaesthetic solution (7–10 ml) is injected both deep and superficial to the external oblique aponeurosis. This is sufficient to provide reliable and consistent postoperative analgesia in patients having additional light general anaesthesia. However, in conscious patients, it is essential to ensure that the injection superficial to the external oblique aponeurosis anaesthetises the skin to be incised. This is best accomplished by asking the surgeon to mark the line of his intended incision and then infiltrating along and slightly beyond this line. Unless the surgeon's mark extends to the pubic tubercle, it is not necessary to infiltrate so far medially or to make a separate injection there. In some instances, it may be preferable to infiltrate the complete shaded area (Fig. 13.8) although this is unnecessary when the surgeon and anaesthetist are used to working together as a team.

Once the cord has been exposed in patients having repair under local anaesthesia alone, the cord and the

for the block to become effective, but postoperative analgesia may last for up to 6 hours (Glasgow 1976).

## Indications

When herniorrhaphy is to be carried out under regional anaesthesia alone, this technique has some advantages over spinal and epidural block in poor-risk cases and outpatients, even though a large dose of local anaesthetic is required. There is little sympathetic block, so significant pulse and blood pressure changes are rare. There is also less disturbance of bladder function, and early ambulation is possible because there is no block of the lower limb muscles. It may be the method of choice for the severe respiratory cripple in whom general anaesthesia is inadvisable and in whom the respiratory muscle paralysis caused by spinal or epidural anaesthesia may be sufficient to precipitate respiratory failure. However, a fraught repair under regional block when the practitioners are only familiar with the procedure performed under general anaesthesia is not to be recommended.

Laparoscopic hernia repair remains controversial. An extraperitoneal approach is generally favoured over an intraperitoneal approach and this can be performed under local anaesthesia (Ferzli et al 1999) but, as with the intraperitoneal approach, general anaesthesia is most commonly employed. Video-assisted percutaneous repairs through small groin incisions may become more widely used and these can be more readily performed under local anaesthesia (Darzi & Nduka 1997).

## Penile block

### Anatomy

Most of the somatic supply of the penis is supplied by the second, third and fourth sacral nerve roots. The fibres run in the dorsal nerve of the penis, which is the terminal branch of the pudendal nerve. The dorsal nerve runs with the artery along the inferior ramus of the pubis, through the suspensory ligament of the penis and under the pubic arch. There it lies in the floor of the suprapubic space, before entering Buck's fascia, the fibrous tissue which invests the corpus cavernosum (Dalens et al 1989) (Fig. 13.9). It supplies the skin and glans. The autonomic supply arises from the inferior hypogastric plexus in the pelvis. Some fibres run with the pudendal nerves, but others accompany the blood vessels to the corpus spongeosum and corpus cavernosum. The base of the penis and scrotum are innervated by

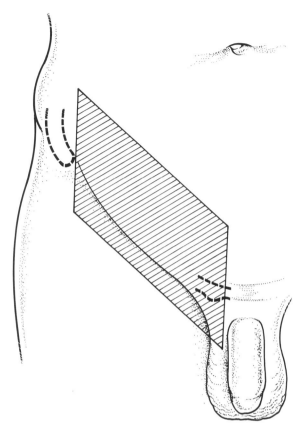

**Fig 13.8** The shaded area should be infiltrated once the primary injections have been made near the anterior superior iliac spine and pubic tubercle

neck of the peritoneal sac should receive separate injections (5 ml) at the level of the deep inguinal ring to block impulses transmitted in the visceral nerves.

Up to 40 ml of solution may be required when performing the operation under local anaesthesia. In the poor-risk patient, 0.5–1.0% plain prilocaine should be used. For the healthy outpatient , 0.5% bupivacaine may be used for the deep injections and 0.25% bupivacaine with epinephrine for the skin infiltration. A total of 40 ml of 0.375% bupivacaine is sufficient for bilateral blocks when using supplementary light general anaesthesia.

Patience, understanding and gentle tissue handling on the part of the surgeon do a great deal to improve the success rate in conscious patients. Small intravenous doses of short-acting agents such as midazolam and alfentanil or a low-dose propofol infusion may also be helpful. If a long-acting local anaesthetic such as bupivacaine is used, at least 20 minutes must be allowed

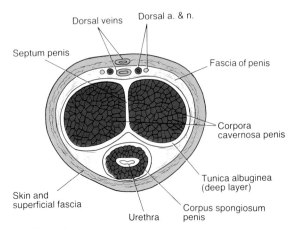

**Fig 13.9** Cross-section of penis to show the position of the dorsal nerves

cutaneous branches of the genitofemoral nerve through its genital branch (Fig. 13.7).

### Technique

Spinal, epidural or caudal techniques may be used for penile surgery, but block of the dorsal nerves and terminal branches of the genitofemoral nerve produces more localised anaesthesia. With the patient supine a finger is placed under the pubic symphysis in the midline. A skin wheal is raised before a 23 g needle 5 cm long is inserted in the midline vertical to the skin to pass under the pubis into the subpubic space. Then, 5 ml of local anaesthetic (0.25–0.5% *plain* bupivacaine) should be injected without resistance on each side of the midline. Alternatively, the needle may be directed in a more caudal direction on to the tough dorsal fascia of the penis and, after careful aspiration, 2–5 ml of anaesthetic solution should be injected without resistance. Forced injection of large volumes of solution, especially in children, within the non-elastic tissues of Buck's fascia, may cause arterial compression and penile gangrene even if no epinephrine has been used (Sara & Lowry 1984). Frequent aspiration is required to avoid intravascular injection in this highly vascular area. *It is imperative that epinephrine is not used.* For complete anaesthesia, another 5–10 ml of solution should be placed in loose subcutaneous tissue in a 'ring' around the base of the penis. Formal subpubic penile block provides better anaesthesia for penile surgery than subcutaneous ring block (Holder et al 1997).

### Indications

This is a useful, simple procedure for reduction of paraphymosis, and for dorsal slit, circumcision or meatotomy. After hypospadias repair, two penile blocks performed at the start and the conclusion of the repair provide better postoperative analgesia than either block alone (Chibber et al 1997).

Penile block gives excellent postoperative pain control, but erection can occur as some of the autonomic supply is unaffected. It is an excellent adjunct to general anaesthesia: it is easier and quicker than spinal or caudal anaesthesia, and avoids motor block, bladder disturbance and central sympathetic block.

## CHOICE OF BLOCK FOR SURGERY TO THE TRUNK

There is no doubt that regional anaesthesia for surgery on the trunk offers many advantages, both during and after operation. Several techniques are available, each with advantages and disadvantages, so the anaesthetist must decide which is the most appropriate. Consideration must be given to several factors, including the skills and experience of the anaesthetist, the availability of adequate monitoring and supervision during and after the procedure, anatomical and physiological features of the individual patient, and the amount of time available. If there are major reasons for avoiding general anaesthesia, even mastectomy may be performed under a field block (Dennison et al 1985).

For *thoracic surgery* the practical choice lies between intercostal, interpleural, paravertebral and thoracic epidural block. Apart from simple procedures on the chest wall, thoracic surgery requires general anaesthesia, with intermittent positive-pressure ventilation, to allow adequate control of respiration and manipulation of the diaphragm. The latter is innervated from the cervical region, so it is unaffected by the above regional techniques. Regional anaesthesia is therefore used as a supplement to general anaesthesia, particularly to provide postoperative pain control. Intercostal block by the surgeon or the anaesthetist is the easiest technique and has a relatively low incidence of serious side effects, but it is limited in efficacy and duration of effect. Cryoanalgesia, applied from within the chest, may be used, or placement of a paravertebral or interpleural catheter considered, but close monitoring of infusions and injections is vital, particularly in the first few postoperative hours because the effects are variable. The best pain control is probably obtained with an epidural infusion, but meticulous monitoring and control of hydration are required.

For *abdominal surgery* the choice lies between subarachnoid, epidural or intercostal block. During upper abdominal procedures, conscious patients will not tolerate large packs or stimulation of the diaphragm, so general anaesthesia with controlled ventilation is required. Regional techniques may be used as supplements to, but virtually never as replacements for, general anaesthesia. For lower abdominal and pelvic procedures, however, excellent anaesthesia and relaxation is obtained with spinal and epidural techniques, and if sedation or light general anaesthesia is required it may be considered to be the supplement. Given adequate postoperative facilities and expertise, epidural anaesthesia is superior to other methods as it is suitable for long surgical procedures, and excellent postoperative pain control can be obtained with top-ups or continuous infusion of local anaesthetic, or with the epidural injection of opioid. If this form of postoperative analgesia is not to be used and if the surgery is sure to be completed in the available time, spinal anaesthesia is preferable because it is quicker to perform, has a more rapid onset and is more effective than epidural anaesthesia.

Intercostal block is useful in abdominal surgery in three situations: first, where spinal or epidural techniques are not possible, because of a major spinal deformity such as spina bifida or ankylosing spondylitis; second, for subcostal incision for open gall bladder surgery, where it is quick and easy to apply at the end of surgery and gives reasonable postoperative analgesia; third, and most important, where sympathetic block may result in dangerous hypotension due to the relative hypovolaemia associated with many acute conditions, such as haematemesis, peritonitis and intestinal obstruction. Spinal and epidural anaesthesia are contraindicated in these conditions, but it should be remembered that sympathetic block, although rare, is possible after posteriorly placed intercostal injections.

The type of regional anaesthesia applicable to *renal surgery* depends to a large extent on the patient's position during surgery. The 'renal position', with the patient on the side and with maximum operating table 'break',

may impair venous return regardless of the anaesthetic technique employed, but the use of spinal or epidural anaesthesia will magnify this problem. This is a situation where unilateral intercostal blocks may offer an advantage.

Low spinal, or lumbar or caudal epidural blocks are all useful in a variety of *gynaecological, urological, perineal* and *anal* procedures. After some of these, for example transurethral prostatectomy, profound postoperative analgesia is not necessary and spinal anaesthesia with an agent of suitable duration is the technique of choice. For anal procedures (but only in those in which sphincter relaxation is surgically acceptable or desirable), low spinal or caudal block may be employed. A short-acting opioid such as alfentanil may be used to supplement general anaesthesia, followed by caudal injection of local anaesthetic at the end of the procedure to provide postoperative analgesia. If the patient is to remain conscious a spinal injection is less painful, quicker in onset and more effective than caudal block, which has a significant failure rate even in expert hands. The main advantage of the caudal approach is that it avoids post-spinal headache, which may be a serious disability in younger patients who would normally mobilise quickly after surgery.

Regional anaesthesia is commonly used for *inguinal hernia repair*. Peripheral nerve block has gained popularity in day-care surgery and for the very frail patient. The advantages include lack of sympathetic block and resulting hypotension, lack of accessory respiratory muscle involvement, no risk of spinal headache and no muscle paralysis of the lower limbs, the patient being able to walk from the table. However, the technique requires careful patient counselling and the co-operation of both patient and surgeon. If the block is performed after the induction of general anaesthesia the discomfort of injection is avoided, minimal general anaesthesia is required thereafter and the advantage of good postoperative pain control is retained. For the patient undergoing penile surgery, regional techniques have much to offer.

## Further Reading

McClure JH, Wildsmith JAW 1991 Conduction blockade for postoperative analgesia. Edward Arnold, London

## References

Ablondi MA, Ryan JF, O'Connell CT, Harley RW 1966 Continuous intercostal nerve blocks for postoperative pain relief. Anesthesia and Analgesia 45: 185–190

Benumof JL, Semenza J 1975 Total spinal anesthesia following intercostal nerve blocks. Anesthesiology 43: 124–125

Bodenham A, Park GR 1990 Plasma concentrations of

bupivacaine after intercostal nerve block in patients after orthotopic liver transplantation. British Journal of Anaesthesia 64: 436–441

Braid DP, Scott DB 1965 The systemic absorption of local anaesthetic drugs. British Journal of Anaesthesia 37: 394–404

Brismar B, Pettersson N, Tokics L, Standberg A, Hedenstierna G 1987 Postoperative analgesia with intrapleural administration of bupivacaine-adrenaline. Acta Anaesthesiologica Scandinavica 31: 515–520

Brodsky JB 1979 Hypotension from intraoperative intercostal nerve blocks. Regional Anesthesia 4/3: 17–18

Chibber AK, Perkins FM, Rabinowitz R, Vogt AW, Hulbert WC 1997 Penile block timing for postoperative analgesia of hypospadias repair in children. Journal of Urology 158: 1156–1159

Conacher ID 1988 Resin injection of thoracic paravertebral spaces. British Journal of Anaesthesia 61: 657–661

Conacher ID, Kokri M 1987 Postoperative paravertebral blocks for thoracic surgery. A radiological appraisal. British Journal of Anaesthesia 59: 155–161

Cottrell WM 1978 Hemodynamic changes after intercostal nerve blocks with bupivacaine–epinephrine solution. Anesthesia and Analgesia 57: 492–495

Coveney E, Weltz CR, Greengrass R et al 1998 Use of paravertebral block anesthesia in the surgical management of breast cancer: experience in 156 cases. Annals of Surgery 227: 496–501

Cronin KD, Davis MJ 1976 Intercostal block for postoperative pain relief. Anaesthesia and Intensive Care 4: 259–261

Crossley AWA 1988 Intercostal catheterisation: an alternative approach to the paravertebral space? Anaesthesia 43: 163–164

Dalens B, Vanneuville G, Dechelotte P 1989 Penile block via the subpubic space in 100 children. Anesthesia and Analgesia 69: 41–45

Danby CA, Adebonojo SA, Moritz DM 1998 Video-assisted talc pleurodesis for malignant pleural effusions utilizing local anesthesia and i.v. sedation. Chest 113: 739–742

Darzi A, Nduka CC 1997 Endoscopically guided percutaneous repair of inguinal hernia through a 2-cm incision. Minihernia repair. Surgical Endoscopy 11: 782–784

Dennison AR, Walkins RM, Ward ME, Lee ECG 1985 Simple mastectomy under local anaesthesia. Annals of the Royal College of Surgeons of England 67: 243–244

Durrani Z, Winnie AP, Ikuta P 1988 Interpleural catheter analgesia for pancreatic pain. Anesthesia and Analgesia 67: 479–481

Eason MJ, Wyatt R 1979 Paravertebral thoracic block – a reappraisal. Anaesthesia 34: 638–642

El-Naggar MA, Bennett B, Raad C, Yogaratnam G 1988 Bilateral intrapleural intercostal nerve block. Anesthesia and Analgesia 67: S57

Engeberg G 1975 Single dose intercostal block for pain relief after upper abdominal surgery. Acta Anaesthesiologica Scandinavica 60 (Supplement): 43–49

Engeberg G 1983 Intercostal block for prevention of pulmonary complications after upper abdominal surgery. Acta Anaesthesiologica Scandinavica 78 (Supplement): 73

Ferzli , Sayad P, Vasisht B 1999 The feasibility of laparoscopic extraperitoneal hernia repair under local anesthesia. Surgical Endoscopy 13: 588–590

Friesen D, Robinson RH 1987 Total spinal anesthesia – a complication of intercostal nerve block. Kansas Medicine 88: 84–96

Gilbert J, Hultman J 1989 Thoracic paravertebral block: a method of pain control. Acta Anaesthesiologica Scandinavica 33: 142–145

Gin T, Chan K, Kan AF, Gregory MA, Wong YC, Oh TE 1990 Effect of adrenaline on venous plasma concentrations of bupivacaine after interpleural administration. British Journal of Anaesthesia 64: 662–666

Glasgow F 1976 Short stay surgery for repair of inguinal hernia. Annals of the Royal College of Surgeons of England 58: 133–139

Glynn CJ, Lloyd JW, Barnard JGW 1980 Cryoanalgesia in the management of pain after thoracotomy. Thorax 35: 325–327

Greengrass R, O'Brien F, Lyerly K et al 1996 Paravertebral block for breast cancer surgery. Canadian Journal of Anaesthesia 43: 858–861

Holder KJ, Peutrell JM, Weir PM 1997 Regional anaesthesia for circumcision. Subcutaneous ring block of the penis and subpubic penile block compared. European Journal of Anesthesiology 14: 495–498

Kambam JR, Hammon J, Parris WCV, Lupinetti FM 1989 Intrapleural analgesia for postthoracotomy pain and blood levels of bupivacaine following intrapleural injection. Canadian Journal of Anaesthesia 36: 106–109

Kaplan J A, Miller E D, Gallagher E G 1975 Post operative analgesia for thoracotomy patients. Anesthesia and Analgesia 54: 773–777

Klein SM, Greengrass RA, Weltz C, Warner DS 1998 Paravertebral somatic nerve block for outpatient inguinal herniorrhaphy: an expanded case report of 22 patients. Regional Anesthesia and Pain Medicine 23: 306–310

Kolvenbach H, Lauven PM, Schneider B, Kunath U 1989 Repetitive intercostal nerve block via catheter for postoperative pain relief after thoracotomy. Thoracic and Cardiovascular Surgeon 37: 273–276

Kvalheim L, Reiestad F 1984 Interpleural catheter in the management of postoperative pain. Anesthesiology 61: A231

Landesberg G, Meretyk S, Lankovsky Z, Shapiro A 1990 Intra-operative intrapleural catheter placement for continuous bupivacaine administration. European Journal of Anaesthesiology 7: 149–152

Lee A, Boon D, Bagshaw P, Kampthorne PA 1990a Randomised double-blind study of interpleural analgesia after cholecystectomy. Anaesthesia 46: 1028–1031

Lee TL, Boey WK, Tan WC 1990b Analgesia and respiratory function following intrapleural bupivacaine after cholecystectomy. Journal of Anesthesiology 4: 20–28

Lonnqvist PA, Hildingsson U 1992 The caudal boundary of the thoracic paravertebral space. A study in human cadavers. Anaesthesia 47: 1051–1052

Lonnqvist PA, McKenzie J, Soni AK, Conacher ID 1995 Paravertebral blockade. Failure rate and complications. Anaesthesia 50: 813–815

McIlvaine WB, Knox RF, Fennessey PV, Goldstein M 1988 Continuous infusion of bupivacaine via intrapleural catheter for analgesia after thoracotomy in children. Anesthesiology 69: 261–264

Matthews PJ, Govenden V 1989 Comparison of continuous paravertebral and extradural infusions of bupivacaine for pain relief after thoracotomy. British Journal of Anaesthesia 62: 204–205

Moore DC 1975 Intercostal nerve block for postoperative somatic pain following surgery of the thorax and upper abdomen. British Journal of Anaesthesia 47: 284–286

Moore DC 1979 Regional block, 4th edn, pp 200–220. CC Thomas, Springfield

Moore DC 1981 Intercostal nerve block: spread of india ink injected to the rib's costal groove. British Journal of Anaesthesia 53: 325–329

Moore DC 1985 Intercostal blockade. British Journal of Anaesthesia 57: 543–544

Moore DC, Mather LE, Bridenbaugh PO 1976 Arterial and venous plasma levels of bupivacaine following epidural and intercostal nerve blocks. Anesthesiology 45: 39–45

Mowbray A, Wong KKS 1988 Low volume intercostal injection. A comparative study in patients and cadavers. Anaesthesia 43: 633–634

Mowbray A, Wong KKS, Murray JM 1987 Intercostal catheterisation. An alternative approach to the paravertebral space. Anaesthesia 42: 958–961

Murphy DF 1983 Continuous intercostal nerve blockade for pain relief following cholecystectomy. British Journal of Anaesthesia 55: 521–524

Nielsen CH 1989 Bleeding after intercostal nerve block in a patient anticoagulated with heparin. Anesthesiology 71: 162–164

Nunn JF, Slavin G 1980 Posterior intercostal nerve block for pain relief after cholecystectomy. British Journal of Anaesthesia 52: 253–260

Oxorn DC, Whatlet GS 1989 Post-cholecystectomy pulmonary function following interpleural bupivacaine and intramuscular pethidine. Anaesthesia and Intensive Care 17: 440–443

Parkinson SK, Mueller JB, Rich TJ, Little WL 1989 Unilateral Horner's syndrome associated with interpleural catheter injection of local anaesthetic. Anesthesia and Analgesia 68: 61–62

Purcell-Jones G, Speedy HM, Justins DM 1987 Upper limb sympathetic blockade following intercostal nerve blocks. Anaesthesia 42: 984–986

Purcell-Jones G, Pither CE, Justins DM 1989 Paravertebral somatic nerve block: a clinical, radiographic, and computed tomographic study in chronic pain patients. Anesthesia and Analgesia 68: 32–39

Reiestad F, Stromskag KE 1986 Interpleural catheter in the management of postoperative pain. A preliminary report. Regional Anesthesia 11: 89–91

Renck H, Johansson A, Aspellin P, Jacobsen H 1984 Multiple intercostal nerve blocks by a single injection – a clinical and radiological investigation. In: Van Kleef J, Burns T, Spierdijk J (eds) Current concepts in regional anaesthesia, pp 1–7. Martinus Nijhoff, Amsterdam

Richardson J, Lonnqvist PA. 1998 Thoracic paravertebral block. British Journal of Anaesthesia 81: 230–238

Richardson J, Sabanathan S, Mearns AJ, Shah R, Goulden C 1995 A prospective randomised comparison of interpleural and paravertebral analgesia in thoracic surgery. British Journal of Anaesthesia 75: 405–408

Richardson J, Sabanathan S, Jones J, Shah RD, Cheema S, Mearns AJ 1999 A prospective, randomised comparison of preoperative and continuous balanced epidural or paravertebral bupivacaine on post-thoracotomy pain, pulmonary function and stress responses. British Journal of Anaesthesia 83: 387–392

Rocco A, Reiestad F, Gudman J, McKay W 1987 Interpleural administration of local anaesthetics for pain relief in patients with multiple rib fractures. Preliminary report. Regional Anesthesia 12: 10–14

Rosenberg PH, Scheinin BMA, Lepantalo MJA, Lindfors O 1987 Continuous intrapleural infusion of bupivacaine for analgesia after thoracotomy. Anesthesiology 67: 811–813

Sabanathan S, Smith PJB, Pradhan GN, Hashimi H, Eng J, Mearns AJ 1988 Continuous intercostal nerve block for pain relief after thoracotomy. Annals of Thoracic Surgery 46: 425–426

Sabanathan S, Mearns AJ, Smith PJB, et al 1990 Efficacy of continuous extrapleural intercostal nerve block on post-thoracotomy pain and pulmonary mechanics. British Journal of Surgery 77: 221–225

Sara CA, Lowry CJ 1984 A complication of circumcision and dorsal nerve block of the penis. Anaesthesia and Intensive Care 13: 79–85

Scott DB, Jebson PJR, Braid DP, Ostengren B, Frisch P 1972 Factors affecting plasma levels of lignocaine and prilocaine. British Journal of Anaesthesia 44: 1040–1049

Scott NB, Mogensen T, Bigler D, Kehlet H 1989 Comparison of the effects of continuous intrapleural vs epidural administration of 0.5% bupivacaine on pain, metabolic response and pulmonary function following cholecystectomy. Acta Anaesthesiologica Scandinavica 33: 535–539

Scott PV 1991 Interpleural regional analgesia: detection of the interpleural space by saline infusion. British Journal of Anaesthesia 66: 131–133

**191**

Seltzer JL, Larijani GE, Goldberg ME, Marr AT 1987 Intrapleural bupivacaine – a kinetic and dynamic evaluation. Anesthesiology 67: 798–800

Skretting P 1981 Hypotension after intercostal nerve block during thoracotomy under general anaesthesia. British Journal of Anaesthesia 53: 527–529

Snowden CP, Bower S, Conacher I 1994 Plasma bupivacaine levels in paravertebral blockade in adults. Anaesthesia 49: 546

Squier RC, Morrow JS, Roman R 1989 Hanging-drop technique for intrapleural analgesia. Anesthesiology 70: 882

VadeBoncouer TR, Riegler FX, Gautt RS, Weinberg GL 1989 A randomized, double-blind comparison of the effects of interpleural bupivacaine and saline on morphine requirements and pulmonary function after cholecystectomy. Anesthesiology 71: 339–343

# 14. Upper limb blocks

## H B J Fischer

Upper limb surgery is often performed under regional anaesthesia using brachial plexus block as the sole peripheral method. Individual peripheral nerve blocks may also be used alone or in combination to produce a restricted field of block according to surgical need. Intravenous regional anaesthesia (IVRA) is also used commonly for short procedures on the forearm or hand. Because each technique has its own limitations in regard to the extent of block and the risk of side-effects, it is important to relate the surgical requirements to the benefits and risks of the intended block (Table 14.1). Local infiltration or peripheral nerve block can be used to supplement brachial plexus techniques, and intravenous sedation or light general anaesthesia may be used in combination with a block. This reduces the delay in starting surgery, while still offering postoperative analgesia from the regional method.

## BRACHIAL PLEXUS ANAESTHESIA

### Anatomy of the plexus (Fig. 14.1)

The brachial plexus innervates the entire upper limb except for the skin over the shoulder which is supplied by the supraclavicular nerves of the cervical plexus. The intercostobrachial nerve ($T_2$) and a branch of $T_3$ (Fig. 14.2) supply the skin of the inner aspect of the upper arm and axilla.

The plexus is formed from the anterior primary rami of the fifth cervical to the first thoracic nerve roots. Contributions occasionally arise from $C_4$ (prefixed) and $T_2$ (postfixed). The *five roots* form *three trunks*, each of which divides into an anterior and a posterior division. The *six divisions* recombine to form *three cords*, which in turn each divide into two terminal

### Table 14.1 Techniques of upper limb block

| Technique | Area blocked | Advantages | Disadvantages |
|---|---|---|---|
| IVRA[a] | Hand, forearm | Simple, low failure rate | Tourniquet pain, risk of toxicity, no prolonged analgesia |
| Interscalene | Shoulder, humerus, elbow, lateral aspect forearm and hand | Blocks deep structures of shoulder and upper arm | $C_8$, $T_1$ often missed, rare risk of serious complications |
| Subclavian perivascular | Whole limb except shoulder | Widest area of block | Risk of pneumothorax, landmarks may be difficult |
| Axillary | Hand, forearm | Easy technique, low risk of complications | Difficult to position painful limb, limited area of block |
| Peripheral nerves | Individual nerve territories | Easy techniques, long duration | Limited area of block, may need multiple injections |

[a]IVRA = intravenous regional anaesthesia.

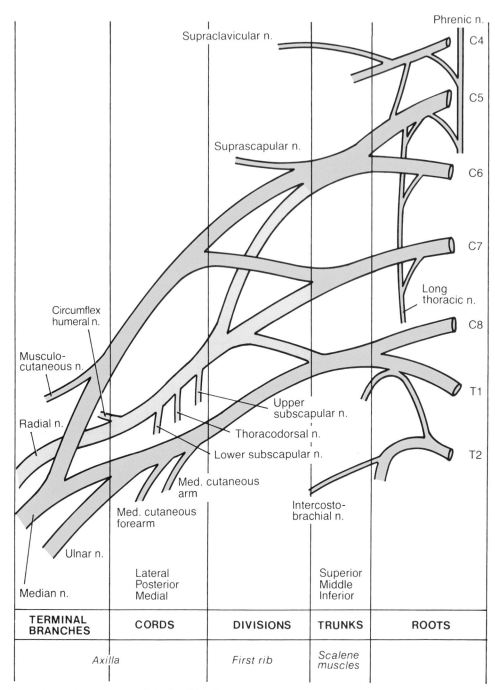

**Fig 14.1** Formation and components of the brachial plexus

branches. The six terminal branches recombine to form the *five terminal nerves* which supply the majority of the upper limb. The proximal branches of the plexus supply the deep structures of the shoulder and thoracic wall. Although the plexus is a complex structure, there is a degree of symmetry in that the plexus originates from five roots and terminates in five peripheral nerves, while the intervening structures – the trunks, anterior and posterior divisions and cords – all occur in groups of three.

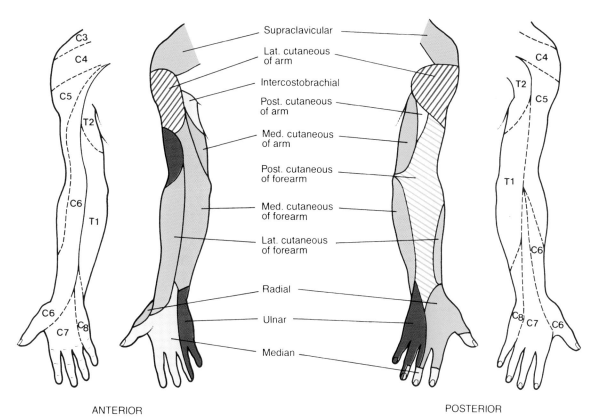

ANTERIOR                    POSTERIOR

**Fig 14.2** Cutaneous innervation and dermatomal maps of the upper limb. The segmental innervation of the deep structures is different from that of the skin: $C_5$ supplies the shoulder, $C_7$ the elbow and $T_1$ the hand

Dermatomal distribution is different from the cutaneous territory of individual nerves because peripheral nerves carry fibres from several roots as a result of interconnections within the plexus. Similarly, the innervation of deep structures is different from that of the overlying skin and subcutaneous tissues (Fig 14.2). For example, the musculocutaneous nerve ($C_5$–$C_7$) supplies the biceps muscle in the upper arm, but the skin of the anterolateral aspect of the forearm.

### Anatomical relations (Figs 14.3 & 14.4)

The *roots* of the brachial plexus lie between the anterior and middle scalene muscles which arise from the transverse processes of the cervical vertebrae and insert into the first rib. The vertebral artery, the stellate ganglion and the cervical epidural space are immediately deep to the plexus. The phrenic nerve ($C_3$–$C_5$) lies between the anterior scalene muscle and the carotid sheath, and the recurrent laryngeal nerve is also close to the roots, between the oesophagus and the trachea.

Superficially, the external jugular vein crosses the interscalene groove, often at the level of the sixth cervical vertebra and cricoid cartilage.

The *trunks* form at the lateral margin of the interscalene groove and are arranged vertically (i.e. superior, middle and inferior) above the first rib. The subclavian artery lies between the inferior trunk and the anterior scalene muscle, whereas the subclavian vein is anterior to the muscle. The cupola of the pleura is inferomedial to the first rib at this level. At the lateral edge of the first rib each trunk divides into two *divisions* which pass behind the clavicle to form the *cords*, which are respectively lateral, posterior and medial to the axillary artery. Each cord divides into two branches at the level of the lateral border of pectoralis minor, and two of the branches combine so that five *terminal nerves* are formed (Table 14.2). The musculocutaneous nerve leaves the plexus high in the axilla and enters the coracobrachialis muscle (Fig. 14.5), where it is liable to remain unblocked when the axillary approach is used.

195

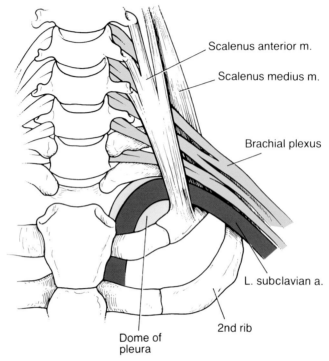

Scalenus anterior m.

Scalenus medius m.

Brachial plexus

L. subclavian a.

2nd rib

Dome of pleura

**Fig 14.3**   Major relations of the brachial plexus

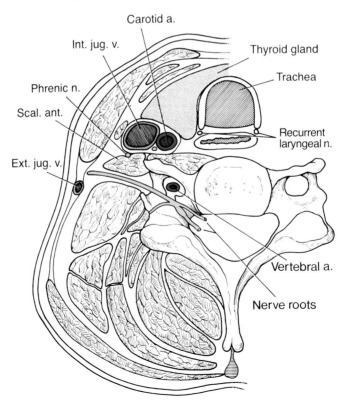

Carotid a.

Int. jug. v.

Thyroid gland

Phrenic n.

Trachea

Scal. ant.

Recurrent laryngeal n.

Ext. jug. v.

Vertebral a.

Nerve roots

**Fig 14.4**   Transverse section of the neck

**Table 14.2** The terminal nerves of the brachial plexus, and their principle branches

| Terminal nerve | Principle sensory branches | Principle motor function |
|---|---|---|
| Axillary (circumflex humeral) | Upper lateral cutaneous nerve of arm | Deltoid and teres minor |
| Radial | Lower lateral cutaneous nerve of arm Posterior cutaneous nerve of forearm Cutaneous nerves to dorsum of hand | Upper arm extensors Forearm extensors Two lumbricals |
| Ulnar | Cutaneous nerves to palm and dorsum of hand | Forearm flexors to $1\frac{1}{2}$ fingers Intrinsic muscles of hand |
| Median | Cutaneous nerves to palmar aspect of hand | Forearm flexors to $3\frac{1}{2}$ fingers Thenar muscles |
| Musculo-cutaneous | Lateral cutaneous nerve of forearm | Upper arm flexors |

N.B. the medial cutaneous nerves of the arm and forearm are branches of the medial cord of the brachial plexus.

### The brachial plexus sheath

A fibrous sheath formed from the prevertebral fascia and the fascial reflections from the two scalene muscles invests the entire plexus. The sheath is contiguous with that of the cervical plexus (so that cervical plexus block can occur with proximal brachial plexus injection techniques), and extends distally to the midpoint of the upper arm. At the level of the first rib, the artery is within the sheath, but the vein is not. Detailed examination by Winnie (1970) has led to a greater understanding of the importance of the sheath in the spread of local anaesthetic proximally and distally from the point of injection. Radiopaque contrast studies in cadavers (Thompson & Rorie 1983) suggested that it might contain thin fascial septa, but the role of such septa in causing delayed or incomplete blocks is debatable, and probably of little clinical significance.

## Techniques of brachial plexus block

Numerous approaches to the plexus have been described, but there are only four major ones currently in widespread use:

1. Interscalene (Winnie 1970)
2. Subclavian perivascular (Winnie & Collins 1964)/ supraclavicular (Patrick 1940)
3. Axillary (de Jong 1961)
4. Infraclavicular (Raj et al 1973).

The distribution of the block achieved differs according to which approach is used (Lanz & Theiss Djankovic 1983). The interscalene approach blocks the proximal components of the plexus, but tends to leave unaffected the $C_8$ and $T_1$ dermatomes, which supply the ulnar aspect of the forearm and hand. The axillary approach preferentially blocks the lower arm and hand, but one or more terminal nerves, often the musculocutaneous and axillary, may be unaffected. The subclavian perivascular technique gives the most complete block because it is performed at the level of the trunks, but it may miss the inferior trunk which has a mixed peripheral nerve/dermatomal pattern. The infraclavicular approach has a similar distribution to the axillary approach, but requires the use of a long insulated needle with a peripheral nerve stimulator. Because the needle must traverse the pectoralis muscles, this block may be uncomfortable for the patient and it will not be described further.

In experienced hands, the choice of technique is determined by the surgical requirements and the preferences of the anaesthetist. For the occasional practitioner, the subclavian perivascular approach is the best compromise between a good distribution of block and a low risk of complications.

### Equipment

The choice between a short-bevel or a conventional hypodermic needle is controversial. Short-bevel or pencil-point regional block needles are said to be preferable to standard hypodermic needles because they may reduce the risk of nerve injury (Selander et al 1977), but a short bevel may cause more damage than a long one if the nerve sheath is penetrated (Rice & McMahon 1992). Nevertheless, the greater 'feel' for different tissue planes provided by a short-bevel needle increases the awareness and accuracy of needle placement, and reduces the likelihood of nerve sheath penetration (Moore et al 1994).

The 'immobile needle' technique (Winnie 1969) uses a short, flexible, intravenous extension set between the syringe and needle. This allows the anaesthetist to position the needle accurately, hold it firmly in position, and so minimise the risk of it being displaced during aspiration and injection.

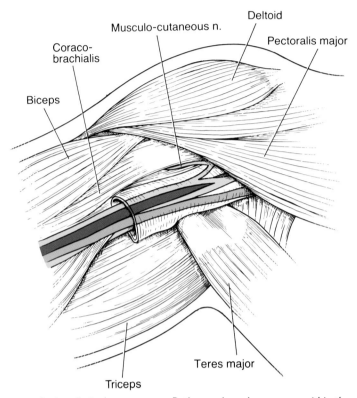

**Fig 14.5**   Position of neurovascular bundle in the upper arm. Both vessels and nerves are within the sheath at this level

A peripheral nerve stimulator is useful as a training aid and to confirm correct needle placement, particularly in sedated or anaesthetised patients and where the anatomical landmarks are difficult to appreciate. The patient must not have received a neuromuscular blocking agent prior to attempted use of a nerve stimulator.

### Drugs and dosage

Prilocaine and lidocaine at 1–2% are both effective where a short duration of block is required, with prilocaine being the drug of choice because of its lower potential for systemic toxicity. However, 1% prilocaine may not provide adequate muscle relaxation unless supplementary peripheral nerve blocks are performed, and the 2% concentration is no longer available. Thus lidocaine will have to be substituted for more profound blocks, but should be used with epinephrine to reduce peak plasma concentrations and provide an adequate duration of action (Wildsmith et al 1977).

Ropivacaine 0.75% and bupivacaine 0.5% are useful if a longer duration of block is required. Ropivacaine has a lower risk of serious systemic toxicity and does not require the addition of epinephrine.

A guide to doses is given in Table 14.3. In children, or frail, elderly patients a reduced dose may be in-

**Table 14.3 Suggested drugs, concentrations and volumes for brachial plexus block in the healthy adult. Doses actually used should reflect features of the individual patient**

| Drug | Plain solution | With epinephrine 1:200 000 |
|---|---|---|
| Prilocaine | 400 mg (40 ml 1%) | Not available |
| Lidocaine | Not advised; risk of toxicity too great with plain solution | 500 mg (33 ml 1.5%) |
| Levobupivacaine | 150 mg (30 ml 0.5%) | Not available |
| Bupivacaine | 150 mg (30 ml 0.5%) | 150 mg (30 ml 0.5%) |
| Ropivacaine | 225–300 mg (30–40 ml 0.75%) | Not available |

dicated. A number of studies show that the volume of solution injected is of prime importance in determining a successful block and 30–40 ml is recommended for adults no matter which approach is used.

### Adjuvant drugs

Opioid drugs and $\alpha_2$-adrenergic agonists have been used to improve the quality and duration of analgesia achieved with local anaesthetics. Results have been difficult to interpret because of the different methodologies used, but a recent study (Bazin et al 1997) showed that adding morphine, sufentanil and buprenorphine to lidocaine significantly prolongs analgesia. Epinephrine reduces systemic absorption of lidocaine and bupivacaine, but does not significantly prolong duration of block of the latter. Clonidine has been shown to prolong brachial plexus blocks in a number of studies (Eisenach et al 1996).

### Latency and duration of block

**The core/mantle concept**  The arrangement of nerves within a plexus, and fibres within a nerve, is not random (Winnie et al 1977). In any peripheral nerve, the fibres supplying the distal structures in its territory lie at the centre or 'core', whereas those supplying the proximal areas are in the outer layer or 'mantle'. Thus when local anaesthetic is deposited around a nerve it will diffuse into, and block, the outer fibres first.

In most mixed peripheral nerves the proportion of sensory and motor fibres is the same in both mantle and core, but this is not the case with the brachial plexus. A large proportion of the core fibres are those providing the rich sensory innervation to the hand, and the mantle fibres are predominantly those providing motor supply to the shoulder and elbow, the skin over the shoulder being supplied by the cervical plexus. The clinical consequence is that the first sign of a successful brachial plexus block is likely to be weakness of either the shoulder or elbow joint. With the proximal methods (interscalene or subclavian) the shoulder joint is usually affected first, and the elbow with the axillary approach. Weakness of joint movement usually progresses from proximal to distal joints and may precede sensory loss.

Whichever technique is used, there is a latent period of about 10–15 minutes before first evidence of block becomes apparent because of the time it takes for drug to diffuse through the considerable coverings of the plexus. The intensity of the block will continue to increase for a further 15–20 minutes. If there is no obvious motor or sensory loss demonstrable within 20 minutes, success is unlikely.

Lidocaine (with epinephrine) and prilocaine typically provide up to 90 minutes of surgical anaesthesia, and 3–4 hours of analgesia, whereas bupivacaine and ropivacaine produce much longer durations. Occasionally, blocks may last for 18–22 hours (Brockway et al 1989), but if such a prolonged duration is needed, a catheter technique (see below) should be used.

### Paraesthesiae and nerve damage

Correct needle placement is usually confirmed by eliciting paraesthesiae within the distribution of the brachial plexus, and the patient should be asked to describe the sensation rather than point to its location to avoid displacing the needle. If the paraesthesiae occur unequivocally within a nerve territory of the upper arm or forearm, no further needle positioning is necessary. The needle should be 'immobilised' to prevent displacement and, after negative aspiration for blood, the injection should be made slowly to avoid distending the sheath too rapidly and causing 'pressure paraesthesiae' which may be uncomfortable. There should be little resistance to flow during injection; severe pain or resistance, or both, suggest that the needle has penetrated a nerve sheath and continued injection will cause nerve damage.

Pre-existing neurological and vascular disease, surgical injury, limb posture, inadequate limb padding and support, tourniquet pressure and ischaemia are all important risk factors for causing nerve damage after upper limb surgery. These factors need to be considered and formal neurophysiological investigation undertaken before the diagnosis of needle or injection neuritis can be made. Symptoms of nerve damage may be apparent immediately postoperatively, but can take a week or more to develop and the duration can vary from 2–3 weeks up to 1–2 years. Full recovery of neurological function is the norm, but in a few rare cases permanent disability can occur.

## Interscalene block

### Clinical indications

This is the most proximal approach to the plexus. The block works preferentially at the roots of the plexus, particularly $C_5$–$C_7$, but the $C_8$ and $T_1$ roots are not blocked reliably. Thus, the skin and deep structures of the shoulder, the upper arm, the elbow and the lateral aspects of the forearm and hand are consistently

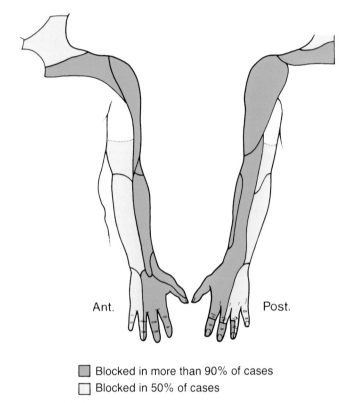

Ant.     Post.

☐ Blocked in more than 90% of cases
☐ Blocked in 50% of cases

**Fig 14.6** Distribution of interscalene block

blocked (Fig. 14.6), while structures in the medial aspect of the forearm and hand may need supplementary nerve block. It is possible to produce partial cervical plexus block with an interscalene block.

### Patient position
The patient lies supine with the head supported by a pillow and the head turned slightly away from the site of needle insertion. The arm should be placed by the patient's side to depress the shoulder slightly. If the posture is exaggerated the neck muscles will be too tense and obscure the interscalene groove.

### Landmarks
The cricoid cartilage is palpated and a line drawn laterally until it crosses the lateral border of the sternomastoid muscle, usually at its midpoint (Fig. 14.7). If this muscle is not obvious, the patient can bring it into prominence by raising the head off the pillow. The index finger of the non-dominant hand is placed immediately posterior

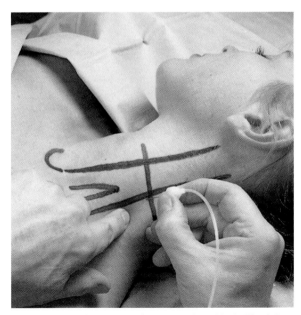

**Fig 14.7** Needle insertion for interscalene block. The left index finger is palpating the interscalene groove

to the border of the sternomastoid where the cricoid line intersects it, and it will then lie on the belly of the anterior scalene muscle. As the finger is moved slightly posterolateral, the interscalene groove is felt as a depression between the two scalene muscles. If the patient is asked to 'sniff' or inhale vigorously, the scalene muscles contract and the groove is accentuated. The external jugular vein often crosses the interscalene groove at the intended point of needle insertion.

## Technique

The groove is identified and a short-bevel needle inserted at the level of the cricoid cartilage, at right angles to the skin in all planes (Fig. 14.7), that is, medial, slightly caudad and posterior (dorsal). If directed horizontally or anteriorly the needle may pass between adjacent transverse processes and enter the vertebral artery or the intervertebral foramen.

The needle is advanced slowly and a distinct 'pop' or loss of resistance may be felt, usually less than 2 cm deep to the skin. Paraesthesiae radiating to the upper arm occur frequently and indicate that the needle is within the plexus sheath. Paraesthesiae detected in the shoulder tip or scapular areas indicate suprascapular or supraclavicular nerve stimulation outside the sheath; an injection at this point would be ineffective. If paraesthesiae are not elicited, the needle should be withdrawn slightly and re-angled more caudally or posteriorly, reviewing the depth and direction of the needle tip frequently during insertion. Alternatively, a peripheral nerve stimulator can be attached to the needle for location of the plexus.

The interscalene groove can be compressed above the needle to promote caudad spread of local anaesthetic, and the injection is made slowly with frequent aspiration.

## Complications

Although relatively easy to perform, interscalene brachial plexus block is associated with rare, but serious, side-effects, which should limit its use by inexperienced practitioners, especially where a less hazardous approach can be used.

**Phrenic nerve block** The ipsilateral hemidiaphragm may be paralysed in almost every case (Urmey et al 1991), but this rarely causes the patient difficulties unless they have significant respiratory disease. The vagus nerve may also be affected, but again without clinical effect.

**Recurrent laryngeal nerve block** Hoarseness is occasionally experienced after interscalene or subclavian perivascular block but is of little consequence, although it is necessary to reassure the patient that this is the case. Bilateral blocks should not be performed because of the adverse effect on laryngeal competence.

**Horner's syndrome** About 50% of interscalene and subclavian perivascular blocks produce this effect and patients should be warned about the effects of facial flushing and unequal pupils.

**Vertebral artery injection** This is a constant risk of the interscalene approach and is potentially very hazardous because small volumes (as little as 1 ml) can cause serious cerebral toxicity.

**Epidural and subarachnoid injection** Serious complications from inadvertent total spinal and high epidural injection have been reported. Careful needle placement and frequent aspiration are essential in avoiding serious complications.

## Subclavian perivascular block

### Clinical indications

This approach anaesthetises the three trunks as they run vertically (superio-inferiorly) across the surface of the first rib (not horizontally, as originally described and often assumed still). At this point the trunks are immediately posterior to the subclavian artery, and within the brachial plexus sheath (see Fig. 14.3). There are fewer components to the plexus at this point than elsewhere and a successful block here provides consistent anaesthesia of the upper limb below the shoulder joint (Fig. 14.8). Occasionally the subclavian artery prevents solution spreading to the inferior trunk and the block may be deficient in the $C_8$–$T_1$ distribution, but this is uncommon if a sufficient volume is injected. Landmarks may be difficult to determine, especially in the obese, and the risk of pneumothorax might detract from its use in patients with severe respiratory disease.

### Position

The patient adopts the same position, described above, as for interscalene block.

### Landmarks

The interscalene groove is identified (see under Interscalene Block and Fig. 14.7) and traced caudally towards the clavicle until the pulse of the subclavian

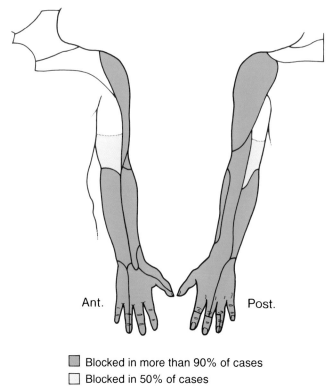

■ Blocked in more than 90% of cases
☐ Blocked in 50% of cases

**Fig 14.8**   Distribution of subclavian perivascular block

artery is palpated, usually at a point posterior to the midpoint of the clavicle. The artery emerges from behind the insertion of scalenus anterior on the first rib and passes beneath the clavicle at its mid-point. If the artery cannot be palpated, the injection is made at the lowest point in the interscalene groove that can be reliably identified.

### Technique

The arterial pulse (or the lowest point of the interscalene groove) is identified and the needle inserted immediately above the palpating finger, between the scalene muscles (Fig 14.9). It is important to align the needle parallel to the midline and in the horizontal plane (in the supine patient) and advance it slowly until paraesthesiae are elicited. It should not be angled medially as this will increase the risk of pneumothorax. As the sheath is penetrated a 'pop' may be felt which helps to confirm correct needle placement. The sheath is rarely more than 2 cm deep to the skin and paraesthesiae usually occur immediately after entering the sheath. If the first rib is contacted or the subclavian artery punctured, the needle should be withdrawn slightly and redirected a

little more posteriorly. Because the artery is within the plexus sheath at this point, intravascular placement indicates close proximity to the plexus.

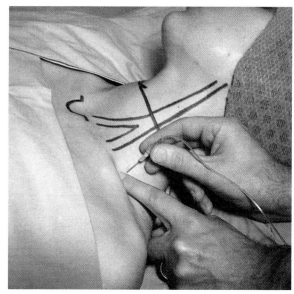

**Fig 14.9**   Needle insertion for subclavian perivascular block

Paraesthesiae usually occur in the distribution of the superior trunk, that is, the lateral aspect of the forearm, because of the vertical arrangement of the trunks. Paraesthesiae in the shoulder area indicate that the suprascapular or supraclavicular nerves have been stimulated, and that the needle lies outside the plexus sheath. If paraesthesiae are difficult to evoke, a peripheral nerve stimulator can be used to produce pulse-synchronous muscle movement. When appropriate responses have been obtained, the injection is made slowly after negative aspiration.

## Complications

**Pneumothorax** This is the main complication of the subclavian perivascular approach, the incidence varying widely from 0.5–25% in different studies. A pneumothorax may remain small and undetected, or increase slowly in size for up to 24 hours before becoming apparent. Cough, chest pain or dyspnoea indicate the need for an erect chest X-ray to confirm the diagnosis.

**Block of adjacent nerves** The major nerves of the neck can all be affected (see under Interscalene Block).

## Axillary block

### Clinical indications

This approach is a safe and relatively simple method of blocking the brachial plexus, although the extent of the block is restricted even when a large volume of local anaesthetic is used. The musculocutaneous and axillary nerves leave the plexus sheath high in the axilla and can remain unblocked in up to 25% of patients by this approach (Fig. 14.10), and the radial nerve, which lies behind the axillary artery, is occasionally missed. Therefore the main indication for axillary brachial plexus block is surgery of the hand and forearm in the distribution of the median and ulnar nerves. If surgery involves the lateral aspects of the forearm and hand, supplementary block of the lateral cutaneous nerve of forearm and radial nerve may be required.

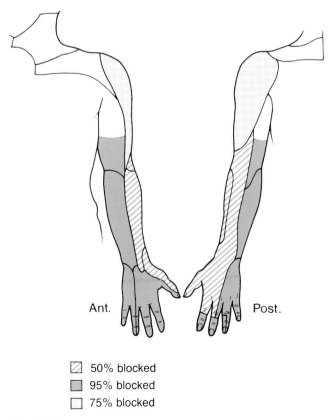

Ant.  Post.

◩ 50% blocked
▨ 95% blocked
☐ 75% blocked

**Fig 14.10**  Distribution of axillary block

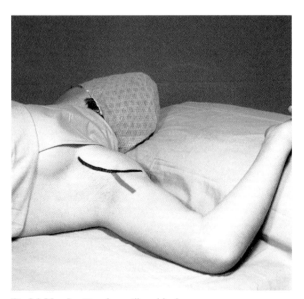

**Fig 14.11**  Position for axillary block

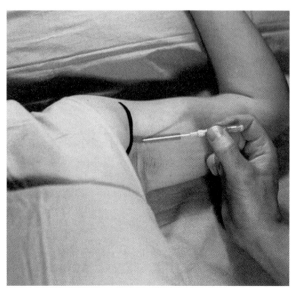

**Fig 14.12**  Alignment of cannula or needle for axillary block

### Position

The patient lies supine with the shoulder abducted to 90° and the elbow flexed to 90° so that the dorsum of the hand lies on the pillow (Fig. 14.11). Over-abduction of the shoulder should be avoided because the arterial pulse may be more difficult to palpate – the patient's hand should not be placed under the head. In patients with pain from trauma or joint disease, the correct position may be difficult to achieve.

### Technique

The axillary arterial pulse is traced medially towards the apex of the axilla. The artery is gently compressed against the humerus with the index finger of the non-dominant hand, at a point approximately level with the lateral border of the pectoralis major muscle. A short-bevel needle is inserted above the artery and immediately proximal to the finger at an angle of 30° to the skin (Fig. 14.12), and slowly advanced until a 'pop' or loss of resistance is felt as it pierces the sheath, which lies quite superficially within the axilla. Paraesthesiae are not always elicited and do not need to be sought for a successful axillary block. If arterial blood is apparent, there are two alternatives: (a) the needle can be deliberately advanced through the posterior wall of the artery until blood cannot be aspirated and the injection made behind the vessel – the transarterial technique (Cockings et al 1987); (b) the needle can be withdrawn and redirected within the sheath after careful negative aspiration. The

transarterial approach was described originally as being highly successful, but this is disputed, and routine puncture of the artery should only be considered if a definite advantage over other methods can be demonstrated.

Many modifications of technique and methods of injecting the local anaesthetic, either as a single, large volume injection or smaller divided doses with the needle being redirected two or more times, have been developed with the aim of increasing the success rates of axillary block. The simplest method, which is consistently successful, is to immobilise the needle once correctly located within the sheath and inject 35–40 ml, after careful aspiration, using digital compression of the axillary sheath distal to the point of injection. The pressure is maintained as the arm is returned to the patient's side and this, together with gentle massage of the solution up into the apex of the axilla, will promote proximal flow of the injectate past the head of humerus, which can obstruct flow when the arm is abducted.

The musculocutaneous nerve can be blocked separately by advancing the needle through the sheath and into the body of coracobrachialis after the main injection is completed and injecting 5–7 ml of the local anaesthetic solution. A further 5 ml can be injected as a subcutaneous wheal to block the branches of the inter-costobrachial nerve if a tourniquet is to be used on the upper arm. These additional measures should produce complete anaesthesia of the upper limb, but an alternative

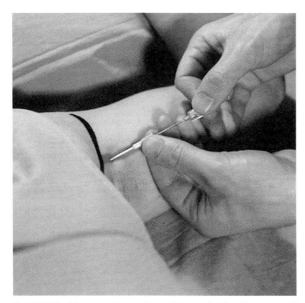

**Fig 14.13** The cannula is advanced once the sheath is entered

approach (and, arguably, a more reliable one) is to perform an axillary block with half the local anaesthetic solution and an interscalene block with the remainder.

### Continuous methods

All three approaches to the brachial plexus can be used to insert an indwelling catheter through which continuous infusions or intermittent top-up injections can be given. This allows the duration of block to be extended to provide prolonged analgesia and sympathetic vasodilatation, and active rehabilitation of the limb. The axillary approach is particularly successful (Figs 14.12 & 14.13). A 20 g intravenous cannula is used and, once the sheath is penetrated and aspiration for blood is negative, it is advanced as the stilette is withdrawn. The cannula should advance freely and, if it does not, should be withdrawn and re-inserted. Once in position, an extension set is connected to the cannula and a dressing applied. The arm is returned to the patient's side and digital compression applied distal to the cannula to encourage proximal flow of the solution.

The security of the indwelling cannula can be difficult to maintain over several days, owing to the wide range of movement at the shoulder and the elasticity of the skin and subcutaneous tissues. A number of specialist 'kits' have been developed for continuous brachial plexus block, but displacement of the cannula or a catheter remains a problem.

### Complications

The axillary technique is associated with fewer serious complications than the other approaches. Intravascular injection and haematoma formation are the main risks. Careful and repeated aspiration for blood will greatly reduce, but not eliminate, the risk of intravascular injection, and if a vessel is punctured it must be compressed for 5 minutes to minimise haematoma formation. Because of this potential for vessel damage, the risks and benefits of this approach must be carefully considered in patients on anticoagulants or with a coagulopathy.

## PERIPHERAL NERVE BLOCKS

Individual peripheral nerve blocks have a limited role in the upper limb compared to brachial plexus block, but are useful supplements for an incomplete brachial plexus block and can also be used with light general anaesthesia to provide prolonged postoperative analgesia after surgery on the hand and forearm. Nerve blocks can be performed singly or in combination at the elbow or the wrist depending on clinical requirements. Blocks at the elbow produce motor and sensory block of the forearm and hand whereas wrist blocks restrict sensory loss to the hand and preserve some motor control of the digits (Table 14.2).

### Equipment

Short-bevel, 22 g regional block needles are recommended for blocks at the elbow, and 3 cm long, 25 g hypodermic needles are suitable for wrist blocks.

A peripheral nerve stimulator can be used to locate those nerves which have a mixed motor and sensory function, and it is especially useful for the radial and median nerves at the elbow.

### Drugs

Bupivacaine and ropivacaine give prolonged analgesia – up to 12 hours – although lidocaine or prilocaine can be used for minor surgical procedures.

### Complications

*Intravascular injection* There are blood vessels in close proximity to the peripheral nerves at both the wrist and elbow and care must be taken to avoid intravascular injection and haematoma formation.

205

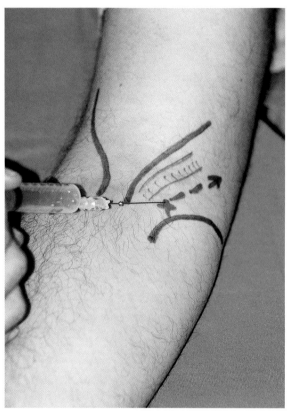

Fig 14.14 Landmarks at the antecubital fossa for the median nerve and medial cutaneous nerve of forearm. The dotted arrow indicates the direction of the subcutaneous injection for the medial cutaneous nerve

**Neural damage** Injury to peripheral nerves during regional anaesthesia is extremely rare (Fischer 1998), although transient symptoms of paraesthesiae may be relatively minor and go unreported. It is important to avoid direct neural contact, which is both extremely painful and potentially damaging to the nerve, and it may be wise to avoid some blocks in the presence of existing nerve compression, for example median nerve block at the wrist for carpal tunnel syndrome. The ulnar nerve is particularly vulnerable to damage in the sulcus of the medial epicondyle of the humerus, and older descriptions of the block which place the needle within the sulcus should not be followed.

## Techniques

### Blocks at the elbow

The medial, lateral and posterior cutaneous nerves of forearm innervate the skin and subcutaneous tissues of

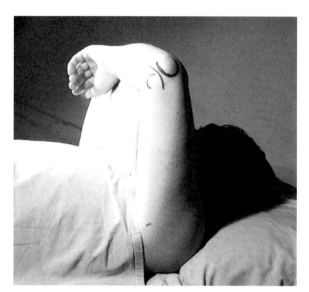

Fig 14.15 Course of ulnar nerve between the medial epicondyle of humerus and olecranon

the forearm, while the median, radial and ulnar nerves are sensory to the hand and motor to the forearm muscles and the intrinsic muscles of the hand (Fig. 14.2). Depending on the clinical requirements, the median and medial cutaneous nerves and the radial and lateral cutaneous nerves are usually blocked together (Fig. 14.14).

**Ulnar nerve** This block can be used in isolation for procedures on the little finger and ulnar aspect of the hand or in combination with median and radial nerve blocks for more extensive analgesia. The nerve lies in the ulnar sulcus of the medial epicondyle (Fig. 14.15) where it is constrained by the medial ligaments of the elbow. The incidence of neuritis is high if the nerve is blocked within the sulcus and the injection should be made 2–3 cm proximal to the epicondyle. With the elbow flexed to 90° and the arm positioned either across the chest or abducted and supinated, the nerve is easily palpated beneath the subcutaneous tissues just proximal to the medial epicondyle, and paraesthesiae are usually elicited during palpation. The needle is inserted 0.5–1 cm and 3–4 ml of local anaesthetic injected.

**Median nerve** The median nerve lies medial to the brachial artery just proximal to the antecubital fossa (Fig. 14.14). After the course of the artery has been identified, a short-bevel needle is inserted just medial to the arterial pulsation until it penetrates the deep fascia, often with a distinct 'pop' approximately 0.5–1 cm beneath the skin. Paraesthesiae may occur, but should not be sought, and 4–5 ml of local anaesthetic are injected. A peripheral nerve stimulator can be used to confirm needle location.

*Medial cutaneous nerve of forearm* This nerve is blocked through the same point of needle insertion by withdrawing the needle until it is superficial to the deep fascia and then redirecting it proximally, parallel to the medial border of the biceps tendon. As the needle is advanced, 5 ml of local anaesthetic is injected subcutaneously. The combination of the two nerve blocks provides sensory block of the medial aspect of the forearm and the lateral aspect of the palm, and motor block of the forearm flexors and intrinsic muscles of the hand.

*Radial nerve* The radial nerve crosses the anterior surface of the lateral epicondyle deep to the brachioradialis. A finger is placed behind the lateral epicondyle to identify the direction of needle insertion, and the needle is inserted lateral to the biceps tendon and directed towards the lateral epicondyle (Fig. 14.16). If paraesthesiae are elicited in the distribution of the radial nerve, the injection is made at that point; otherwise the needle is advanced until it contacts the epicondyle. It is then withdrawn slightly and a 10 ml injection made in a fanwise pattern. If a peripheral nerve stimulator is used, extension of the fingers and abduction of the thumb indicate successful nerve location.

*Lateral cutaneous nerve of forearm* This is the sensory continuation of the musculocutaneous nerve. It is usually blocked in tandem with the radial nerve to provide both sensory and motor block to the lateral aspect of the forearm and hand (dorsal surface). The needle is withdrawn after completion of the radial block and redirected proximally in the subcutaneous tissues parallel to the lateral border of the biceps tendon, 5 ml of local anaesthetic is injected as the needle is advanced.

*Posterior cutaneous nerve of forearm* This is sensory to the posterior aspect of the forearm and is easily blocked by injecting 5 ml of local anaesthetic subcutaneously from the posterior border of the lateral epicondyle of the humerus to the olecranon process.

## Blocks at the wrist
These have limited use, but may be useful for minor surgery to the hand.

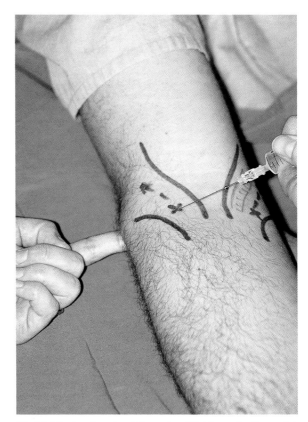

**Fig 14.16** Landmarks at the antecubital fossa for the radial nerve and lateral cutaneous nerve of forearm. The dotted arrow indicates the direction of the subcutaneous injection for the lateral cutaneous nerve

*Ulnar nerve* Block at the wrist is more difficult than at the elbow and has no advantages over the elbow block.

*Median nerve* The nerve enters the hand deep to the flexor retinaculum, lateral to the tendon of palmaris longus and medial to flexor carpi radialis (Fig. 14.17). The needle is inserted about 1 cm medial to flexor carpi radialis and 1 cm proximal to the flexor skin crease of the wrist to a depth of about 1 cm. The retinaculum may offer some resistance to the needle advancement. Paraesthesiae are elicited and 2–3 ml of local anaesthetic injected with a further 1ml injected subcutaneously as the needle is withdrawn to block the superficial palmar branch.

*Radial nerve* A subcutaneous injection of 5–7 ml of local anaesthetic across the dorsal surface of the wrist at the level of the ulnar styloid process (Fig. 14.18) blocks the terminal dorsal branches of the nerve which supply the radial two-thirds of the hand up to the distal phalanges (Fig. 14.2).

207

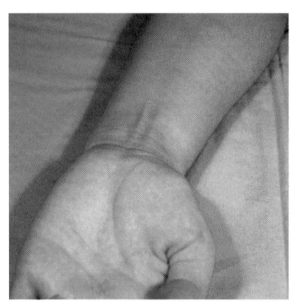

**Fig 14.17** The groove between the tendons of palmaris longus and flexor carpi radialis marks the point of insertion for median nerve block at the wrist

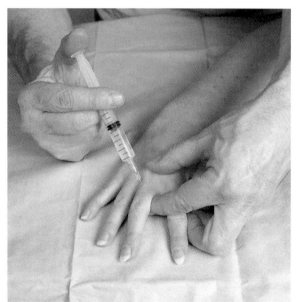

**Fig 14.19** Digital nerve block

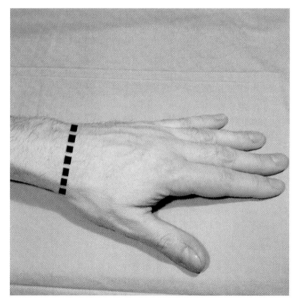

**Fig 14.18** Line of subcutaneous infiltration for radial nerve block at the wrist

*Digital nerve blocks* (Fig. 14.19) These blocks, somewhat inaccurately referred to as 'ring' block, are very effective for minor surgery to the fingers. Each digit is innervated by two dorsal and two palmar nerves which are blocked by injecting 2–3 ml of local anaesthetic into the web space either side of the digit. The injection is made either in the vertical plane, advancing the needle from the dorsal skin surface towards the palmar aspect of the hand, or in the horizontal plane, injecting the same volume of local anaesthetic as the needle is slowly advanced towards the metacarpophalangeal joint. Local anaesthetics containing vasoconstrictor (e.g. epinephrine) must not be used because of the risk of prolonged ischaemia. Furthermore, excessive volumes of local anaesthetic may cause vascular compression, and should be avoided.

## INTRAVENOUS REGIONAL ANAESTHESIA (IVRA)

Bier originally described the intravenous injection of local anaesthetic into an exsanguinated limb in 1908, but his method has been modified over the years and the technique currently used is based on the method described by Holmes in 1963. IVRA is a reliable and successful method of upper limb anaesthesia, but its success depends on the intravenous injection of a large dose of local anaesthetic. The use of bupivacaine by inexperienced clinicians in combination with unreliable equipment resulted in fatal complications (Heath 1982). The use of bupivacaine is now contraindicated in IVRA.

## Clinical indications

IVRA provides sensory and motor block in the forearm and hand with up to 98% success and is suitable for surgery distal to the elbow with a tourniquet time of about 1 hour. Tourniquet pain is difficult to prevent and limits the duration of surgery, although prolonged use of IVRA has been reported. The simplicity, high success rate and speed of recovery of limb function following tourniquet deflation mean that the technique is suited to use in the day-surgery unit and accident and emergency department in experienced hands. A major limitation of IVRA is the lack of any analgesia once the tourniquet is deflated, but this can be overcome by supplementation with peripheral nerve blocks.

## Contraindications

IVRA is contraindicated for patients in whom ischaemia would cause significant problems – sickle cell trait, Raynauds disease and significant soft tissue injury or infection – because tissue necrosis may occur. Severe cardiac disease (cardiac failure, heart block, severe hypertension) is also a contraindication.

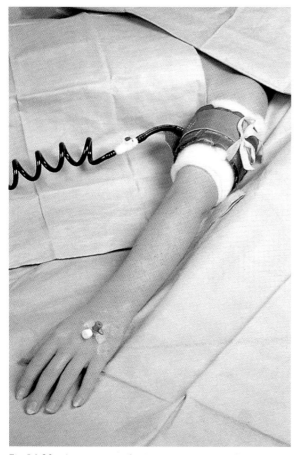

**Fig 14.20** Arrangement for intravenous regional anaesthesia (IVRA)

## Tourniquet equipment

A variety of tourniquet designs are available with either manual or automatic inflation and single or double cuffs. For simplicity and safety, a manual pump with high-pressure tubing and accurate pressure gauge leading to a single orthopaedic tourniquet is recommended (Fig. 14.20), and this equipment must be maintained properly and calibrated regularly. Double cuffs have been recommended as a means of avoiding pain from the tourniquet, but this is often not achieved and there is a risk of confusion when inflating and deflating the cuffs in the correct sequence. Sphygmomanometer cuffs, of any design, must *never* be used.

## Drugs and doses

A fit adult usually requires 40 ml, with smaller volumes being administered for elderly patients or children. Preservative-free prilocaine 0.5% has long been considered the agent of choice, but this preparation has been withdrawn recently on commercial grounds. The clinician is left with the option of using preservative-free lidocaine 0.5%, or carefully diluting the 1% solution of prilocaine which unfortunately contains preservative and is therefore not ideal.

Opioid drugs such as morphine, pethidine and fentanyl have been used as adjuvants, but do not improve analgesia, and result in drowsiness and nausea after tourniquet release.

## Technique

Despite the apparent simplicity of the technique, the usual precautions for managing the potentially serious complications of regional anaesthesia must be observed:

- venous access established in the other arm
- a full range of resuscitation equipment and drugs immediately available
- the patient fasted prior to the block
- the tourniquet checked beforehand and the inflation pressure monitored during use
- the block performed by an experienced clinician who is responsible for monitoring the patient during the procedure.

The intravenous cannula in the opposite arm is checked for patency before a 20 g cannula is inserted into a vein on the dorsum of the hand or the distal part of the forearm of the limb to be blocked. Scalp vein or other infusion needles are not recommended because of the increased risk of vessel wall puncture and displacement. The tourniquet is placed securely on the upper arm and is adequately padded to prevent damage to the skin.

The patient's blood pressure is measured before the limb is exsanguinated by applying an Esmarch bandage firmly from fingers to tourniquet, care being taken not to displace the cannula. After removal of the Esmarch bandage, the limb should appear pallid with no evidence of arterial pulsation or venous congestion. If the limb has been traumatised and the patient cannot tolerate application of the bandage, the limb should be elevated and the brachial artery compressed for 2 minutes, just distal to the tourniquet, before the tourniquet is inflated to 100 mmHg above the patient's systolic pressure. It is important to assess the limb for adequate exsanguination because patchy sensory block and inadequate muscle relaxation may be a problem, especially with large muscular arms, and venous bleeding can interfere with the surgery. If necessary, the process should be repeated with a slightly higher tourniquet inflation pressure.

Once satisfactory exsanguination is achieved, the local anaesthetic is injected slowly over 2–3 minutes through the intravenous cannula. There will be rapid onset of paraesthesiae and a blotchy appearance to the skin, with full sensory block occurring within 10 minutes, although motor block may take a further 10 minutes to develop. Rapid or forceful injection must be avoided because it can generate high intravenous pressure and force the drug beyond the tourniquet into the systemic circulation. The tourniquet inflation pressure should be continuously monitored throughout the duration of the block, and the tourniquet should remain inflated for a minimum of 20 minutes after the injection, even if surgery is completed sooner. Circumoral tingling, tinnitus and drowsiness may occur after tourniquet

deflation, and occasionally bradycardia and hypotension may be observed, indicating that minor systemic toxicity can occur even with 0.5% prilocaine. The patient must be kept under close supervision for 30 minutes after tourniquet deflation.

## Complications

### Systemic toxicity

Serious sequelae have not been reported when the technique is performed correctly using prilocaine, but the risk of systemic toxicity due to failure of equipment or a faulty technique is always present. Local anaesthetic can be forced beneath the tourniquet into the systemic circulation if the cannula is placed in a proximal forearm or antecubital fossa vein, or if the injection is made rapidly or with force (Haasio et al 1989). Inadvertent tourniquet deflation can occur with inadequate supervision of the equipment or inexperienced personnel. This technique should not be used by inexperienced doctors, unfamiliar with the hazards of regional anaesthesia and untrained in its management. It is not suitable for single operator-anaesthetist use, and the patient should always be attended by a trained doctor, experienced in the technique and solely responsible for the patient's care.

### Tourniquet compression injury

Nerve damage due to inappropriate tourniquet application is uncommon, but it is important to pad the arm before applying the tourniquet and to position the cuff carefully over the mid-part of the upper limb, avoiding the epicondyles of the humerus. Duration of tourniquet time is not directly related to the risk of nerve damage, but the pain from direct pressure of the cuff as well as from ischaemia usually limits duration to about 1 hour.

## Further Reading

Winnie AP 1983 Perivascular techniques of brachial plexus block. Plexus anaesthesia, vol.1. Schultz, Copenhagen

Brown DL, Bridenbaugh LD 1998 Upper limb block. In: Cousins MJ, Bridenbaugh PO (eds) Neural blockade in clinical anesthesia and management of pain, 3rd edn, pp 345-371. Lippincott-Raven, Philadelphia

Pinnock CAP, Fischer HBJ, Jones RP 1996 Peripheral nerve blockade. pp 107–139. Churchill Livingstone, Edinburgh

## References

Bazin JE, Massoni C, Bruelle P, Fenies V, Groselier D, Schoeffler P 1997 The addition of opioids to local anaesthetics in brachial plexus block: the comparative effects of morphine, buprenorphine and sufentanil. Anaesthesia 52: 858–862

Brockway MS, Winter AW, Wildsmith JAW 1989 Prolonged brachial plexus block with 0.42% bupivacaine. British Journal of Anaesthesia 63: 604–605

Cockings E, Moore PL, Lewis RC 1987 Transarterial brachial plexus blockade using high doses of 1.5% mepivacaine. Regional Anesthesia 12: 159–164 de Jong R 1961 Axillary block of the brachial plexus. Anesthesiology 22: 215–225

Eisenach JC, De Kock M, Klimscha W 1996 Alpha2 agonists for regional anesthesia. Anesthesiology 85: 655–674

Fischer HBJ 1998 Regional Anaesthesia – before or after general anaesthesia? [Editorial] Anaesthesia 53: 727–729

Haasio J, Hiippala S, Rosenberg PH 1989 Intravenous regional anaesthesia of the arm: effect of the technique of exsanguination on the quality of anaesthesia and prilocaine plasma concentrations. Anaesthesia 44: 19–21

Heath ML 1982 Deaths after intravenous regional anaesthesia [Editorial] British Medical Journal 285: 913–914

Holmes C McK 1963 Intravenous regional anaesthesia: a useful method of producing analgesia of the limbs. Lancet 1: 245–247

Lanz E, Theiss Djankovic D 1983 The extent of blockade following various techniques of brachial plexus block. Anesthesia and Analgesia 62: 55–58

Moore DC, Mulroy MF, Thompson GE 1994 Peripheral nerve damage and regional anaesthesia British Journal of Anaesthesia 73: 435–436

Patrick J 1940 The technique of brachial plexus block anaesthesia. British Journal of Surgery 27: 734

Raj R, Montgomery S, Nettles D, Jenkins M 1973 Infraclavicular brachial plexus block: a new approach. Anesthesia and Analgesia 52: 897–904

Rice ASC, McMahon SB 1992 Peripheral nerve injury caused by injection needles used in regional anaesthesia: influence of bevel configuration, studied in a rat model. British Journal of Anaesthesia 69: 433–438

Selander D, Dhuner KG, Lundborg G 1977 Peripheral nerve injury due to injection needles used for regional anaesthesia. An experimental study of the acute affects of needle point trauma. Acta Anaesthesiologica Scandinavica 21: 182–188

Thompson G, Rorie D 1983 Functional anatomy of the brachial plexus sheath. Anesthesiology 59: 117–122

Urmey WF, Talts KH, Sharrock NE 1991 One hundred percent incidence of hemidiaphragmatic paresis associated with interscalene brachial plexus anesthesia as diagnosed by ultrasonography. Anesthesia and Analgesia 72: 498–503

Wildsmith JAW, Tucker GT, Cooper S, Scott DB, Covino GB 1977 Plasma concentrations after interscalene brachial plexus block. British Journal of Anaesthesia 49: 461–466

Winnie AP 1969 An 'immobile needle' for nerve block. Anesthesiology 31: 577–578

Winnie AP 1970 Interscalene brachial plexus block. Anesthesia and Analgesia 49: 455–466

Winnie AP, Collins VJ 1964 The subclavian perivascular technique of brachial plexus anaesthesia. Anesthesiology 25: 353–363

Winnie AP, Tay CH, Patel KP, Ramamurthy S, Durrani Z. 1977 Pharmacokinetics of local anesthetics during plexus blocks. Anesthesia and Analgesia 56: 852–861

# 15. Lower limb blocks

## W A Macrae and D M Coventry

While most regional techniques have become more widely used in recent years, lower limb blocks have not enjoyed quite the same increase in popularity. Many anaesthetists feel that the techniques are complicated, difficult and unreliable, and that too much detailed anatomy has to be learnt before the blocks can be attempted. Spinal and epidural methods offer straightforward single-needle techniques for anaesthesia of the lower limb, whereas multiple injections are required to block the nerves more peripherally. However, the view that all nerve blocks of the lower limb are difficult and unreliable is incorrect. The aim of this chapter is to present simple techniques which give consistent results and may be used routinely. It is hoped that this approach will persuade the reader to include lower limb nerve blocks in his or her repertoire. Only brief reference will be made to techniques which have not been found so useful in routine clinical practice.

## GENERAL CONSIDERATIONS

### Anatomy

Some knowledge of anatomy is essential for the performance of nerve blocks in the lower limb, but no attempt will be made to describe the complete course of each nerve or to describe its anatomical relations because only comparatively small areas need to be understood in detail. The anatomy described is sufficient to permit reliable identification of each nerve.

### Lumbosacral plexus (Fig. 15.1)

The nerve supply of the lower limb is from the lumbosacral plexus, which is formed from the anterior primary rami of the second lumbar to the third sacral roots. Each root divides into an anterior and posterior division, and these divisions then join and branch to form the individual nerves.

### Cutaneous innervation

Whereas knowledge of *dermatomal* distribution in the lower limb is needed for the proper use of spinal and epidural blocks, it is the *cutaneous* distribution of the various nerves (Fig. 15.2) which determines the practical application of peripheral nerve block. This cutaneous distribution varies. For example, the junction between the areas supplied by the saphenous (femoral) and the superficial peroneal (sciatic) nerves can be anywhere between the upper edge of the medial malleolus and the big toe. Such variation must be borne in mind if an operation is to be performed near the edge of the distribution of a nerve. It is essential to test carefully and block the nerve supplying the adjacent area if necessary.

### Innervation of deep structures

The sensory nerve supply to deep tissues has not been as well elucidated as that of the skin. It is generally safe to assume that muscle and bones are supplied by the same peripheral nerves as the skin overlying them, but joints generally have a more complex nerve supply and receive innervation from all the nerves supplying structures around them. For example, the hip and knee joints are supplied by femoral, sciatic and obturator nerves, and the ankle is supplied by branches of both femoral and sciatic nerves. As in the upper limb, the dermatomal innervation of *deep* structures is quite different from that of the skin. The foot is supplied by the lower roots ($S_3$–$S_4$) and the upper parts of the limb by the upper roots ($L_1$–$L_2$).

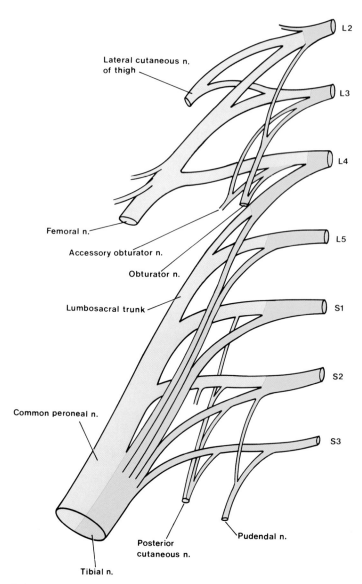

**Fig 15.1** The lumbosacral plexus

## Factors influencing choice of technique

The art of anaesthesia lies in giving each patient the most suitable anaesthetic for each operation. The choice of technique depends on the variables considered in the first section of this book, but a few points apply particularly to the use of local anaesthesia in the lower limb.

### The patient

Peripheral nerve blocks have advantages in patients with cardiovascular disease because the extensive sympathetic block which may be associated with spinal or epidural anaesthesia is avoided (Fanelli et al 1998). Spinal and epidural anaesthesia may also be contra-indicated or complicated by spinal disease associated with the lower limb condition requiring surgery, or by the position of the patient who may, for example, be in fixed traction and cannot be moved until anaesthesia has been induced. Conversely, a peripheral nerve block will be impossible to perform if a plaster of Paris cast covers the injection site. Many lower limb nerves are blocked at points where they lie close to arteries. If the latter are affected by peripheral vascular disease it is important to avoid needle trauma to them.

A relatively large volume of local anaesthetic is required for major lower limb blocks. If bilateral femoral and sciatic nerve blocks were to be performed at the hip, as much as 80 ml of local anaesthetic could be required, and this, in standard concentrations, could amount to a potentially toxic dose. It must be stressed that systemic concentrations after these blocks tend to be low (Misra et al 1991, Robison et al 1991, Connolly et al 2000), and that toxicity is not a common problem. However, if factors are present which make such large doses particularly undesirable, a technique requiring a smaller dose of drug, such as a spinal, may be preferable.

The patient's wishes must be taken into account. Most patients will accept regional anaesthesia if it is properly explained to them, and if it is accepted practice in the unit. However, patients who are disturbed by injections or who are to undergo bilateral procedures are far more likely to accept the single injection required for a spinal or epidural than a technique involving multiple injections.

### The operation

Obviously, the operation dictates what sort of block is appropriate. For most orthopaedic operations on the leg, a tourniquet is used and the block must eliminate pain from the tourniquet as well as from the operative site. If tourniquet discomfort does develop, it must be dealt with promptly and effectively before the patient's response disrupts the operation. Sedation, even with an opioid analgesic, may not be adequate and recourse to a light general anaesthetic may well be necessary, although many of the benefits of a nerve block for a peripheral procedure are then lost.

### The time factor

Sciatic and femoral nerve blocks take a relatively long time because the patient has to be positioned twice and two separate injections are required. The blocks take between 15 and 30 minutes to become effective so, if speed is important, a spinal anaesthetic is a better choice.

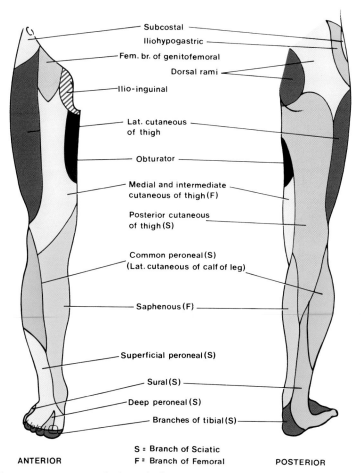

Subcostal
Iliohypogastric
Fem. br. of genitofemoral
Dorsal rami
Ilio-inguinal
Lat. cutaneous of thigh
Obturator
Medial and intermediate cutaneous of thigh (F)
Posterior cutaneous of thigh (S)
Common peroneal (S) (Lat. cutaneous of calf of leg)
Saphenous (F)
Superficial peroneal (S)
Sural (S)
Deep peroneal (S)
Branches of tibial (S)

S = Branch of Sciatic
F = Branch of Femoral

ANTERIOR                    POSTERIOR

**Fig 15.2** Distribution of cutaneous nerves in the lower limb

When lower limb blocks are being performed it is particularly important to organise the operating list to take this time factor into account, otherwise delay will occur and the anaesthetist will become unpopular. Having the support and co-operation of colleagues is as important as knowing where to put the needle.

### Broad recommendations

Choice of block for operations on the lower limb in the average patient is not difficult. The most useful blocks are undoubtedly epidurals and spinals. They are adaptable to almost all operations on the lower limb, and are so easy to perform and so reliable that they are an essential part of every anaesthetist's repertoire. They are the methods of choice for hip and knee surgery and operations involving the femoral shaft, and are also useful for bilateral operations below the knee.

However, nerve blocks have their place. For skin grafts from the thigh, block of the femoral nerve and the lateral cutaneous nerve are useful. For unilateral varicose veins, femoral nerve block, together with local infiltration to the groin, is often adequate (Vloka et al 1997). For unilateral operations below the knee, femoral and sciatic nerve blocks are, in the opinion of many, the methods of choice.

Individual nerve blocks are also useful in the diagnosis and treatment of chronic pain and every anaesthetist involved in such work should be familiar with the commoner lower limb nerve blocks.

### Technical aspects

The general principles of technique for blocks of the major nerves of the lower limb (factors such as choice of equipment, aseptic technique and the dosage, latency and duration of drugs) are much the same as for the brachial plexus (see Ch.14). Lidocaine 1.5% and bupivacaine 0.5%, with or without epinephrine, are suitable for most lower limb blocks. Prilocaine at 1–2% has much to commend it in many situations, while ropivacaine at 0.5–0.75% may be a safer alternative to bupivacaine when prolonged block is required (Greengrass et al 1998). Stimulators are used widely for location of the sciatic nerve because it is so deeply situated.

The *siting of the tourniquet* should also be discussed. For operations on the knee, it must be applied to the thigh, but, for operations on the ankle and foot, it may be applied to the calf. This position is widely used in some Scandinavian countries, and has been used by the authors for many years without any problems, although the precise position is important. If it is placed too high, there may be pressure on the common peroneal nerve as it winds around the neck of the fibula or on the saphenous nerve where it lies on the anteromedial surface of the tibia just below the knee. If the tourniquet is too low, it will be in the surgeon's way. The advantage of placing the tourniquet on the middle of the calf (see Fig. 15.12) for operations on the ankle and foot is that nerve block at the knee will provide anaesthesia for both the tourniquet and the operation (Fig. 15.2)

## LUMBAR PLEXUS BLOCKS

A number of approaches, both anterior and posterior, to the lumbar plexus have been described (Hanna et al 1993), all with the essential aim of blocking both femoral and obturator nerves with a single injection. However, the evidence is that the posterior approaches are the most effective (Parkinson et al 1989), there being little to choose (in terms of efficacy) between block at the $L_2$–$L_3$ (Hanna et al 1993) or the $L_4$–$L_5$ levels (Chayen et al 1976). The latter is also known as the 'psoas compartment' block and has two potential advantages: the components of the plexus are somewhat closer together at that level; and the landmarks are rather better defined.

### Psoas compartment block

#### Anatomy

The lumbar plexus is formed by the ventral rami of the first three and major part of the fourth lumbar nerves (Fig. 15.1). After emerging from the lateral foramina of the vertebral column, the nerves run inferolaterally and are first located within the posterior part of the psoas major muscle (see Fig. 21.9). This muscle is enclosed in a fascial sheath limited medially by the bodies of the lumbar vertebrae, and posteriorly by the lumbar transverse processes, ligaments and quadratus lumborum. The femoral and lateral cutaneous nerves emerge from the lateral, and the obturator nerve from the medial aspects of psoas, respectively. After emerging from psoas, the nerves lie in a fascial compartment between it and quadratus lumborum. Local anaesthetic injected into psoas, or into the potential space between psoas and quadratus lumborum, should block all three nerves.

#### Clinical application

Lumbar plexus block is frequently combined with sciatic nerve block to provide analgesia of the whole lower limb in situations when central nerve block is contraindicated. It may be used as the sole technique for femoral neck surgery or be combined with a general anaesthetic to provide postoperative analgesia. This combination is particularly useful for prolonged revision hip surgery. Although there is usually good cardio-vascular stability, it is worth noting that epidural spread can occur and appears more common with the psoas compartment approach (Parkinson et al 1989), particularly in children (Dalens et al 1988). Parkinson and colleagues (1989) noted one block as high as $T_6$, but this may have been related to the relatively large dose of local anaesthetic used (0.5 ml kg$^{-1}$). Hanna and colleagues (1993) believe that as little as 10 ml will block the lumbar plexus without the risk of epidural spread, but volumes of 25–30 ml are more commonly used.

### Technique

The patient is positioned in the lateral decubitus position with the operative side uppermost. Initially, the fourth lumbar spine is identified from its relationship to the iliac crests. A point 3 cm caudad to this, and 5 cm lateral to the midline, is marked and the skin and subcutaneous tissue infiltrated with local anaesthetic. A 21 g, 100 mm, short-bevelled insulated needle is attached to a nerve stimulator and advanced perpendicular to all planes until the transverse process of $L_5$ is located at a depth of approximately 5 cm. The needle is then withdrawn and advanced with progressively increased cephalad angulation until it 'glides' above the transverse process. It is then advanced further, until contractions of the quadriceps femoris muscle are elicited, usually 1–2 cm deeper than the transverse process. The injection of 25–30 ml of local anaesthetic solution will usually produce complete block within 15 minutes.

## NERVE BLOCK AT THE HIP

## Femoral nerve block

### Anatomy (Fig. 15.3)

The femoral nerve ($L_2$–$L_4$) runs down the posterolateral wall of the pelvis behind the fascia iliaca, lying on the psoas and iliacus muscles. The femoral artery and vein lie anterior to the fascia iliaca, which sweeps downwards and forwards from the posterior and lateral walls of the pelvis and blends with the inguinal ligament. As the vessels pass behind the inguinal ligament they become invested in a fascial sheath. The femoral nerve lies *behind and lateral* to this sheath and, unlike the vessels, is not

within it. All three are deep to the fascia lata, but unfortunately the exact position of the nerve in relation to the artery is inconstant. It may be close to the sheath or several centimetres lateral to it, as well as being more deeply placed. Just below the inguinal ligament the nerve divides into several branches. Because of these factors, femoral nerve block is not as easy as may be thought. Moore (1965a) states that when sciatic and femoral nerve blocks are combined, and found to be inadequate, it is usually the femoral nerve which has been missed.

### Clinical application

It is important to stress that, although femoral nerve block is not always easy, it is a useful technique, and well worth mastering. The majority of incisions for varicose vein surgery are made within its distribution and it may be used alone or in combination with block of the lateral cutaneous nerve for the taking of skin grafts from the thigh. It is suitable for many orthopaedic operations on the leg and foot and can provide analgesia for a fracture of the upper part of the femoral shaft.

### Technique (Fig. 15.4)

A line drawn between the anterior superior iliac spine and the pubic tubercle marks the position of the inguinal ligament. The femoral artery is palpated as it passes behind the midpoint of the ligament. The needle is inserted just below the ligament, 1 cm lateral to the artery, parallel with the course of the nerve, but inclined superiorly at an angle of about 45°. A 'click' is felt as the needle passes through the fascia lata, and it should be advanced with a gentle probing motion until a second 'click' is noted as the needle penetrates the fascia iliaca. The needle is advanced further until paraesthesiae are obtained. When a nerve stimulator is used, quadriceps contraction with 'patellar tap' should be elicited with a current of 0.5 mA or less. If the needle has been inserted to a depth of 3 or 4 cm without finding the nerve, it should be withdrawn and the direction changed slightly, either medial or lateral. Once the nerve is located, the needle is immobilised and an aspiration test performed before 15–20 ml of local anaesthetic solution is injected.

## Lateral cutaneous nerve of thigh

### Anatomy

The lateral cutaneous nerve of the thigh (lateral femoral cutaneous nerve) ($L_2$–$L_3$) runs forward in a

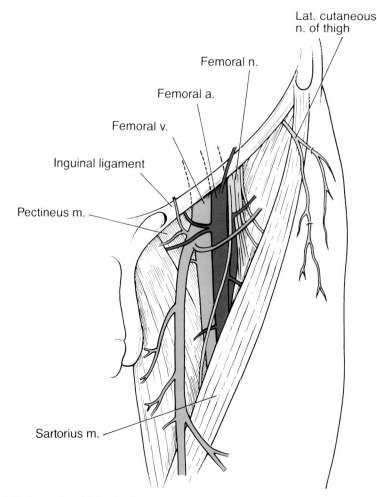

**Fig 15.3** Positions of the femoral and lateral cutaneous nerves

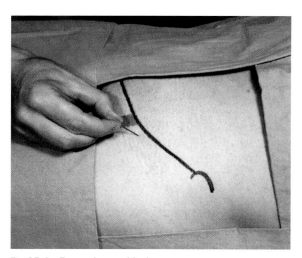

**Fig 15.4** Femoral nerve block

curve on the iliacus muscle outside the pelvic viscera and fascia iliaca. Anteriorly, it passes behind the inguinal ligament to enter the thigh deep to the fascia lata, 1–2 cm medial to the anterior superior iliac spine (Fig. 15.3). In the thigh, it divides into two branches, anterior and posterior, which pierce the fascia lata about 10 cm below the anterior superior iliac spine and supply the skin of the lateral aspect of the thigh.

## Clinical application
The block is usually combined with others to provide anaesthesia of the lower limb. Because the lateral aspect of the thigh is used frequently as a skin graft donor site, this block is a useful adjunct to general anaesthesia for skin harvesting and provides excellent postoperative analgesia. However, it should only be used as the sole

anaesthetic technique if the donor site is small and lies well within the distribution of the nerve.

## Technique

The nerve is blocked where it emerges below the inguinal ligament. The patient lies supine and the anterior superior iliac spine is palpated and marked. The needle is introduced perpendicularly through the skin 1 cm medial to, and 2 cm below, the anterior superior iliac spine. After passing through skin and subcutaneous tissue, slight resistance to needle advancement is felt and then a 'click' as the needle passes through the fascia lata. After aspiration, 2 ml local anaesthetic solution is injected. The needle tip is then withdrawn into the subcutaneous tissues, redirected laterally and advanced deep to the fascia lata where it will be approximately 1 cm from the original injection site. A further 2 ml of local anaesthetic is then injected. This process is repeated medial to the original injection site.

This is a fairly easy block with a high success rate although, like many blocks, it can be difficult in obese patients because the key to success is to insert the needle into the correct tissue plane. In these patients the following procedure may aid correct needle placement. Once the needle tip is in the subcutaneous tissues, a finger is placed on the skin either side of the needle shaft. When these two fingers are moved from side to side, the needle will move with the subcutaneous tissues, but once it has penetrated the fascia lata it will be anchored in place.

## Obturator nerve block

The obturator nerve ($L_2$–$L_4$) slants down the side wall of the pelvis to the upper part of the obturator foramen, through which it passes into the thigh. In the foramen, it divides into anterior and posterior branches. The obturator nerve sends branches to the hip and knee joints and supplies a variable area of skin on the inside of the thigh. It also supplies the adductor muscles. Block of the obturator nerve is both difficult and uncomfortable, sometimes painful, for the patient. The success rate even in experienced hands is poor (Moore 1965b) and the block is of little value on its own. It is used occasionally to complement sciatic and femoral nerve blocks for knee operations, but a spinal, an epidural or a lumbar plexus block are more useful.

## The 'three-in-one' block

### The sheath concept

This interesting variation on femoral nerve block was first described by Winnie and colleagues (1973). The aim is to block the femoral, lateral cutaneous and obturator nerves with a single injection. The principle upon which the block is based is that these nerves are branches of the lumbar plexus and lie sandwiched between the same muscles and fascia. If a large volume of local anaesthetic is injected into this musculofascial plane, it will spread centrally to affect all three nerves. The original description (Winnie et al 1973) showed that such spread could be demonstrated radiographically after femoral injection. However, other studies have failed to confirm satisfactory spread to all three nerves, in particular to the obturator nerve. Block appears to occur primarily by spread of local anaesthetic between the iliacus and psoas muscles and under the fascia iliaca and only rarely by proximal contact with the lumbar plexus (Capdevila et al 1998).

### Clinical application

Using the 'three-in-one' approach, Lang and colleagues (1993) demonstrated block of the obturator nerve in only 4% of patients, despite producing successful femoral and lateral cutaneous blocks. Parkinson and colleagues (1989) were unable to demonstrate obturator block with this approach in any patient when motor block was evaluated specifically. Thus the 'three-in-one' block would seem most useful for surgical procedures in the distribution of the femoral and lateral cutaneous nerves, and not those involving a significant obturator component, such as hip dislocation or femoral neck surgery. It can, therefore, be used to provide tourniquet analgesia when combined with sciatic nerve block for operations below the knee, and can be used alone for some varicose vein surgery and for the harvesting of split skin grafts from the thigh. It would appear more appropriate to use a posterior approach to the lumbar plexus (see above) when surgery to areas involving the obturator nerve is anticipated.

### Technique (Fig. 15.5)

'Three-in-one' block is essentially a modification of femoral nerve block. The nerve is identified as described above, after which the needle should be held firmly to prevent it moving. Firm pressure is applied distal to the needle with the thumb in order to prevent

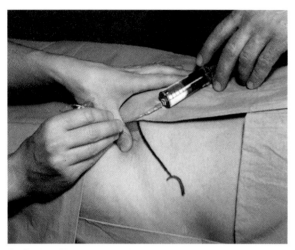

**Fig 15.5** 'Three-in-one' block

peripheral spread, and the local anaesthetic is injected after an aspiration test. It is best if an assistant holds the syringe and injects the drug while the anaesthetist holds the needle with one hand and presses below it with the other.

In the original paper (Winnie et al 1973), a 20 ml volume of local anaesthetic was said to be adequate to block all three nerves, but many anaesthetists now find that at least 25–30 ml is needed to ensure block of femoral and lateral cutaneous nerves.

## Sciatic nerve block

### Anatomy

The sciatic nerve is the largest nerve in the body. It starts in the pelvis as the continuation of the sacral plexus (Fig. 15.1) and passes from the pelvis into the buttock through the greater sciatic foramen. At this point, it is accompanied by the posterior cutaneous nerve of the thigh, which can be thought of as a branch of the sciatic.

After emerging from the greater sciatic foramen, the nerve is just posterior to the acetabulum and the head of the femur. It lies on the muscles around the hip joint and is covered by gluteus maximus. It then runs vertically downwards in the hamstring compartment of the thigh to reach the popliteal fossa, where it divides into common peroneal and tibial branches (see Fig. 15.9). Occasionally, this division occurs much higher in the thigh. The tibial nerve passes vertically downwards through the calf to supply the heel and sole of the foot. The common peroneal nerve winds diagonally across the popliteal fossa to the lateral part of the calf before

descending to the foot where its branches innervate the dorsal structures. The sural nerve is formed from components of both tibial and common peroneal branches and supplies the lateral border of the foot (see Fig.15.9).

### Clinical application

Block of the nerve in the buttock is easy and reliable. It produces anaesthesia of the back of the thigh because the posterior cutaneous nerve lies close to the sciatic and is blocked by the same injection. It also provides anaesthesia of the anterolateral part of the leg and most of the foot. In combination with femoral or saphenous nerve block, it provides anaesthesia for the whole of the leg below the knee. It causes motor block of the hamstrings as well as of the muscles of the lower leg.

### Techniques

Five methods have been described for blocking the sciatic nerve at the level of the hip joint:

1. Posterior approach (of Labat)
2. Anterior approach (Beck 1963)
3. Supine block (Raj et al 1975)
4. Lateral approach (Guardini et al 1985)
5. Parasacral approach (Morris et al 1997).

The easiest block with the highest success rate is undoubtedly the posterior approach. However, the anterior approach can be useful if the patient is in pain and cannot be moved. The supine, lateral and parasacral approaches will not be described.

***Posterior approach*** (Fig. 15.6) Correct positioning is vital if this block is to be carried out effectively. The patient lies with the side to be blocked uppermost. The lower leg is straight and the upper leg is flexed at the hip and knee so that the thigh is at right angles to the body. The greater trochanter is palpated and its upper border marked. The iliac crest is traced posteriorly and the posterior superior iliac spine is marked. Between these two points a line is drawn and from its midpoint a perpendicular is dropped. The point for needle insertion is about 5 cm along this perpendicular, and its position can be checked by drawing a line between the coccyx and the top of the greater trochanter. The needle is inserted where the two lines intersect.

After skin cleansing, local anaesthetic is infiltrated into the skin and muscle. Using a nerve stimulator set to deliver 2 mA, the anaesthetist inserts a 100 mm, 21 g needle at right angles to the skin and advances it until

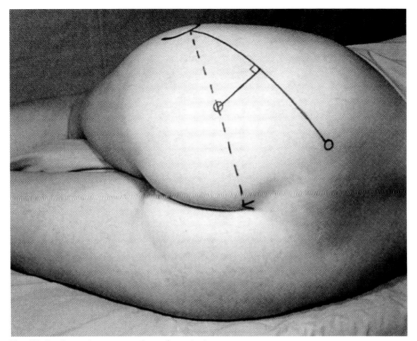

**Fig 15.6**  Posterior approach to the sciatic nerve

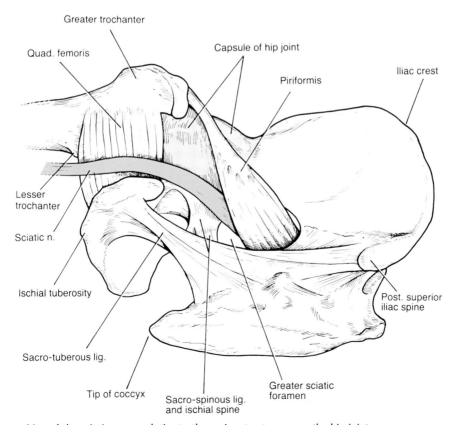

Greater trochanter

Quad. femoris

Capsule of hip joint

Piriformis

Iliac crest

Lesser trochanter

Sciatic n.

Ischial tuberosity

Post. superior iliac spine

Sacro-tuberous lig.

Tip of coccyx

Sacro-spinous lig. and ischial spine

Greater sciatic foramen

**Fig 15.7**  The position of the sciatic nerve relative to the major structures near the hip joint

221

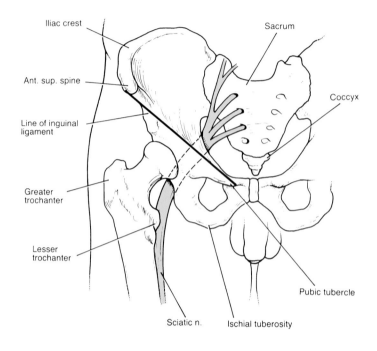

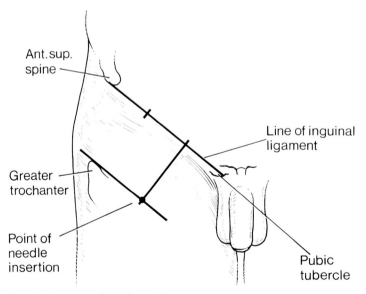

**Fig 15.8** Landmarks for the anterior approach to the sciatic nerve

contraction in the hamstring muscles is elicited. At this point the current is reduced to about 0.5 mA, and the needle advanced slightly further until contraction is elicited in gastrocnemius. This causes plantar flexion of the foot, usually without hamstring contraction. If dorsal flexion at the ankle occurs, it is preferable to withdraw the needle a few centimetres and redirect the needle slightly more medially until plantar flexion is elicited.

If bone is encountered without muscle contraction, the needle is withdrawn and redirected medially or laterally until a motor response is obtained. While inserting the needle, the anaesthetist should try to imagine the anatomy of the pelvis underneath (Fig. 15.7). The sciatic nerve is emerging through the greater sciatic foramen, which forms a bony arch, and if this arch can be 'visualised', block of the nerve will become easier. Once the final position is obtained, the needle is held firmly and 20 ml of local anaesthetic is injected.

*Anterior approach* (Fig. 15.8) For this the patient lies supine. The anterior superior iliac spine and the pubic tubercle are palpated and marked, and a line is drawn between them to represent the inguinal ligament. This line is divided into three equal parts and a perpendicular dropped from the junction of the medial and middle thirds. A line is then drawn from the top of the greater trochanter parallel to the line of the inguinal ligament and the point where it meets the perpendicular is the point of needle insertion. This overlies the lesser trochanter on the inner aspect of the femur, and at this level the sciatic nerve lies close behind the acetabulum and the head of the femur. The anterior approach requires a fairly long needle. In most cases a 150 mm, 21 g insulated needle is used.

After skin cleansing, a wheal of local anaesthetic is raised, the needle is inserted and directed slightly laterally so that it strikes the medial surface of the femur. It is then withdrawn and 'walked' off the femur so that it passes medial to the femoral head. Some anaesthetists believe that if the needle is inserted 5 cm deeper than

its point of contact with the femur it will lie very close to the nerve, and that if the local anaesthetic can be injected easily and without resistance, a good block will result. However, this is not always the case and it is better to use a nerve stimulator, and elicit plantar flexion of the foot. Computerised tomography (Charlton et al 1987) has shown that the sciatic nerve often lies more laterally behind the femur than was previously appreciated. Thus, when using the classical landmarks described above, it may be impossible to bring the tip of the needle close enough to the nerve. Use of a more medial insertion point with more lateral direction of the needle may lead to a higher success rate, but recent cadaver studies have suggested that *internal* rotation of the hip may be more helpful (Vloka et al 2001). After careful aspiration, 20 ml of local anaesthetic is injected.

## NERVE BLOCK AT THE KNEE

### Sciatic nerve (popliteal fossa) block

Block of the sciatic nerve in the popliteal fossa anaesthetises the foot and most of the leg, although complete block of both of the major terminal nerves

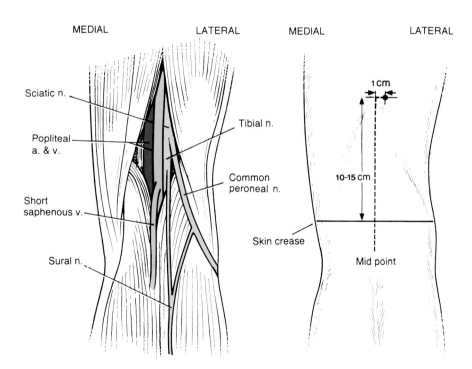

**Fig 15.9** Sciatic nerve block in the popliteal fossa. The perpendicular from the skin crease is extended to overlie the apex of the fossa

223

may be less consistent than a posterior approach at the hip (Kilpatrick et al 1992). Its advantage is that widespread motor block above the knee is avoided making it more suitable for many patients and for day surgery. When positioning is a problem, a lateral approach can be considered, but will not be described further here (Hadzic & Vloka 1998).

### Technique (Fig. 15.9)

The patient lies prone and the leg is gently lifted to flex the knee joint so that the tendons of the biceps femoris (laterally) and semimembranosus with semitendinosus (medially) stand out. A line is drawn in the flexion crease between these tendons and from the middle of this line a perpendicular is drawn upwards for 10–15 cm to the apex of the fossa. The point of needle insertion is 1 cm lateral to the top of this perpendicular, because the sciatic nerve does not lie in the middle of the popliteal fossa, but slightly to the lateral side. Using a nerve stimulator, the anaesthetist inserts a 50 mm, 22 g insulated needle parallel to the perpendicular, pointing it upwards at 30–45° and gently advancing it until a motor response in the foot is elicited. The nerve normally lies 3–5 cm deep to the skin. If no response is obtained, the needle is withdrawn almost to the skin, and redirected slightly laterally or medially. It is important to make only small changes in direction because the nerve may otherwise be missed. The most complete block of both terminal nerves appears to be obtained by eliciting either dorsiflexion, inversion or a combination of inversion/plantar flexion of the foot with the current at or below 0.5 mA (Benzon et al 1997).

## Saphenous nerve block

The saphenous nerve (Fig. 15.10) is the terminal branch of the femoral nerve and supplies the skin of the anteromedial aspect of the leg. The lower border of the area supplied by this nerve is variable. Because most operations on the ankle and foot require a tourniquet, saphenous nerve block can be used to provide complete analgesia for a mid-calf tourniquet.

The nerve runs down through the thigh in the adductor canal under the sartorius muscle. It pierces the fascia lata between the tendons of sartorius and gracilis on the inner aspect of the knee joint and becomes subcutaneous. In thin people, the nerve can often be rolled under the fingers where it lies on the medial aspect of the head of the tibia, about 2 cm below the lower border of the patella. The long saphenous

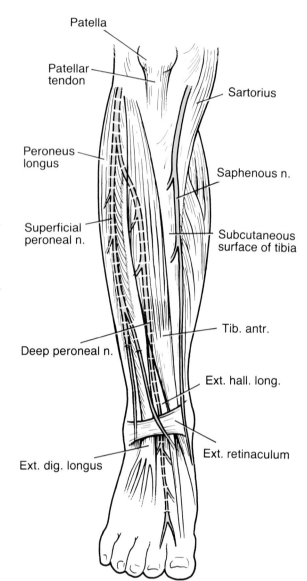

**Fig 15.10** Nerves on the anterior aspect of the leg and foot

vein is a close relation here and is a useful landmark. The nerve is blocked by infiltrating 10 ml of local anaesthetic into the subcutaneous tissues at this point. The proximity of the vein makes aspiration particularly important.

## DISTAL BLOCKS OF THE LOWER LIMB
## Ankle block

In order to anaesthetise the foot by injecting at the level of the ankle, it is necessary to block five nerves. They are the saphenous nerve (the terminal branch of

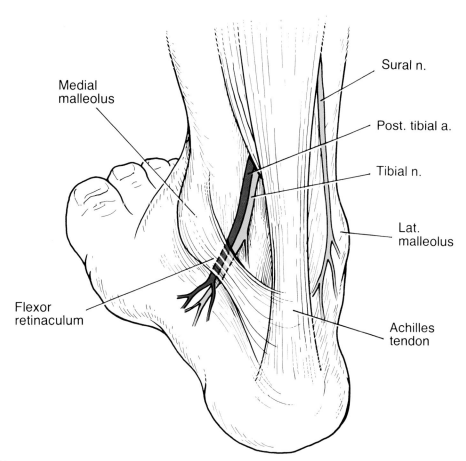

**Fig 15.11** Nerves on the posterior aspect of the ankle joint

the femoral nerve) and four nerves derived from the sciatic: the tibial, sural, superficial peroneal and deep peroneal nerves. Ankle block, although technically straightforward, has very limited use. It is uncomfortable for the patient because multiple injections are required and incomplete blocks occur with depressing regularity. Although anatomical knowledge may help reduce the number of injections, most procedures will require tibial nerve block along with at least one other. As most procedures on the foot require a tourniquet, ankle block is only really appropriate either to supplement incomplete proximal blocks or for postoperative analgesia.

The saphenous nerve is blocked just above, and slightly anterior, to the medial malleolus (Fig. 15.10); the tibial nerve immediately behind the medial malleolus and deep to the posterior tibial artery (Fig. 15.11); the sural behind the lateral malleolus (Fig. 15.11); the deep peroneal between the tendons of tibialis anterior and extensor digitorum longus on the anterior aspect

of the ankle (Fig. 15.10); and the superficial peroneal nerve by infiltrating subcutaneously across the anterior aspect of the ankle joint (Fig. 15.10).

The important landmark of the tibial artery may be absent and a more distal bony landmark, the sustentaculum tali, provides a much more useful site for accurate tibial nerve block (Wassef 1991). The sustentaculum tali is felt as a bony ridge 1–2 cm distal to the medial malleolus. The needle is inserted perpendicularly at a point inferior and posterior to this ridge and an injection of 5–8 ml of local anaesthetic injected. There should be no resistance to injection.

## Digital nerve block

Digital nerve block is a simple, safe, effective and extremely useful technique and is probably underused, especially as a means of postoperative analgesia. After operations on the toes in which periosteum is damaged (e.g. osteotomy or nail-bed ablation), postoperative

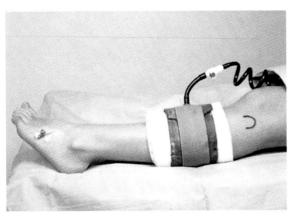

**Fig 15.12**  Intravenous regional anaesthesia in the lower limb. The head of the fibula has been marked. Note that the tourniquet is well below that level

pain can be severe and out of all proportion to the scale of the procedure. Even if a general anaesthetic is used for the operation itself, a digital nerve block with 0.5% *plain* bupivacaine can provide analgesia for more than 12 hours. The technique is essentially the same as described for the upper limb (see Ch.14).

## Intravenous regional anaesthesia (IVRA)

IVRA (Fig. 15.12) is not as widely used for lower limb procedures as it is for those in the upper limb (see Ch. 14). Although this may be because conditions for which it is suited are seen less often in the lower limb, it is more probably because the technique is not considered to be practical. The large dose of local anaesthetic required when the tourniquet is placed on the thigh can result in a significant incidence of problems due to systemic toxicity, yet operative and tourniquet pain are very frequent (Valli et al 1987). If the tourniquet is placed at mid-calf level the dose of drug used is the same as in the upper limb and the technique is identical in every respect (see Ch. 14). However, tourniquet discomfort can still be a problem and some workers find that anaesthesia is not as reliable as in the upper limb (Valli & Rosenberg 1986, Fagg 1987). This suggests that case selection is very important for the use of this technique.

## Local anaesthesia for knee arthroscopy

Spinal and epidural blocks are the most convenient techniques for operations on the knee. Lumbar plexus block combined with sciatic block at the hip is an alternative. Femoral nerve block, on its own, is insufficient.

For arthroscopy alone, or for operations carried out through the arthroscope, a simple infiltration technique can be used. This has the advantage that both general anaesthesia and central neural blocks are avoided, so it is particularly suitable for day patients. It is vital that the surgeon and anaesthetist work together for this technique to be effective. The anaesthetist must know where the surgeon intends to insert the irrigating needles, the arthroscope and any other instrument.

The skin and deeper tissues at the entry portals are infiltrated with local anaesthetic (0.5% prilocaine with 1:200 000 epinephrine). A 20 ml volume of solution is normally sufficient. A 19 g needle is then inserted into the knee joint and 50 ml of the same local anaesthetic solution is injected. The knee is passively flexed and extended a few times to spread the local anaesthetic, and after 10 minutes the procedure can start. No tourniquet is used because the epinephrine provides excellent operating conditions and additional analgesia for a tourniquet is therefore unnecessary. If the knee is irrigated with standard solutions of local anaesthetic there is no loss of anaesthesia, but if an effusion is present it is wise to drain it prior to injection of any solution to avoid dilution and to improve the surgeon's view.

This technique can be used satisfactorily for the great majority of patients undergoing arthroscopy, but it is contraindicated in certain groups. Those with severe osteoarthritis of the hip will require spinal or epidural anaesthesia to allow the surgeon to manipulate both joints during the arthroscopy. It may be impossible to provide satisfactory analgesia in patients with widespread scarring of the knee due to injury or previous surgery. Finally, infiltration may be unsuitable for patients with an acutely painful knee. Spasm of the quadriceps muscles may make it difficult to perform the block, and for the surgeon to perform a satisfactory arthroscopy. However, it may be possible to improve the situation by performing a femoral nerve block in addition to the local infiltration. If these limitations are borne in mind the block can be used successfully for a wide range of arthroscopic procedures (Buckley et al 1989).

## Continuous infusion techniques

One of the great advantages of peripheral block techniques is the ability to extend the excellent analgesia into the postoperative period. With bupivacaine and ropivacaine, even a single injection will last in excess of 14 hours and sometimes as long as 24 hours. Many procedures carried out on the lower limb, such as knee replacement or amputation surgery, are associated with considerable pain for at least the first 48 hours and benefit significantly from continuation of local anaesthetic block using peripheral nerve catheter techniques. In some situations, this may also facilitate active rehabilitation and physiotherapy, and encourage earlier mobilisation and restoration of limb function. The effectiveness of infusion analgesia, and of repeated bolus injections, will generally depend on the innervation of the surgical area involved. Often careful selection of the site of infusion will provide excellent analgesia particularly if combined initially with an isolated block of other appropriate nerves. The postoperative analgesia may be enhanced further, if necessary, by the use of non-steroidal anti-inflammatory drugs. This obviates the need to use opioids with their well-recognised side-effects.

## Continuous sciatic block

This technique is possible at a number of sites in the lower limb. The traditional posterior approach, as described earlier in this chapter, is a useful site for catheter insertion and infusion for procedures carried out below the knee, in particular below knee amputation (Connolly & Coventry 1998). The sciatic block is performed with a 110 mm, 18 g needle and cannula through which a catheter can then be inserted. The catheter placement can be facilitated by creating space with an initial injection of 20 ml of local anaesthetic solution through the needle side arm (Contiplex D catheter set, B. Braun Medical). The catheter can usually be inserted 5–10 cm before the cannula is removed and carefully secured to skin with a clear adhesive dressing and tape. A femoral nerve block is added to complete surgical anaesthesia and the sciatic infusion continued postoperatively using ropivacaine 0.2% at a rate of about 6 ml h$^{-1}$.

The continuous parasacral approach has also been described for similar cases, using an insulated Tuohy needle for catheter placement and a subsequent infusion of bupivacaine 0.1% at a rate of 8 ml h$^{-1}$ (Morris & Lang 1997). For surgery around the foot and ankle, the sciatic nerve catheter can be placed in the popliteal fossa (Singelyn et al 1997).

## Continuous lumbar plexus or femoral block

The applicability of a single infusion for postoperative analgesia for most surgery of the hip or knee is less clear, because each joint has a multiple innervation from femoral, obturator and sciatic nerves. This is further complicated by the debate over exactly which nerves are commonly blocked by the various approaches to the lumbar plexus. In addition, the incision for hip arthroplasty may extend into the lower thoracic ($T_{12}$) dermatome or curve into the sacral innervation of the buttock. It is therefore unlikely that a single infusion will provide complete postoperative pain control for many of these procedures, but may make a highly significant contribution to improving the quality of analgesia and reducing opioid requirements. Serpell and colleagues (1991) have shown that continuous femoral nerve block is useful for controlling pain after knee surgery. Mansour and Bennetts (1996), on the other hand, concluded that additional sciatic nerve block was essential for successful immediate postoperative analgesia, but longer-term pain control could be achieved by continuous lumbar plexus block alone using a femoral approach.

Providing continuous analgesia after major hip surgery is a more contentious issue with few appropriate, controlled studies available. Typically, obturator nerve block is used to relieve hip pain, but the anterior hip capsule is innervated by branches of the femoral nerve, and the posterior capsule by branches of sciatic and superior gluteal nerves (Birnbaum et al 1997). In addition, the majority of incisions are made within the lateral cutaneous territory, with overlap into sacral and lower thoracic ($T_{12}$) roots. Although all these nerves need to be blocked to provide complete surgical anaesthesia, the posterior approaches to the lumbar plexus can be used to provide excellent postoperative analgesia. They provide more reliable block of all the principal lumbar plexus nerves, in particular the obturator nerve, which is not blocked consistently by the femoral approach (Parkinson et al 1989, Capdevila et al 1998). In the majority of cases the plexus can be reached by the posterior approaches described earlier, using a 110 mm, 18 g cannula and catheter (e.g. the Contiplex D system, B. Braun Medical). The initial injection of 30 ml ropivacaine 0.75% through the needle should create space to facilitate catheter insertion. Subsequent infusion of ropivacaine 0.2% at a rate of about 6 ml h$^{-1}$ can then be used to prolong analgesia in the postoperative period. Owing to the dose of local anaesthetic used for this block, it would be inappropriate to combine it with other blocks if subsequent infusion is contemplated.

# References

Beck GP 1963 Anterior approach to sciatic nerve block. Anesthesiology 24: 222

Benzon HT, Kim C, Benzon H et al 1997 Correlation between evoked motor responses of the sciatic nerve and sensory blockade. Anesthesiology 87: 547–552

Birnbaum K, Prescher A, Hessler S, Heller KD 1997 The sensory innervation of the hip joint – an anatomical study. Surgical and Radiologic Anatomy 19: 371–375

Buckley JR, Hood GM, Macrae W 1989 Arthroscopy under local anaesthesia. Journal of Bone and Joint Surgery 71B: 126–127

Capdevila X, Biboulet P, Bouregba M, Barthelet Y, Rubenovitch J, d'Athis F 1998 Comparison of the 3-in-1 and fascia iliaca compartment blocks in adults: clinical and radiographic analysis. Anesthesia and Analgesia 86: 1039–1044

Charlton JE, Nicholls BJ, White E 1987 Anterior and lateral approaches to the sciatic nerve: a study using computerized tomography. British Journal of Anaesthesia 59: 127P

Chayen D, Nathan H, Chayen M 1976 The psoas compartment block. Anesthesiology 45:95–99

Connolly C, Coventry DM 1998 Combined sciatic/femoral block followed by sciatic infusion of ropivacaine 2 mg/ml for below knee amputation; a feasibility study. Regional Anesthesia 23 (Supplement): 81

Dalens B, Tanguy A, Vanneuville G 1988. Lumbar plexus block in children. A comparison of two procedures in 50 patients. Anesthesia and Analgesia 67: 750–758

Fagg P 1987 Intravenous regional anaesthesia for lower limb orthopaedic surgery. Annals of the Royal College of Surgeons of England 69: 274–275

Fanelli G, Casati A, Aldegheri G et al 1998. Cardiovascular effects of two different regional anaesthetic techniques for unilateral leg surgery. Acta Anaesthesiologica Scandinavica 42: 80–84

Greengrass RA, Klein SM, D'Ercole FJ, Gleason DG, Shimer CL, Steele SM 1998. Lumbar plexus and sciatic nerve block for knee arthroplasty: comparison of ropivacaine and bupivacaine. Canadian Journal of Anaesthesia 45:1094–1096

Guardini R, Waldron BA, Wallace WA 1985 Sciatic nerve block: a new lateral approach. Acta Anaesthesiologica Scandinavica 29: 515–519

Hadzic A, Vloka JD 1998 A comparison of the posterior versus lateral approaches to block of the sciatic nerve in the popliteal fossa. Anesthesiology 88: 1480–1486

Hanna MH, Peat SJ, D'Costa F 1993 Lumbar plexus block: an anatomical study. Anaesthesia 48: 675–678

Kilpatrick A, Coventry DM, Todd JG 1992 A comparison of two approaches to sciatic nerve block. Anaesthesia 47: 155–157

Lang SA, Yip RW, Chang PC, Gerard MA 1993 The femoral 3-in-1 block revisited. Journal of Clinical Anesthesiology 5:292–296

Mansour NY, Bennetts FE 1996 An observational study of combined continuous lumbar plexus and single-shot sciatic nerve blocks for post-knee surgery analgesia. Regional Anesthesia 21: 287–291

Misra U, Priddie AK, McClymont C, Bower S 1991 Plasma concentrations of bupivacaine following combined sciatic and femoral 3-in-1 nerve block in open knee surgery. British Journal of Anaesthesia 66: 310–313

Moore D C 1965a Regional block, 4th edn, p 287. CC Thomas, Springfield

Moore D C 1965b Regional block, 4th edn, p 293. CC Thomas, Springfield

Morris GF, Lang SA 1997 Continuous parasacral sciatic nerve block: two case reports. Regional Anesthesia 22: 469–472

Morris GF, Lang SA, Dust WN, Van der Wal M 1997 The parasacral sciatic nerve block. Regional Anesthesia 22: 223–228

Parkinson SK, Mueller JB, Little WL, Bailey SL 1989. Extent of blockade with various approaches to the lumbar plexus. Anesthesia and Analgesia 68: 243–248

Raj PP, Parks RI, Watson TD, Jenkins MT 1975 New single position supine approach to sciatic–femoral nerve block. Anesthesia and Analgesia 54: 489

Robison C, Ray DC, McKeown DW, Buchan AS 1991 Effect of adrenaline on plasma concentrations of bupivacaine following lower limb nerve block. British Journal of Anaesthesia 66: 228–231

Serpell MG, Millar FA, Thomson MF 1991 Comparison of lumbar plexus block versus conventional opioid analgesia after total knee replacement. Anaesthesia 46: 275–277

Singelyn FJ, Aye F, Gouverneur JM 1997 Continuous popliteal-sciatic nerve block: an original technique to provide postoperative analgesia after foot surgery. Anesthesia & Analgesia 84: 383–386

Valli H, Rosenberg PH 1986 Intravenous regional anesthesia below the knee. Anaesthesia 41: 1196–1201

Valli H, Rosenberg PH, Hekali R 1987 Comparison of lidocaine and prilocaine for intravenous regional anesthesia of the whole lower extremity. Regional Anesthesia 12: 128–134

Vloka JD, Hadzic A, Mulcare R, Lesser JB, Kitain E, Thys DM 1997 Femoral nerve block versus spinal anesthesia for out-patients undergoing long saphenous vein stripping surgery. Anesthesia and Analgesia 84: 749–752

Vloka JD, Hadzic A, April E, Thys DM 2001 Anterior approach to the sciatic nerve: the effects of leg rotation. Anesthesia and Analgesia 92: 460–462

Wassef MR 1991 Posterior tibial nerve block. A new approach using the bony landmark of the sustentaculum tali. Anaesthesia 46: 841–844

Winnie A P, Ramamurthy S, Durrani Z 1973 The inguinal paravascular technic of lumbar plexus anesthesia: the '3 in 1 block'. Anesthesia and Analgesia 52: 989–996

# 16. Head, neck and airway blocks

## N G Smart and S Hickey

Regional nerve blocks, performed by the dental, maxillofacial, ophthalmic or ear, nose and throat surgeon have an established place as the sole anaesthetics for relatively minor operations on the head and neck. General anaesthesia would be quite inappropriate for such surgery, and the size of the workload, particularly in dentistry, is such that there are insufficient properly trained anaesthetists to provide a service. Because specialist anaesthetists have traditionally been involved only in the management of the more major procedures, they have tended to limit themselves to the use of general anaesthesia. The relative complexity of the innervation of the head and neck has also limited the extent to which anaesthetists have explored the possibilities of regional anaesthesia in this area, even though most have personally experienced its benefits during a visit to the dentist. In fact, blocks in this region of the body can contribute significant analgesia both during and after the procedure, so that it is very worthwhile for the anaesthetist to acquire the necessary techniques.

## INNERVATION OF THE HEAD AND NECK

The structures of the head and neck are supplied by a relatively large number of nerves – the twelve cranial and the first four cervical nerves. However, many of these subserve very specialised sensory or secretory functions which are of no relevance to nerve block for surgery. For that purpose, the most important nerves are those that supply the skin (Fig. 16.1) and the structures of the airway, so their anatomy will be described in detail. Fortunately, the nerves which serve somatic function contain either sensory or motor fibres only: thus sensory block can be produced without motor paralysis. This is a distinct advantage with intra-oral

blocks because the muscles maintaining and controlling the airway remain unaffected.

## Trigeminal nerve (Figs 16.2 & 16.3)

This, the fifth and largest of the cranial nerves, supplies the muscles of mastication and is also the principle sensory nerve of the head, supplying:

- The skin of the face and the anterior half of the head (the mask area);
- The mucous membranes of the nose, sinuses, mouth and anterior two thirds of the tongue;
- The teeth and the temporomandibular joint;
- The contents of the orbit (except the retina); and
- Part of the dura.

The *trigeminal ganglion* (also known as *semilunar or Gasserian*) lies in the middle cranial fossa in a recess near the apex of the petrous temporal bone. At the ganglion, the sensory component of the nerve divides into three, each with a discrete area of distribution (Fig. 16.1).

### Ophthalmic nerve

The ophthalmic nerve enters the orbit through the superior orbital fissure and divides into three main branches.

1. The *frontal nerve* has two terminal cutaneous branches. The *supraorbital nerve* emerges from the supraorbital foramen, turns upwards and supplies the upper eyelid, the forehead and upper anterior part of the scalp as far as the vertex. The *supratrochlear nerve* emerges at the supraorbital margin, a finger's breadth from the midline, to supply the paramedian part of the forehead and the medial part of the upper eyelid.
2. The *nasociliary nerve* also has two terminal branches. The *infratrochlear nerve* emerges from the orbit just

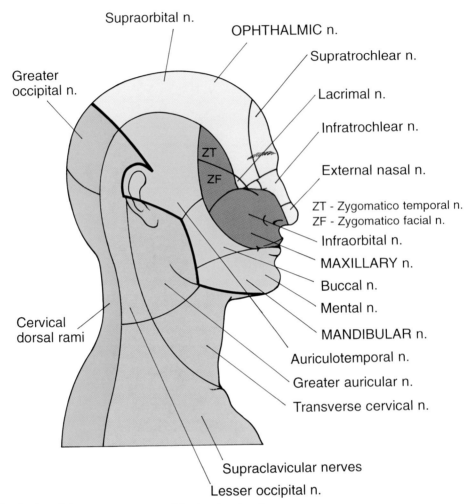

**Fig 16.1** Distribution of the cutaneous nerves of the head and neck

above the medial palpebral ligament to supply the medial parts of the eyelids and the root of the nose. The *anterior ethmoidal nerve* leaves the orbit through the anterior ethmoidal foramen. It gives off *internal nasal branches* to the mucous membrane of the adjacent lateral and septal nasal walls, and then emerges between the nasal bone and the lateral nasal cartilage as the *external nasal nerve*, to supply the skin of the lower half of the dorsum of the nose.

**3.** The *lacrimal nerve* terminates in the *palpebral branch*, which pierces and supplies the lateral part of the upper eyelid.

### Maxillary nerve

The maxillary nerve leaves the cranium through the foramen rotundum, crosses the pterygopalatine fossa anterior to the lateral pterygoid plate, and enters the orbit through the inferior orbital fissure. The relevant terminal cutaneous branches are as follows:

1. The *infraorbital nerve*, which emerges from the infraorbital foramen beneath the orbicularis oculi muscle and supplies the skin and mucous membrane of the upper lip, the lower eyelid, the skin between them and that on the side of the nose.

2. The *zygomaticofacial nerve*, which leaves the orbit through the zygomaticofacial foramen, and supplies skin over the bony part of the cheek.

3. The *zygomaticotemporal nerve*, which emerges from the temporal surface of the zygomatic bone to supply the skin over the anterior part of the temple.

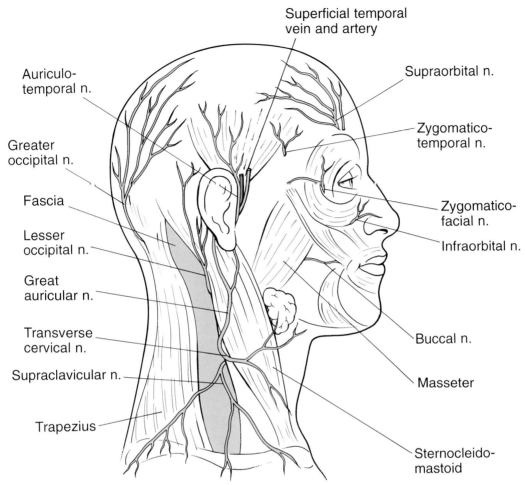

**Fig 16.2** Positions of the nerves of the right side of the scalp, face and neck. Note that the superficial branches of the cervical plexus emerge together from the midpoint of the posterior border of sternocleidomastoid, and that the branches of the facial nerve have been omitted from the area in front of the ear for clarity

*Mandibular nerve*

The mandibular nerve leaves the skull through the foramen ovale accompanied by the motor root of the trigeminal nerve, and crosses the pterygopalatine fossa posterior to the lateral pterygoid plate, but anterior to the neck of the mandible. There it divides into a small anterior (mostly motor) and a large posterior (mostly sensory) division. An important sensory branch of the *anterior division* is the *buccal nerve*, which supplies the skin over and the mucous membrane deep to the buccinator muscle. The *posterior division* trunk has three main branches:

1. The *auriculotemporal nerve* hooks round the posterior surface of the neck of the mandible, lying close to the superficial temporal vessels and the parotid gland, and supplies the skin of the temple and the superior two-thirds of the anterior aspect of the ear.

2. The *inferior dental nerve* enters the mandibular foramen on the medial surface of the ramus of the mandible. Within the mandible it gives off branches to the teeth and gums, and finally exits through the mental foramen as the *mental nerve*, supplying the skin of the chin, and the skin and mucous membrane of the lower lip.

3. The *lingual nerve* runs between the medial pterygoid muscle and the ramus of the mandible and is covered only by mucous membrane at the level of the third molar. It supplies the mucous membrane of the anterior two-thirds of the tongue and the adjacent parts of the floor of the mouth and gum.

231

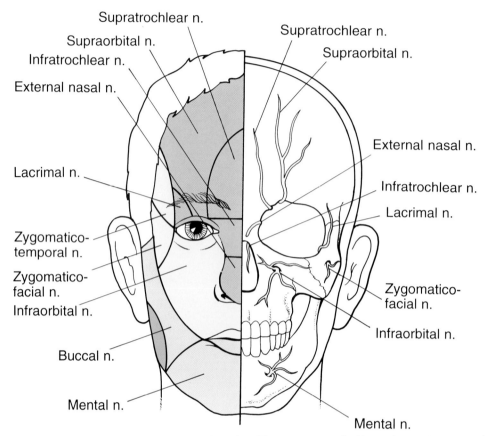

**Fig 16.3** Cutaneous branches of the trigeminal nerve branches. The territory supplied by each nerve is seen on the left while the positions of the major nerves are marked on the right. Note the straight-line relationship between the supraorbital, infraorbital and mental foramina

Thus, the trigeminal nerve supplies all of the skin of the face, except for the area over the parotid gland and the angle of the mandible, which is supplied by the great auricular nerve (see below). It is important to note that the landmarks identifying the three main terminal cutaneous branches of the trigeminal nerve, the supraorbital foramen, the infraorbital foramen and the mental foramen, all lie in a straight line (Fig. 16.3).

## Facial nerve

As it traverses the parotid gland in front of the ear, the facial (seventh) nerve divides into five main branches – temporal, zygomatic, buccal, mandibular and cervical – which radiate out to supply the muscles of expression in the respective parts of the face. The mandibular branch runs forward below the angle of the mandible before turning upwards and forwards to supply the angle of the mouth.

## Glossopharyngeal nerve

The glossopharyngeal (ninth) nerve supplies sensation to the posterior third of the tongue, the pharynx, palatine tonsil, part of the soft palate and the anterior surface of the epiglottis. It emerges from the skull through the jugular foramen and descends between the internal carotid artery and the internal jugular vein. It curves round the lateral surface of the stylopharyngeus muscle and passes with it into the pharynx between the superior and middle constrictor muscles. Here it lies deep to the mucous membrane of the lower part of the tonsillar fossa, and then passes forwards into the tongue.

## Vagus nerve

The vagus (tenth) nerve also emerges from the skull through the jugular foramen. The *pharyngeal branch* arises immediately below the skull and runs between the internal and external carotid arteries to form, with the glossopharyngeal nerve, a large part of the pharyngeal plexus innervating the pharyngeal wall.

There are two other branches of particular interest. First, the *superior laryngeal nerve* arises from the inferior ganglion of the vagus and runs downwards, forwards and medially to cross in front of the greater horn of the hyoid bone where it divides into two. The *internal branch* pierces the thyrohyoid membrane to supply the mucous membrane of the larynx (including the posterior surface of the epiglottis) down to the level of the vocal cords, while the *external branch* is the motor nerve to the cricothyroid muscle. Second, the *recurrent laryngeal nerve* loops under the aorta on the right, and the sub-clavian artery on the left, ascends in the groove between the trachea and the oesophagus and enters the larynx posteriorly, deep to the inferior border of the inferior constrictor muscle. It supplies the mucous membrane of the larynx below the vocal cords and all the muscles of the larynx except cricothyroid.

## Hypoglossal nerve

The hypoglossal (twelfth) nerve is the motor nerve to the tongue. From the base of the skull, where it is closely related to the glossopharyngeal and vagus nerves, it passes between the internal jugular vein and the internal carotid artery, and curves downwards and forwards to the base of the tongue.

## Cervical nerves (Figs 16.1 & 16.2)

The dorsal rami of $C_2$–$C_4$ supply the skin of the back of the neck and, through the medial branch of the dorsal ramus of $C_2$ (the *greater occipital nerve*), the scalp. This, the thickest cutaneous nerve in the body, crosses the suboccipital triangle and pierces semispinalis capitis. It supplies the scalp as far as the vertex.

The ventral rami of $C_1$–$C_4$ form the cervical plexus, which may be divided into two parts. The *deep cervical plexus* lies posterior to the internal jugular vein and the prevertebral fascia, and extends inferiorly from the root of the auricle to the superior border of the thyroid cartilage. It gives rise to the *phrenic nerve* and smaller branches which innervate the muscles and other deep structures of the neck.

The *superficial cervical plexus* has a number of cutaneous branches and these emerge from behind the mid-portion of the sternomastoid muscle, from where they are distributed widely. The *lesser occipital nerve* supplies the skin over the mastoid process, and the *great auricular nerve* the skin on both surfaces of the ear and over the angle of the mandible. The *transverse cervical nerve* passes forwards across the superficial surface of sternomastoid and supplies most of the skin on the side and front of the neck. Finally, the supraclavicular nerves radiate out to supply skin of the chest and shoulder down to the level of the second rib – the 'cape' area.

## CLINICAL APPLICATION

Techniques have been described for blocking the main trunks and branches of all the cranial nerves, not just those mentioned above. However, many of these methods involve injection near the base of the skull, require very detailed knowledge of anatomy, and are technically difficult. These issues, together with lack of well-defined clinical need and concerns about safety, mean that major cranial nerve blocks are used rarely. Even with the more distal blocks it is important that these points are kept clearly in mind, especially the safety issue.

## Safety

The close proximity of the major nerves to other important structures in the area below the base of the skull means that major complications can be produced all too easily. Accidental intra-arterial injection of as little as 1 ml of local anaesthetic will produce major CNS toxicity, and even if arterial puncture is identified it may lead to a significant haematoma. Subarachnoid spread of local anaesthetic from injection into the dural cuff around a cranial nerve will also produce con-sequences out of proportion to the dose involved. The more proximal the injection, the more likely it is that both sensory and motor nerves to the airway will be affected, with consequent risk of obstruction or aspiration. Thus essential pre-requisites are intravenous access for all but the most peripheral of these methods, use of appropriate monitoring equipment, and the ready availability of resuscitation equipment.

Similar concerns apply to the classical technique of 'deep' cervical plexus block. Diaphragmatic paralysis is inevitable, and careful needle angulation is needed to avoid injection into the vertebral artery, or the epidural or subarachnoid spaces. Cervical epidural block, and even high spinal anaesthesia, have been applied to head and neck surgery, but the potential problems and availability of alternative methods mean that such techniques are rarely used.

Nerve damage from needle trauma may be influenced by bevel configuration. Animal studies suggest long-bevel needles are associated with a lower long-term incidence of nerve injury (Rice & McMahon 1992) and the American Dental Association recommends their use. Short-bevel needles are useful for some blocks because they allow better appreciation of tissue planes, but they offer little advantage in the mouth and the relative bluntness makes them more painful. Intra-oral blocks can be performed using standard hypodermic syringes and needles, but it is worth the regular user becoming proficient with the dental cartridge system because this is very suited to these methods.

## Indications

Head and neck blocks, used alone or in combination with general anaesthesia, can benefit patients in a range of clinical situations.

- *Postoperative pain control.* The longer acting agents can produce prolonged analgesia, reducing the need for systemic analgesics and improving patient comfort. For example, auricular nerve block facilitates early ambulation and discharge home with minimal systemic upset in children undergoing pinnaplasty.
- *Sole anaesthetic technique.* Many elderly patients presenting for excision of basal or squamous cell carcinomas of the face are debilitated and poor risks for general anaesthesia. Infiltration techniques tend to distend the skin and distort the local anatomy, making surgery difficult. Peripheral nerve blocks offer an effective, simple and safe alternative. Major resections and reconstruction under regional block have also been reported (Neill 1996).
- *Awake intubation.* Regional block allows instrumentation of the airway and endotracheal intubation in the patient with a difficult airway prior to induction of general anaesthesia.
- *Chronic pain relief.* Neurolytic blocks have been shown to decrease patient dependence on opioid analgesics and improve quality of life (Lipton 1989, Neill 1992).
- *Carotid artery surgery.* Cervical plexus block preserves consciousness and allows assessment of the cerebral circulation when the carotid artery is clamped (Davies et al 1993). This method of anaesthesia is used com-

monly in the USA, but controversy exists as to whether outcome is improved.

## SUGGESTED TECHNIQUES

## The trigeminal nerve and its branches

The trigeminal nerve system can be blocked at several points along its course, but the distal blocks have more favourable risk/benefit profiles. The terminal branches are more easily identified (Fig. 16.3) and so can be blocked more consistently, while their greater separation from the major subcranial structures means that accidental misplacement of the injectate has less serious consequences.

### Trigeminal ganglion block

Trigeminal ganglion block is technically difficult and requires radiographic control. Its use is largely confined to specialist units dealing with intractable trigeminal neuralgia and cancer pain. The reader is referred to more specialised texts for its description (Murphy 1988, Bonica 1990).

### Branches of the ophthalmic nerve

Block of the *supraorbital and supratrochlear nerves* is useful for surgery of the forehead and the scalp as far as the vertex. The important bony landmark is the supraorbital foramen, which is palpable on the superior orbital rim at a point immediately above the ipsilateral pupil when the patient gazes straight ahead. A single subcutaneous injection of 3–4 ml of local anaesthetic, starting in the midline at the root of the nose and directed laterally above the eyebrow as far as the supraorbital foramen, will block both nerves.

The landmark for *external nasal nerve* block is the junction of the lateral nasal cartilage and nasal bone. Injection of 2 ml of local anaesthetic immediately lateral to the midline anaesthetises the apex and vestibule of the nose. The *infratrochlear nerve* can be blocked by an infiltration of 1–2 ml of solution, starting at the superomedial border of the orbit and moving towards, but stopping just short of, the medial palpebral ligament, which results in anaesthesia of the nose around the medial angle of the eye. When bilateral external nasal and infratrochlear nerve blocks are combined with bilateral infraorbital nerve blocks (see below), superficial surgery on the nose can be performed. However, if the surgery involves the skeleton or mucosa of the nose, anaesthesia of the nasal cavity (see below) is required also.

An infiltration starting at the zygomatic foramen and directed upwards along the lateral margin of the orbit anaesthetises the lateral part of the upper eyelid supplied by the *lacrimal nerve*. When this is combined with supraorbital and supratrochlear nerve block, surgery on the entire upper eyelid is possible.

## The nasal cavity

Topical analgesia is simple to perform and quite safe provided that it is remembered that local anaesthetic uptake from mucosal surfaces is rapid and extensive. Total uptake can be reduced if the local anaesthetic is confined to the intended site of action by applying it with soaked cotton pledgets, but it is essential that the *total* dose administered is kept under review, particularly when several blocks are combined. Cocaine

10%, to a maximum of 1.5 mg kg$^{-1}$ (but see the discussion in Ch. 5 & 6 on weight-related doses), has long been the traditional drug for this method because its local anaesthetic action is accompanied by intense vasoconstriction which improves the surgical field. However, large doses of cocaine are associated with severe hypertension and arrhythmia, and lidocaine, in standard doses, is a safer alternative. For this use it can be combined with a vasoconstrictor such as phenylephrine 0.25% to reduce both systemic uptake of drug and surgical bleeding.

The *anterior ethmoidal nerve* is blocked by inserting a pledget parallel to the bridge of the nose, backwards and upwards as far as the superior border of the nasal cavity. Similarly, *sphenopalatine ganglion* block is achieved by passing pledgets along the upper borders of the inferior and middle turbinates to the posterior wall of the pharynx.

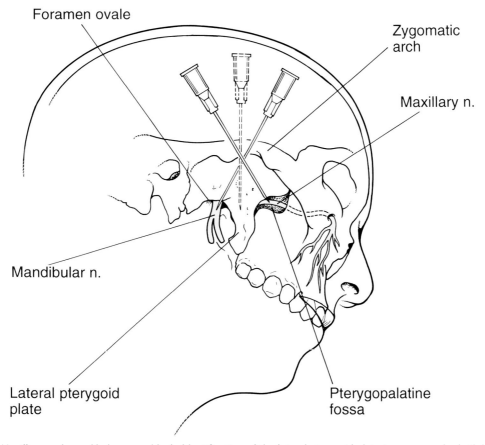

**Fig 16.4** Maxillary and mandibular nerve block. Identification of the lateral pterygoid plate is necessary for both blocks, but subsequent angulation of the needle is different: the maxillary nerve is found anterosuperiorly and the mandibular posteriorly. (Adapted from Murphy 1988)

## The maxillary nerve and its branches

It is possible to block the main trunk of the maxillary nerve in the pterygopalatine fossa, using a lateral approach (Fig. 16.4). The superficial landmarks are the midpoint of the zygomatic arch and the notch between the condyle and the coronoid process of the mandible. The notch is accentuated as the mouth is opened and closed. A 22 g, 9 cm short-bevel needle is inserted perpendicular to the skin, through the notch below the midpoint of the zygomatic arch. The needle is advanced through the masseter and temporalis muscles until the tip contacts the lateral pterygoid plate, usually at a depth of about 4 cm. It is then redirected superiorly and anteriorly until bony resistance is lost, when it is advanced a further 1 cm. The tip will then lie in the pterygopalatine fossa and in close proximity to the mandibular nerve. Injection of 4 ml of solution, without eliciting paraesthesiae and after very careful aspiration tests, will produce anaesthesia of the whole of the maxilla. However, the potential complications (as outlined above) of such a proximal technique make this an unwise method for the inexperienced, particularly when much of the area can be blocked using simpler and safer distal procedures.

The *infraorbital nerve* can be approached either percutaneously or, preferably, from within the mouth. Accidental entry to the infraorbital foramen, with the attendant hazards of damage to the artery, nerve or floor of the orbit, is less likely by the latter route. A 27 g dental needle is inserted just lateral to the lateral incisor tooth, and advanced upwards through the upper buccal sulcus towards the infraorbital foramen, taking care to stop short of the infraorbital rim and so avoid damage to the eye. Then 1 ml of local anaesthetic is injected in the vicinity of the foramen, but the needle should not be allowed to enter the canal. Widespread anaesthesia (of the lower eyelid, cheek, lateral nose, ala, and upper lip) results. This technically simple and relatively safe nerve block is a valuable and commonly used method for superficial plastic surgery.

The zygomatic foramen, 1–2 cm lateral to the lower lateral margin of the orbit, is the landmark for block of both the *zygomaticofacial* and *zygomaticotemporal nerves*. The zygomaticofacial nerve emerges from the foramen itself (Fig. 16.3) while the zygomaticotemporal nerve pierces the temporal fascia approximately 2 cm above this point. Infiltration of 2 ml of local anaesthetic at each site produces anaesthesia in the distribution shown in Fig. 16.1.

## The mandibular nerve and its branches

Extensive analgesia (the temple, auricle, external auditory meatus, cheek, lower lip, tongue, gums and mandible) results from block of the main trunk of the mandibular nerve where it lies in the infratemporal fossa (Fig. 16.4). As with the maxillary nerve, the clinical value of mandibular nerve block is limited by complications, but it is undoubtedly useful in patients with widespread pain associated with intra-oral malignancy. However, the occasional user will be able to achieve much, and with a greater margin of safety, by blocking the more distal branches of the nerve (see later).

The landmarks, and the needle insertion point, are the same as for maxillary nerve block, but once the needle contacts the lateral pterygoid plate it is redirected posteriorly until bony contact is lost. At this point paraesthesiae in the distribution of the nerve confirm correct needle position, but the needle should not be advanced much beyond the depth of the lateral pterygoid plate because of the risk of pharyngeal puncture. Fortunately, paraesthesiae are not essential because local anaesthetic injected just beyond the lateral pterygoid plate will reach the nerve by diffusion.

***Inferior dental and lingual nerves*** The inferior dental foramen lies in the centre of the medial aspect of the vertical ramus of the mandible. It may be located by palpating the concavity of the retromolar trigone with the index finger, the nail identifying the medial ridge. With the barrel of the syringe resting on the contra-lateral premolar, the needle is inserted parallel to the occlusal surface just beyond the midpoint of the palpating finger. As the injection (2 ml) is made, the syringe is swung across to allow the needle to be inserted a further 2 cm parallel to the horizontal ramus of the mandible. The injection will anaesthetise both nerves.

***The buccal nerve*** This is also blocked using an intra-oral approach. A 27 g dental needle is inserted into the mucous membrane of the cheek, level with the occlusive plane of the first mandibular molar, and advanced posteriorly towards the external oblique ridge of the mandibular ramus. Infiltration of 2 ml of local anaesthetic between the needle entry point and the ridge will block the nerve.

***The mental nerve*** Block of this nerve requires identification of the mental foramen, the position of which varies with age and dentition. In the young adult it is situated below the first premolar tooth half-way between the gum margin and the lower border of the body of the mandible, but with advancing age the foramen 'moves' superiorly and posteriorly. The opening is often difficult to palpate, but its position may be confirmed using the straight-line relationship with the other foramina (Fig. 16.3). A 25 g needle is introduced extra-orally through the skin of the lower lip, below and in front of the second premolar tooth. It is directed towards the foramen, around which 1–2 ml of local anaesthetic should be infiltrated. It is neither necessary nor desirable for the needle to enter the foramen.

**The auriculotemporal nerve** This nerve is associated closely with the superficial temporal artery and vein in front of the ear. Using the pulsation of the artery just above the temporomandibular joint as a landmark, the nerve can be blocked by infiltration of 2–3 ml of local anaesthetic around the vessels. Branches of the facial nerve lie close by and facial paresis may result also.

## Cervical nerves

### Deep cervical plexus block (Fig. 16.5)

Deep cervical plexus block is a paravertebral block of $C_2$–$C_4$. With the patient lying supine, and the head turned to the opposite side, the tip of the mastoid process and Chassaignac's tubercle (the anterior tubercle on the transverse process of the sixth cervical vertebra) are marked (Fig. 16.5). A line is drawn from the posterior margin of the mastoid process to Chassaignac's tubercle.

The transverse processes of $C_2$, $C_3$, and $C_4$ all lie on this line and can usually be palpated, with that of $C_2$ located approximately 1.5 cm below the tip of the mastoid process, and those of $C_3$ (needle position in Fig 16.5) and $C_4$ found at further 1.5 cm intervals. The needle should be inserted in a caudal direction towards each transverse process to ensure that the epidural or subarachnoid spaces or the vertebral artery are not entered accidentally.

Deep cervical plexus block was originally described using three separate injections, one at the level of each of the three relevant vertebrae. However, a single injection at $C_4$ is equally effective because the cervical nerve roots are contained in a continuous sheath between the scalenus anterior and scalenus medius muscles (Winnie et al 1975), which allows the local anaesthetic to spread to all components of the plexus. A 22 g needle is inserted through the skin at the $C_4$ level on the line noted above, and then directed slightly caudad. Usually, the transverse process of $C_4$ is contacted at a depth of 1.5–3 cm, and paraesthesiae are obtained. Prior to injection of 10–15 ml of local anaesthetic, careful aspiration is essential to exclude vascular puncture or entry to the subarachnoid space. Accidental injection of local anaesthetic into the vertebral artery (which lies close by in the transverse foramen) results in immediate convulsions, while spread to the epidural or subarachnoid spaces produces cardiorespiratory collapse of slower onset. Paralysis of the diaphragm is a consequence of phrenic nerve block, so bilateral blocks are contraindicated.

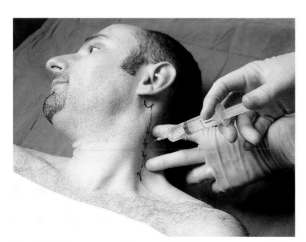

**Fig 16.5** Deep cervical plexus block. The crosses mark the tips of the transverse processes of the cervical vertebrae. The needle has been inserted at $C_3$

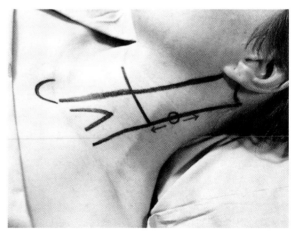

**Fig 16.6** Landmarks for superficial cervical plexus block. The circle marks the point of needle insertion, and the arrows mark the direction in which solution should spread

### Superficial cervical plexus block (Fig. 16.6)

Block of the superficial branches of the cervical plexus anaesthetises the skin, but not the deeper structures, of the anterolateral aspect of the neck from the mandible above to below the clavicle. Technically easy to perform, there is little risk of blocking the phrenic or recurrent laryngeal nerves, so bilateral blocks are not contra-indicated. The main landmark is the sternocleidomastoid muscle, which can be accentuated if the supine patient is asked to lift the head from the pillow. All four branches of the plexus emerge from behind the midpoint of sternocleidomastoid (approximately 1–2 cm above the point at which the external jugular vein crosses it). With the head turned to the opposite side 5–10 ml of local anaesthetic is injected subcutaneously along the posterior border of the muscle in cranial and caudal directions from the midpoint of the muscle.

### Great auricular nerve block

The great auricular nerve can be blocked selectively by injecting 2–3 ml of local anaesthetic in a straight line running anteriorly and posteriorly from the tip of the mastoid process. Its area of distribution to the ear is also included as part of superficial cervical plexus block.

### Greater occipital nerve block

The simplest technique for blocking this nerve is to infiltrate 10 ml of local anaesthetic superficially on a line running between the mastoid process and the greater occipital protuberance. The lesser occipital nerve is blocked simultaneously. Greater occipital nerve block is useful in the diagnosis and treatment of occipital neuralgia and can be combined with lesser occipital, auriculotemporal, supraorbital and supratrochlear nerve blocks to produce surgical anaesthesia of the scalp in a 'skull cap' distribution.

## Regional anaesthesia of the ear

The posterior surface of the ear and the lower third of the anterior surface are supplied by the great auricular nerve and, often, the lesser occipital nerve (see above). Both nerves are branches of the cervical plexus. The superior two-thirds of the anterior surface is supplied by the auriculotemporal nerve. Block of these nerves allows extensive surgery from otoplasty and wedge resection to amputation. Anaesthesia of the concha may be inadequate, but it can be reinforced by subcutaneous infiltration of 2–3 ml of local anaesthetic posteriorly through the conchal cartilage. In children, postoperative nausea and vomiting may be reduced by block of the auricular branch of the vagus. This requires infiltration of 2 ml of local anaesthetic at the bony-cartilaginous junction of the external auditory meatus.

## Awake intubation

A discussion on the indications for awake fibreoptic tracheal intubation is outside the scope of this book. However, this technique is becoming more widespread in both the elective and emergency situations, and knowledge of how to anaesthetise the airway adequately is essential for those practising it (Morris 1994). Local anaesthesia of the airway does render the patient at risk of aspiration and this must be taken into account if the patient has a full stomach, or if blood or pus is present in the nasal or oral cavities.

Individual block of the nerves which supply the upper airway is not practical, so a technique which uses predominantly topical anaesthesia is recommended. Pretreatment with a drying agent (e.g. glycopyrrolate 0.4 mg i.v.) improves the anaesthesia obtained from topical application of local anaesthetic, and having the patient in the sitting position helps prevent the tongue from falling backwards. Block of one or both nasal cavities is then performed as described previously. Anaesthesia of the nasopharynx can be supplemented using a nasopharyngeal airway covered in lidocaine gel (5%), and the posterior pharyngeal wall is anaesthetised using a 10% lidocaine spray (10 mg per metered dose) aimed directly at the back of the mouth.

The pressure receptors at the root of the tongue which initiate the gag reflex are submucosal and not blocked reliably by topical anaesthesia. It has been suggested that this problem can be overcome by performing bilateral glossopharyngeal nerve block (injecting 2 ml of local anaesthetic into the base of the anterior tonsillar pillar (Benumof 1991), although there may be little advantage over 'gargle and spray' topical anaesthesia (Sitzman et al 1997).

The larynx is blocked using a *cricothyroid puncture*. The cricothyroid membrane is identified and a skin bleb raised over it. A 20 g cannula, attached to a syringe containing 4 ml of the 4% topical preparation of lidocaine (note that this is *not* suitable for skin infiltration), is inserted through the cricothyroid membrane in the midline (Fig. 16.7). Aspiration of air confirms the correct position. The stilette of the cannula is then removed to

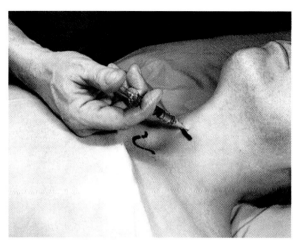

**Fig 16.7** Cricothyroid puncture

avoid damage to the posterior tracheal wall during injection. The patient is asked to breathe out maximally and the local anaesthetic administered as two, 2 ml injections. This will cause the patient to breathe in deeply and cough, thus coating the trachea and larynx.

The superior laryngeal nerve can be blocked specifically by applying a cotton ball soaked in 4% lidocaine to the pyriform fossa using Krause's forceps. Alternatively an external approach can be used. A suitable needle is passed in a posteromedial direction to make contact with the greater cornu of the hyoid, and then walked off it caudally. A loss of resistance may be appreciated as the needle penetrates the thyrohyoid membrane: 3 ml of 2% lidocaine is then injected.

## Regional anaesthesia for carotid endarterectomy (contributed by Dr Alastair Nimmo, Edinburgh)

Carotid endarterectomy is a procedure which presents a significant challenge to the anaesthetist, and it has been argued that regional anaesthesia in an awake or lightly sedated patient can contribute to reduced morbidity (Stoneham & Knighton 1999). Certainly, it enables repeated, virtually continuous, neurological assessment to be performed during the operation as an indication of the adequacy of cerebral perfusion during cross clamping of the carotid artery.

The operation is performed in the territory of the cervical plexus, and three regional anaesthetic techniques have been used – cervical epidural anaesthesia, cervical plexus block or local infiltration alone. Local infiltration alone is less likely to produce satisfactory anaesthesia than the others and cervical plexus block is the commonest method used. It may be achieved by either the deep or superficial approach (perhaps best by a combination of the two) performed as described above using bupivacaine at 0.375% or 0.5%. If both blocks are performed together, care must be taken not to exceed a safe total dose.

Occasionally, supplementary infiltration of the skin and subcutaneous tissues by the surgeon may be required if the block is incomplete. Unfortunately, even an effective cervical plexus block may not be sufficient because surgical retraction on the mandible often results in pain in the jaw, teeth or ear which local infiltration under the mandible may not relieve. Routine use of an inferior dental nerve block is perhaps the most effective approach (Bourke & Thomas 1998). Pain, presumably transmitted through either sympathetic or vagal fibres, is also common during dissection around the carotid artery. It may be prevented if the surgeon carefully injects 1–2 ml of local anaesthetic into the carotid sheath at an early stage. To minimise the risk of toxicity, all these supplementary injections are best performed using prilocaine 1%.

Heavy premedication and long-acting sedative and analgesic drugs should be avoided. Low-dose infusions of propofol and remifentanil (approximately $100\ \mu g\ h^{-1}$) may be started before the blocks are performed, and then adjusted to ensure that the patient is lightly sedated, but readily responsive during surgery. A transparent surgical drape may be used to prevent the patient feeling claustrophobic.

## References

Benumof JL 1991 Management of the difficult airway. Anesthesiology 75: 1087–1110

Bonica JJ 1990 Neurolytic blockade and hypophysectomy. In: Bonica JJ (ed) Management of pain, 2nd edn, pp 1980–2039. Lea and Febiger, Philadelphia

Bourke DL, Thomas P 1998 Mandibular nerve block in addition to cervical plexus block for carotid endarterectomy. Anesthesia and Analgesia 87: 1034–1036

Davies MJ, Mooney PH, Scott DA, et al. 1993 Neurologic changes during carotid endarterectomy under cervical block predict a high risk of postoperative stroke. Anesthesiology 78: 829–833

Lipton S 1989 Pain relief in active patients with cancer – the early use of nerve blocks improves the quality of life. British Medical Journal 298: 37–38.

Morris IR 1994 Fibreoptic intubation. Canadian Journal of Anaesthesia 41: 996–1007

Murphy TM 1988 Somatic block of head and neck. In: Cousins MJ, Bridenbough PO (eds) Neural blockade in clinical anaesthesia and management of pain, 2nd edn, pp 537–558. JB Lippincott, Philadelphia

Neill RS 1992 Terminal care of intraoral cancer. European Journal of Pain 13: 8–11

Neill RS 1996 Regional anaesthesia in ophthalmology and otorhinolaryngology. In: Brown DL (ed) Regional anaesthesia and analgesia, pp 487–494. WB Saunders, Philadelphia

Rice ASC, McMahon SB 1992 Peripheral nerve injury caused by injection needles used in anaesthesia; influence of bevel configuration, studied in a rat model. British Journal of Anaesthesia 69: 433–438

Sitzman BT, Rich GF, Rockwell JJ et al 1997 Local anesthetic administration for awake direct laryngoscopy. Anesthesiology 86: 34–40

Stoneham MD, Knighton JD 1999 Regional anaesthesia for carotid endarterectomy. British Journal of Anaesthesia 82: 910–919

Winnie AP, Ramamurthy S, Durrani Z, Radonjic R 1975 Interscalene cervical plexus block; a single injection technique. Anesthesia and Analgesia 54: 370–375

# 17. Eye blocks

## A P Rubin

Many minor operations on the lids or conjunctiva may be performed with topical or infiltration anaesthesia, and, increasingly, even cataract surgery is being performed using topical administration alone. However, most ophthalmic surgery requires akinesia (immobility) of the globe and, often, a reduction in intra-ocular pressure in addition to sensory block. To produce both analgesia and akinesia, local anaesthetic must be injected into the orbit to block not only the sensory nerves, but also the motor nerves to the extraocular muscles (the four recti and the two obliques), the orbicularis oculi and the levator palpebrae superioris. The traditional method for this is retrobulbar block, which has been used for more than 100 years (Knapp 1884) and involves injection of local anaesthetic inside the cone formed behind the eye by the rectus muscles.

Originally, retrobulbar block was combined with facial nerve block to ensure paralysis of the orbicularis oculi muscle. However, with the newer peribulbar block (Davis & Mandel 1986), which involves an injection *outside* the muscle cone, local anaesthetic will spread to the eyelids to block the nerve supply to the orbicularis oculi muscle as well as blocking the nerves within the orbit. A yet newer technique, currently being used more frequently, is the sub-Tenon's fascia block (Stevens 1992), in which a blunt cannula is placed deep to the conjunctiva and Tenon's fascia, from where the local anaesthetic spreads backwards towards the intraconal structures.

## ANATOMY OF THE ORBIT

The globe lies in the front half of the orbit (Fig. 17.1) and is about 2.3–2.5 cm long (the axial length), with the 'equator' being about half-way back. Myopic eyes may be longer with thinner sclera, and thus be at greater risk of perforation by a needle.

The orbit itself is a cone-shaped cavity with its apex placed posteromedially and its base being the quadrilateral anterior opening bounded by the orbital margins (Fig. 17.2). The medial wall is parallel to the sagittal plane, but the lateral wall is angled inwards at 45°. The roof is horizontal, but the floor slopes upwards, front to back, at about 10°. The globe may be closer to the roof than the floor of the orbit.

The four rectus muscles arise from the annulus of Zinn at the back of the orbit (Fig. 17.3), and are inserted into the globe just anterior to its equator (Fig. 17.1). The muscle cone is thought of as forming a boundary between two compartments, the central (*retrobulbar*) and the peripheral (*peribulbar*) spaces (Fig. 17.1). Although these spaces are similar to the epidural space and brachial plexus sheath in containing connective tissue septa and blood vessels, the orbital fat is continuous between the two and solutions spread freely from one to the other. Within the cone is the optic nerve, the trunk of the ophthalmic artery, the ciliary ganglion and the nerves to the muscles. All of these structures are vulnerable to damage secondary to direct trauma, decreased blood supply or compression. Such problems are best avoided by using short needles, which cannot be inserted too far into the orbit. The inferotemporal, nasal and superotemporal segments are the least vascular and it is usual to make injections in these areas (Hamilton 1998).

The sensory supply of the orbit is provided by the lacrimal, frontal and nasociliary branches of the ophthalmic division of the trigeminal nerve, each of which enters the orbit through the superior orbital fissure (Fig. 17.3). Autonomic fibres run from the ciliary ganglion, which is situated within the cone, near to the orbital apex. The oculomotor (the third cranial) nerve supplies the superior, inferior and medial rectus muscles

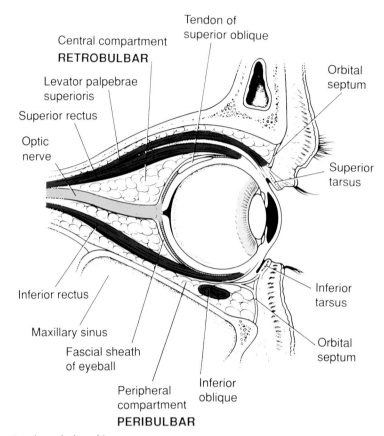

**Fig 17.1**   Vertical section through the orbit

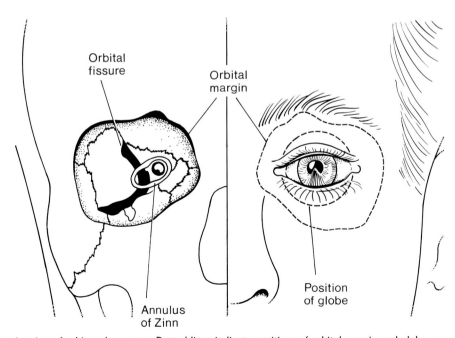

**Fig 17.2**   Anterior view of orbit and contents. Dotted lines indicate positions of orbital margin and globe

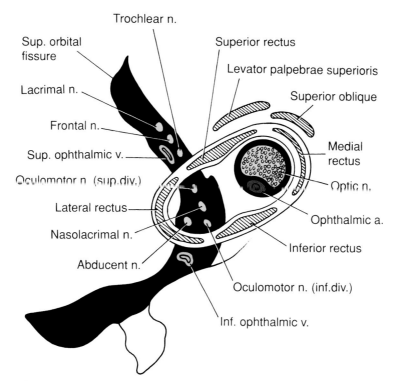

**Fig 17.3**  Structures at the apex of the orbit

as well as the inferior oblique and levator palpebrae superioris; the trochlear (fourth) nerve supplies the superior oblique; the abducent (sixth) nerve supplies the lateral rectus; and the facial (seventh) nerve the orbicularis oculi. After traversing the stylohyoid foramen the facial nerve passes through the parotid gland, and its temporal and zygomatic branches innervate the orbicularis oculi muscle.

## GENERAL MANAGEMENT

### Indications

In adults, most ophthalmic surgery may be performed under regional anaesthesia, the limiting factor being the ability of the patient to lie comfortably and still for the requisite time. It is particularly applicable to cataract and glaucoma surgery, and facilitates day-stay care. Rapid discharge with good analgesia is possible, and is associated with less emetic and other side effects (Williams et al 1995).

### Contraindications

These methods are less suitable for prolonged surgery, or for use in younger adults and children. The patients should accept the technique and be able to lie fairly flat, without obvious risk of coughing or sneezing. They should not suffer from involuntary movements, claustrophobia, dementia or pathological anxiety. For patients on warfarin, the INR should be within the therapeutic range, which is determined by the condition for which the patient is being anticoagulated (Joint College Guidelines 2001).

### Preparation of the patient

There is debate as to the degree of preoperative assessment and investigation required. Many would wish to see a complete history and physical examination followed by all relevant investigations. However, the trend is to use nurse assessment and to reduce the number of investigations to a minimum, leaving the anaesthetist to concentrate on the high-risk patients. It has been suggested that the 'stress-free' surgery (which regional anaesthesia produces) reduces the risk of cardiovascular complications (Barker et al 1990, Glantz et al 2000).

Full discussion of the proposed technique should allay the patient's anxiety and most will accept it once they are reassured that they will not feel any pain during the block or the operation, and that they will not see

243

anything frightening. Although the issue may be controversial, it is no longer routine to fast the patient in many units (Maltby & Hamilton 1993, Steeds & Mather 2001). The risk of serious reactions (such as central, perineural spread of drug or systemic toxicity), which may result in a risk of aspiration of gastric contents, is extremely low and the patients feel better if they are allowed a modest oral intake. Also the management of diabetic patients, who make up about 15% of the cataract population, is simplified because they can remain on their normal regimens. The bladder should be empty, and premedication is rarely required in this predominantly elderly population.

## Monitoring

A pulse oximeter, electrocardiograph and blood pressure recorder should be used. Intravenous access should be secured and full resuscitation equipment and drugs available.

## General principles

The patient must be kept in a comfortable position at all times, using pillows and padding as required. A pillow under the knees helps to remove strain on the back, and the neck must also be supported and comfortable. Sedation is rarely required, but the anxious may benefit from small doses of midazolam (1 mg), with or without an analgesic (e.g. 200 μg alfentanil), usually given prior to performance of the block.

Every care should be taken to ensure that the local anaesthetic technique is as painless as possible. This may be achieved by the use of very fine, sharp needles, the preliminary injection of warmed local anaesthetic solution diluted in ten times its volume of balanced salt solution (Bloom et al 1984, Korbon et al 1987), very slow injection, gentle technique, and constant explanation and reassurance. Injections through the conjunctiva, which is easily anaesthetised with topical solution, are less painful than through the skin, and also are less likely to produce subcutaneous haemorrhage.

Agreement with the surgeon on the degree of akinesia required will determine the conduct of the block and the desired end result. In the last few years, with improvements in surgical equipment and technique, full akinesia has become less essential, and some surgeons will even perform cataract surgery with topical anaesthesia alone, and without akinesia. The anaesthetist or an assistant must remain in direct physical contact with the patient at all times to monitor vital signs, to act as a medium for communication of any distress, and to provide reassurance.

## Local anaesthetic solutions

### Topical

Proxymetacaine 0.5% or benoxinate 0.4% are preferred because they do not 'sting' as much as tetracaine (amethocaine) 1%. Once the cornea is anaesthetised, tetracaine, which lasts longer and produces more intense analgesia, may be used.

### Injection

High concentrations of local anaesthetic are required to produce motor as well as sensory block. The most commonly used solution is a mixture of equal parts of 2% lidocaine and 0.75% bupivacaine (Feibel 1985, Hamilton et al 1988). The theory (Gotta 1990) is that the lidocaine acts more quickly while the bupivacaine gives an adequate duration. It is usual to add hyaluronidase 7.5 IU ml$^{-1}$ (Thomson 1988) to improve diffusion of the fluid through the fat-filled spaces of the orbit. Epinephrine is rarely used now, because sufficient duration may be achieved without it. Some anaesthetists use lidocaine or prilocaine, often with a vasoconstrictor, if the surgical time is predictably short. The advantage of the medium duration agents is that the anaesthesia and akinesia wear off more quickly and the cornea does not have to be protected with a pad and shield for as long.

## TECHNIQUES
## Orbital (akinetic) regional block

Although *peribulbar* and *retrobulbar* block have been considered as separate techniques previously, the injection is made into the same adipose tissue compartment and the difference is merely a matter of needle direction and depth of insertion (Figs 17.4 & 17.5). Most of the structures to be blocked are in a central location within the cone, so the more central blocks work more quickly and effectively (Hamilton et al 1988). The more peripheral blocks usually take longer to work, require larger volumes of local anaesthetic, and more injections. It is now usual to combine elements of both techniques. The preferred route of injection is through the conjunctiva, which is easily anaesthetised topically. However, if the patient has a deep-set eye, a narrow

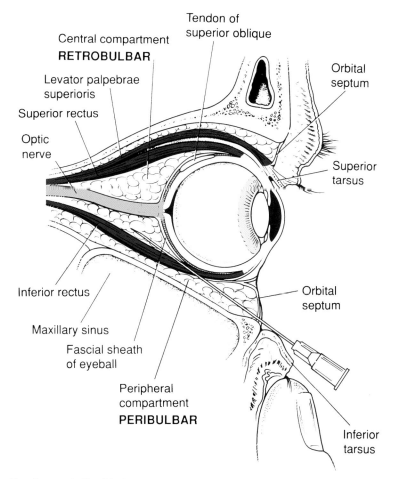

**Fig 17.4**  Needle position for retrobulbar block

palpebral fissure, or is unable to stop screwing up the eye, the transcutaneous approach may be safer.

With the patient supine and looking straight ahead, the conjunctiva is anaesthetised topically, and the lower eyelid pulled downwards and outwards; about 1 ml of 0.2% lidocaine (2% lidocaine mixed with ten times its volume of balanced salt solution) is injected through a 1 cm, 30 g needle in the inferotemporal region of the inferior conjunctival fornix. The needle is inserted at a tangent to the globe, and the injection should be made into the fat so as not to 'lift' the conjunctiva. This injection should be painless and make the subsequent injections equally painless.

About 2 minutes later, a sharp, 2.5 cm, 25 g disposable needle is inserted through the same point, initially tangential to the globe (Fig. 17.6), but then parallel to the orbital floor (Fig. 17.7). A more temporal approach reduces the chance of damaging, or injecting

into, the inferior oblique muscle. The bevel of the needle should face the globe to reduce the risk of perforation. The injection may be made at a depth of 2–2.5 cm ('peribulbar') or the needle, once the tip has passed the equator, may be angled upwards and inwards to enter the more central region just behind the globe ('shallow retrobulbar') (Hamilton 1996). In order to avoid possible damage to the optic nerve, which lies medially, the needle should not cross the plane of the lateral edge of the iris.

After careful aspiration, up to 5 ml of solution should be injected very slowly. There should be no pain or resistance. The upper lid may be seen to fill and drop (ptosis), and this is a good sign. The pressure within the globe must be assessed. When this is normal, the globe feels soft and moves freely within the orbit, and there should be no proptosis, although there may be some 'filling' of the lower lid with solution, and some sub-conjunctival swelling (chemosis). If either is excessive, the

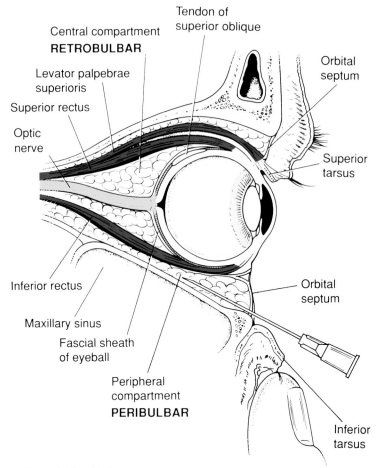

**Fig 17.5** Needle position for peribulbar block

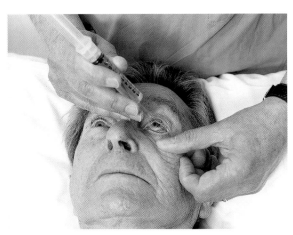

**Fig 17.6** Initial needle angulation for inferotemporal component of an orbital block

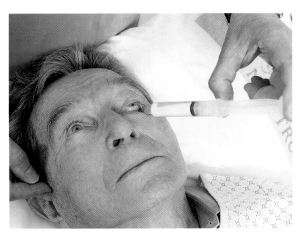

**Fig 17.7** Final needle position for inferotemporal component of an orbital block

needle should be repositioned and the injection continued. If the pressure increases, the injection should be stopped.

Great care should be taken to choose the least vascular areas, to withdraw the needle very carefully and to apply gentle pressure on the closed eye immediately after injection to control any potential haemorrhage. The anaesthetised cornea must be protected from possible damage at all times, and kept moist. A pressure device such as the Honan balloon (Davidson et al 1979) is usually applied over the closed, padded eye after injection to aid dispersion of the solution and to reduce the intraocular pressure.

Within 5 minutes, significant akinesia should be apparent. If there is failure to block the medial rectus or the orbicularis oculi, the same needle may be inserted through the conjunctiva between the caruncle and the skin of the medial canthus, and directed straight back parallel to the medial orbital wall (Fig. 17.8) into the nasal (medial) compartment (Hustead et al 1994). Between 3 and 5 ml of local anaesthetic is injected at a depth of 1.5–2 cm. Some of the solution will remain deep to the medial orbital septum (Figs. 17.4 & 17.5) and improve the peribulbar block, while some will come forwards through foramina above and below the septum to fill the eyelids and block the orbicularis oculi. If the needle is inserted too far there is a risk of it entering the central space. The optic nerve may then be damaged or the injection made into its sheath.

If the first inferotemporal injection was made central to the muscle cone, and is followed by the nasal injection, anaesthesia will be adequate in about 98% of cases. However, if the first injection was peripheral to the cone, about 25% of patients will require a further injection if full akinesia is required. The site of this injection depends on the clinical deficiency. If the medial rectus or orbicularis oculi remain unblocked, a nasal injection is required, while failure to block adequately the superior rectus or levator palpebrae superioris may justify a superotemporal injection through the upper eye lid, level with the lateral edge of the iris (Fig. 17.9). The superotemporal injection must go upwards towards the orbital roof to avoid the globe because there is only

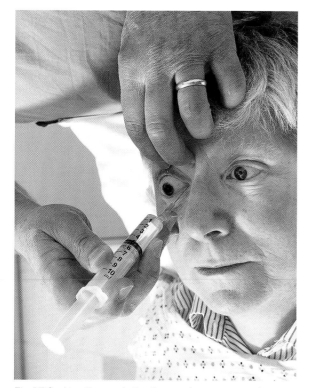

**Fig 17.8** Needle angulation for nasal component of an orbital block

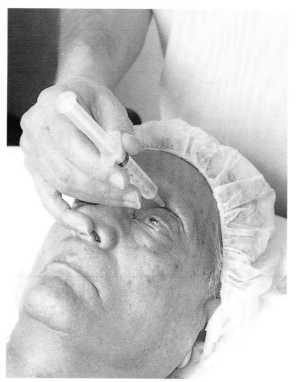

**Fig 17.9** Superotemporal supplementation of an orbital block through the upper eyelid

247

limited space between it and the orbital roof. If there is failure to block several muscles, the inferotemporal injection should be repeated.

These subsequent injections should be painless because the initial one is likely to produce adequate anaesthesia, if not total akinesia. Each injection should be followed by a period of firm pressure, and adequate akinesia and low intraocular pressure achieved before the patient is offered for surgery. It must be stressed that every additional injection carries risks so no attempt should be made to produce akinesia in excess of the surgical requirements.

### Complications (Hamilton 1998)

Chemosis (subconjunctival oedema) may follow injections, but is not usually of any concern and usually disappears with pressure. The most common complication is *haemorrhage*. Venous haemorrhage is usually mild and, while unsightly, is easily controlled whereas arterial haemorrhage may be dramatic, causing proptosis, extensive subconjunctival and lid haematomata, and a dramatic increase in intraocular pressure. It often necessitates postponement of surgery (Fiebel 1985, Morgan et al 1988). The high pressure may compromise the circulation to the retina and urgent decompression by lateral canthotomy may be required.

*Globe perforation* is an ever present risk, but is probably more likely in long, myopic eyes. The long eye has a thinner sclera and may have an irregular outline (staphylomata). The needle should be inserted tangentially to the globe, and should move freely in the orbital fat without rotating the globe with it. Pain and resistance to either needle advancement or injection are warning signs. Diagnosis may be difficult and early management in a vitreoretinal unit will improve the likelihood of a better visual result.

*Damage to the optic nerve* might result from direct trauma, injection into the nerve sheath or the ischaemic consequences of the pressure of the injection.

*Myotoxicity* may follow the use of high concentrations of local anaesthetic (e.g. 4% lidocaine), or direct injection into a muscle, and may result in muscle palsy (Rainin & Carlson 1985).

*Systemic consequences* include confusion, convulsions, loss of consciousness, and respiratory or cardiac arrest. They can result from systemic local anaesthetic toxicity, injection of local anaesthetic into the optic nerve sheath or retrograde arterial flow.

Vasovagal or allergic reactions are also possible.

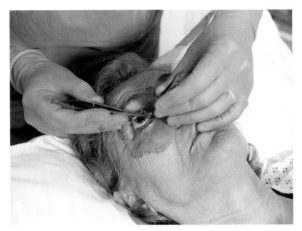

**Fig 17.10** Site of initial conjunctival incision for sub-Tenon's fascia block

## Non-akinetic methods

These methods have become much more practical with improvements in surgical technique and a decreasingly invasive approach to cataract surgery. The debate is whether the risk of complications of the surgery in the presence of possible eye movement is greater than the small risk of complications of orbital regional blocks.

### Topical anaesthesia

This simple method is growing in popularity (Grabow 1993). The use of topical anaesthetic alone means that the eye will be fully mobile so a considerable degree of patient co-operation and surgical dexterity is necessary. Up to 31% of patients report pain (Fukasaku & Marron 1994), usually associated with contact with the unanaesthetised iris. This figure seems to be unacceptably high.

### Subconjunctival anaesthesia

A small amount of local anaesthetic is injected subconjunctivally in the perilimbal region and produces good analgesia without akinesia, but even with this technique, a case of globe perforation has been reported (Yanoff & Redovan 1990).

### Sub-Tenon's fascia block

This is a technique (Stevens 1992) which is growing rapidly in popularity, and is comparatively simple, reliable and relatively safe because it avoids sharp needles. After good topical anaesthesia of the conjunctiva, with the eye looking upwards and outwards, the conjunctiva is grasped with a non-toothed forceps (Fig 17.10). A small 'button-hole' incision is made with blunt spring scissors about 10 mm from the limbus in the inferonasal portion of the conjunctiva and Tenon's fascia. Bare sclera is seen in the depth of the incision. The distal conjunctival edge is held up and the blunt curved cannula, with loaded syringe attached, is passed into the sub-Tenon's fascia space, following the curve of the globe on the nasal side and stopping posterior to the equator, usually at a depth of about 1.5–2.0 cm (Fig. 17.11). If resistance is felt, a little of the solution may be injected to facilitate advancement of the cannula. Up to 5 ml of solution may be injected, the degree of akinesia achieved depending on volume. The local anaesthetic tracks backwards into the central space where it acts rather like a retrobulbar injection. Pressure should be applied over the eye for a few minutes after the injection.

Haemorrhage and conjunctival chemosis are the only common complications (Roman et al 1997), but the technique might be contraindicated in glaucoma patients where the preservation of the normal conjunctiva is important.

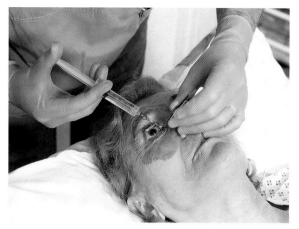

**Fig 17.11**  Cannula for sub-Tenon's fascia block partially inserted

## References

Barker JP, Robinson PN, Vafidis GC, Hart GR, Sapsed-Byrne S, Hall GM 1990 Local analgesia prevents the cortisol and glycaemic responses to cataract surgery. British Journal of Anaesthesia 64: 442–445

Bloom LH, Scheie HG, Yanoff M 1984 The warming of local anesthetic agents to decrease discomfort. Ophthalmic Surgery 15: 603

Davidson B, Kratz RP, Mazzocco T R, Maloney WF 1979 An evaluation of the Honan intraocular pressure reducer. Journal of the American Intraocular Implant Society 5: 237

Davis DB II, Mandel MR 1986 Posterior peribulbar anesthesia; an alternative to retrobulbar anesthesia. Journal of Cataract and Refractive Surgery 12: 182–184

Feibel RM 1985 Current concepts in retrobulbar anesthesia. Survey of Ophthalmology 30: 102–110

Fukasaku H, Marron J 1994 Pinpoint anesthesia: a new approach to local ocular anesthesia. Journal of Cataract and Refractive Surgery 20: 468–471

Glantz I, Drenger B, Gozal Y 2000 Perioperative myocardial ischaemia in cataract surgery patients: general versus local anesthesia. Anesthesia and Analgesia 91: 1415–1419

Gotta AW 1990 The pharmacology of local anesthetics used in ophthalmic surgery. In: Zahl K, Meltzer MA (eds) Regional anesthesia for intraocular surgery. Ophthalmic Clinics of North America, Vol 3, No 1

Grabow HB (1993) Topical anaesthesia for cataract surgery. European Journal of Implant and Refractive Surgery 5: 20–24

Hamilton RC 1996 Retrobulbar block revisited and revised. Journal of Cataract and Refractive Surgery 22: 1147–1150

Hamilton RC 1998 Complications of ophthalmic regional anesthesia. Ophthalmology Clinics of North America 11: 99–114

Hamilton RC, Gimbel HV, Strunin L 1988 Regional anaesthesia for 12 000 cataract extraction and intraocular lens implantation procedures. Canadian Journal of Anaesthesia 35: 615–623

Hustead RF, Hamilton RC, Loken RG 1994 Periocular local anesthesia: medial orbital as an alternative to superior nasal injection. Journal of Cataract and Refractive Surgery 20: 197–201

Joint College Guidelines, Local Anaesthesia for Intraocular Surgery. The Royal College of Anaesthetists and The Royal College of Ophthalmologists, 2001

Knapp H 1884 On cocaine and its use in ophthalmic and general surgery. Archives of Ophthalmology 13: 402–448

Korbon GA, Hurley DP, Williams GS 1987 pH-adjusted lidocaine does not 'sting'. Anesthesiology 66: 855–856

Maltby JR, Hamilton RC 1993 Preoperative fasting guidelines for cataract surgery under regional anaesthesia [Letter] British Journal of Anaesthesia 71: 167

Morgan CM, Schatz H, Vine AK, Cantrill HL, Davidorf FH, Gitter KA, Rudich R 1988 Ocular complications associated with retrobulbar injections. Ophthalmology 95: 660–665

Rainin EA, Carlson BM 1985 Postoperative diplopia and ptosis: A clinical hypothesis based on the myotoxicity of local anesthetics. Archives of Ophthalmology 103: 1337–1339

Roman SJ, Chong Sit DA, Boureau CM, Auclin FX, Ullern MM 1997 Sub-Tenon's anaesthesia: an efficient and safe technique. British Journal of Ophthalmology 81: 673–676

Steeds C, Mather SJ. 2001 Fasting regimens for regional ophthalmic anaesthesia; a survey of members of the British Ophthalmic Anaesthesia Society. Anaesthesia, 56: 638

Stevens JD 1992 A new local anaesthesia technique for cataract extraction by one quadrant sub-Tenon's infiltration. British Journal of Ophthalmology 76: 670–674

Thomson I 1988 Addition of hyaluronidase to lignocaine with adrenaline for retrobulbar anesthesia in the surgery of senile cataract. British Journal of Ophthalmology 72: 700

Williams N, Strunin A, Heriot W 1995 Pain and vomiting after vitreoretinal surgery: a potential role for local anaesthesia. Anaesthesia and Intensive Care 23: 444–448

Yanoff M, Redovan EG 1990 Anterior eyewall perforation during subconjunctival cataract block. Ophthalmic Surgery 21: 362–363

# 18. Regional anaesthesia in obstetrics

## J H McClure

Regional analgesia in obstetrics is an art based on a science. The science involves knowledge of the anatomy of the nervous system and reproductive tract, the physiology of pregnancy and the pharmacology of local anaesthetics. The anaesthetist learns the art with experience on the labour ward, performing regional techniques, assessing their results and learning how to modify them in the best interests of the mother and her baby. There is no short cut to this experience which is, in large measure, the justification for having specialists in obstetric anaesthesia. It was originally James Young Simpson's hope (Simpson 1848) that 'local anaesthesia' could be used as an alternative to general anaesthesia, but this was not realised in obstetric practice until 1900 when Oskar Kreis used spinal anaesthesia during operative vaginal delivery (Kreis 1900). Sacral epidural analgesia with procaine was used during labour by Stoekel, but he warned of the risk of 'impairing the force of labour' (Stoeckel 1909).

Regional analgesia, especially lumbar epidural block, is now widely available for mothers in labour and there are several reasons for its popularity. The main alternative methods of analgesia – parenteral and inhalational – have the potential for producing maternal and fetal central nervous system depression. In the mother this can range from amnesia for the birth of her child, to confusion and disorientation such that she loses the ability to co-operate with attendant staff. In the neonate, the effect can extend from mild neurobehavioural abnormalities, detectable only by sophisticated testing (Scanlon et al 1974, 1978, Hollmen et al 1978, Amiel-Tison et al 1982, Brockhurst et al 2000), to severe respiratory depression with failure to initiate normal respiration at birth. Regional analgesia in obstetrics offers the possibility of maternal pain relief without clouding of consciousness or neonatal depression and it has minimal effect on the uterine blood flow or the fetus itself (Joupila et al 1978a, b, Hollmen et al 1982, Halpern et al 1998). There are those who believe, as Stoeckel did, that labour is prolonged, particularly if high doses of local anaesthetic drug are used, due to an adverse effect on mobility and pelvic muscle tone. However, modern epidural analgesia during labour should preserve the mobility of the mother. This not only improves maternal satisfaction (Murphy et al 1991), but may also reduce the incidence of forceps delivery (Van Steenberge et al 1987).

The majority of elective and emergency operative procedures are now performed under epidural or spinal anaesthesia. The reduction in the number of general anaesthetics given in obstetrics has almost certainly contributed to the reduction in maternal deaths due to anaesthesia in the UK (Reports on Confidential Enquiries into Maternal Deaths in the UK 1985–96). The pregnant mother has high expectations for good pain relief in labour, and for optimal regional anaesthesia, should she require an operative delivery. It is crucial that her expectations are realistic and that she is able to make informed decisions about her care before the pain of labour interferes with decision making. The issue of consent for epidural analgesia is highly topical and ideally this should be discussed, and consent obtained, in the antenatal period when the risks and benefits can be explained rationally. The anaesthetist cannot guarantee complete pain relief and it is imperative that strategies are in place in the event of partial or complete failure of regional block.

## ANATOMY AND PHYSIOLOGY
### Innervation

The pain of uterine contractions is transmitted via visceral afferent fibres to the sympathetic chain and then to the first lumbar, twelfth and eleventh thoracic segments of the spinal cord (Fig. 18.1). This pain is felt in the lower abdomen and the back. Back pain may be very severe and may extend into the sacral area if the fetal head persists in the occipito-posterior (O-P) position and presses on the lumbosacral plexus and other structures in the pelvis. The pain of the second stage is transmitted via the pudendal nerves to the second, third and fourth sacral segments of the spinal cord. The ilio-inguinal nerves, the genital branches of the genitofemoral nerves and the perineal branch of the posterior nerve of thigh may also be involved in the transmission of pain during the second stage. This may explain, in part, the poor quality of anaesthesia obtained with pudendal nerve block alone.

## Epidural space

The epidural space is filled with fat, connective tissue, and a venous plexus which may become distended in late pregnancy. In the non-pregnant patient, there is normally a negative pressure in the epidural space, which is influenced by the intrathoracic pressure. The observed pressure may reflect indentation of the dura by the needle or catheter (Aitkenhead et al 1979). Raised venous pressure due to caval compression or advanced pregnancy increases epidural pressure, as does the sitting position and the second stage of labour (Galbert & Marx 1974). It is, therefore, not surprising that Usubiaga and colleagues (1967) failed to demonstrate a 'negative' epidural pressure in mothers undergoing Caesarean section. Venous distension and the humoral effects of progesterone reduce the compliance of the epidural space and are thought to cause the enhanced epidural drug spread seen in the pregnant patient (Datta et al 1983, Fagraeus et al 1983, Park 1988).

## Aortocaval occlusion

Aortocaval occlusion occurs in all women at term, though not all will have symptoms of the 'supine hypotensive syndrome of pregnancy' (Holmes 1960). The gravid uterus compresses the vena cava and aorta against the lumbar spine, causing blood to flow via the paravertebral and

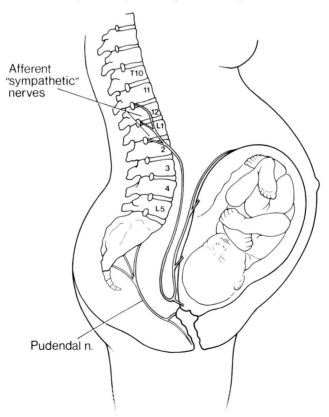

**Fig 18.1**   Innervation of the uterus and birth canal

azygous system of veins, and resulting in a reduction in venous return to the right heart and reduced uterine blood flow (Kerr et al 1964, Lees et al 1967). Lateral tilt may partially relieve the compression, but the full lateral position may be required in some cases, particularly when the uterus is large (Kinsella et al 1992). In the presence of aortocaval occlusion, systemic arterial blood pressure may, to some extent, be maintained by compensatory vasoconstriction, but regional anaesthesia will block the latter. Hypotension will ensue unless scrupulous attention is paid to the patient's position, and to the maintenance of the circulation with vasoconstrictors or fluid.

### Preloading with intravenous fluid

The technique of preloading (Ramanathan et al 1983) with 500 ml to 1 litre of crystalloid solution is commonly used before a central block is established, but it is controversial and is often ineffective in preventing hypotension (Jackson et al 1995). Preloading may even be hazardous in patients with cardiac disease and reduced left ventricular compliance. If hypotension does occur it is better to treat it with a vasopressor, for example 3–6 mg intravenous boluses of ephedrine or 20–40 µg boluses of phenylephrine (Ramanathan et al 1984, Ramanathan & Grant 1988, Taylor & Tunstall 1991). Fluid preloading should not be confused with, or regarded as a substitute for, the absolute requirement to maintain an adequate circulating volume. Hypovolaemia is very poorly tolerated in the presence of sympathetic block and should be treated by volume replacement.

## LOCAL ANAESTHETIC TECHNIQUES
## Infiltration anaesthesia

Infiltration with local anaesthetic is widely used to anaesthetise the perineum before episiotomy or repair of a perineal tear. Lidocaine at 1% concentration is usually the agent of choice and care must be taken with the total dose administered in this very vascular area. Twenty millilitres (200 mg) is the officially recommended maximum dose (Ch. 5). The addition of 1:200 000 epinephrine reduces the speed of systemic absorption and allows a larger dose of lidocaine (500 mg) to be given, but systemic epinephrine effects may become apparent. Caesarean section may also be performed under infiltration anaesthesia and is considered later.

## Paracervical block

This block has largely disappeared from clinical practice in obstetrics because of the risk of fetal bradycardia secondary to rapid uptake of local anaesthetic into the fetal circulation (Cibils 1976, Greiss et al 1976), but it is still used in some gynaecological procedures. The visceral afferent fibres from the uterus are blocked by injecting 10 ml of 1% lidocaine on each side of the cervix below the mucosa of the lateral vaginal fornix. A guarded needle (Fig. 18.2) is used and the injections should be made at '4' and '8 o'clock', avoiding the uterine arteries and the fetal head. The duration of analgesia is limited to between 30 minutes and 1 hour, so the blocks may have to be repeated.

## Pudendal nerve block

Bilateral pudendal nerve block may be used in the second stage of labour to reduce the discomfort of forceps delivery in the absence of epidural or spinal block. Additional infiltration of the perineum and labia is required to block the branches of the ilio-inguinal and genitofemoral nerves. This block is generally performed immediately prior to forceps delivery by the obstetrician using the vaginal route and 1% lidocaine. The transvaginal approach requires a guarded needle (Fig. 18.2) to protect the vagina and the fetal head when the ischial spine is being located. The guide of the needle should be placed medial to the ischial spine at its point of attachment to the sacrospinous ligament. The needle is inserted and an initial dose of 5 ml of 1% lidocaine is injected when the needle pierces the vagina. The needle is advanced until a 'pop' indicates that it has penetrated the sacrospinous ligament, then a further 5 ml is injected. The procedure is repeated on the other side. Good anaesthesia is not always guaranteed and a minimum of 5 minutes should be allowed for the local anaesthetic to take effect (Hutchins 1980).

## EPIDURAL ANALGESIA IN LABOUR
## Caudal analgesia

Caudal block, performed through the sacral hiatus, is discussed in Chapter 12. It has largely been superseded by lumbar epidural anaesthesia in obstetrics, but it is of historical interest (Stoekel 1909, Hingson & Edwards 1943). It may still be of benefit in the rare patient in whom lumbar epidural block is impossible, or who is

253

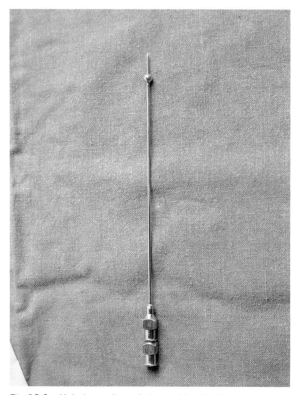 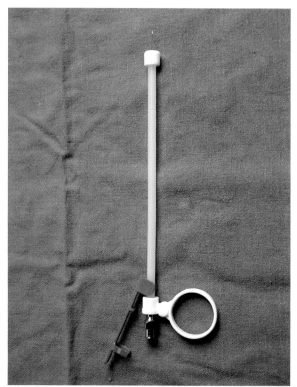

**Fig 18.2**   Kobak needle and disposable sheathed needle

distressed by pain, arising from the sacral roots, which has not been helped by repeated lumbar epidural local anaesthetic injection. The use of lumbar epidural opioids has significantly reduced the need for such supplementary sacral block because these opioids act on the sacral as well as the lumbar segments of the spinal cord.

## Lumbar epidural analgesia

Ideally, a lumbar epidural catheter should be sited before the mother is in a distressed state. This allows informed consent to be obtained, and the anaesthetist's task is easier and safer if the mother is co-operative and able to flex her spine in the sitting or lateral position. Accurate placement of an epidural catheter in the mother who is in acute distress requires a degree of skill and dexterity which only comes with great practice. A small dose of intravenous meperidine (pethidine) and a skilled midwife may help in the most distressed and unco-operative mothers.

### Management of the second stage of labour

If an epidural block is fully effective in the sacral segments, the effectiveness of the bearing-down reflex will be reduced by block of the afferent side of the reflex. However, the actual ability to bear down should be unimpaired because the diaphragm and abdominal muscles produce this effort. Most obstetricians now consider that it is acceptable to let the second stage continue for longer than the notional one hour limit and allow the fetal head to descend through the pelvis by uterine action before active 'pushing' is begun.

## Techniques

Better mobility during labour, increasingly demanded by mothers, has been shown to improve maternal satisfaction and enhance personal autonomy (Collis et al 1995). Such mobility can be achieved with epidural analgesia if low concentrations of local anaesthetic are used, or with a combined spinal–epidural (CSE) technique. It remains to be seen which of these two methods is superior. Increased mobility does not, however, decrease the incidence of forceps or Caesarean delivery (Russell and Reynolds 1996).

Continuous infusion epidural analgesia was very popular in the 1980s because it avoided the painful intervals, which sometimes occurred when there was a delay in administering a 'top-up' injection. However, a fixed-dose infusion does not allow for individual variability and causes an unacceptable degree of motor block in some patients. The situation has changed since then in that midwives are now authorised to give top-ups, and patient-controlled epidural analgesia (PCEA) pumps are more widely available. As a result, it is possible to adjust the dosage and timing of top-ups, and thus to ensure mobility for the individual patient during labour (Collis et al 1999).

### Intermittent injection technique

The classical teaching in the 1970s was to administer a 'test dose' of 4 ml of 2% lidocaine *with or without* 1:200 000 epinephrine to exclude intravascular or intrathecal placement of the epidural catheter, followed by a loading dose of 6–8 ml of 0.25% or 0.5% bupivacaine. This inevitably led to a degree of motor block of the lower limbs. Top-up injections were given subsequently on demand. This intermittent injection technique is a form of patient-controlled analgesia and it allows for individual variability in analgesic requirements throughout labour. However, it may lead to painful intervals if top-up injections are not immediately forthcoming or if the mother delays her request until she is in acute pain.

### Continuous infusion epidural analgesia (CIEA)

The introduction of accurate and reliable volumetric pumps, and concern about painful intervals, led to the development of CIEA, which reduced the frequency of these intervals and the number of top-up injections required. However, there is a high incidence of motor block if local anaesthetic alone is used to maintain analgesia (Thorburn & Moir 1981, Van Steenberge et al 1987, Murphy et al 1991). The introduction of less concentrated solutions of bupivacaine (e.g. 0.08% combined with fentanyl $2 \mu g \, ml^{-1}$) reduced both the intensity of motor block and the number of supplementary injections required (Jones et al 1989, Russell & Reynolds 1993). Some infusions may result in unilateral block, presumably due to lateral placement of the catheter, and if this cannot be resolved by withdrawing the catheter by 1–2 cm and the mother lying on her unblocked side, the infusion should be abandoned and converted to a bolus technique. Lateral eye catheters are less likely to cause unilateral blocks during CIEA than end-hole catheters (Dickson et al 1997).

### Patient-controlled epidural analgesia (PCEA)

A loading dose of local anaesthetic *with or without* opioid is followed by PCEA. A low-dose background infusion may also be given. This combines the benefits of the bolus and CIEA techniques, and has the additional bonus that the mother feels in control (Gambling et al 1988, Purdie et al 1992). PCEA pumps can be programmed to give 4–6 ml boluses of dilute anaesthetic, with or without an opioid, on demand (usually with a 15 minute 'lock-out' time) and a low-dose background infusion (around $4–6 \, ml \, h^{-1}$). A limit can be set on the hourly consumption also. The use of small bolus doses appears to avoid the risk of hypotension.

### 'Mobile' epidural

The use of low doses of local anaesthetic (e.g. 15 ml of 0.1% bupivacaine or 8–10 ml of 0.2% ropivacaine) combined with an opioid allows mobility, which improves both maternal satisfaction and the likelihood of spontaneous vaginal delivery (Murphy et al 1991, Writer et al 1998). The standard bolus dose acts as a 'test dose' each time it is given, which acts as a safeguard even if there is no reason to suspect intravenous placement of the catheter. Intravenous placement of the catheter should be considered if there is failure to establish or maintain satisfactory analgesia. A formal 'test dose' is recommended if a greater dose of local anaesthetic is administered subsequently, as in the event of a more profound block being required for Caesarean section or forceps delivery. The development of significant motor block after 15 ml 0.1% bupivacaine or 8–10 ml 0.2% ropivacaine should lead to suspicion of subarachnoid placement of the catheter.

Midwives in the UK are permitted to give intermittent epidural injections with a mixture of dilute local anaesthetics and opioid, provided it is from a premixed bag clearly labelled and identified for use in an individual patient.

### Combined spinal–epidural analgesia (CSEA)

This technique was first described by Soresi in 1937, and it has since been adapted to provide good quality analgesia with minimal effect on motor power (Collis et al 1994, Morgan 1995). A choice of three methods is available.

1. *Two interspace.* The first report of CSEA in obstetric anaesthesia was by Brownridge (1981) who placed the epidural catheter first at the $L_1–L_2$ interspace

followed by a spinal block performed at the $L_3$–$L_4$ interspace. There is the theoretical risk of cutting the epidural catheter with the spinal needle, but this risk is negligible with an atraumatic pencil-point spinal needle.

2. *Needle-through-needle, single interspace* (Carrie 1990). The needle-through-needle technique popularised by Carrie and Donald (1991) requires a 12 cm pencil-point spinal needle to be introduced through a 10 cm Tuohy epidural needle. There is a risk of subsequently advancing the epidural catheter through the hole in the dura (Robbins et al 1995).

3. *'Double-barrel' needle* (Turner & Reifenberg 1995). These special needles were designed to ensure dural puncture is separated from epidural catheter placement. They are not in widespread use.

Combined spinal–epidural techniques have been the subject of an extensive review by Cook (2000). There is some concern about loss of the sense of proprioception (Buggy et al 1994) and the risk of meningitis (Harding et al 1994). The technique of CSEA in labour offers the advantage of being able to give a small initial intrathecal dose of local anaesthetic and opioid (2.5 mg bupivacaine and 25 µg fentanyl) which results in almost immediate onset of analgesia without loss of motor power. The intrathecal dose has a duration of approximately one hour and subsequent epidural top-up injections of dilute bupivacaine (15 ml 0.1%) and fentanyl (2 µg ml$^{-1}$) are then given. It is recommended that mothers are supervised and assisted by midwifery or auxiliary nursing staff when walking because of the possible risk of a fall. The high degree of mobility offered by this technique results in high maternal satisfaction, but it has yet to be determined whether it reduces the incidence of instrumental delivery or offers any other advantage over a low-dose epidural (Collis et al 1994, Price et al 1998).

## ANALGESIC DRUGS

## Local anaesthetic drugs

The pharmacology of the local anaesthetic drugs has been considered in Chapter 6.

### Lidocaine

Lidocaine at 1% concentration is most commonly used for local infiltration and peripheral blocks because of its rapid onset time. A dose of 300–500 mg of 2% lidocaine (15–30 ml) is necessary for epidural anaesthesia for Caesarean section. This is a large dose, which may produce systemic toxicity. For this reason, it is normally used with 1:200 000 epinephrine. This reduces the speed of absorption and, hence, the plasma concentration. Lidocaine is not suitable for continuous epidural analgesia in labour because it produces a high incidence of motor block. Lidocaine 2% *with or without* 1:200 000 epinephrine is still used in some centres as a 'test dose' and may also be used if epidural analgesia is to be converted to a more dense anaesthetic block in the event of Caesarean section or forceps delivery.

### Bupivacaine

Bupivacaine hydrochloride, which is a racemic mixture of the S and R isomers of the butyl form of the pipecholylxylidine group of local anaesthetics, is still the most commonly used drug for epidural analgesia in labour. Compared with lidocaine, bupivacaine causes significantly less motor block when given in equipotent doses and is therefore a better agent for use during labour. The onset time of bupivacaine is slower than lidocaine and the duration of action is longer, but these variables depend on the dose given.

### Levobupivacaine

The pure S isomer of bupivacaine is less cardiotoxic than the racemic mixture and is equipotent in terms of analgesia and motor block (Reynolds 1997). It is theoretically safer than racemic bupivacaine if a large dose is to be administered.

### Ropivacaine

Concern about the cardiotoxicity of racemic bupivacaine led to the 0.75% concentration (7.5 mg ml$^{-1}$) being withdrawn from epidural use in obstetrics, and a search for safer alternatives when profound neural block is required. Ropivacaine is the propyl form of the pipecholylxylidines and is produced as a single isomer (S). It is less cardiotoxic than bupivacaine and is available in 2 mg ml$^{-1}$ and 7.5 mg ml$^{-1}$ concentrations for use in obstetric epidural analgesia and anaesthesia (McClure 1996).

Ropivacaine also exhibits greater sensory–motor separation compared with equi-analgesic doses of bupivacaine (Zaric et al 1996). The reduced intensity of motor block seen with ropivacaine increases maternal mobility and satisfaction, and the likelihood of a spontaneous vertex delivery (Writer et al 1998).

## Chloroprocaine

Chloroprocaine 3% (20–25 ml) provides rapid onset of epidural anaesthesia within 5–10 minutes, should a rapid profound block be required. The duration of action is short (30–60 minutes) and additional top-up injections of an alternative local anaesthetic may be required as the block regresses. 2-chloroprocaine was associated with neurological toxicity when formulated with bisulphite as a preservative. A new bisulphite-free preparation with a high pH appears to have reduced this risk, but subarachnoid administration is still contraindicated because of the risk of neurotoxicity (Gissen et al 1984). Chloroprocaine is not available in the UK.

## Minimum local analgesic concentration (MLAC)

MLAC is a term introduced by Columb and Lyons (1995) to measure clinical potency and is considered equivalent to the $EC_{50}$, that is, the median concentration of a local anaesthetic that will provide adequate epidural analgesia in 50% of mothers during the first stage of labour. The measurement allows comparison of different drugs and the effect of adding other agents such as opioids. The MLAC increases as labour progresses and initial studies have shown that racemic bupivacaine is equipotent to levobupivacaine and that the MLAC of bupivacaine is reduced by the addition of fentanyl and sufentanil (Lyons et al 1998, Capogna et al 1998, Polley et al 1999).

The MLAC of ropivacaine is 40% greater than the MLAC of bupivacaine in the first stage of labour, but this observation is clinically irrelevant (Polley et al 1999). It is a drug's overall profile in terms of therapeutic indices which is important to the clinician. The relevant ratios in respect of a local anaesthetic are the analgesic/toxicity ratio and the analgesic/motor block ratio and, to date, these have not been directly compared (D'Angelo & James 1999).

## Opioids

It quickly became apparent that morphine and other opioids, when used alone, were insufficient to provide satisfactory analgesia in labour (Husemeyer et al 1980, Heytens et al 1987), and balanced epidural analgesia (a mixture of local anaesthetic and opioid) has been in use since the early 1980s. Epidural diamorphine

(Lowson et al 1995), meperidine (Perris & Malins 1981), fentanyl (Jones et al 1989) and sufentanil (Van Steenberge et al 1987, Russell & Reynolds 1993) are all currently used in combination with dilute bupivacaine in labour. Some anaesthetists favour the regular routine use of a combination to reduce the tendency to develop a progressive increase in motor block during CIEA or after a number of top-up injections. Others reserve the administration of opioid to improve a patchy block, a unilateral block or deficient sacral analgesia or to alleviate back pain. In the UK, the most commonly used epidural opioid is fentanyl, probably because it has featured the most frequently in published studies. It is used during labour as a bolus dose of 50 µg or up to 30 µg h$^{-1}$ by infusion.

## $\alpha_2$-adrenergic agonists

### Clonidine

Clonidine is an $\alpha_2$-adrenergic agonist and may be used in combination with epidural local anaesthetics and opioids (O'Meara & Gin 1993). Side-effects are sedation and hypotension, but these are minimal when the dose is limited to 50 µg (Claes et al 1998).

## INDICATIONS FOR EPIDURAL BLOCK IN LABOUR

### Pain relief

The primary indication for lumbar epidural analgesia in labour is the relief of pain, and for this it is unsurpassed. Barely 60% of women are satisfied with the pain relief afforded by carefully given parenteral and inhalational methods (Beazley et al 1967), but most centres which have established epidural services claim satisfactory analgesia in about 90% of cases. The pain from persisting O-P position requires either a greater spread of local anaesthetic within the epidural space to cover the sacral roots or the addition of an opioid to the local anaesthetic (Reynolds & O'Sullivan 1989).

### Pre-eclamptic toxaemia

The blood pressure of toxaemic patients is particularly sensitive to circulating catecholamines. Thus patients with mild, untreated pre-eclampsia may show abrupt increases in blood pressure, particularly during uterine contractions. Patients with more severe pre-eclampsia will have been controlled with antihypertensive drugs in the antenatal period, but the blood pressure may 'break through' this control during labour. However, it is a mistake to try to control the blood pressure with the epidural block alone and additional antihypertensive therapy is necessary.

## Vaginal breech delivery

Although obstetricians are increasingly favouring elective Caesarean section for breech presentations, some babies are still delivered vaginally. These patients sometimes have an uncontrollable urge to bear down before the cervix is fully dilated. This can cause severe oedema and bruising of the cervix, making delivery difficult. The main risk to the infant is damage to the after-coming head, which may be delivered precipitously through a tight pelvic floor, and this may result in intracranial haemorrhage if the infant is premature. Both these problems are admirably managed with epidural analgesia because it prevents uncontrolled bearing-down and the obstetrician can gently control delivery of the head. Earlier fears that epidural analgesia would increase the incidence of breech extraction, with its high incidence of morbidity and mortality, have proved to be unfounded.

## Multiple pregnancy

During vaginal delivery the second twin may be at risk from uterine inertia, cord compression or partial separation of the placenta, and modern obstetric opinion favours expediting its delivery. Oxytocin can be used to stimulate the flagging uterus, but if spontaneous delivery does not take place soon, forceps, an assisted breech delivery or even Caesarean section may be required. An effective epidural allows the obstetrician to proceed immediately with the method of his choice without the risks associated with general anaesthesia in these circumstances.

## Premature infants

Many of the above remarks about breech deliveries also apply to premature infants presenting by the vertex. Delivery tends to be precipitate and this increases the risk of intracranial haemorrhage. Epidural analgesia, by abolishing the bearing-down reflex, permits a slow, controlled delivery and avoids the need to give the mother systemic analgesics which may depress the premature infant.

## Diabetes mellitus

Diabetic mothers have reduced placental function and their babies consequently have a high perinatal mortality rate. If elective Caesarean section is not planned, labour is usually induced at 37–38 weeks and babies of diabetic mothers benefit from epidural anaesthesia for the same reasons as premature babies.

## Cardiovascular disease

It is impossible to generalise about heart disease because of the wide variety of congenital and acquired conditions that can be seen, and all cases should be discussed with a cardiologist, particularly those patients with fixed cardiac output conditions. However, if a patient is to have a vaginal delivery, most of the adverse factors are best treated by a carefully given lumbar epidural block, although the first dose of local anaesthetic should be small because hypotension is more likely. The block allows labour to be augmented without maternal distress and, when extended to the sacral segments, it prevents uncontrolled bearing-down in the second stage which can result in Valsalva manoeuvres. Furthermore, vasodilatation due to the epidural block helps to accommodate the increase in venous return which occurs in the third stage as caval occlusion is released and the uterus contracts after delivery. Oxytocin is a safer alternative to ergometrine in the second stage in these patients.

The obstetric anaesthetist is now seeing an increasing number of women who have artificial heart valves. Their cardiac function is often extremely good, but they are usually receiving long-term anticoagulant therapy in pregnancy, often with low molecular weight (LMW) heparin. The decisions as to when this therapy should be stopped and normal coagulation restored in labour, and when to allow central neural block to be performed, can only be made in close consultation with the obstetrician, haematologist and cardiologist.

The use of regional anaesthesia for Caesarean section in the rare patient with severe cardiac disease is contentious, and each case should be considered individually. Hypotension is much more likely with the high block required for surgery, particularly in fixed cardiac output conditions, and there may be sudden changes in haemodynamics. Many anaesthetists would consider light, muscle relaxant augmented general anaesthesia with full invasive cardiovascular monitoring the technique of choice for these patients.

## Respiratory disease

Few patients now come to the labour ward with severe disease of the lower respiratory tract. The most likely exceptions are those with asthma or an acute infection. These patients are likely to be very distressed during hyperventilation and Valsalva manoeuvres, and they find lumbar epidural analgesia very helpful.

For Caesarean section, mild respiratory disease has little effect on the choice between general and regional anaesthesia. In more severe cases, the choice depends largely on the degree of productive cough suffered by the patient. Although some might advocate regional block, general anaesthesia avoids the distress of being unable to cough effectively when the abdominal muscles are relaxed due to central neural block and when the abdomen is open during surgery. However, an epidural started at the end of the operation helps the patient to cough effectively afterwards.

## Inco-ordinate uterine action

This is a condition in which painful, but ineffective, uterine contractions produce slow dilatation of the cervix and, eventually, an exhausted patient. It is often associated with maternal vomiting, dehydration, ketosis and indications of fetal distress. Oxytocin administration, combined with epidural analgesia, may secure a vaginal delivery and save the patient an emergency Caesarean section (Moir & Willocks 1967, Maltau & Anderson 1975).

## CONTRAINDICATIONS TO EPIDURAL BLOCK IN LABOUR

It is customary to classify certain conditions as 'absolute' or 'relative' contraindications to epidural anaesthesia in obstetrics. 'Absolute' contraindications include a bleeding diathesis, whether iatrogenic or due to disease, refusal by the patient to accept the technique, skin sepsis near the needle entry site, and inadequate facilities for caring for the patient after the epidural has been performed. 'Relative' contraindications include conditions in which the risk–benefit ratio is less favourable than usual. Full explanation and discussion with the patient is essential.

## Bleeding diathesis

This is most commonly caused by anticoagulant therapy, but may also be due to a platelet or coagulation factor deficiency. The subject is considered fully in Chapter 7. LMW heparin presents a relatively new risk in obstetric epidural analgesia and each maternity unit should develop a strategy for managing the thrombophilic patient who has been taking LMW heparin during pregnancy (Horlocker & Wedel 1998).

## Hypotension and hypovolaemia

These conditions must always be treated, and the underlying cause determined, before an epidural is performed, since any sympathetic block reduces the patient's ability to compensate for them.

## Neurological disease

Multiple sclerosis is no longer considered to contraindicate epidural block in obstetrics though some neurologists still express anxiety about spinal anaesthesia (Bader et al 1988, Confavreux et al 1998). The evidence for central neural block causing an acute demyelinating episode is lacking and there seems no obvious reason why the epidural injection of local anaesthetic should worsen this condition. It seems unreasonable to deprive patients with static neurological disease the benefits of an epidural if it is indicated. However, a full explanation should be given to the patient and informed consent obtained. It is increasingly the case that the patient has researched the available literature in great detail beforehand.

## Previous back trouble or spinal surgery

There is no reason why epidural anaesthesia *per se* should exacerbate previous problems. However, the removal of bony landmarks during previous spinal surgery, or subsequent skin scarring, may make identification of the epidural space difficult. Access to operation notes and radiographs may be helpful in such cases. After spinal surgery – especially some types of spinal fusion – adhesions may form in the epidural space, making the spread and effectiveness of the local anaesthetic unpredictable, and this possibility should be fully discussed with the patient beforehand. However, Daley and colleagues (1990) have shown that epidural block is almost as effective in patients who have undergone lumbar spinal surgery as in those who have not. If the epidural block is inadequate or the epidural space cannot be found, a spinal may be successful.

## Uterine scar

A uterine scar from a previous hysterotomy or Caesarean section may rupture during labour. The use of epidural block in these cases is controversial because any pain associated with uterine rupture may be concealed. However, pain is a relatively rare warning of scar rupture, and other clinical features, such as fetal distress and vaginal bleeding, are more common. All such patients require meticulous maternal and fetal monitoring whether an epidural is used or not.

## MANAGING INCOMPLETE EPIDURAL ANALGESIA IN LABOUR

A strategy should be in place for ensuring rapid assessment and correction of inadequate analgesia. The upper and lower levels of the block should be defined and any evidence of unilateral spread or a missed segment noted. An additional top-up injection of local anaesthetic is then given, and this may include an opioid such as fentanyl (e.g. 15 ml of 0.1% bupivacaine and 30 μg fentanyl). The dressing over the puncture site should be inspected for leakage at this time and, in cases of unilateral spread, the mother should be encouraged to lie on her unblocked side, though the evidence that this is beneficial is poor (Merry et al 1983). The block should then be reassessed within 15 minutes, and if it is still deficient the catheter should be inspected at its point of insertion (a number are inadvertently pulled out). If a unilateral block persists, the catheter should be withdrawn 1–2 cm if this is feasible. A further top-up of local anaesthetic solution may be given at this stage (either the same dose or a stronger solution), but if all these measures fail the catheter should be resited.

## IMMEDIATE COMPLICATIONS OF EPIDURAL ANALGESIA

### Hypotension

The causes and management of hypotension are considered fully in Chapter 8. In obstetrics, it is important that aortocaval compression is avoided by utilising left lateral tilt or the full lateral position if necessary. Early use of a vasoconstrictor (e.g. boluses of intravenous ephedrine 3 mg or phenylephrine 20–40 μg) is recommended in addition to intravenous Hartmann's solution. Oxygen should be administered, particularly if there is fetal bradycardia.

## Dural puncture

Most maternity units quote an incidence of less than 1% for this unfortunate complication, but the puncture hole created by a Tuohy needle is likely to result in post-dural puncture headache in over 50% of obstetric patients. There are two strategies of management.

1. The needle is withdrawn and the epidural catheter resited at an adjacent interspace. Care should be taken to ensure the catheter has not entered the subarachnoid space through the hole created previously. An extensive block is sometimes observed, presumably due to local anaesthetic gaining access to the cerebrospinal fluid through the hole in the dura. A carefully observed test dose is essential after a dural puncture. The patient who has had a recognised dural tap with a Tuohy needle is a special case and is very likely to require a dural blood patch. An infusion of 0.9% saline into the epidural space, a high fluid intake and bed rest will help to control symptoms until this can be done.
2. The 'epidural' catheter may be threaded into the subarachnoid space and analgesia provided by continuous spinal anaesthesia. Small doses of local anaesthetic (2.5 mg bupivacaine, i.e. 1 ml of 0.25% solution) with or without opioid (12.5–25 μg fentanyl) are required to provide continuous analgesia. Only an anaesthetist should give these injections.

## Systemic toxicity

Toxicity secondary to a significant plasma concentration of local anaesthetic is most commonly due to accidental injection into an epidural vein. It is usually self-limiting, provided the injection of local anaesthetic is stopped immediately, but any specific problem should be treated quickly. General resuscitative measures include maintenance of the airway and placing the patient in the lateral or recovery position in order to avoid the risk of regurgitation and aspiration. Oxygen should be administered and convulsions controlled with a small dose of thiopental or midazolam. The epidural may be resited if the episode of systemic toxicity was brief and treatment was instituted quickly without having to resort to general anaesthesia and Caesarean section.

## Accidental total spinal block

This is a life-threatening emergency and requires prompt recognition and treatment to avoid permanent sequelae. Treatment consists of immediate administration of oxygen and assisted respiration with a tight fitting face-mask if necessary. Aortocaval compression should be relieved and cardiopulmonary resuscitation commenced if the mother is unconscious. The airway should be secured with tracheal intubation and consideration should be given to administering an intravenous induction agent to ensure unconsciousness. Bradycardia, if present, should be treated with atropine and the circulation supported with ephedrine (3 mg aliquots) or dilute epinephrine 1:100 000 (10 µg ml$^{-1}$) as an intravenous infusion. Emergency Caesarean section is indicated if there is a total spinal block as this condition presents a major risk to the mother and fetus. Respiratory and circulatory support, and general anaesthesia, should be maintained until the effects of the spinal anaesthetic begin to wear off.

## LATE COMPLICATIONS OF EPIDURAL ANAESTHESIA

### Backache

Retrospective surveys have found an association between epidural analgesia in labour and postpartum backache (MacArthur et al 1990, 1992, Russell et al 1993, MacLeod et al 1995) and, although the association was not confirmed in prospective cohort studies (Macarthur et al 1997, Russell & Reynolds 1998), most obstetric anaesthetists will warn mothers of this possibility. Backache is generally short-lived and may be related to poor posture during the second stage of labour with acute flexion of the hips and spine in the presence of motor and sensory block.

### Headache

Unfortunately, post-dural puncture headache (PDPH) has its highest incidence in women of child-bearing age, and newly delivered women are especially prone to this complication. A severe headache, which is worse when the patient is sitting or standing, is particularly distressing because it interferes with the mother's attempts to feed and care for her new baby. The incidence is related to spinal needle size, and is 3–10% in this population, even with 26 g needles. Smaller gauge needles have been produced (Carrie & Collins 1991), but they are more difficult to use (Flaatten et al 1989, Dahl et al 1990). Atraumatic or 'pencil-point' tip needles (24 g and 27 g) are now in common use and they have

reduced the incidence of PDPH to less than 2% (Cesarini et al 1990, Carrie & Donald 1991, Reid & Thorburn 1991). This is one reason why spinal anaesthesia has regained its popularity as the anaesthetic of choice for elective Caesarean section. However, the risk of PDPH has not been eliminated and it is reassuring to know that dural blood patch is an effective remedy if bed rest, increased fluid intake and analgesics are unsuccessful. All patients who have had central neural block should be followed-up the day after delivery. They should be aware of the small risk of headache and report it if it proves troublesome. Prevention is better than cure and good training in epidural and spinal anaesthetic techniques should reduce the risk.

## Neurological deficit

This requires expert neurological assessment, and care must be taken to exclude peripheral nerve injury due to an obstetrical cause (Scott & Hibbard 1990). It is crucial that any pre-existing neurological deficit is carefully documented, and the risk–benefit balance assessed, before a central neural block is performed.

## REGIONAL ANAESTHESIA FOR CAESAREAN SECTION

### Infiltration anaesthesia

Caesarean section can be performed under local infiltration, and large volumes (100 ml) of 0.5% lidocaine with 1:200 000 epinephrine may be used, although many would advocate doubling this volume and halving the concentration by adding an equal volume of 0.9% saline. However, in the developed world few obstetricians, and even fewer anaesthetists, have seen or administered infiltration anaesthesia for Caesarean section, although its use in the developing world may be life-saving. Careful infiltration of all layers of the abdomen using a 25 g spinal needle, and gentle surgical technique, are both absolute requirements. The midline skin, the subcutaneous tissues, the anterior, lateral and posterior rectus sheath, and the peritoneum should each be infiltrated as surgery progresses (Ranney & Stanage 1975). A Pfannenstiel incision is not appropriate for use with this technique because of the greater surgical dissection required.

**261**

## Central neural block

Aortocaval compression must be avoided at all times in the presence of widespread sympathetic block, secondary to epidural or spinal anaesthesia extending up to the midthoracic dermatomes. A solid or inflatable wedge (Carrie 1982) must be placed under a flank to ensure displacement of the uterus to the side.

A block extending from $T_6$ to $S_5$ is required for Caesarean section, but it is also essential that the neural block is complete and intense. The *extent* of epidural spread is generally easy to define by light pinprick or application of cold, but the *intensity* of block is more difficult to assess. Some indication of intensity of block may be given by observing the degree of motor block and the response to a vigorous pinch of the skin of the lower abdomen. Visceral sensation is never completely abolished because the peritoneum is innervated by the vagus nerves, which remain unblocked, and mothers should be warned that pressure and tugging sensations may be felt. Exteriorisation of the uterus after delivery should be avoided, particularly if epidural anaesthesia is used.

Compared with epidural anaesthesia, spinal (intrathecal) anaesthesia is more intense and extensive, and a more reliable sacral block is produced. For this reason, many obstetric units favour this technique for both elective and urgent Caesarean section, provided that severe fetal distress is not present. A significant number of labour epidurals are intensified by topping-up with concentrated local anaesthetic to allow Caesarean section to proceed in the event of fetal distress or failure to progress in labour.

### Spinal anaesthesia

A dose of 2.5–3.0 ml of heavy bupivacaine, given at the $L_3$–$L_4$ interspace, will provide the midthoracic block necessary for Caesarean section. The patient should be in the sitting or lateral position for the injection, then turned to the supine wedged position immediately afterwards. It is crucial that the upper part of the thoracic spine remains higher than the point of injection of the hyperbaric solution when the patient is either in the lateral or supine wedged position. This is in order to ensure that the local anaesthetic spreads into the lowest part ($T_6$) of the thoracic curve of the spine, but does not extend cephalad to the upper thoracic or cervical regions. The gradient of the upper part of the thoracic spine can be increased by placing a pillow under the

shoulders and two or three pillows under the head. A small dose of opioid, for example 300 μg diamorphine, may be added to improve postoperative pain control, provided an appropriate level of patient care and monitoring is available after surgery. Spinal block to the $T_6$ level should also be obtained for a trial of forceps delivery because emergency Caesarean section may be necessary if the trial fails.

Some anaesthetists still prefer to use 2.5–3.0 ml of plain bupivacaine, though the range of upper dermatomal spread is wider and the extent of the block is therefore unpredictable (Carrie & O'Sullivan 1984). Spinal anaesthesia, because of its speed of onset, may also be used for emergency Caesarean section, provided that profound fetal distress is not present. The decision requires full discussion of the degree of urgency with the obstetrician. Spinal anaesthesia may now be the technique of choice for Caesarean section in severe pre-eclampsia (Hood & Curry 1999, Sharwood-Smith et al 1999), but if the patient has received a therapeutic dose of magnesium, hypotension may result. Magnesium can be antagonised by calcium and the hypotension usually responds to ephedrine (James 1998).

### Combined spinal–epidural anaesthesia (CSEA)

This combines the advantages of two central blocks: rapid onset of a dense block from the spinal, and continuous anaesthesia or analgesia from the epidural. Three CSEA techniques are described earlier in this chapter. The intrathecal dose used in CSEA can be smaller than that used for spinal anaesthesia alone because it is supplemented, and eventually superseded, by epidural drug administration. This results in a reduced incidence of hypotension. The risk of intrathecal placement of the epidural catheter should always be considered and only small, divided doses of local anaesthetic should be given (Robbins et al 1995).

## Epidural anaesthesia

Epidural anaesthesia may be used for elective Caesarean section, and an epidural already in use for analgesia may be augmented in the event of a Caesarean section, forceps delivery or manual removal of placenta being required. If an epidural is being started *de novo*, a minimum of 30 minutes should be allowed between its insertion and the start of surgery. A shorter period of time may suffice if a dense block has developed during labour, perhaps as a result of a long-running continuous infusion. However, the current practice is to provide less intense epidural block during labour so plenty of time should be allowed for the development of a block adequate for surgery.

The drugs most commonly used for epidural anaesthesia are 0.5% bupivacaine or 2% lidocaine with 1:200 000 epinephrine (Howell et al 1990). Fentanyl at 50–75 µg is often added (Noble et al 1991). Recently, 7.5 mg ml$^{-1}$ ropivacaine has become available and it also provides good surgical anaesthesia (Irested et al 1997, Morton et al 1997). The risk of systemic toxicity dictates that all large doses of local anaesthetic should be preceded by a test dose and given incrementally. A suitable regimen consists of a 5 ml test dose followed by three, 5 ml aliquots of 0.5% bupivacaine, or 2% lidocaine with epinephrine. The total volume can be reduced, depending on the intensity of block seen during labour.

A total dose of 20 ml of 7.5 mg ml$^{-1}$ ropivacaine has been found to give good conditions for Caesarean section with less risk of cardiotoxicity than a comparable dose of bupivacaine (Irested et al 1997, Morton et al 1997). Levobupivacaine is also less cardiotoxic than racemic bupivacaine (Bader et al 1999). The addition of an epidural opioid improves the quality of the block achieved with local anaesthetic alone. Some anaesthetists vary the position of the patient with each increment in order to ensure spread, but it is doubtful if this is necessary (Norris & Dewan 1987).

## Immediate complications

### Hypotension

Hypotension may be sudden in onset, particularly after spinal anaesthesia and may cause severe nausea and vomiting in the mother. The risk can be reduced by careful positioning to ensure there is adequate lateral tilt and elevation of the head and shoulders on pillows. This prevents spread of heavy bupivacaine to the upper thoracic spine. Many anaesthetists administer 500 ml to 1 litre of crystalloid and/or prophylactic intravenous ephedrine (Gutsche 1976, Kang et al 1982) in mothers who are not pre-eclamptic.

### Respiratory distress or depression

A potential disadvantage of spinal anaesthesia is the possibility of respiratory distress or depression due to an extensive block. In the non-pregnant patient, even a block which produces paralysis of all the intercostal muscles leaves the innervation of the diaphragm ($C_3$–$C_5$) unaffected, and consequently the patient has adequate respiratory reserve. However, in the recumbent, pregnant patient at term the gravid uterus may hinder diaphragmatic respiration. In addition, paralysis of the abdominal muscles reduces the ability to cough effectively and may produce respiratory distress or embarrassment (Gamil 1989). In practice this only proves a problem in the patient with significant respiratory disease or a chronic cough with copious sputum production.

### Inadequate block

If the block is found to be inadequate before surgery, and time is available, a further dose of local anaesthetic may be given, for example 5 ml of 0.5% bupivacaine, 2% lidocaine with epinephrine or 7.5 mg ml$^{-1}$ ropivacaine. The risk of systemic toxicity must always be considered, but the use of an incremental administration technique and awareness of the total recommended dose of each local anaesthetic drug should reduce this risk to a minimum. Alternatively, the epidural block may be replaced or supplemented by a spinal anaesthetic. A reduced dose of spinal anaesthetic drug compared to that used in spinal anaesthesia *de novo* is generally required.

If the block is found to be inadequate during surgery, a strategy should be used that is familiar to the anaesthetist and agreed beforehand with the patient. Any discomfort which is not tolerated by the patient should result in immediate induction of general anaesthesia. Depending on the degree of discomfort, further local anaesthetic can be given through the epidural catheter or local infiltration of a safe dose of anaesthetic carried out by the obstetrician. Oxygen and nitrous oxide can be given by face-mask, and isoflurane may be added if necessary. An opioid such as fentanyl can be given intravenously with appropriate warning to the paediatrician if it is administered before delivery. There is no place for a benzodiazepine unless the mother is without pain and is merely anxious.

# References

Aitkenhead AR, Hothersall AP Gilmour DG, Ledingham IMcA 1979 Dural dimpling in the dog. Anaesthesia 34: 14–19

Amiel-Tison C, Barrier G, Shnider S, Levinson G, Hughes SC, Stefani SJ 1982 A new neurologic and adaptive capacity scoring system for evaluating obstetric medications in full-term newborns. Anesthesiology 56: 340–350

Bader AM, Hunt CO, Datta S, Naulty JS, Ostheimer GW 1988 Anesthesia for the obstetric patient with multiple sclerosis. Journal of Clinical Anesthesia 1: 21–24

Bader AM, Tsen LC, Camann WR, Nephew E, Datta S 1999 Clinical effects and maternal and fetal plasma concentrations of 0.5% epidural levobupivacaine versus bupivacaine for Cesarean delivery. Anesthesiology 90: 1596–1601

Brockhurst NJ, Littleford JA, Halpern SH 2000 The neurologic and adaptive capacity score. A systematic review of its use in obstetric anesthesia research. Anesthesiology 92: 237–246

Brownridge P 1981 Epidural and subarachnoid analgesia for elective Caesarean section. Anaesthesia 36: 70

Buggy D, Hughes N, Gardiner J 1994 Posterior column sensory impairment during ambulatory extradural analgesia in labour. British Journal of Anaesthesia 73: 540–543

Capogna D, Celleno D, Lyons G, Columb M, Fusco P 1998 Minimum local analgesic concentration of extradural bupivacaine increases with the progression of labour. British Journal of Anaesthesia 80: 11–13

Carrie LES 1982 An inflatable obstetric anaesthetic 'wedge'. Anaesthesia 37: 745–747

Carrie LES 1990 Extradural, spinal and combined block for obstetric surgical anaesthesia. British Journal of Anaesthesia 65: 225–233

Carrie LES, Collins PD 1991 29-gauge spinal needles. British Journal of Anaesthesia 66: 145–146

Carrie LES, Donald F 1991 A 26-gauge pencil-point needle for combined-epidural anaesthesia for Caesarean section. Anaesthesia 46: 230–231

Carrie LES, O'Sullivan GM 1984 Subarachnoid bupivacaine 0.5% for Caesarean section. European Journal of Anaesthesia 1: 275–283

Cesarini M, Torrielli R, Lahaye F, Mene JM, Cabiro C 1990 Sprotte needle for intrathecal anaesthesia for Caesarean section: incidence of postdural puncture headache. Anaesthesia 45: 656–658

Cibils LA 1976 Response of human uterine arteries to local anesthetics. American Journal of Obstetrics and Gynecology 126: 202–210

Claes B, Soetens M, Van Zundert A, Datta S 1998 Clonidine added to bupivacaine–epinephrine–sufentanil improves epidural analgesia during childbirth Regional Anesthesia and Pain Management 23: 540–547

Collis RE, Baxandall ML, Srikantharajah ID, Edge G, Kadim MY, Morgan BM 1994 Combined spinal epidural (CSE) analgesia; technique, management, and outcome in 300 mothers. International Journal of Obstetric Anesthesia 3: 75–81

Collis RE, Davies DWL, Aveling W 1995 Randomised comparison of combined spinal–epidural and standard epidural analgesia in labour. The Lancet 345: 1413–1416

Collis RE, Plaat FS, Morgan BM 1999 Comparison of midwife top-ups, continuous infusion and patient-controlled epidural analgesia for maintaining mobility after a low-dose combined spinal–epidural. British Journal of Anaesthesia 82: 233–236

Columb MO, Lyons G 1995 Determination of the minimum local analgesic concentrations of epidural bupivacaine and lidocaine in labor. Anesthesia and Analgesia 81: 833–837

Confavreux C, Hutchinson M, Hours MM, Cortinovis-Tourniaire P, Moreau T 1998 Rate of pregnancy-related relapse in multiple sclerosis. Pregnancy in Multiple Sclerosis Group. New England Journal of Medicine 339: 285–291

Cook TM 2000 Combined spinal–epidural techniques. Anaesthesia 55: 42–64

Dahl JB, Schultz P, Anker-Moller E, Christensen EF, Staunstrup HG, Carlsson P 1990 Spinal anaesthesia in young patients using a 29-gauge needle: technical considerations and an evaluation of postoperative complaints compared with general anaesthesia. British Journal of Anaesthesia 64: 178–182

Daley MD, Rolbin SH, Hew EM, Morningstar BA, Stewart JA 1990 Epidural anesthesia for obstetrics after spinal surgery. Regional Anesthesia 15: 280–284

D'Angelo R, James RL 1999 Is ropivacaine less potent than bupivacaine? Anesthesiology 90: 941–943

Datta S, Lambert DH, Gregus J, Gissen AJ, Covino BG 1983 Differential sensitivities of mammalian nerve fibers during pregnancy. Anesthesia and Analgesia 62: 1070–1072

Dickson MAS, Moores C, McClure JH 1997 Comparison of single, end-holed and multi-orifice extradural catheters when used for continuous infusion of local anaesthetic during labour. British Journal of Anaesthesia 79: 297–300

Fagraeus L, Urban BJ, Bromage PR 1983 Spread of epidural analgesia in early pregnancy. Anesthesiology 58: 184–187

Flaatten H, Rodt SA, Vamnes J, Rosland J, Koller ME 1989 Postdural puncture headache. A comparison between 26- and 29-gauge needles in young patients. Anaesthesia 44: 147–149

Galbert MW, Marx GF 1974 Extradural pressures in the parturient patient. Anesthesiology 40: 449–502

Gambling DR, McMorland GH, Yu P, Lazlo G 1988 A comparison of patient-controlled epidural analgesia and intermittent 'top-ups' during labour. Anesthesia and Analgesia 35: 249–254

Gamil M 1989 Serial peak expiratory flow rates in mothers during Caesarean section under extradural anaesthesia. British Journal of Anaesthesia 62: 415–418

Gissen AJ, Datta S, Lambert D 1984 The chloroprocaine controversy. II. Is chloroprocaine neurotoxic? Regional Anesthesia 9: 135–145

Greiss FC, Still JG, Anderson SG 1976 Effects of local anesthetic agents on the uterine vasculature and myometrium. American Journal of Obstetrics and Gynecology 124: 889–898

Gutsche B 1976 Prophylactic ephedrine preceding spinal analgesia for Cesarean section. Anesthesiology 45: 462–465

Halpern SH, Leighton BL, Ohnsson A, Barrett JF, Rice A 1998 Effect of epidural vs parenteral opioid analgesia on the progress of labor: a meta-analysis. Journal of the American Medical Association 280: 2105–2110

Harding SA, Collis RE, Morgan BM 1994 Meningitis after combined spinal–extradural anaesthesia in obstetrics. British Journal of Anaesthesia 73: 545–547

Heytens L, Cammu H, Camu F 1987 Extradural analgesia during labour using alfentanil. British Journal of Anaesthesia 59: 331–337

Hingson RA, Edwards WB 1943 Continuous caudal analgesia. An analysis of the first ten thousand confinements thus managed with the report of the authors' first thousand cases. Journal of the American Medical Association 123: 538–546

Hollmen A I, Jouppila R, Koivisto M et al 1978 Neurological activity of infants following anesthesia for Caesarean section. Anesthesiology 48: 350–356

Hollmen AI, Jouppila R, Jouppila P, Koivula A, Vierola H 1982 Effect of extradural analgesia using bupivacaine and 2-chloroprocaine on intervillous blood flow during normal labour. British Journal of Anaesthesia 54: 837–842

Holmes F 1960 Incidence of the supine hypotensive syndrome in late pregnancy. A clinical study in 500 subjects. Journal of Obstetrics and Gynaecology 67: 274–275

Hood DD, Curry R 1999 Spinal versus epidural anesthesia for cesarean section in severely pre-eclamptic patients; a retrospective survey. Anesthesiology 90: 1276–1282

Horlocker TT, Wedel DJ 1998 Spinal and epidural blockade and perioperative low molecular weight heparin: Smooth sailing on the Titanic. Anesthesia and Analgesia 86: 1153–1156

Howell P, Davies W, Wrigley M, Tan P, Morgan B 1990 Comparison of four local extradural anaesthetic solutions for elective Caesarean section. British Journal of Anaesthesia 65: 648–653

Husemeyer RP, O'Connor MC, Davenport HT 1980 Failure of epidural morphine to relieve pain in labour. Anaesthesia 35: 161–163

Hutchins CJ 1980 Spinal analgesia for instrumental delivery. A comparison with pudendal nerve block. Anaesthesia 35: 376–377

Irestedt L, Emanuelsson B-M, Ekblom A, Olofsson C, Reventlid H 1997 Ropivacaine 7.5 mg/ml for elective Caesarean section. A clinical and pharmacokinetic comparison of 150 mg and 187.5 mg. Acta Anaesthesiologica Scandinavica 41: 1149–1156

Jackson R, Reid JA, Thorburn J 1995 Volume preloading is not essential to prevent spinal induced hypotension at Caesarean section. British Journal of Anaesthesia 75: 262–265

James MFM 1998 Magnesium in obstetric anaesthesia. International Journal of Obstetric Anesthesia 7: 115–123

Jones G, Paul DL, Elton RA, McClure JH 1989 Comparison of bupivacaine and bupivacaine with fentanyl in continuous extradural analgesia during labour. British Journal of Anaesthesia 63: 254–259

Jouppila R, Jouppila P, Kuikka J, Hollmen A 1978a Placental blood flow during Caesarean section under lumbar extradural analgesia. British Journal of Anaesthesia 50: 275–279

Jouppila R, Jouppila P, Hollmen A, Kuikka J 1978b Effect of segmental extradural analgesia on placental blood flow during normal labour. British Journal of Anaesthesia 50: 563–567

Kang YG, Abouleish E, Caritis S 1982 Prophylactic intravenous ephedrine infusion during spinal anesthesia for Cesarean section. Anesthesia and Analgesia 61: 839–842

Kerr MG, Scott DB, Samuel E 1964 Studies of the inferior vena cava in late pregnancy. British Medical Journal 1: 532–533

Kinsella SM, Whitwam JG, Spencer JA 1992 Reducing aortocaval compression: how much is enough? British Medical Journal 305: 539–540

Kreis O. 1900 Uber Medullarnarkose bei Gebarenden. Zentralbl F Gynaekol 24: 724

Lees MM, Scott DB, Kerr MG, Taylor SH 1967 The circulatory effects of recumbent postural change in late pregnancy. Clinical Science 32: 453–465

Lowson SM, Eggers KA, Warwick JP, Moore WJ, Thomas TA 1995 Epidural infusions of bupivacaine and diamorphine in labour. Anaesthesia 50: 420–422

Lyons G, Columb M, Wilson RC, Johnson RV 1998 Epidural pain relief in labour: potencies of levobupivacaine and racemic bupivacaine. British Journal of Anaesthesia 81: 899–901

Macarthur AJ, Macarthur C, Weeks SK 1997 Is epidural anesthesia in labor associated with chronic low back pain? A prospective cohort study. Anesthesia and Analgesia 85: 1066–1070

MacArthur C, Lewis M, Knox EG, Crawford JS 1990 Epidural anaesthesia and long term backache after childbirth. British Medical Journal 301: 9–12

MacArthur C, Lewis M, Knox EG 1992 Investigation of long-term problems after obstetric epidural anaesthesia. British Medical Journal 304: 1279–1282

MacLeod J, Macintyre C, McClure JH, Whitfield A 1995 Backache and epidural analgesia. A retrospective survey of mothers 1 year after childbirth. International Journal of Obstetric Anesthesia 4: 21–25

McClure JH 1996 Ropivacaine. British Journal of Anaesthesia 76: 300–307

Maltau JM, Anderson HT 1975 Epidural anaesthesia as an alternative to Caesarean section in the treatment of prolonged exhaustive labour. Acta Anaesthesiologica Scandinavica 19: 349–354

Merry AF, Cross JA, Mayadeo SV, Wild CJ 1983 Posture and the spread of extradural analgesia in labour. British Journal of Anaesthesia 55: 303–307

Moir DD, Willocks J 1967 Management of inco-ordinate uterine action under continuous epidural analgesia. British Medical Journal iii: 396–400

Morgan BM 1995 'Walking' epidurals in labour. Anaesthesia 50: 839–840

Morton CJ, Bloomfield S, Magnusson A, Jozwiak H, McClure JH 1997 Ropivacaine 0.75% for extradural anaesthesia in elective Caesarean section: An open clinical and pharmacokinetic study in mother and neonate. British Journal of Anaesthesia 79: 3–8

Murphy JD, Henderson K, Bowden MI, Lewis M, Cooper GM 1991 Bupivacaine versus bupivacaine plus fentanyl for epidural analgesia: effect on maternal satisfaction. British Medical Journal 302: 564–567

Noble DW, Morrison LM, Brockway MS, McClure JH 1991 Epinephrine, fentanyl or epinephrine and fentanyl as adjuncts to bupivacaine for extradural anaesthesia in elective Caesarean section. British Journal of Anaesthesia 66: 645–650

Norris MC, Dewan DM 1987 Effect of gravity on the spread of extradural anaesthesia for Caesarean section. British Journal of Anaesthesia 59: 338–341

O'Meara ME, Gin T 1993 Comparison of 0.125% bupivacaine with 0.125% bupivacaine and clonidine as extradural analgesia in the first stage of labour. British Journal of Anaesthesia 71: 651–656

Park WY 1988 Factors influencing the distribution of local anaesthetics in the epidural space. Regional Anesthesia 13: 49–57

Perris BW, Malins AF 1981 Pain relief in labour using epidural pethidine and epinephrine. Anaesthesia 36: 631–633

Polley LS, Columb MO, Naughton NN, Wagner DS, Cosmas JMV 1999 Relative analgesic potencies of ropivacaine and bupivacaine for epidural analgesia in labor. Anesthesiology 90: 944–950

Price C, Lafreniere L, Brosnan C, Findley I 1998 Regional analgesia in early active labour: combined spinal–epidural vs. epidural. Anaesthesia 53: 951–955

Purdie J, Reid J, Thorburn J, Asbury AJ 1992 Continuous extradural analgesia: Comparison of midwife top-ups, continuous infusions and patient controlled administration. British Journal of Anaesthesia 68: 580–584

Ramanathan S, Grant GJ 1988 Vasopressor therapy for hypotension due to epidural anesthesia Caesarean section. Acta Anaesthesiologica Scandinavica 32: 559–565

Ramanathan S, Masih A, Rock I, Chalon J, Turndorf H 1983 Maternal and fetal effects of prophylactic hydration with crystalloids or colloids before epidural anesthesia. Anesthesia and Analgesia 62: 673–678

Ramanathan S, Friedman S, Moss P, Arisnendy J, Turndorf H 1984 Phenylephrine for the treatment of maternal hypotension due to epidural anesthesia. Anesthesia and Analgesia 63: 262

Ranney B, Stanage WF 1975 Advantages of local anesthesia for Cesarean section. Obstetrics and Gynecology 45: 163–167

Reid JA, Thorburn J 1991 Headache after spinal anaesthesia. British Journal of Anaesthesia 67: 674–677

Reports on Confidential Enquiries into Maternal Deaths in the United Kingdom. 1985–96 Four Triennial Reports. HMSO & TSO, London

Reynolds F 1997 Does the left hand know what the right hand is doing? An appraisal of single enantiomer local anaesthetics. International Journal of Obstetric Anesthesia 6: 257–269

Reynolds F, O'Sullivan G 1989 Epidural fentanyl and perineal pain in labour. Anaesthesia 44: 341–344

Robbins PM, Fernando R, Lim GH 1995 Accidental intrathecal insertion of an extradural catheter during combined spinal–extradural anaesthesia for Caesarean section. British Journal of Anaesthesia 75: 355–357

Russell R, Reynolds F 1993 Epidural infusions for nulliparous women in labour. A randomised double-blind comparison of fentanyl/bupivacaine and sufentanil/bupivacaine. Anaesthesia 48: 856–861

Russell R, Reynolds F 1996 Epidural infusion of low-dose bupivacaine and opioid in labour. Does reducing motor block increase the spontaneous delivery rate? Anaesthesia 51: 266–273

Russell R, Reynolds F 1998 Epidural analgesia and chronic backache. Anesthesia and Analgesia 87: 747–748

Russell R, Groves P, Taub N, O'Dowd J, Reynolds F 1993 Assessing long-term backache after childbirth. British Medical Journal 306: 1299–1303

Scanlon JW, Brown WU, Weiss JB, Alper MH 1974 Neurobehavioral responses of newborn infants after maternal epidural anesthesia. Anesthesiology 40: 121–128

Scott DB, Hibbard BM 1990 Serious non-fatal complications associated with extradural block in obstetric practice. British Journal of Anaesthesia 64: 537–541

Sharwood-Smith G, Clark V, Watson E 1999 Regional anaesthesia for Caesarean section in severe pre-eclampsia: spinal anaesthesia is the preferred choice. International Journal of Obstetric Anesthesia 8: 85–89

Simpson JY 1848 Local anaesthesia, notes on its production by chloroform etc. in the lower animals and in man. Lancet ii 39–42

Soresi AL 1937 Episubdural anesthesia. Anesthesia and Analgesia 16: 306–310

Stoeckel W 1909 Uber sakrale Anaesthesie. Zentralbl F Gynaekol 33: 1

Taylor JC, Tunstall ME 1991 Dosage of phenylephrine in spinal anaesthesia for Caesarean section. Anaesthesia 46: 314–316

Thorburn J, Moir DD 1981 Extradural analgesia: the influence of volume and concentration of bupivacaine on the mode of delivery, analgesic efficacy and motor block. British Journal of Anaesthesia 53: 933–939

Turner MA, Reifenberg NA 1995 Combined spinal–epidural anaesthesia. The single space double-barrel technique. International Journal of Obstetric Anesthesia 4: 158–160

Usubiaga JE, Wikinski JA, Usubiaga LE 1967 Epidural pressure and its relation to spread of anaesthetic solutions in the epidural space. Anesthesia and Analgesia 46: 440–446

Van Steenberge A, Debroux HC, Noorduin H 1987 Extradural bupivacaine with sufentanil for vaginal delivery. British Journal of Anaesthesia 59: 1518–1522

Writer WDR, Stienstra R, Eddleston JM et al 1998 Neonatal outcome and mode of delivery after epidural analgesia for labour with ropivacaine and bupivacaine: a prospective meta-analysis. British Journal of Anaesthesia 81: 713–717

Zaric D, Nydahl P, Philipson L, Samuelsson L, Heierson A, Axelsson K 1996 The effect of continuous lumbar epidural infusion of ropivacaine ( 0.1%, 0.2% and 0.3% ) and 0.25% bupivacaine on sensory and motor blockade in volunteers – a double-blind study. Regional Anesthesia 21: 14–25

# 19. Regional anaesthesia in children

## A R Lloyd-Thomas

Regional anaesthesia is now firmly placed at the heart of paediatric anaesthesia (Aynsley-Green et al 1995, de Lima et al 1996). However, it differs from adult practice in that it is almost always performed in combination with general anaesthesia rather than as an alternative to it. Indeed, as a general rule, it would be neither safe nor possible to attempt regional blocks in the awake child.

### NEUROBIOLOGY OF PAIN

In outline, the pain pathway is much the same in children as in adults (see Ch. 3). However, there are important functional differences.

- The receptive fields of individual neurones may be much larger (Fitzgerald 1994), implying less accurate pain localisation in the immature nervous system.
- Activity in non-nociceptive fibres (A$\delta$) can, in the neonate, activate neurones in dorsal horn laminae which are predominantly nociceptive in the adult (Jennings & Fitzgerald 1996).
- Descending inhibitory pathways are less well developed, allowing unmodulated nociceptive input to the spinal cord (Kar & Quirion 1995).
- There may be differences in the proportion of subclasses of opioid receptors in neonates, and this may contribute to their reduced ability to modulate nociceptive transmission (Andrews & Fitzgerald 1994).

The above factors suggest that younger patients may experience more pain than adults. In addition, it is very likely that later response to pain in children can be affected adversely by previous inadequate control of pain, for example, during and after circumcision (Taddio et al 1995, 1997). All of this information argues strongly for the use of regional anaesthesia, whenever possible, in the anaesthetic management of children.

Injury results in repetitive C-fibre activation which, through spinal cord NMDA and neurokinin receptors, gives rise to the development of secondary hyperalgesia, increasing the patient's perception of pain (Wall 1988). Regional anaesthesia will reduce this C-fibre activity, thereby inhibiting the development of hyperalgesia (LaMotte et al 1991).

### LOCAL ANAESTHETIC PHARMACOLOGY

In general terms, the principles of local anaesthetic pharmacology outlined in Chapters 4–6 apply as much to children as adults. However, several reports of toxicity (Ved et al 1993, Maxwell et al 1994), especially in association with continuous infusion (Agarwal et al 1992, Berde 1992, McCloskey et al 1992, Larsson et al 1994), indicate that children, particularly neonates and infants, need separate consideration.

#### Metabolism and clearance

There is a paucity of data on the metabolism of local anaesthetic drugs in neonates, but what information there is suggests that the capacity of the liver to deal with these drugs is limited in comparison with older children (Eyres 1995). The elimination half-lives of the local anaesthetics are longer in neonates and infants than in adults (Mazoit et al 1988). This is true of bupivacaine, even though its clearance is relatively greater, because its volume of distribution is also much larger (Weston & Bourchier 1995).

#### Risk of toxicity

The risk of toxicity after a local anaesthetic injection is dependent upon many factors (Ch. 5 & 6), no matter what the age of the patient, but some specific ones need to be considered, especially in the very young. Most obviously, there is the problem of adjusting the dose used to the size of the patient, even without allowing for the impact of certain physiological differences. Rate of rise of plasma concentration is proportional to cardiac output which is higher (relatively) in neonates, and this effect will be increased by the slower metabolism noted above. The immaturity of the blood–brain barrier (Eyres 1995) may be relevant, although the practice of performing blocks *after* the administration of general anaesthesia will obscure the early features of systemic toxicity.

Whatever the underlying factors, there is no doubt that plasma concentrations are influenced by the age of the recipient, and concentrations of local anaesthetics associated with the risk of toxicity have been reported after ilio-inguinal and caudal block in infants, despite apparently conservative doses (Smith et al 1996, Luz et al 1998). Although the actual plasma concentration is not the only factor in the generation of toxicity, the general principle of using conservative doses in young patients should be followed. With this approach, 'single shot' injections are likely to be safe, but cumulation remains a significant hazard in neonates and infants receiving continuous infusions (Cheung et al 1997, Peutrell et al 1997).

## Treatment of toxicity

Systemic toxicity from local anaesthetic drugs results in progressive depression of central nervous and cardiovascular systems with readily recognisable symptoms and signs (Table 19.1). However, the prior administration of general anaesthesia means that there will be no obvious warning features, and that cardiac arrhythmias or cardiovascular collapse may be the first manifestation of toxicity. Extrasystoles, broadening of the QRS complex,

ventricular tachycardia and fibrillation may all occur, especially with the longer acting agents (De la Coussaye et al 1992, Maxwell et al 1994) (Table 19.1).

Basic life support, with correction of any acidosis, is the first stage of management. Central nervous toxicity (convulsions) can be treated with diazepam or midazolam, but a short period of neuromuscular block, with ventilatory support, may help to reduce the acidaemia consequent upon convulsive activity (Dalens 1995). By contrast, cardiovascular toxicity is more difficult to treat. Bupivacaine toxicity is complex and several therapeutic options have been described, including epinephrine, bretylium and amiodarone (Eyres 1995). Intravenous phenytoin 5 mg kg$^{-1}$, repeated at 5 min intervals to a maximum of 15 mg kg$^{-1}$, has been effective in aborting bupivacaine-induced ventricular tachyarrhythmias in two neonates (Maxwell et al 1994).

## Prevention of toxicity

Attention to technique and use of appropriate doses (see below) should ensure the lowest risk of local anaesthetic toxicity, and some important general principles regarding the performance of regional blocks in children are worth emphasising (see Table 19.2). The value of a test dose is reduced by the concurrent administration of general anaesthesia, which also reduces the sensitivity of epinephrine as a test-dose marker (Desparmet et al 1990). Slow careful injection with repeated aspiration is the hallmark of good practice. Ropivacaine (Ivani et al 1998) and levobupivacaine may produce less cardiovascular toxicity and further data are required on the side-effects of these drugs in young patients.

---

**Table 19.1** Signs of central nervous system toxicity from local anaesthetic drugs (Peutrell & Hughes 1995)

| Early signs | Late signs |
|---|---|
| • Somnolence | • Perioral paraesthesiae |
| • Heaviness of the head | • Tinnitus |
| • Impaired postural control | • Visual disturbance |
| | • Dysarthria |
| | • Convulsions |

---

**Table 19.2** Basic recommendations for the safe conduct of local anaesthetic injections in children

1. Aspirate prior to each injection
2. Evaluate the effect of a test dose of 0.5–1.0 ml, containing epinephrine*
3. Inject slowly over a period of approximately 90 seconds
4. Repeat aspirations should be performed during the course of the injection
5. Stop the injection if any abnormal signs or symptoms occur

***Do not** use epinephrine injections when contraindicated, e.g. dorsal penile block, digital block or other extremity block where vasoconstriction may result in ischaemia.

## Local anaesthetic doses in children

Making recommendations about 'safe' doses in children is difficult. Adult recommendations are based on the results of clinical studies, but these are relatively rare in children, particularly across the whole paediatric population range from the neonate to the teenager. Age, body weight and height have all been used as a basis for dosage, but weight has generally been adopted as the standard. However, the uncritical application of 'ml kg$^{-1}$' regimens has potential pitfalls, which have been emphasised in Chapters 5 and 6.

## PERIPHERAL TECHNIQUES

### Topical application

The eutectic mixture of local anaesthetics (EMLA) is an oil-in-water emulsion of equal amounts of the base forms of lidocaine and prilocaine. In this formulation these agents can penetrate the skin and produce cutaneous analgesia. EMLA cream has to be applied to the skin for at least 1 hour to be fully effective (Arendt-Nielsen & Bjerring 1988), but it enables venepuncture to be performed painlessly in almost every case, and it has made this procedure much less traumatic for both child and anaesthetist. EMLA has also been used for neonatal circumcision, skin grafts and the insertion of grommets through the eardrum in older children.

Amethocaine gel (4%) is an alternative to EMLA and has the advantage of a more rapid onset time – 30 to 60 minutes (Dunnett 1996).

## Wound infiltration

In neonates and infants, wound infiltration is very valuable for reducing the requirement for deep anaesthesia and postoperative analgesia (Shenfield et al 1995) and, in older children undergoing ambulatory surgery, it can be as reliable as peripheral or central blocks. A dose of 1.25 mg kg$^{-1}$ bupivacaine (0.5 ml kg$^{-1}$ of 0.25% solution, or 0.25 ml kg$^{-1}$ of 0.5% solution) should not be exceeded (see Ch. 5).

## Peripheral nerve blocks

Peripheral blocks (Table 19.3) are the mainstay of analgesic management for paediatric ambulatory surgery. They are suitable for peripheral or body surface surgery (e.g. paraumbilical block for umbilical hernia repair) (Courreges et al 1997). They also avoid the dangers and side-effects of central block. For example, plexus and compartment blocks provide good unilateral analgesia, maintain sensory and motor function in the contralateral limb and avoid disturbing urinary function.

Peripheral blocks require special care in children because the child under general anaesthesia cannot give warning of needle trauma to the nerve or intraneural injection. The use of a short-bevelled needle

**Table 19.3** Dose ranges of local anaesthetic agents for various common blocks. The upper limits quoted should not be exceeded

| Block name | Dose of bupivacaine 0.25% | Block | Operations |
|---|---|---|---|
| Axillary | 0.4–0.6 ml kg$^{-1}$ | Brachial plexus | Arm and hand surgery |
| Intercostal | Max 0.8 ml kg$^{-1}$ with 1:200 000 epinephrine | Intercostal 1–6 Intercostal 6–12 | Thoracotomy Abdominal surgery |
| Inguinal | 0.4–0.6 ml kg$^{-1}$ | Ilio-inguinal Iliohypogastric | Inguinal hernia Orchidopexy |
| Penile | 0.2 ml kg$^{-1}$ | Dorsal penile | Circumcision Meatoplasty |
| Femoral | 0.4–0.6 ml kg$^{-1}$ | Femoral | Femoral fracture Surgery to femur |
| Fascia iliaca compartment | 0.8 ml kg$^{-1}$ | Femoral Obturator Lateral cutaneous | Femoral surgery |

improves the 'feel' as it is advanced through the tissues, while a short extension catheter between the syringe and needle prevents dislodgment of the needle when solution is injected.

## Ilio-inguinal–iliohypogastric block

The needle is inserted at a point one quarter of the distance along a line from the anterior superior iliac spine to the umbilicus. It is advanced until loss of resistance is felt, indicating penetration of the external oblique aponeurosis. Local anaesthetic is injected with the needle directed laterally towards the iliac crest and then medially towards the inguinal ligament. A second injection may be made lateral to the pubic tubercle. Alternatively, a spinal needle can be inserted through the block needle and advanced subcutaneously to the same point. Injection on withdrawal of the needle will deposit local anaesthetic along the line of the incision.

## Penile block

The penis is drawn downwards, the pubic symphysis identified and the skin marked on either side, 0.5–1.0 cm from the midline, at the root of the penis. From these points, the needle is directed medially and caudally, inferior to the pubic ramus, until there is a characteristic 'give' as Scarpa's fascia is pierced. This will be at a depth of 0.5–3.0 cm, depending upon the size of the patient. A *plain* solution of local anaesthetic *must* be used. There should be no resistance to injection. This block is unsuitable for major penile surgery such as hypospadias and it is less reliable than a caudal epidural injection for circumcision.

## Axillary brachial plexus block

The artery is immobilised between two fingers of the non-dominant hand and a needle is advanced until it enters the axillary sheath. This may be very difficult to detect in infants.

Several hours of analgesia may be produced by a single injection of bupivacaine, but if prolonged analgesia is required, a conventional 22 g intravenous cannula can be inserted. It is advanced towards the axillary artery until it is judged to be just short of the vessel. It should then be in the sheath and, if correctly positioned, it will be easy to advance. Any resistance indicates inaccurate placement. An infusion of bupivacaine 0.125%, 0.25–0.5 mg kg$^{-1}$ h$^{-1}$ (0.2–0.4 ml kg$^{-1}$ h$^{-1}$), can be continued as long as necessary.

The supraclavicular approach to the plexus should only be undertaken by anaesthetists with considerable experience. Other standard upper limb blocks can be performed as needed in children (see Dalens 1995).

## Lower limb blocks

Blocks of the femoral nerve (McNicol 1986), fascia iliaca compartment (Doyle et al 1997), lateral cutaneous nerve of thigh (McNicol 1986), sciatic nerve (McNicol 1985) and other standard peripheral lower limb blocks can all be performed in children. However, they are very specialised techniques and caudal epidural injection is probably more reliable in less experienced hands.

## Intercostal block

Percutaneous intercostal blocks are technically easy to perform, but they are associated with the very significant risk of pneumothorax, especially in children less than 10 years old. Moreover, the failure rate may be as high as 25%. They may be used for the placement of chest drains and for inpatients with fractured ribs. They should be performed in the mid-axillary line, where the inner intercostal muscles separate the nerve from the parietal pleura, so that the likelihood of pneumothorax is reduced. They should only be performed by experienced practitioners.

A safer and more reliable technique is to place an epidural catheter adjacent to the intercostal neurovascular bundle, under direct vision, at the time of operation. This is especially useful following surgery for the harvesting of costal cartilage. A loading dose of bupivacaine 0.25% at 1.25 mg kg$^{-1}$ (0.5 ml kg$^{-1}$), is followed by an infusion of bupivacaine 0.125% at 0.25 mg kg$^{-1}$ h$^{-1}$ (0.2 ml kg$^{-1}$ h$^{-1}$). See also Table 19.3.

## Interpleural block

This can be used in cases where analgesia of the thoracic cavity is required (for which peripheral blocks would be inadequate), but where there may be concerns about performing thoracic epidural block, for example, in neonates and infants. The percutaneous approach cannot be recommended because there is a significant risk of pneumothorax (Dalens 1995), but a catheter can be placed under direct vision by the surgeon (Tobias et al 1993b). Absorption of local anaesthetic is rapid after interpleural block so there is real potential for systemic toxicity. However, Giaufrc and colleagues (1995), using an infusion of bupivacaine 0.1% at a rate of

0.5–1.0 ml kg$^{-1}$ h$^{-1}$ for up to 48 hours, were able to provide satisfactory analgesia, with no signs of toxicity. Other infusion regimens have been described (Stayer et al 1995, Semsroth et al 1996).

A single-dose regimen can also be effective. Weston and Bourchier (1995) gave a single interpleural dose of bupivacaine at 2 mg kg$^{-1}$ to very-low-birth-weight babies and obtained good analgesia without producing toxic plasma concentrations. It is vital to the success of inter-pleural block that the catheter is correctly sited at the time of operation (it must be well away from chest drains) and that the patient is in the supine position, so that local anaesthetic collects in the paravertebral gutter, which lies just lateral to the paravertebral space. At this point, the intercostal nerve is immediately posterior to the pleura (Fig. 19.1), and the local anaesthetic has only a short distance to diffuse to exert its effect.

## Paravertebral block

This technique is useful for chest surgery, and it has also been shown to be as effective as epidural block for renal surgery in children (Lonnquist & Olsson, 1994). It has the advantage that there is no risk of spinal cord trauma, but pneumothorax and spinal anaesthesia are possible complications. Diffusion of local anaesthetic to the epidural space occurs in up to 70% of cases and this may be an important site of action (Purcell-Jones et al 1989).

The patient should be placed prone and a line drawn between the two thoracic spinous processes at the level to be blocked. A second, parallel line is drawn, on the side to be blocked, at a distance equal to the space between the two spinous processes. A short-bevelled, or Tuohy, needle of appropriate size is inserted on this line at a point level with the inferior border of the upper spinous process, and advanced until loss of resistance to liquid is felt (Fig. 19.1). A single injection may be made or a catheter inserted through the needle. Alternatively, the catheter can be introduced under direct vision by the surgeon at thoracotomy (Karmakar et al 1996).

Eng and Sabanathan (1992) infused 0.5% bupivacaine at a rate of 0.2 ml kg$^{-1}$ h$^{-1}$ for up to 5 days in children between the ages of 7 and 16 years who had undergone thoracotomy, and obtained excellent analgesia. However, this dose rate (equivalent to 1 mg kg$^{-1}$ h$^{-1}$) would result in significant accumulation and toxicity if used in neonates or infants. Indeed, Karmakar and colleagues (1996) reported potentially toxic plasma concentrations

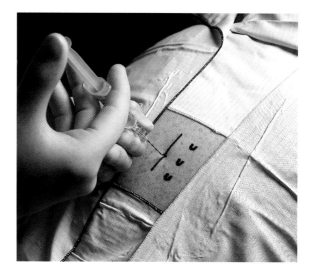

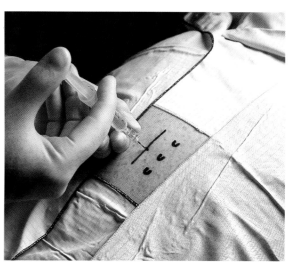

**Fig 19.1** (A) Needle insertion for paravertebral block in a child. (B) Location of paravertebral space by loss of resistance to liquid

of up to 3.14 μg ml$^{-1}$ in infants who received half that dose for up to 48 hours, so a further reduction in dosage is clearly necessary in this age group. Cheung and colleagues (1997) found that plasma concentrations remained within safe limits in neonates and infants when bupivacaine 0.125% with epinephrine 1:400 000 was infused at a rate of 0.25 mg kg$^{-1}$ h$^{-1}$, (0.2 ml kg$^{-1}$ h$^{-1}$), but the analgesia was less effective, with up to 18% of patients needing opioid supplements. Nevertheless, it is better to accept the need for supplementation than to risk local anaesthetic toxicity.

## CENTRAL TECHNIQUES

Caudal epidural block has been widely used in paediatric practice for many years, but only since the late 1980s have the lumbar and thoracic approaches to the epidural space gained in popularity. However, all specialised UK paediatric centres now use continuous epidural analgesia routinely, even in neonates and infants (de Lima et al 1996). These central blocks provide excellent pain control – and this is their main advantage – but they may, in addition, reduce the stress response to surgery (Wolf et al 1993) and improve postoperative respiratory function. The latter may be of value in high-risk neonates and infants undergoing major surgery.

## Caudal block

### Equipment

A 21 g, 38 mm cannula allows easy injection from a 10 or 20 ml syringe and is long enough to reach the sacrococcygeal ligament in all but the most obese child. The 23 g, 25 mm size is more suitable for neonates and small infants. Needles of corresponding size may be used if a single injection is all that is required. Dalens and Hasanaoui (1989) found that use of the short-bevelled design resulted in the lowest incidence of intravascular placement, but this was not confirmed in a subsequent study (Newman et al 1996).

### Technique

The child is turned into the left lateral position (for the right-handed anaesthetist). Accurate location of the sacral cornua is essential for success, and it is important to realise that these bony protuberences, which represent the unfused laminae of the fifth sacral segment, appear to be more cephalad than in the adult. They are palpated best by moving the left thumb up and down across the base of the sacrum (Fig. 19.2) and they can be thought of as forming the base of an isosceles triangle whose apex points cephalad. The apex is formed by the fusion of the sacral bones in the midline and the area of the triangle is filled by the sacrococcygeal ligament (Fig. 19.3).

When the cornua have been identified, the thumb is moved cephalad so that it lies over the apex of the triangle. The cannula is inserted immediately caudad to the thumb at an angle of about 40° (Fig. 19.4), and when it has penetrated the skin and subcutaneous fat it meets the resistance of the sacrococcygeal ligament. As it passes through the ligament into the sacral canal, a distinct loss of resistance is felt. The cannula should be inserted close to the apex of the triangle because the sacral cavity is comparatively deep at that point and it is easier to appreciate that the cavity has been entered. The cannula may then be advanced gently up the sacral canal. However, if a needle is used, no attempt should be made to advance it because this increases the risk of intravascular placement.

If blood appears at the hub, the cannula should be withdrawn until the flow ceases, and the lumen cleared with saline. Aspiration may then produce blood-stained saline, but as long as frank blood does not appear, local anaesthetic may be injected. If a needle is used, aspiration tests for blood sometimes give false negative results because the vessel wall is sucked onto the needle bevel. This risk can be minimised by the prior injection of 1 ml of solution to distend the vein, followed by

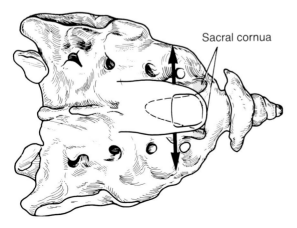

**Fig 19.2** Identification of sacral cornua using sideways movement of the thumb

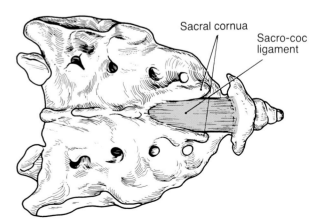

**Fig 19.3** Sacrococcygeal ligament

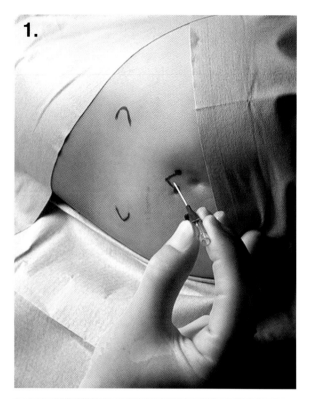

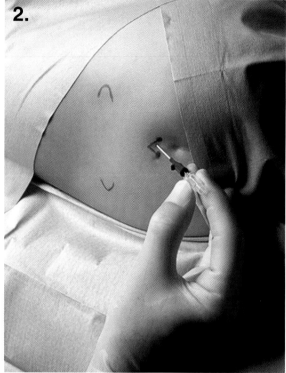

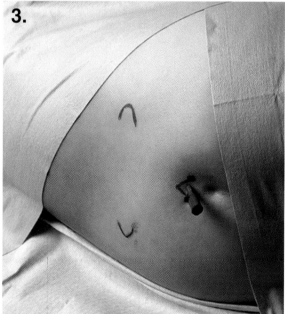

Fig 19.4   Cannula insertion for caudal block in a child

The dose regimen for paediatric caudal anaesthesia is well established (Table 19.4). Recently, $2\,mg\,kg^{-1}$ of ropivacaine ($1.0\,ml\,kg^{-1}$ of 0.2% solution) has been used by single caudal injection and was found to have a longer duration of action than bupivacaine (Ivani et al 1998). As well as being highly effective, the technique has a good safety record, the incidence of complications (0.7 per 1000 cases), being the lowest for any central block (Giaufre et al 1996).

The straighter spinal column and less dense packing of the epidural space by fat and fibrous tissue allows catheters to be threaded up to the thoracic region from gentle aspiration. The appearance of blood is not an indication for abandoning the block as long as the needle or cannula can be repositioned satisfactorily.

| Table 19.4  Paediatric caudal dosages | | |
|---|---|---|
| | Loading dose bupivacaine 0.25% plain (ml kg$^{-1}$) | Infusion dose bupivacaine 0.125% plain (ml kg$^{-1}$ h$^{-1}$) |
| **Neonates** | | |
| Low (L$_5$ – S$_5$) | 0.5 | 0.16–0.2 |
| High (T$_{12}$ – S$_5$) | 0.8 | 0.16–0.2 |
| **Infants & Children** | | |
| Low (L$_5$ – S$_5$) | 0.6 | 0.32–0.4 |
| High (T$_{12}$ – S$_5$) | 0.8–1 | 0.32–0.4 |

the sacral hiatus. This provides thoracic segmental analgesia, yet avoids the hazards associated with introducing a needle at the thoracic level (Bosenberg et al 1988). In the immature sacrum, the epidural space may also be reached by an $S_2$–$S_3$ intervertebral approach (Busoni & Sarti 1987).

## Epidural block

The epidural space may be approached by the lumbar or thoracic routes in children and is popular for a wide range of paediatric surgery (Dalens & Chrysostome 1991, Porter 1993, Tobias et al 1993a, Webster et al 1993, Luz et al 1996, Peutrell et al 1997).

### Identifying the epidural space

The technique for identification of the epidural space has been the subject of much debate in the literature, following reports of complications associated with the use of air for loss of resistance (LOR) (Sethna & Berde 1993). Dalens and Chrysostome (1991) noted incomplete analgesia after LOR to air, but more serious sequelae, including fatalities possibly secondary to venous air embolism, have been reported by Flandin-Blety and Barrier (1995) in a retrospective survey of epidural analgesia in paediatric patients. In a review of adult practice, Saberski and co-workers (1997) identified wide-ranging complications (pneumocephalus, spinal cord and nerve root compression, subcutaneous emphysema, venous air embolism, incomplete analgesia and paraesthesia) after the use of air. However, in many of the cases cited in both these papers there were basic failures of technique which, if avoided, could have prevented the complications described. Nevertheless, in paediatric practice, air does present potential hazards not seen in adults. It is easier to inject rapidly relatively large volumes, and the incidence of venous air embolism is known to be associated with both the volume injected and the rate of injection (Sethna & Berde 1993). Moreover, intracardiac communications with variable right-to-left shunt (the foramen ovale is patent in 50% of children up to 5 years of age) allow air to cross into the arterial circulation. The low venous epidural pressure makes detection of inadvertent venous cannulation difficult, so air can enter the circulation readily, even when the injection pressure is low. The only disadvantage to saline is that it can make dural puncture harder to detect, but well-described methods exist for confirmation in cases of doubt. Provided that standard techniques

are followed carefully, and repeated attempts to identify the epidural space are avoided, the incidence of complications related to venous air embolism is low, but avoiding air injection altogether will minimise the risk of accidents.

The prevention of inadvertent dural puncture requires not only a sensitive method for detecting loss of resistance, but also a careful technique because the epidural space in neonates and infants may be as little as 5 mm from the skin (Hasan et al 1994). Dural puncture is rare in experienced hands, but if it does occur, postdural puncture headache may require treatment with a dural blood patch. In children, persistent cerebrospinal fluid leakage may present with atypical symptoms such as orthostatic nausea and dizziness (McHale & O'Donovan 1997).

### Equipment

Packs specially designed for paediatric use are commercially available (Portex, UK). The 18 g and 19 g, Huber tip, Tuohy needles are 50 mm long and have graduations at 5 mm intervals. The '18 g' catheter has the standard three helically placed eyes. This design has a much lower incidence of kinking and occlusion, and is now used in all ages (Fig. 19.5). Technical complications are common during postoperative infusions

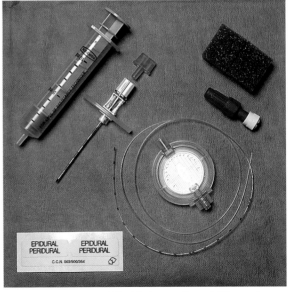

**Fig 19.5** Half-length 18 g Tuohy needle and 21 g catheter for paediatric epidural analgesia

when catheters with a single end hole are used (Lloyd-Thomas & Howard 1994).

## Technique

The narrowness of the epidural space in the child influences the approach to it and the method of needle insertion. The paramedian approach with cephalad angulation is preferred because the needle enters the epidural space obliquely and the risk of dural puncture is reduced. The landmarks and technique (Fig. 19.6) are the same as for the adult (see Ch. 11). Epidural catheters should be sited as close as possible to the dermatomes to be blocked in order to ensure effective anaesthesia. This can be difficult to achieve in children, but is vital if an epidural infusion is to be used in the postoperative period, especially if local anaesthetics are to be infused without supplementation (Berde 1994). Infusions should not exceed the maximum recommendations in Table 19.5 . Attempts to compensate for a catheter which is less than ideally placed by increasing the infusion rate is hazardous. If analgesia is inadequate an opioid supplement should be added.

## Dosage

**Loading doses** Berde (1992) has outlined safe loading doses for epidural administration (Table 19.5). Unlike

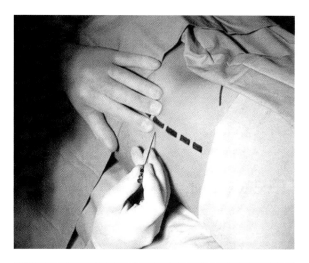

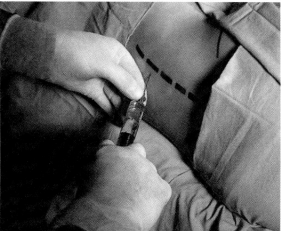

**Fig 19.6** Epidural needle insertion using the paramedian approach in a child

the situation in adults, haemodynamic stability is the norm during the onset of an epidural block in children up to the age of 8–10 years (Murat et al 1987), and left ventricular function, as assessed by M-mode echocardiography, is unaffected. However, mild decreases in mean blood pressure and heart rate may be seen (Tsuji et al 1996).

**Continuous infusions** A regimen for these is given in Table 19.5. During epidural bupivacaine infusions, linear pharmacokinetics are seen for up to 50 hours, after which marked increases in plasma concentrations can occur. These rapid increases may be seen much earlier in infants (6–12 hours) if high infusion rates are used. In young infants, even an infusion of bupivacaine 0.25% at 0.38 mg kg$^{-1}$ h$^{-1}$ (0.15 ml kg$^{-1}$ h$^{-1}$), may result

**Table 19.5** Dose ranges[a] of local anaesthetic for epidural use (Berde 1992, Eyres 1995)

| | Loading dose bupivacaine 0.25% plain (ml kg$^{-1}$) | Infusion dose bupivacaine 0.125% plain (ml kg$^{-1}$ h$^{-1}$) |
|---|---|---|
| **Neonates** | | |
| Lumbar | 0.8–1 | 0.16–0.2 |
| Thoracic | 0.8 | 0.16–0.2 |
| **Infants & Children**[b] | | |
| Lumbar | 0.8–1 | 0.32–0.4 |
| Thoracic | 0.8 | 0.32–0.4 |

[a]The dose actually used should be the lowest consistent with adequate analgesia and should be titrated to the desired clinical effect. The upper limits quoted should not be exceeded. Epinephrine (1:200 000) given with the loading dose will minimise peak plasma concentrations of local anaesthetic.
[b]Infants and children are best managed with a mixture of local anaesthetic and opioid. Preservative-free morphine (10 μg ml$^{-1}$) should be added to the infusate. The morphine infusion rate should not exceed 5 μg kg$^{-1}$ h$^{-1}$

in significant accumulation after 32 hours (Peutrell et al 1997).

The better toxicity profile of ropivacaine should give this agent an advantage in epidural analgesia. However, Moriarty (1997) found that an epidural infusion of ropivacaine 0.25%, given at 0.8–1.6 mg kg$^{-1}$ h$^{-1}$ (0.3–0.6 ml kg$^{-1}$ h$^{-1}$), was unsatisfactory as a sole analgesic (supplementary paracetamol and NSAIDs were required), although the absence of motor block was an advantage. Further data on this drug is awaited.

### Epidural opioids

The addition of an opioid to an epidural infusion can enhance the quality of analgesia. Successful segmental analgesia with lipophilic opioids (e.g. fentanyl) requires that the catheter tip lies adjacent to the dermatomes to be blocked (Berde 1994), and unless this can be achieved, it is not segmentally effective (Campbell et al 1992). In contrast, hydrophilic opioids such as morphine enter the cerebrospinal fluid (CSF), so catheter position is less critical (Rosen & Rosen, 1989). In paediatric epidurals therefore, where it is difficult to be certain of the catheter position, preservative-free morphine may be the logical choice.

Morphine (Rosen & Rosen 1989), diamorphine (Lloyd-Thomas 1993) and fentanyl (Wood et al 1994) are the opioids most studied in children. In a randomised study, Kart and co-workers (1997) found that a bupivacaine/fentanyl infusion gave better analgesia than intermittent morphine injections, and the incidence of side-effects was similar for both techniques. It has been shown that local anaesthetics are an essential component in the control of movement-induced pain (Dahl et al 1992), and the lack of bupivacaine in the morphine group may account for the analgesic differences described. However, in another study (Carr et al 1998), the addition of bupivacaine to fentanyl was not found to enhance analgesia.

The disadvantage of epidural opioids is the increase in unwanted effects, such as urinary retention, pruritus, nausea, vomiting and respiratory depression (Wilson & Lloyd-Thomas 1993; Wood et al 1994, Kart et al 1997). The likelihood of side effects is increased in older children, especially urinary retention (Lloyd-Thomas 1993). The impact of side-effects can be minimised by restricting the opioid dose, ensuring adequate post-operative fluids, using naloxone early (for pruritus and retention, 0.5 µg kg$^{-1}$ repeated at 10 min intervals to a maximum of 2 µg kg$^{-1}$) and catheterising older children at the time of operation (Berde 1994).

The incidence of respiratory depression in patients receiving epidural opioids is less than 1% when management is by a pain control team (Lloyd-Thomas & Howard 1994), although sedation and slight reduction in respiratory rate are more common (6.5%). Infusion analgesia probably has a more predictable effect on respiration than large intermittent bolus doses (Bozkurt et al 1997). Not all opioids are effective as supplements to epidural blocks. For example, tramadol has little effect when given with bupivacaine for hypospadias repair (Prosser et al 1997).

When epidural opioid infusions are used in children, a dose of morphine given at 5 µg kg$^{-1}$ h$^{-1}$ or fentanyl at 0.4 µg kg$^{-1}$ h$^{-1}$ should not be exceeded (Berde 1994).

### Complications

Carefully conducted regional anaesthesia is effective and safe (Giaufre et al 1996). However, as any technique increases in popularity, complications will be observed and reported ( Cohen et al 1993, Dunwoody et al 1997, Larsson et al 1997, McHale & O'Donovan 1997, Meunier et al 1997).

Nurses must be aware that sensory block increases the risk of *compression neuropraxia*, and frequent turning should be part of the nursing care of all patients with epidural blocks (Cohen et al 1993).

The possibility that *compartment syndrome* may be masked by an epidural block has been a long-standing concern in orthopaedic surgery (Dunwoody et al 1997). The author's personal approach to this problem is to administer an epidural for the surgery, but to use intra-venous morphine (patient or nurse controlled) in the postoperative period.

Although the overall incidence of infection is very low (Strafford et al 1995), *epidural abscess* is a cause for concern (Larsson et al 1997, Meunier et al 1997). Epidural catheter puncture points must be inspected regularly and antibiotic therapy given, and the catheter removed, at the first sign of infection.

## Spinal block

Spinal anaesthesia has gained in popularity for infants of less than 44 weeks postconceptual age – a group known to be at risk of postoperative apnoea after general anaesthesia (Malviya et al 1993). The incidence of this complication can be reduced by the use of spinal anaesthesia, though apnoea can still occur (Tobias et al 1998). The success rate of spinal anaesthesia in these patients is variable, with some authors reporting a need for supplementation (general anaesthesia or ketamine) in up to 45% of patients (Webster et al 1991). However, if supplementation is given, the advantage of the spinal is lost because the risk of apnoea becomes the same as if a full general anaesthetic had been administered.

Spinal anaesthesia has the advantage of producing low plasma concentrations of local anaesthetic, with consequent minimal risk of systemic toxicity (Beauvoir et al 1996).

### Technique

Skin at the intended puncture site should be anaesthetised by either topical application or local infiltration. The insertion of a paediatric lumbar puncture needle of appropriate size may be facilitated by making first a small incision in the skin. Kokki and colleagues (1998) found that hyperbaric bupivacaine (0.5% in 8% glucose) at a dose of 0.3–0.5 mg kg$^{-1}$ (0.06–0.1 ml kg$^{-1}$) gave a higher success rate than the same dose of the isobaric solution, but tetracaine 1% at 0.8 mg kg$^{-1}$ (0.08 ml kg$^{-1}$) (Webster 1991) is probably better than either, owing to its longer duration of action (Mahe & Ecoffey 1988).

Spinal anaesthesia has also been described for use in older children (Kokki et al 1998).

## $\alpha_2$-adrenoceptor agonists and NMDA antagonists

Increased understanding of spinal cord 'wind-up' phenomena and the development of hyperalgesia has focused interest on producing analgesia with $\alpha_2$-adrenoceptor agonists and NMDA antagonists.

### Clonidine

There is a close correlation between analgesia and the lumbar CSF concentration of clonidine, with 0.130 µg ml$^{-1}$ required for adequate analgesia when it is used as the sole agent (Eyres 1995). A much lower dose of clonidine is effective when combined with other analgesics. Caudal epidural clonidine at 1 µg kg$^{-1}$ (Jamali et al 1994), 1.5 µg kg$^{-1}$ (Constant et al 1998) or 2 µg kg$^{-1}$ (Lee & Rubin 1994, Cook et al 1995) combined with local anaesthetics, will double the duration of analgesia when compared to local anaesthesia alone. The place of this drug in paediatric analgesia is not yet clear, but for further information the reader is referred to more detailed sources (Hayashi & Maze 1993, Eisenach et al 1996, Kamibayashi & Maze 1996, Sandler 1996).

### Ketamine

In children, epidural administration of preservative-free ketamine (0.5 mg kg$^{-1}$), an NMDA antagonist, increased the duration of caudal analgesia (bupivacaine 0.25%), measured as the time to first request for analgesia, from a median of 3.2 hours to 12.5 hours (Cook et al 1995). Increasing the dose of preservative-free ketamine to 1 mg kg$^{-1}$ further prolonged the analgesia (16.5 hours), but at the expense of behavioural side-effects (Semple et al 1996). There is no clinical evidence of serious behavioural side-effects when doses of less than 500 µg kg$^{-1}$ are employed.

## CONCLUSION

Regional anaesthesia has 'come of age' in paediatric anaesthesia with many children benefiting from sophisticated management. Now that the basic techniques have been validated, the next step will be to refine the drug combinations to produce optimal analgesia.

## References

Agarwal R, Gutlove DP, Lockhart CH 1992 Seizures occuring in pediatric patients receiving continuous infusion of bupivacaine. Anesthesia and Analgesia 75: 284–286

Andrews K, Fitzgerald M 1994 The cutaneous withdrawal reflex in human neonates: sensitization, receptive fields, and the effects of contralateral stimulation. Pain 56: 95–101

Arendt-Nielsen L, Bjerring P 1988 Laser-induced pain for evaluation of local analgesia: a comparison of topical application (EMLA) and local injection (Lidocaine). Anesthesia and Analgesia 67: 115–123

Aynsley-Green A, Lloyd-Thomas AR, Ward-Platt MP 1995 Paediatric pain. In: Aynsley-Green A, Ward-Platt MP, Lloyd-Thomas AR (eds.) Clinical paediatrics: stress and pain in infancy and childhood, 3 edn, pp. ix–xi. Ballière, London

Beauvoir C, Rochette A, Desch G, D'Athis F 1996 Spinal anaesthesia in newborns: total and free bupivacaine plasma concentration. Paediatric Anaesthesia 6: 195–199

Berde CB 1992 Convulsions associated with pediatric regional anesthesia. Anesthesia and Analgesia 75: 164–166

Berde CB 1994 Epidural analgesia in children. Canadian Journal of Anaesthesia 41: 555–560

Bosenberg AT, Bland BAR, Schulte-Steinberg O, Downing JW (1988) Thoracic epidural anesthesia via caudal route in infants. Anesthesiology 69: 265–269

Bozkurt P, Kaya G, Yeker Y 1997 Single-injection lumbar

epidural morphine for postoperative analgesia in children. Regional Anesthesia 22: 212–217

Busoni P, Sarti A 1987 Sacral intervertebral epidural block. Anesthesiology 67: 993–995

Campbell FA, Yentis SM, Fear DW, Bissonnette B. 1992 Analgesic efficacy and safety of a caudal bupivacaine–fentanyl mixture in children. Canadian Journal of Anaesthesia 39: 661–664

Carr AS, Fear DW, Sikich N, Bissonnette B 1998 Bupivacaine 0.125% produces motor block and weakness with fentanyl epidural analgesia in children. Canadian Journal of Anaesthesia 45: 1054–1060

Cheung SLW, Booker PD, Franks R, Pozzi M 1997 Serum concentrations of bupivacaine during prolonged continuous paravertebral infusion in young infants. British Journal of Anaesthesia 79: 9–13

Cohen DE, Van Duker B, Siegel S, Keon TP 1993 Common peroneal nerve palsy associated with epidural analgesia. Anesthesia and Analgesia 76: 429–431

Constant I, Gall O, Gouyet L, Chauvin M, Murat I 1998 Addition of clonidine or fentanyl to local anaesthetics prolongs the duration of surgical analgesia after single shot caudal block in children. British Journal of Anaesthesia 80: 294–298

Cook B, Grubb DJ, Aldridge LA, Doyle E 1995 Comparison of the effects of adrenaline, clonidine and ketamine on the duration of caudal analgesia produced by bupivacaine in children. British Journal of Anaesthesia 75: 698–701

Courreges P, Poddevin F, Lecoutre D 1997 Para-umbilical block: a new concept for regional anaesthesia in children. Paediatric Anaesthesia 7: 211–214

Dahl JB, Rosenberg J, Hansen BL, Hjortso N-C, Kehlet H 1992 Differential analgesic effects of low-dose epidural morphine and morphine–bupivacaine at rest and during mobilization after major abdominal surgery. Anesthesia and Analgesia 74: 362–365

Dalens B 1995 Regional anesthesia in infants, children and adolescents, 1st edn. Williams and Wilkins/Waverley Europe, London

Dalens B, Chrysostome Y 1991 Intervertebral epidural anaesthesia in paediatric surgery: success rate and adverse effects in 650 consecutive procedures. Paediatric Anaesthesia 1: 107–117

Dalens B, Hasanaoui A 1989 Caudal anesthesia in pediatric surgery: success rate and adverse events in 750 consecutive patients. Anesthesia and Analgesia 68: 83–89

De la Coussaye JE, Brugada J, Allessia MA 1992 Electrophysiological and arrythmogenic effects of bupivacaine. Anesthesiology 77: 132–141

de Lima J, Lloyd-Thomas AR, Howard RF, Sumner E, Quinn TM 1996 Anaesthetists perceptions of and prescribing for infant and neonatal pain. British Medical Journal 313: 787

Desparmet J, Mateo J, Ecoffen C, Mazoit X 1990 Efficacy of an epidural test dose in children anesthetized with halothane. Anesthesiology 72: 249–251

Doyle E, Morton NS, McNicol LR 1997 Plasma bupivacaine levels after fascia iliaca compartment block with and without adrenaline. Paediatric Anaesthesia 7: 121–124

Dunnett SR 1996 A study to compare the speed of onset, degree and duration of anaesthesia produced by Ametop Gel, EMLA cream and placebo gel in negroid skin type. In: Wolfsen AD, McCafferty DF (eds) Amethocaine Gel – a New Development in Effective Percutaneous Local Anaesthesia, 1st edn, pp. 52–59. RSM Press, London

Dunwoody JM, Reichert CC, Brown KL 1997 Compartment syndrome associated with bupivacaine and fentanyl epidural. Journal of Pediatric Orthopedics 17: 285–288

Eisenach JC, De Kock M, Klimscha W 1996 Alpha2-adrenergic agonists for regional anesthesia. A clinical review of clonidine (1984–1995). Anesthesiology 85: 655–674

Eng J, Sabanathan S 1992 Continuous paravertebral block for post-thoracotomy analgesia in children. Journal of Pediatric Surgery 27: 556–557

Eyres RL 1995 Local anaesthetic agents in infancy. Paediatric Anaesthesia 5: 213–218

Fitzgerald M 1994 Neurobiology of fetal and neonatal pain. In: Wall, P.D. and Melzack, R., (eds) Textbook of Pain, 3rd edn, pp. 153–163. Churchill Livingstone, London

Flandin-Blety C, Barrier G 1995 Accidents following extradural analgesia in children. The results of a retrospective study. Paediatric Anaesthesia 5: 41–46

Giaufre E, Gruguerolle B, Rastello C, Coquet M, Lorec AM 1995 New regimen for interpleural block in children. Paediatric Anaesthesia 5: 125–128

Giaufre E, Dalens B, Gombert A 1996 Epidemiology and morbidity of regional anesthesia in children: a one-year prospective survey of the French-Language Society of Paediatric Anesthesiologists. Anesthesia and Analgesia 83: 904–912

Hasan MA, Howard RF, Lloyd-Thomas AR 1994 Depth of epidural space in children. Anaesthesia 66: 1085–1086

Hayashi Y, Maze M 1993 Alpha2 adrenoceptor agonists and anaesthesia. British Journal of Anaesthesia 71: 108–118

Ivani G, Mereto N, Lampugnani E, De Negris P, Torre M, Mattioli G, Jasonni V, Lonnqvist PA 1998 Ropivacaine in paediatric surgery: preliminary results. Paediatric Anaesthesia 8: 127–129

Jamali S, Monin S, Begon C, Dubousset AM, Ecoffey C 1994 Clonidine in pediatric caudal anesthesia. Anesthesia and Analgesia 78: 663–666

Jennings E, Fitzgerald M 1996 C-fos can be induced in the neonatal rat spinal cord by both noxious and innocuous stimulation. Pain 68: 301–306

Kamibayashi T, Maze M 1996 Perioperative use of alpha-2 adrenergic agonists. [Review] Current Opinion in Anaesthesia 9, 323–327

Kar S, Quirion R 1995 Neuropeptide receptors in developing and adult rat spinal cord: an in vitro quantitative autoradiography study of calcitonin gene-related peptide, neurokinins, b-opioid, galanin, somatostatin, neurotension and vasoactive intestinal polypeptide receptors. Journal of Comparative Neurology 354, 253–281

Karmakar MK, Booker PD, Franks R, Pozzi M 1996 Continuous extrapleural paravertebral infusion of bupivacaine for post-thoracotomy analgesia in young infants. British Journal of Anaesthesia 76: 811–815

Kart T, Walther-Larsen S, Svejborg TF, Feilberg V, Eriksen K, Rasmussen M 1997 Comparison of continuous epidural infusion of fentanyl and bupivacaine with intermittent epidural administration of morphine for post-operative pain management in children. Acta Anaesthesiologica Scandinavica 41: 461–465

Kokki H, Tuovinen K, Hendolin H 1998 Spinal anaesthesia for paediatric day-case surgery: a double blind, randomized, parallel group, prospective comparison of isobaric and hyperbaric bupivacaine. British Journal of Anaesthesia 81: 502–506

LaMotte RH, Shain CN, Simone DA, Tsai E-F 1991 Neurogenic hyperalgesia: psychophysical studies of underlying mechanisms. Journal of Neurophysiology 66: 190–211

Larsson BA, Olsson GL, Lonnqvist PA 1994 Plasma concentrations of bupivacaine in young infants after continuous epidural infusion. Paediatric Anaesthesia 4: 159–162

Larsson BA, Lundeberg S, Olsson GL 1997 Epidural abscess in a one-year-old boy after continuous epidural analgesia. Anesthesia and Analgesia 84: 1245–1247

Lee JJ, Rubin AP 1994 Comparison of a bupivacaine–clonidine mixture with plain bupivacaine for caudal analgesia in children. British Journal of Anaesthesia 72: 258–262

Lloyd-Thomas A 1993 An acute pain service for children. Anaesthesie Loco-Regional 2, 71–77

Lloyd-Thomas AR, Howard RF 1994 A pain service for children. Paediatric Anaesthesia 4: 3–15

Lonnquist PA, Olsson GL 1994 Paravertebral versus epidural block in children. Effects on postoperative morphine requirements after renal surgery. Acta Anaesthesiologica Scandinavica 38: 346–349

Luz G, Innerhofer P, Buchmann B, Frischhut B, Menardi G, Benzer A 1996 Bupivacaine plasma concentrations during continuous epidural anaesthesia in infants and children. Anesthesia and Analgesia 82: 231 234

Luz G, Wieser CH, Innerhofer P, Frischhut B, Ulmer H, Benzer A 1998 Free and total bupivacaine plasma concentrations after continuous epidural anaesthesia in infants and children. Paediatric Anaesthesia 8: 473–478

Mahe V, Ecoffey C 1988 Spinal anesthesia with isobaric bupivacaine in infants. Anesthesiology 68: 601–603

Malviya S, Swartz J, Lerman J 1993 Are all pre-term infants younger than 60 weeks postconceptual age at risk for postanesthetic apnea? Anesthesiology 78: 1076–1081

Maxwell LG, Martin LD, Yaster M 1994 Bupivacaine-induced cardiac toxicity in neonates: successful treatment with intravenous phenytoin. Anesthesiology 80: 682–686

Mazoit JX, Denson DD, Samii K 1988 Pharmacokinetics of bupivacaine following caudal anesthesia in infants. Anesthesiology 68: 387–391

McCloskey JJ, Haun SE, Deshpande JK 1992 Bupivacaine toxicity secondary to continuous caudal epidural infusion in children. Anesthesia and Analgesia 75: 287–290

McHale J, O'Donovan FC 1997 Post-dural puncture symptoms in a child. Anaesthesia 52: 688–690

McNicol LR 1985 Sciatic nerve block for children. Sciatic nerve block by the anterior approach for postoperative pain relief. Anaesthesia 40: 410–414

McNicol LR 1986 Lower limb blocks for children. Lateral cutaneous and femoral nerve blocks for postoperative pain relief in paediatric practice. Anaesthesia 41: 27–31

Meunier JF, Norwood P, Dartayet B, Dubousset A-M, Ecoffey C 1997 Skin abscess with lumbar epidural catheterization in infants: is it dangerous? Report of two cases. Anesthesia and Analgesia 84: 1248–1249

Moriarty A 1997 Use of ropivacaine in post-operative infusions [Letter]. Paediatric Anaesthesia 7: 478–178

Murat I, Delleur MM, Esteve C, Egu JF, Raynaud P, Saint-Maurice C 1987 Continuous extradural anaesthesia in children: clinical and haemodynamic implications. British Journal of Anaesthesia 69: 1441–1450

Newman PJ, Bushnell TG, Radford P 1996 The effect of needle size and type in paediatric caudal analgesia. Paediatric Anaesthesia 6: 459–461

Peutrell JM, Holder K, Gregory M 1997 Plasma bupivacaine concentrations associated with continuous extradural infusions in babies. British Journal of Anaesthesia 78: 160–162

Peutrell JM, Hughes DG 1995 A grand-mal convulsion in a child in association with a continuous infusion of bupivacaine Anaesthesia 50: 563–564

Porter F 1993 Pain assessment in children: infants. In: Schechter NL., Berde CB, Yaster M (eds) Pain in Infants, Children and Adolescents, pp. 87–96. Williams and Wilkins, Baltimore

Prosser DP, Davis A, Booker PD, Murray A 1997 Caudal tramadol for postoperative analgesia in paediatric hypospadias surgery. British Journal of Anaesthesia 79: 293–296

Purcell-Jones G, Pither CE, Justins DM 1989 Paravertebral somatic nerve block: a clinical, radiographic and computed tomographic study in chronic pain patients. Anesthesia and Analgesia 68: 32–39

Rosen KR, Rosen DA 1989 Caudal epidural morphine for control of pain following open heart surgery in children. Anesthesiology 70: 418–421

Saberski LR, Kondamuri S, Osinubi OYO 1997 Identification

of the epidural space: is loss of resistance to air a safe technique? [Review] Regional Anesthesia 22: 3–15

Sandler AN 1996 The role of clonidine and alpha2-agonists for post-operative analgesia. [Editorial] Canadian Journal of Anaesthesia 43: 1191–1194

Semple D, Findlow D, Aldridge LM, Doyle E 1996 The optimal dose of ketamine for caudal epidural blockade in children. Anaesthesia 51: 1170–1172

Semsroth M, Plattnew O, Horcher E 1996 Effective pain relief with continuous intrapleural bupivacaine after thoracotomy in infants and children. Paediatric Anaesthesia 6: 303–310

Sethna NF, Berde CB 1993 Venous air embolism during identification of the epidural space in children [Editorial] Anesthesia and Analgesia 76: 925–927

Shenfield O, Eldar I, Lotan G, Avigad I, Goldwasser B 1995 Intraoperative irrigation with bupivacaine for analgesia after orchidopexy and herniorrhaphy in children. Journal of Urology 153: 185–187

Smith T, Moratin P, Wulf H 1996 Smaller children have greater bupivacaine plasma concentrations after ilioinguinal block. British Journal of Anaesthesia 76: 452–455

Stayer SA, Pasquariello CA, Schwartz RE, Balsara RK, Lear BR 1995 The safety of continuous pleural lignocaine after thoracotomy in children and adolescents. Paediatric Anaesthesia 5: 307–310

Strafford MA, Wilder RT, Berde CB 1995 The risk of infection from epidural analgesia in children: a review of 1620 cases. Anesthesia and Analgesia 80: 234–238

Taddio A, Goldbach M, Ipp M, Stevens B, Koren G 1995 Effects of neonatal circumcision on pain responses during vaccination in boys. Lancet 345: 291–292

Taddio A, Katz J, Illersich AL, Curran G 1997 Effect of neonatal circumcision in pain response during subsequent routine vaccination. Lancet 349: 599–603

Tobias JD, Lowe S, O'Dell N, Holcomb GWI 1993a Thoracic epidural anaesthesia in infants and children. Canadian Journal of Anaesthesia 40: 879–882

Tobias JD, Martin LD, Oakes L, Rao B, Wetzel RC 1993b Post-operative analgesia following thoracotomy in children: interpleural catheters. Journal of Pediatric Surgery 28: 1466–1470

Tobias JD, Burd RS, Helikson MA 1998 Apnea following spinal anaesthesia in two former pre-term infants. Canadian Journal of Anaesthesia 45: 985–989

Tsuji MH, Horigome H, Yamashita M 1996 Left ventricular functions are not impaired after lumbar epidural anaesthesia in young children. Paediatric Anaesthesia 6: 405–409

Ved SA, Pinosky M, Nicodemus H 1993 Ventricular tachycardia and brief cardiovascular collapse in two infants after caudal anesthesia using a bupivacaine–epinephrine solution. Anesthesiology 79: 1121–1123

Wall PD 1988 The prevention of postoperative pain. Pain 33: 289–290

Webster AC, McKishnie JD, Kenyon CF, Marshall DG 1991 Spinal anaesthesia for inguinal hernia repair in high-risk neonates. Canadian Journal of Anaesthesia 38: 281–286

Webster AC, McKishnie JD, Reid WD 1993 Lumbar epidural anaesthesia for inguinal hernia repair in low birth weight infants. Canadian Journal of Anaesthesia 40: 670–675

Weston PJ, Bourchier D 1995 The pharmacokinetics of bupivacaine following interpleural nerve block in infants of very low birthweight. Paediatric Anaesthesia 5: 219–222

Wilson PTJ, Lloyd-Thomas AR 1993 An audit of extradural infusion analgesia in children using bupivacaine and diamorphine. Anaesthesia 48: 718–723

Wolf AR, Eyres RL, Laussen PC, Edwards J, Stanley IJ, Row P, Simon L 1993 Effects of extradural analgesia on stress responses to abdominal surgery in infants. British Journal of Anaesthesia 70: 654–660

Wood CE, Goresky GV, Klassen KA, Kuwahara B, Neil SG 1994 Complications of continuous epidural infusions for postoperative analgesia in children. Canadian Journal of Anaesthesia 41: 613–620

# 20. Postoperative pain and audit

## J D R Connolly and G A McLeod

Of all the many reasons advanced for the greater use of regional anaesthesia (see Ch. 2), perhaps the one accepted most commonly is better control of postoperative pain. Despite huge advances in the understanding of pain mechanisms, wider interest in its treatment, and the development of new methods of delivering analgesic drugs, many patients still receive inadequate management. Both the joint working party of the Royal College of Surgeons of England and the then College of Anaesthetists (1990), and the Acute Pain Management Guidelines Panel (1992) in the United States, recognised that there had been widespread failure in pain relief, noting that this not only contributes to patient discomfort, but also prolongs recovery from surgery. Since then, there has been significant interest in managing acute pain, notably the establishment of Acute Pain Teams to co-ordinate treatment. However, patients in the USA continue to cite fear of pain as their primary preoperative worry, with up to three-quarters of them still suffering pain after surgery (Warfield & Kalm 1995), and there is evidence that matters are no better in the UK (Connolly 1998).

## Factors influencing postoperative pain

A number of important factors have been shown to influence the occurrence, intensity and duration of postoperative pain.

## Attitude of medical and nursing staff

Traditionally, nursing staff have been notoriously reluctant to treat pain (Foott 1978), probably because they feared that effective doses of opioid drugs would cause respiratory depression. Medical staff, having prescribed the postoperative analgesia, were content to leave its administration to nurses and were rarely present to witness its effects at first hand. Consequently, neither profession took full responsibility for the provision of analgesia. The result, in the words of one surgical patient, was that '*the one place in the country where you can get least relief is a hospital itself*' (MacInnes 1976).

The situation has not been helped by our terminology. The commonly used expression 'pain relief' actually invites us to wait until pain has occurred before it is treated. 'Pain prevention' or, at the very least, 'pain control' should be the aim of those responsible for postoperative analgesia (Armitage 1989).

### The patient's attitude

Many patients still believe that pain after surgery is inevitable and that it must be endured on the '*no pain, no gain*' principle. Often such patients do not request pain relief and, occasionally, they may not even admit that pain has occurred until afterwards.

### The preoperative visit

Realistic education, with a full explanation of the methods of pain control available, will encourage co-operation and improve the patient's feeling of control. Formal studies of the provision of 'procedural' and 'instructional' information have shown considerable benefits on postoperative pain (Peck 1986).

### Site of the surgical wound

Some operations are intrinsically more painful than others: upper abdominal more than lower abdominal; knee replacement more than hip replacement; and long incisions more than short ones.

## Anaesthetic management

One cause of particularly acute patient distress is recovering consciousness after surgery under general anaesthesia in severe pain because the method of postoperative pain control has not yet been implemented. Such distress is best avoided if the analgesic method is an integral part of the anaesthetic technique used for the actual surgery. This approach should be an essential component of modern practice, no matter what type of analgesia is to be used, but a regional method will provide a period of particularly high quality pain control. The analgesia will extend seamlessly into the postoperative period and act as a foundation for other, sequential analgesic methods, although it is important to start their administration *before* the block regresses.

## Quality of postoperative care

Careful attention to general comfort, the maintenance of good fluid balance and the regular assessment of pain all contribute to its control. The use of a simple visual analogue or verbal rating system is an essential component of modern postoperative care because it enables treatment to be tailored to the individual patient (Gould et al 1992).

## CONTROLLING THE POSTOPERATIVE PERIOD

Although the potential for wider use of regional techniques to improve postoperative pain control is acknowledged, there are those who question whether the objective benefits justify the resources used, or whether there is any significant contribution to surgical outcome. Kehlet (1996) believes that the better pain control provided by regional anaesthesia should be seen as a means to an end (early and rapid remobilisation after surgery) rather than an end in itself. This approach requires that the postoperative period is managed proactively, and the control of pain, while humane and important, is but one of several factors involved in the delivery of high quality, economic health care (Table 20.1). As in the management of pain alone, education is important. Patients are not only told what to expect, but they are also given 'goals' which allow them to contribute to, and even control, their own progress. An example, for a patient undergoing total hip replacement, is shown in Table 20.2. Such a multimodal approach

**Table 20.1** Managing the postoperative period

| | |
|---|---|
| Preoperative education | |
| Attenuation of the stress response | Improved |
| Optimum pain control | convalescence & |
| Early exercise | outcome |
| Enteral nutrition | |

**Table 20.2** Expected progress of patients undergoing total hip replacement

| | | |
|---|---|---|
| 1. | Assessment at preoperative unit 2–4 weeks prior to surgery. Plan outlined. | |
| 2. | Hospital admission during the afternoon before surgery | |
| 3. | Day 0 | Operation |
| 4. | Day 1 | Dressing reduced |
| | | Patient mobilised |
| 5. | Day 2 | Bladder catheter removed |
| | | Wound exposed |
| | | Walking with help |
| 6 | Day 3 | Walking on crutches unaided |
| | | Climbing stairs |
| | | Check X-ray |
| 7. | Day 4 | Discharge home |

has been shown to shorten the time to discharge after retropubic prostatectomy (Carpenter et al 1994).

Even within this multimodal approach to postoperative care it must be recognised that the pain control itself should be multimodal. The more major the surgery the more likely it is that any attempt to control pain by using one drug by one route will fail or lead to complications. The combination of an opioid with a local anaesthetic is more effective than either alone (McQuay et al 1988) and it is well known that nonsteroidal anti-inflammatory drugs (NSAIDs) reduce morphine requirements. Developments of agents with entirely different mechanisms of analgesia (e.g. $\alpha_2$ agonists and NMDA antagonists) will add further to the systemic options in the future. However, local and regional techniques still produce the best quality of analgesia, and their safe and proper administration should be part of the armamentarium of every anaesthetist who wishes to deliver high quality pain control. As surgery becomes more major, the techniques required become more complex (Table 20.3). Conversely, as time after surgery elapses, the degree of pain, and thus the need for analgesics, diminishes.

## REGIONAL TECHNIQUES AFTER SURGERY

### General principles

There are very few, if any, surgical procedures where the use of a local or regional technique of some kind will not contribute to greater patient comfort in the postoperative period. Specific details of injection techniques have been described in the previous chapters, but the important principles of their use for postoperative pain management must be emphasised.

1. The technique chosen must produce analgesia of the wound. This may seem self-evident, but does require careful consideration of the anatomy of the nerve supply to the wound. When a central block is used the segmental levels of both somatic and autonomic innervation must be identified, and the catheter sited appropriately. Similarly, effective use of peripheral blocks requires a good knowledge of their distribution.

2. If the block is to be performed whilst the patient is anaesthetised, he or she must be informed in advance that the relevant part of the body may be numb on recovery of consciousness.

3. Similarly, if long-acting local anaesthetics are used it is important that the nursing staff are aware that there will be a lack of sensation in the distribution of the block. Long-acting agents should be used with particular care in day-surgery patients.

4. Follow-up analgesia must be timed for administration before the time of regression of the block so that the patient does not experience a complete lack of pain control. As already stated, medical and nursing staff can be reluctant to administer analgesic drugs to patients who are *not in pain*, and their education is an essential part of any pain service.

5. The complexity of patient management produced by the regional technique should be appropriate to the clinical situation. For example, a continuous epidural infusion can contribute much after surgical repair of the abdominal aorta, and the level of monitoring will be the same no matter what the analgesic method. However, the patient who has received a femoro-distal bypass graft may not suffer a great deal of postoperative pain particularly if ischaemia has been relieved, and management may be unnecessarily complicated by the presence of an epidural infusion.

### Wound infiltration

Simple infiltration of the wound at the end of the operation is a useful, but often neglected method. All layers of the wound, including muscles in fascial sheaths, must be injected. Bupivacaine given at 2.5 mg ml$^{-1}$ can give good pain control for 6 hours or more, depending on the site of the wound and the volume used. The method is particularly useful for herniorrhaphy (Ryan et al 1984). The infiltration is usually performed by the surgeon, but he or she often requires a gentle reminder from the anaesthetist to perform it, and a brisker reminder to aspirate before injecting to prevent intravascular injection.

The effects of wound infiltration may be prolonged by continuous infusion through an implanted catheter system. Occasional reports of the use of this approach have appeared (Levack et al 1986), but it has never achieved great popularity.

### Peripheral nerve blocks

Many hours of freedom from pain can be provided by blocking peripheral nerves at the level of the wrist, elbow, ankle or knee joints using a long-acting drug. After the effect has regressed, patients often need only minor oral analgesics. Although these blocks may not provide sufficient analgesia for the actual operation, they may be used to supplement a general anaesthetic or a more major nerve block technique. Ankle block has a widespread reputation for difficulty, but it is a straightforward method for providing analgesia after forefoot surgery, although all five nerves must be blocked because of the overlap between them (Schuman 1976). An alternative for toe surgery is a mid-tarsal block (Sharrock et al 1986).

### Major nerve and plexus block

#### Upper limb

Brachial plexus block can provide prolonged pain control as well as good operating conditions. A long-acting local anaesthetic may, after a single injection, provide good analgesia for up to 12 hours, and continuous infusion techniques, using an indwelling catheter, can extend this for much longer (Selander 1977, Valashsky & Aronson 1980, Kaasio et al 1990). Maintenance of both sterility and catheter placement can be a challenge, but the benefits are worth it in the appropriate case.

285

Brachial plexus block can be performed at a number of levels and the distribution of block produced by each is somewhat different (Ch. 14). Thus, this is an example of where the injection technique used should be related carefully to the site of the operation. Axillary block is ideal for elbow and hand surgery, but will produce little if any effect on the shoulder joint for which the interscalene route is best.

### Thoracic nerve block

*Paravertebral block* will produce *unilateral* segmental analgesia, particularly of the chest wall, and can be used after breast, thoracic or upper abdominal procedures. As with lumbar plexus block, which may indeed simply be a variety of paravertebral block, a catheter may be used to prolong analgesia by bolus administration or continuous infusion (Schuleman et al 1989, Catala et al 1996).

*Intercostal block* is time consuming, carries a small risk of pneumothorax, and requires a relatively large dose of drug. However, injection of the 6th to the 11th intercostal nerves using small doses of bupivacaine at 12-hourly intervals has been shown to provide good continuous analgesia (Kavanagh et al 1994). It is a useful technique in patients who are very frail or in whom opioids are contraindicated.

*Interpleural block* enjoyed great popularity after it was first introduced (Kvalheim & Reiestad 1984), but its use seems to have declined. Perhaps its most useful indication was a subcostal incision for cholecystectomy, but laparoscopic cholecystectomy has largely displaced the open operation. In addition, relatively large doses of local anaesthetic are required, yet the analgesia varies in quality (El-Baz & Faber 1988), and most workers feel that the technique is inferior to epidural analgesia.

### Lower limb block

*Lumbar plexus block*, by the posterior approach, provides good analgesia after hip arthroplasty, and the continuous technique has been shown to be effective in reducing morphine demands (Spansberg et al 1996, Vaghadia et al 1987). To produce complete analgesia of the leg both sciatic and femoral nerves must be blocked, but the effect of a single injection can last for 24 hours or longer and be as effective as any other technique.

Catheter techniques have been used for sciatic (Smith et al 1984), femoral (Hirst et al 1996), 'three-in-one' (Edwards & Wright 1992) and even popliteal nerve blocks (Singelyn et al 1997). As with other methods, it is important to maintain the placement of the catheter and ensure that a method appropriate to the source of pain is used.

## Central nerve block

Specific peripheral (major and minor) nerve blocks can provide excellent, localised pain control and are well tolerated by patients. They are particularly useful for early postoperative physiotherapy after orthopaedic procedures and avoid the need for large doses of opioids to cover such procedures. However, each technique has to be learned, and practised frequently to maintain expertise. Analgesic techniques which use the spinal or epidural route have the advantage that they can be applied to a very wide range of surgery at different levels of the body. However, it is particularly important that the block affects the dermatomes which are the source of the painful stimuli (see Ch. 11 & Fig. 11.18).

### Epidural analgesia

Widely used, thoroughly investigated, flexible and widespread in application, epidural analgesia is considered by many to be the 'gold standard' for control of postoperative pain. Epidural anaesthesia is a major part of modern practice, being used by the lumbar route for lower limb surgery, at the lower thoracic level for lower abdominal surgery, and upper thoracic level for upper abdominal and thoracic surgery. The caudal approach can be used for perineal surgery in adults and more widespread procedures in children, and cervical epidural block has a small role in specialist situations. It only takes a small modification in technique to extend the analgesia well into the postoperative period. Properly managed, this can provide a wide range of benefits (Ch. 2).

However, the technique is not without its disadvantages, dangers even, and the approach must be meticulous, with an appropriate level of nursing supervision for as long as the block is effective. The provision of extended postoperative analgesia by continuous epidural block will only be achieved safely if all aspects are managed actively. This has been discussed in Chapter 11, but some important points bear repeating:

- The catheter must be placed at an appropriate level in the epidural space to ensure that the nerves supplying the wound, and other sources of postoperative discomfort such as drain sites, are blocked;

- Nursing and junior medical staff must have precise instructions on the action to be taken in the event of analgesia becoming inadequate or complications developing;
- Combinations of local anaesthetic and opioid drugs increase effectiveness and reduce complications.

Unfortunately, there is no unanimity on the optimum volume and concentration of local anaesthetic to be used, let alone which is the best opioid to add to it. However, it is strongly recommended that every department should agree on a standard 'mixture' for continuous epidurals, and audit its use regularly.

The identification, over 20 years ago, of opioid receptors in the spinal cord generated enthusiasm for the provision of high quality 'peripheral' analgesia without the problems associated with epidural local anaesthetic administration. However, this early enthusiasm was tempered by occasional cases of respiratory depression, and the much more frequent problem of pruritus. When opioids are used alone this can be so severe as to make the patient request discontinuation of the epidural. Nausea, vomiting and retention of urine may also occur. In more recent years it has been established that entirely different classes of drug have analgesic actions at spinal cord level. These include the $\alpha_2$ agonists clonidine and dexmedetomidine, the NMDA antagonist ketamine, and the benzodiazepine midazolam. Evidence on their local toxicity is incomplete and their efficacy is mixed. These approaches offer intriguing avenues for future development, but cannot be recommended for routine practice as yet.

### The subarachnoid route

Although spinal anaesthesia is used extensively for surgery to the lower half of the body, it is not widely used to provide postoperative analgesia *per se*, unless an opioid is given at the same time as the local anaesthetic prior to surgery. Most available opioid drugs have been used in this way, although it is particularly important that they are in preservative-free form to avoid nerve damage. Fentanyl 5–25 µg, morphine 0.1–0.3 mg, and diamorphine 0.25–1 mg are the most commonly used. Fentanyl will produce 1–6 hours of analgesia, and morphine and diamorphine 8–24 hours. This combined technique has the advantage of 'smoothing out' the transition between the profound block produced by the local anaesthetic, and the establishment of adequate systemic analgesia. Unfortunately, concerns about

respiratory depression often delay the administration of systemic opioid and result in a period of poor pain control.

The availability of fine bore plastic catheters opened up the possibility of the more widespread use of 'spinal' analgesia, but problems with the cauda equina syndrome (Rigler et al 1991) rapidly reduced the enthusiasm for their use. More recently, there has been some re-evaluation of the use of the catheter spinal technique and its use in surgery and postoperative pain control. Low-dose infusions of bupivacaine, with and without morphine, have been used to provide analgesia for 24–48 hours after lower limb surgery (Bachmann et al 1997). At the present time, this method of pain control has not been fully evaluated and cannot be recommended for routine use, but it may have advantages worthy of further investigation in the future.

## AUDITING THE EFFECT

The provision of better pain control is one of the more readily conceded advantages of regional anaesthesia, yet the overall benefit has been questioned (Kehlet 1996). Many research projects have demonstrated physiological benefits of the 'regional' approach, but such projects, essential though they are to development, are always undertaken in relatively small, carefully defined groups of patients whose management is closely supervised by the investigators. These constraints are, of course, essential in this type of research, although the recent publication of a meta-analysis (Rodgers et al 2000) has confirmed that the benefits extend to reduced mortality and major morbidity. However, it is important to confirm that these benefits are attained in routine practice.

Any improvement in quality of care in a modern healthcare system must demonstrate its worth and, in the current climate, its clinical benefits must be balanced against costs. An ageing population, increasing patient expectations and widespread variations in practice all influence decision making. Audit is becoming central to the culture of healthcare, allowing not only identification of problem clinical areas, but also measuring local practice against clinical guidelines and outside standards.

Audit in regional anaesthesia has tended to focus on activity and safety. Many departments record their use of regional techniques in the operating theatre and labour ward. However, there is rarely any attempt to relate the data obtained to standards of individual or departmental practice. There is even less use of audit as a force for improving clinical outcome by relating local practice to accepted standards or the results of other centres.

## The audit cycle

There are a number of well-defined stages in audit (Crombie et al 1997).

1. *Identification of a clinical problem.* A simple audit of activity is important to demonstrate that trainees are given adequate opportunities to learn regional techniques and that consultants are maintaining their expertise. However, determining whether the techniques make a difference to patient outcome is a much more major challenge. Increasingly this 'outcome' must include a cost–benefit component. Occasionally, observation of local clinical practice will demonstrate that a particular aspect needs review.

2. *Definition of standards for comparison.* In many areas of medical practice, standards agreed at national level are available for comparison, but this is not generally so in anaesthesia. It is important that a declared standard is realistic and obtainable, but capable of being modified through successive audit cycles. There may have to be a compromise between the clinical importance, practicality and acceptability of the project, but it should not be to such a degree that it simply validates current practice and prevents change.

3. *Collection of data.* Proper management of the audit process is central to success. Individual anaesthetists may usefully audit their own practice, and this can ensure accurate data collection, but it may be cumbersome and time consuming with larger projects. Any serious consideration of the impact of a clinical intervention on outcome in anaesthesia requires a multidisciplinary approach and collaboration with more groups than just our surgical colleagues. One individual should take responsibility for data collection, and the 'pain nurse', being the central individual of most 'pain teams', is the ideal person. Much of the data collected will enable the efficacy of the pain control provided to patients to be quantified, and simple pain charts for bedside use keep the data-collection process simple.

4. *Comparison with standards.* The lack of defined national standards of postoperative pain control causes some difficulty currently, but the introduction of standard formats for audits (e.g. the Royal College of Anaesthetists audit 'recipe' book) should allow comparisons to develop between different centres.

5. *Accounting for differences.* Differences between local and standard practice should be presented to all interested parties, and the reasons for any difference explored fully. There must be some mechanism for assessing whether any change in practice produces an appropriate improvement, especially if the change requires a restructuring of priorities and resources.

6. *Implementing change.* Simple awareness of the outcome of an audit can persuade staff of the need for change, but that change may still require careful management. The implementation of continuous epidural analgesia after surgery requires that all staff are trained in its use. If this does not happen, the result may well be a deterioration, rather than an improvement, in patient outcome. Ideally, the audit should stimulate discussion and ideas so that the whole team moves together, implementing an evidence-based change.

7. *Evaluating the impact.* Once the change has been implemented, it is important to repeat the audit after a period of time to ensure that the expected benefits have been gained.

## Audit in regional anaesthesia

Audit in regional anaesthesia is not yet highly developed, but there are a number of examples which are relevant, some of them performed at quite a simple level.

### Prevalence of audit

Smith and colleagues (1999) found that over half of all Australian obstetric anaesthesia departments were not collecting any audit data. Of those departments which were collecting some data, 18 reported that there had been an improvement in patient care, and 13 reported that the benefits outweighed the costs involved. However, only 6 departments (9% in total) had performed a complete audit cycle and it was concluded that Australian obstetric anaesthesia audit strategies were inadequate for the development of a national minimal data set. Given the rarity of major problems in modern anaesthesia, it is essential that estimates of their incidence are based on reviews of large numbers of patients, something which can only be achieved at national level. It is almost certain that similar findings would apply in many other countries, and relate to very different uses of regional techniques.

## Introduction of pain services

Probably because the introduction of Acute Pain Services required allocation of resources, and occurred at the time when audit was becoming widespread, this area provides examples of complete, well-conducted audit cycles.

Gould and colleagues (1992) studied current practice in a general surgical ward setting. This was then, in sequence, followed by the introduction of pain assessment charts, an algorithm for use of intramuscular analgesia, greater use of local anaesthetic wound infiltration, a postoperative pain information sheet and, finally, patient controlled analgesia (PCA). A continuing audit process of over 2000 patients showed improvements in pain relief at every stage. A review of a similar process, involving over 2700 patients in several different types of UK hospital (Harmer & Davies 1998), showed that the approach was generally applicable. The incidence of severe pain on movement decreased from 37% to 13% and there was a comparable reduction in the incidence of nausea and vomiting. A similar survey of the effect of audit in 23 hospitals in the USA (Miaskowski et al 1999) showed that patients managed by a pain service had lower post-operative pain scores, were more satisfied with their management, had less side-effects and were discharged sooner from hospital. Such early discharge is a very positive outcome and demonstrates the power of properly applied audit.

## Use of regional anaesthesia

The Swedish Association of Anaesthesia and Intensive Care attempted to assess the use of central neural techniques, and to evaluate the risk of complications (Holmstrom et al 1997). Subarachnoid block was pre-ferred for shorter surgical procedures, such as Caesarean section and urological surgery, whereas epidural block (or combined spinal/epidural block) was chosen when severe postoperative pain could be anticipated. A note-worthy finding of this study was that an improved registry of complications was needed.

## Training in regional anaesthesia

The increasing use of personal log-books during training allows a detailed record of an individual's practical experience, including that of regional anaesthesia. An American survey, comparing residency programme training reports, showed an increase in the use of regional techniques between 1980 and 1990 from 21.3% to 29.8% respectively, primarily because of a doubling

in the use of epidural block (Kopazc & Bridenbaugh 1993).

Although the considerable variability among programmes caused some concern, the report did attempt to identify how much experience is required for a successful block. If a 90% success rate is desired, 45 and 60 attempts at spinal and epidural block respectively, may be necessary. Such data are crucially important for individuals, departments and organisations that supervise training.

## The safety of regional anaesthesia

The possibility of neurological complications after regional anaesthesia is a long-standing concern, but identification of the true incidence again requires large numbers of patients. Auroy and colleagues (1997) have reported the largest prospective analysis, and compli-cations were attributed, fully or partially, to regional anaesthesia in 89 out of 100 000 blocks. Twenty-six out of 32 cardiac arrests occurred during spinal anaesthesia, an incidence six times greater than for any other form of regional technique. Of the 34 neurological compli-cations (radiculopathy, cauda equina syndrome, paraplegia), two-thirds were associated with either paraesthesia during needle puncture (n = 19) or pain during injection (n = 2), suggesting nerve trauma as the cause. Twelve patients had neurological sequelae of spinal anaesthesia, nine of them having received hyperbaric lidocaine. Convulsions, attributed to increased plasma concentrations of local anaesthetic drug, occurred in 23 patients, although none suffered a cardiac arrest. The incidence of convulsions associated with limb blocks was seven times higher than that for epidurals. Such detailed data as these are rare and yet they form an essential component of the risk–benefit analysis when the anaesthetist is deciding on a particular anaesthetic technique.

## Measuring quality

This discussion has taken up the challenge of demonstrating that regional techniques, particularly in the context of postoperative pain management, can have a beneficial effect on outcome. It is clear that audit in regional anaesthetic practice requires much develop-ment if we are to be able to assess properly the risk of side-effects or prove the benefits. Furthermore, changes in management, prompted by audit and directed at con-verting potential benefits into real ones, will be worthless unless these benefits have actually been delivered to the patient. An audit by a multidisciplinary group (anaesthetists, epidemiologists and health policy researchers) in Scotland has shown that this may not be the case (McLeod et al 2001).

The group used verbal ratings of pain from 560 patients to categorise them into four predetermined groups, using the overall pain experience as an outcome. They found that 33% of patients received 'excellent' pain control, a proportion which is unlikely to be improved upon by any future development in drugs or technology. Conversely, 36% had a variable or poor experience of pain control. Indeed, 4% of patients never achieved pain relief with the epidural, and the technique was abandoned. Further, a quarter of patients had to have the epidural removed because of technical problems (12%) or because of premature discharge from the high dependency unit due to pressure on beds (13%). Thus the audit showed that the true efficacy of the method cannot begin to be assessed until all associated factors have been addressed and all problems solved.

## The future of audit in regional anaesthesia

There are many pressures for audit to become an integral component of clinical practice. However, there is concern that the majority of projects are small and unco-ordinated. There is a need for national organisations to agree on the essential data to be collected, to use the currently available evidence to persuade individuals and departments that this work is worthwhile, and then use the data to evaluate the benefit of the techniques involved.

## References

Acute Pain Management Guidelines Panel 1992 Acute pain management: operative or medical procedures and trauma. US Public Health Service Agency for Healthcare Policy and Research, Publication 92–0032

Armitage EN 1989 Postoperative pain – prevention or relief? British Journal of Anaesthesia 63: 136–138

Auroy Y, Narchi P, Messiah A, Litt L, Rouvier B, Samii K 1997 Serious complications related to regional anesthesia: results of a prospective survey in France. Anesthesiology 87: 479–486

Bachmann M, Laasko E, Niemi L, Rosenberg PH, Pitkamen M 1997 Intrathecal infusion of bupivacaine with or without morphine for post-operative analgesia after hip and knee arthroplasty. British Journal of Anaesthesia 78: 666–670

Carpenter RL, Liu SS, Mulroy MF, Weissmann RM, Olsson GL 1994 Multimodal approach to optimise recovery shortens time to discharge after retropubic prostatectomy. Anesthesiology 81: 3A–A1025

Catala E, Casas JL, Unzueja MC, Diaz X, Aliaga L, Landeira JM 1996 Continuous infusion is superior to bolus doses with thoracic paravertebral blocks after thoracotomies. Journal of Cardiothoracic and Vascular Anesthesia 10: 586–588

Connolly JDR 1998 Musgrave Park Hospital Audit. [Personal communication]

Crombie I, Davies HTO, Abraham SCS, du V Fleurie C 1997 The audit handbook: improving healthcare through clinical audit. J Wiley & Sons, Chichester

Edwards ND, Wright EM 1992 Continuous low dose 3-in-1 nerve blockade for post-operative pain relief after total knee replacement. Anesthesia and Analgesia 75: 265–267

El-Baz N, Faber LP 1988 Intrapleural infusion of local anesthetics: a word of caution. Anesthesiology 68: 809–810

Foott S 1978 Personal view. British Medical Journal 2: 950

Gould TH, Crosby DL, Harmer M et al 1992 Policy for controlling pain after surgery: effect of sequential changes in management. British Medical Journal 314: 1187–1193

Harmer M, Davies KA 1998 The effect of education, assessment and a standardised prescription on postoperative pain management. The value of clinical audit in the establishment of acute pain services. Anaesthesia 53: 424–430

Hirst GC, Lang SA, Dust WN, Cassidy JD, Yip RW 1996 Femoral nerve block. Single injection versus continuous infusion for total knee arthroplasty. Regional Anaesthesia 21: 292–297

Holmstrom B, Rawal N, Arner S 1997 The use of central regional anesthesia techniques in Sweden: results of a nationwide survey. Swedish Association of Anesthesia and Intensive care. Acta Anaesthesiologica Scandinavica 41: 565–572

Kaasio J, Tuominen M, Rosenberg PR 1990 Continuous interscalene brachial plexus block during and after shoulder surgery. Annales Chirurgici et Gynaecological 79: 103–107

Kavanagh BP, Katz J, Sandler AM 1994 Pain control after thoracic surgery: a review of current techniques. Anesthesiology 81: 737–782

Kehlet H 1996 ISRA Congress, Auckland. [Personal communication]

Kopacz DJ, Bridenbaugh LD 1993 Are anesthesia residency programs failing regional anesthesia? The past, present, and future. Regional Anaesthesia 18: 84–87

Kvalheim L, Reiestad F 1984 Interpleural catheter in the management of postoperative pain. Anesthesiology 61: A231

Levack ID, Holmes JD, Robertson GS 1986 Abdominal wound perfusion for the relief of postoperative pain. British Journal of Anaesthesia 58: 615–619

MacInnes C 1976 Cancer ward. New Society (April 29): 232–234

McLeod GA, Davies HTO, Munnoch N, Bannister J, Macrae W 2001 Postoperative pain relief using thoracic epidural analgesia: outstanding success and disappointing failures. Anaesthesia 56: 75–81

McQuay HJ, Carroll D, Moore RA 1988 Postoperative orthopaedic pain – the effect of opiate premedication and local anaesthetic blocks. Pain 33: 291–295

Miaskowski C, Crews J, Ready LB, Paul SM, Ginsberg B 1999 Anesthesia-based pain services improve the quality of postoperative pain management. Pain 80: 23–29

Peck CL 1986 Psychological factors in acute pain management. In: Cousins MJ, Phillips GD (eds) Clinics in critical care medicine: acute pain management, pp 251–274. Churchill Livingstone, New York

Rigler ML, Drasner K, Krejac TC et al 1991 Cauda equina syndrome after continuous spinal anesthesia. Anesthesia and Analgesia 72: 275–281

Rodgers A, Walker N, Schug S et al 2000 Reduction of postoperative mortality with epidural or spinal anaesthesia: results from overview of randomised trials. British Medical Journal 321: 1493–1497

Royal College of Surgeons of England and the College of Anaesthetists 1990 Report of the working party on Pain after Surgery. London: Commission on the provision of Surgical Services

Ryan JA, Adye BA, Jolly PC, Mulroy MF 1984 Outpatient inguinal herniorhaphy with both regional and local anesthesia. American Journal of Surgery 148: 313–316

Schuleman S, Sharp T, Gilbert TJ 1989 Continuous thoracic paravertebral block. Journal of Cardiothoracic Anesthesia 3 (5 Supplement 1): 54–59

Schuman DJ 1976 Ankle block anesthesia for foot surgery. Anesthesiology 44: 342

Selander D 1977 Catheter technique in axillary plexus block. Presentation of a new method. Acta Anaesthesiologica Scandinavica 21: 324–329

Sharrock NE, Waller JF, Fierro LE 1986 Midtarsal block for surgery of the forefoot. British Journal of Anaesthesia 58: 37–41

Singelyn FJ, Aye F, Gouverneur JM 1997 Continuous popliteal sciatic nerve block: an original technique to provide post-operative analgesia after foot surgery. Anesthesia and Analgesia 84: 383–386

Smith BE, Fischer HBJ, Scott PV 1984 Continuous sciatic nerve block. Anaesthesia 39: 155–157

Smith SJ, Cyna AM, Simmons SW 1999 A survey of Australasian obstetric anaesthesia audit. Anaesthesia and Intensive Care 27: 391–395

Spansberg NL, Anher-Moller E, Dahl JB, Schultz P, Chistensen EF 1996 The value of continuous blockade of the lumbar plexus as an adjunct to acetylsalicylic acid for pain relief after surgery for femoral neck fractures. European Journal of Anaesthesiology 13: 410–412

Vaghadia H, Kapnoudhis P, Jenkins LC, Taylor D 1987 Continuous lumbosacral block using a Tuohy needle and catheter technique. Canadian Journal of Anaesthesia 34: 455–458

Valashsky E, Aronson HB 1980 Continuous interscalene brachial plexus block for surgical operations on the hand.[Letter] Anesthesiology 53: 356

Warfield CA, Kalm CH 1995 Acute pain management programmes in US hospitals and experiences and attitudes amongst US adults. Anesthesiology 83: 1090–1094

# 21. Pain and autonomic nerve block

## D M Justins

The sympathetic nervous system has been the target for pain relieving techniques since the early part of the 20th century, although sympathetic block is now used much less frequently than in the past. This is a consequence of a number of factors, two of the most important being a better understanding of the mechanisms of pain and a realisation that the role of the sympathetic nervous system in pain may have been overemphasised (Schott 1998). This has led to a reappraisal of the role of neural block in the management of chronic pain, and the development of more logical treatments using systemic medication, stimulation techniques, physical therapy and psychological approaches (Boas 1998). Analysis of the evidence for effectiveness of sympathetic block in pain management has revealed a large amount of anecdote and an absence of randomised controlled trials (Kozin 1992, Kingery 1997).

It is not fully understood how the sympathetic nervous system is involved in the pathophysiology of some painful states, or why sympathetic block relieves pain. Pain relief may result from the interruption of afferent nociceptive fibres which accompany the autonomic nerves. This is the mechanism by which an obstetric epidural relieves labour pain and by which coeliac plexus block relieves the visceral pain caused by carcinoma of the pancreas. In other cases, the mode of action may be more complex and be linked to the interruption of sympathetic efferent activity which contributes to the perpetuation of some painful conditions (the so-called 'sympathetically maintained' pain). Another mode of action of sympathetic block may involve disruption of reflex control systems so that peripheral or central sensory processing is altered. Finally, sympathetic block causes peripheral vasodilatation and this may relieve ischaemic pain and facilitate the healing of painful skin ulcers.

## GENERAL PRINCIPLES

### Indications for sympathetic block

#### Peripheral vascular disease
Sympathetic blocks may be used for the following.

1. *Acute vascular disorders*: post-traumatic vasospasm; acute arterial or venous occlusion; cold injury; inadvertent intra-arterial injection of drugs, for example, thiopental or contaminated drugs of abuse.
2. *Chronic vasospastic conditions*: Raynaud's syndrome; acrocyanosis; livedo reticularis; sequelae of spinal cord injury or disease (e.g. polio).
3. *Chronic obliterative arterial diseases*: thromboangiitis obliterans (Buerger's disease); atherosclerosis.
4. *Perioperative purposes*: microvascular surgery; arteriovenous fistula formation for dialysis.

However, there are no controlled trials of chemical sympathectomy in peripheral vascular disease and much of the evidence is anecdotal (Gordon et al 1994). It is difficult to predict the result of a block in patients with atherosclerosis. Neurolytic lumbar sympathetic blocks have been claimed to relieve rest pain and improve healing of skin ulcers in about 65–75% of patients with atherosclerosis, although the procedure is of much less benefit for claudication. The traditional explanation for this is that sympathectomy increases skin blood flow, but does not improve nutritive blood flow to muscles. However, Gleim and colleagues (1995) disagree with this view and they reported significant immediate and long-term improvements in painless walking distance after neurolytic lumbar sympathetic block. The benefit may last for 6–9 months and during this time the patient may develop collateral circulation. The results are comparable to surgical sympathectomy, but with reduced morbidity and mortality. If amputation is necessary, a preoperative sympathetic block may aid in defining the limits of tissue viability and also facilitate healing of the stump, but there is little evidence to support the commonly held view that preoperative epidural block diminishes the incidence of stump or phantom pain after amputation (Nikolajsen & Jensen 2001). Established stump or phantom pain is occasionally helped by sympathetic block, but treatment is generally difficult and unsatisfactory.

## Visceral pain

Afferent nociceptive fibres from the viscera accompany sympathetic nerves. Sympathetic block interrupts these pathways, and also the efferent viscero-visceral reflexes so that ischaemia and spasm are relieved. Situations in which the blocks may be considered are as follows.

1. *Abdominal cancer.* Neurolytic coeliac plexus block produces partial to complete pain relief which lasts for the remainder of life in about 70–90% of patients with pain arising from carcinoma of the pancreas, stomach, gall bladder or liver (Brown et al 1987, Eisenberg et al 1995). Mercadante (1993) compared coeliac plexus block with conventional analgesics in a series of 20 patients and showed beneficial effects with both approaches, although the incidence of side-effects was higher in the systemic analgesia group. The pain of other abdominal malignancies and rectal tenesmus due to pelvic carcinoma may also be helped (Bristow & Foster 1988). Neurolytic superior hypogastric plexus blocks have been used for chronic pelvic pain associated with cancer (Plancarte et al 1990a, Leon-Casasola et al 1993). Block of the ganglion impar at the inferior end of the sacrum has been used for perineal pain in cancer.

2. *Chronic non-malignant abdominal pain.* This does not respond as well, and the results of coeliac plexus block for chronic pancreatitis are disappointing. Unilateral sympathetic block at the $L_1$ level is sometimes helpful in the loin-pain haematuria syndrome. It has been claimed that some chronic perineal pain syndromes respond to bilateral lumbar sympathetic block, and superior hypogastric block has been used for chronic non-malignant pelvic pain syndromes.

3. *Acute abdominal pain.* There may be some benefit in the pain of pancreatitis and ureteric colic, but this is usually managed with systemic analgesics.

4. *Cardiac pain.* The pain of acute myocardial infarction, and intractable angina, is eased by upper thoracic sympathetic or stellate ganglion block. Stellate ganglion block was used for intractable angina before cardiac by-pass surgery was developed and there is now renewed interest in this treatment. Endoscopic transthoracic sympathectomy was found to be beneficial in an uncontrolled trial involving 24 patients with severe angina (Wettervik et al 1995).

5. *Perioperative purposes.* Anaesthesia for upper abdominal surgery may be achieved using a combination of coeliac plexus and intercostal nerve blocks.

## Hyperhidrosis

Sympathetic blocks produce anhidrosis and patients with hyperhidrosis may be referred for sympathectomy. Before neuroablative sympathetic blocks are considered the patient should have a thorough trial of conservative treatment. Side-effects such as Horner's syndrome are common if neurolytic procedures are attempted. Endoscopic transthoracic sympathectomy of the upper limb is a safe and effective alternative to open cervical sympathectomy in the management of hyperhidrosis of the upper limb, as well as in vasospastic conditions and sympathetically maintained pain (Byrne et al 1990).

## Neuropathic pain

The aetiology of neuropathic pain (Ch. 3) may be metabolic, ischaemic, hereditary, compressive, traumatic, toxic, infectious or immune mediated (Woolf & Mannion 1999). Typically, there are sensory deficits, abnormal sensations (e.g. paraesthesiae) and pain. In some cases the pain may be maintained by sympathetic efferent activity or by circulating catecholamines. After partial nerve injury, both injured and uninjured axons become sensitive to circulating catecholamines and to nor-epinephrine released from postganglionic sympathetic terminals (Woolf & Mannion 1999). The cell bodies of sensory neurones in the dorsal root ganglion also come under the closer influence of sympathetic axons after nerve injury, so that sympathetic activity may be capable of initiating or maintaining activity in sensory fibres (McLachlan et al 1993). This pain can be described as sympathetically maintained pain.

Unfortunately, there is a lack of strong evidence for the effectiveness of sympathetic block in neuropathic pain (Kozin 1992, Kingery 1997, Boas 1998) and, as mentioned above, it appears that the role of the sympathetic nervous system in these situations has been overemphasised (Schott 1998). The present lack of evidence may reflect the poor quality of existing trials which often report on a heterogeneous group of patients with ill-defined clinical conditions. Blocks have been used inappropriately as a single modality treatment for conditions which require multidisciplinary management. Examples of neuropathic pain include the following.

***Acute herpes zoster*** There have been claims that sympathetic blocks reduce pain and promote healing during the acute phase, but suggestions that the incidence of post-herpetic neuralgia can be reduced remain unproven (Hogan 1993, Ali 1995). Certainly, sympathetic blocks are of unproven value in established postherpetic neuralgia (Wu et al 2000).

***Carcinomatous neuropathy*** Invasion by carcinoma, particularly of the brachial or lumbar plexus, and carcinoma of head and neck may produce a neuropathic pain which is partially responsive to sympathetic block.

***Complex Regional Pain Syndromes (CRPS)*** Causalgia and reflex sympathetic dystrophy (RSD) were the terms used to describe two poorly understood disorders which usually present with pain accompanied by various combinations of sensory disturbance, motor abnormality, swelling, and vasomotor, sudomotor and trophic changes. Causalgia followed major nerve injury, and RSD followed a variety of other causes. The term 'reflex sympathetic dystrophy' is now considered particularly misleading and new terminology has been introduced. In essence reflex sympathetic dystrophy has been renamed CRPS Type I and causalgia has become CRPS Type II (Merskey & Bogduk 1994, Walker & Cousins 1997).

The diagnostic criteria for CRPS Type I (Merskey & Bogduk 1994) are:

1. The presence of an initiating noxious event, or a cause of immobilisation;
2. Continuing pain, allodynia, or hyperalgesia in which the pain is disproportionate to any inciting event;
3. Evidence at some time of oedema, changes in skin blood flow or abnormal sudomotor activity in the region of the pain;
4. No other conditions which would account for the degree of pain and dysfunction should be present.

Criteria 2–4 must be satisfied.
The diagnostic criteria for CRPS Type II are:

1. the presence of continuing pain, allodynia, or hyperalgesia after a nerve injury, not necessarily limited to the distribution of the injured nerve;

2. Evidence at some time of oedema, changes in skin blood flow or abnormal sudomotor activity in the region of the pain;
3. No other conditions which would account for the degree of pain and dysfunction should be present.

All three criteria must be satisfied.

When sympathetic involvement is proven or suspected, it is widely believed that aggressive therapy, including sympathetic nerve blocks, should be initiated as soon as possible. Unfortunately, a successful result is not inevitable and some cases remain intractable despite every therapeutic endeavour. Perhaps the most important contribution of the blocks is to reduce pain and facilitate physiotherapy (Charlton 1990). Resolution becomes less likely once dystrophic changes are established and the conditions can follow an unremitting course of increasing pain and disability. Local anaesthetic sympathetic blocks have been shown to be superior to conservative therapy in an uncontrolled series of RSD patients (Wang et al 1985). Continuous upper limb somatic and sympathetic block can be established using an infusion administered through a brachial plexus catheter. This technique has been used in the treatment of RSD and after reconstructive microvascular surgery (Manriquez & Pallares 1978).

Undoubtedly, occasional patients with neuropathic pain or CRPS do benefit from sympathetic blocks, but the identification of these patients is difficult and many questions about the pathology remain to be answered. There are no clear guidelines on the indications for different techniques, and the optimal frequency, interval and duration of treatment have not been established. (Schutzer et al 1984, Kozin 1992, Kingery 1997, Schott 1998)

### Other indications

In addition to those conditions detailed above, others which have been suggested for sympathetic block include: stellate ganglion block for Bell's palsy, quinine toxicity, retinal artery occlusion, and certain types of acute hearing loss.

## Contraindications to sympathetic block

***Prolongation of coagulation*** There is significant risk of damage to blood vessels with many of these techniques because the sympathetic trunks are deeply placed and close to major blood vessels. A large haematoma may be produced if there is a coagulation disorder.

**Local infection or neoplasm** Needles should not be inserted through infected or neoplastic tissue because there is a risk of spread to deeper structures.

**Anatomical or vascular anomalies** Anatomical distortion (e.g. pressure from a tumour or spinal scoliosis) may make the block more difficult and reduce the success rate. Anomalous vessels increase the risk of accidental needle puncture.

**Hypovolaemia** Splanchnic, coeliac and bilateral lumbar sympathetic blocks can precipitate marked hypotension.

**Inadequate facilities** Full facilities for resuscitation and radiographic control of the procedures must be available (see below).

## Clinical application of sympathetic blocks

It is not appropriate to employ sympathetic block as the sole therapy for the management of pain. Comprehensive assessment and a multidisciplinary approach utilising treatments such as systemic medication, physical therapy, stimulation techniques (e.g. TENS) and psychological approaches are essential in addition to the neural block. There are circumstances in which the main responsibility of the anaesthetist is to perform the sympathetic block while other aspects of management are co-ordinated by another doctor. Examples are a lumbar sympathectomy for a patient with peripheral vascular disease or a coeliac plexus block for a patient with carcinoma of the pancreas. It is important for the anaesthetist to work as a part of the team in such instances.

*Diagnostic blocks* can be used to differentiate between somatic and visceral pain, to identify a sympathetic component, to assess whether blood flow increases, or if sweating decreases. If an attempt is being made to define the sympathetic contribution to any particular pain syndrome the diagnostic block must be a pure sympathetic block without any accompanying somatic block. This can only be achieved with precise interruption of the sympathetic chain. Neither epidural injections nor intravenous regional techniques with local anaesthetic or guanethidine are selective and they do not help in the diagnosis of a sympathetically maintained pain. An image intensifier is mandatory to confirm precise needle position and the spread of injected solution. Objective signs of sympathetic block must be identified using changes in skin temperature or conductivity, or tests of sweat production with ninhydrin, cobalt blue or starch iodine. Skin temperature can be tested by touch, surface thermometer or thermal-sensitive strips with a liquid crystal display. When a limb has been blocked, dilated veins become visible and the increase in blood flow can be measured using a Doppler flow probe or venous plethysmography (Breivik et al 1998). The occurrence of Horner's syndrome does not confirm that there is sympathetic block in the arm.

False positive results may be due to spread of solution to adjacent somatic nerves or into the epidural space, systemic effects of absorbed local anaesthetic taken up from the injection site, or the placebo response. False negative results may follow an incomplete or inappropriate block and inadequate assessment before or after the block. A complete sympathetic block is difficult to achieve (Malmqvist et al 1987). Many patients will have both sympathetic and somatic components to their pain. There is no clear correlation between the degree or duration of pain relief and the actual period of sympathetic block, and the same patient may show variable responses on different occasions. Some patients demonstrate unexpected or unusual responses, such as contralateral or delayed blocks, and some pain is made worse (Purcell-Jones & Justins 1988).

*Intravenous testing* by intravenous administration of the α-adrenergic blocking drug phentolamine has been suggested as a test of sympathetic involvement in chronic pain and as a predictor of the outcome of sympathetic neural block (Arner 1991, Raja et al 1991). However, there are uncertainties about the sensitivity, specificity and reliability of this test.

*A prognostic block* can be used to demonstrate to the patient the effect on pain, blood flow or sweating, but there may be poor correlation between the result of the prognostic block and the outcome of any subsequent surgical or neuroablative procedure. A local anaesthetic block produces wider disruption of nerve function. If neuroablation is to be based upon the results of prognostic blocks, more than one should be performed and a consistent response demonstrated. Sometimes the prognostic block will produce an increase in pain or an increase in limb temperature, which the patient finds uncomfortable and unacceptable.

*Therapeutic blocks* may be performed with local anaesthetics, neurolytic chemicals such as phenol or alcohol, neuroablative techniques such as radiofrequency lesioning, or with drugs such as guanethidine and bretylium in intravenous regional techniques. Neurolytic blocks are indicated primarily for painful abdominal cancer and peripheral vascular disease, and should be used with great caution and reluctance in all other conditions. Local anaesthetic sympathetic blocks have been reported as being superior to conservative therapy in a series of RSD patients (Wang et al 1985). Axillary brachial plexus block produced better results than stellate ganglion block in a series of patients with upper limb RSD (Defalque 1984). There are no clear guidelines as to the indications for different techniques and the optimal frequency and duration of treatment have not been established.

## Essential requirements for sympathetic block

1. The performance of sympathetic blocks requires a full understanding of the relevant anatomy and the pathophysiology of the underlying condition. The complications of sympathetic blocks can be very serious.
2. Informed consent must be obtained before the block is performed so that the patient has a full understanding of what is planned and what the block aims to achieve.
3. Resuscitation equipment must be immediately available.
4. Secure venous access is essential for all patients, and facilities for the treatment of hypotension must be available. An intravenous fluid pre-load of crystalloid solution is usually given for all bilateral blocks (splanchnic, coeliac, lumbar sympathetic, superior hypogastric).
5. Patients may experience some discomfort when the blocks are being performed and many practitioners employ sedation with drugs such as midazolam and alfentanil in addition to infiltration with local anaesthetic. General anaesthesia is rarely necessary. It has been argued that nerve damage could go unrecognised in an anaesthetised patient who is unable to speak or respond.
6. Constant monitoring should include regular measurement of blood pressure and pulse oximetry. Oxygen desaturation may occur during sedation, especially when the patient is in the prone position.
7. Radiological control in the form of an image intensifier, ultrasound or computed tomography (CT) scanner is mandatory for splanchnic, coeliac, lumbar sympathetic blocks and superior hypogastric blocks. Whenever possible a permanent print should be made and filed in the patient's notes, most especially for any neurolytic procedure. The image intensifier allows a faster, safer procedure, overcomes the problem of variable anatomical landmarks, allows precise needle placement, demonstrates the spread of injected solution and reveals inadvertent intravascular injection even when aspiration tests have been negative. With accurate needle placement small volumes of neurolytic solution can be used, thereby minimising the risk of complications.
8. An aseptic technique is essential.

## Neurolytic solutions for sympathetic blocks

A number of different solutions will destroy nerves, but phenol and alcohol are used most commonly for neurolytic sympathetic blocks.

*Phenol* destroys all nerve fibre types by protein denaturation. It is not selective and will destroy both motor and sensory nerves although the fibres can regenerate so the blocks should not be regarded as permanent. The strongest aqueous solution is 6.6%, but higher concentrations can be obtained using an oily base such as X-ray contrast medium and this is recommended. Contact with somatic nerves may cause neuritis. Toxic reactions may occur if a dose of 600 mg is exceeded in a 70 kg man.

*Alcohol* has a similar non-selective destructive action on nerves, but it produces a very high incidence of neuritis and is usually reserved for coeliac plexus block where the large injection volumes preclude the safe use of phenol.

## SYMPATHETIC BLOCK TECHNIQUES
## Stellate ganglion block

### Anatomy

The stellate (cervico-thoracic) ganglion is formed by the fusion of the inferior cervical and first thoracic sympathetic ganglia. It lies anterior to the transverse process of the seventh cervical and first thoracic vertebrae and the neck of the first rib (Fig. 21.1). It is anterior to the prevertebral fascia, may be covered in its

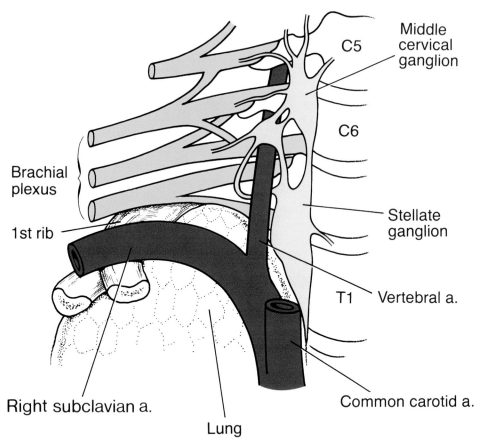

**Fig 21.1**   Position of the stellate ganglion. Note that, at the level of injection (C$_6$), the vertebral artery is a posterior relation

lower parts by the dome of the pleura, and lies posterior to the carotid sheath. The sympathetic outflow to the upper limb is derived predominantly from the T$_2$ and T$_3$ ganglia, so a stellate ganglion block which results in a Horner's syndrome does not guarantee that the arm supply has also been blocked. Confirmation of an effective block in the arm should be obtained by temperature measurements.

*Technique*
A number of approaches to the stellate ganglion have been described, but the simplest and most satisfactory is the anterior paratracheal. With the patient in the supine position, the head is extended and a point is marked 2–3 cm above and 2 cm lateral to the suprasternal notch. Pressure is applied with two fingers in the groove between the trachea and the carotid sheath (Fig. 21.2). In a very thin patient it may be possible to feel the transverse process of C$_6$, which lies at the level of the cricoid cartilage. A 23 g, 30 mm needle is inserted

directly backwards to pass between the trachea and the carotid sheath until it strikes the transverse process of C$_6$, some 2.5–3 cm from the skin. The needle should then be withdrawn 2–3 mm so that the tip lies anterior to the prevertebral fascia and the longus colli muscle. The needle is fixed in this position with one hand, whilst an aspiration test is performed. A test dose should be injected, and then 10–15 ml of solution is injected slowly, with repeated aspiration tests. The use of a short catheter between needle and syringe allows an assistant to perform the injection while the needle is kept 'immobile'. The patient should be instructed not to talk or swallow during the injection, but to raise a hand as a signal to stop if the injection is painful. If the needle is in the correct fascial plane, there should be slight resistance to injection, but no swelling should be apparent. To produce full sympathetic block of the upper limb the solution must extend to the T$_3$ ganglion and volumes larger than 10 ml may be necessary. Although it is often done, there may be little advantage

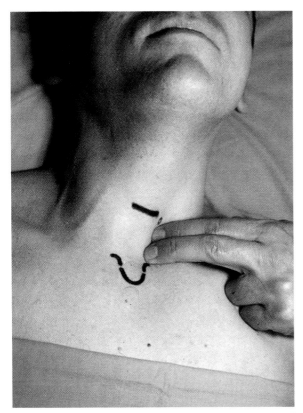

**Fig 21.2** Landmarks for stellate ganglion block. The cricoid cartilage and the tip of the transverse process of $C_6$ have been marked

in sitting the patient to aid spread to the thoracic ganglia (Hardy & Wells 1987, Hogan et al 1992).

**Other approaches** Lateral and posterior approaches should only be used when the anterior approach is difficult because of anatomical distortion. These techniques have a much higher incidence of complications, including epidural and intrathecal injection.

## Choice of solution

Lidocaine 1% is suitable for a diagnostic block, but bupivacaine 0.25% or 0.5% is preferred for other blocks. Continuous infusion on to the stellate ganglion has been described using the classic anterior paratracheal technique to insert a catheter (e.g. an epidural catheter). Bupivacaine 0.25% can be infused at up to 8 ml h$^{-1}$ to maintain sympathetic block in the arm (Owen-Falkenberg & Olsen 1992).

Neurolytic stellate ganglion blocks are potentially very hazardous and should be performed only by an experienced practitioner. If this technique is used, very small volumes (less than 1 ml) containing radiopaque medium can be injected under X-ray control to ensure that surrounding structures are not damaged (Racz & Holubec 1989). A technique for producing radiofrequency lesions has been described by Geurts and Stolker (1993), but transthoracic endoscopic techniques are safer and more predictable.

### Complications

**Systemic toxicity** The stellate ganglion is closely related to several major blood vessels, particularly the vertebral artery. Intra-arterial injection of even a minute dose of local anaesthetic will produce immediate and startling signs of central toxicity because the drug is delivered directly to the brain.

**Vaso-vagal reactions** They are readily triggered from the neck and these should be distinguished from local anaesthetic toxicity. The patient becomes anxious, pale, sweaty and nauseated, with bradycardia and hypotension. Withdrawal of the needle and elevation of the legs is usually sufficient treatment.

**Horner's syndrome** Unilateral meiosis, ptosis and enophthalmos are inevitable results of successful stellate ganglion block and the patient must be warned of this beforehand. Conjunctival vasodilatation and unilateral nasal congestion will also occur. No special treatment is required, although the meiosis may be reversed with 10% phenylephrine drops.

**Other nerve block** If the injection is in the wrong tissue plane, the local anaesthetic may affect the roots of the *brachial plexus*. No treatment is required, but the block may lead to diagnostic and prognostic confusion. *Phrenic nerve block* will occur if the solution is injected too far anteriorly, but this rarely causes any problems. However, *spinal or epidural injection* will cause significant problems and may occur if the needle passes between the transverse processes of the adjacent vertebrae. Finally, local anaesthetic solution may also spread to cause recurrent laryngeal nerve palsy with *hoarseness*. The patient should be warned that this is a possible complication.

**Tissue damage** The dome of the pleura rises above the first rib and is closely related to the ganglion. The patient becomes vulnerable to a *pneumothorax* if the needle is inserted in a caudad direction. The oesophagus is also vulnerable to damage by a misplaced needle, and *intercostal neuralgia*, manifesting as severe chest wall pain, has been described after stellate ganglion block (McCallum & Glynn 1986).

*Bilateral stellate blocks should never be performed because of the risk of pneumothorax, phrenic nerve block and recurrent laryngeal nerve palsy.*

## Thoracic sympathetic block

The upper thoracic sympathetic ganglia rest against the heads of the ribs and are covered by the pleura. The lower two or three are on the sides of the vertebral bodies. The thoracic sympathetic trunk runs between the ganglia and just in front of the somatic nerves. The very close relationship between somatic and sympathetic nerves means that any solution injected near the sympathetic nerves will also spread to the somatic roots. For this reason there are only very limited applications for upper thoracic sympathetic block. Direct vision endoscopic surgical techniques offer a more certain result.

### Technique

For an upper thoracic sympathetic block the patient should lie prone. Under image intensifier control the appropriate vertebral level is identified and a spinal needle is inserted 4–5 cm lateral to the spinous process, midway between the transverse processes. The needle is directed cephalad and medially on to the more cephalad transverse process of that level. The needle is then withdrawn and redirected caudad to the transverse process and towards the side of the vertebral body. The lateral view is checked to ensure that the needle tracks cephalad to the vertebral foramen to avoid the emerging somatic nerve. The needle is advanced until the tip is immediately beside the vertebral body, anterior to the vertebral foramen and next to the anterior aspect of the neck of the rib. Injection should be limited to 2–3 ml, and neurolytic solutions should be used with extreme caution for non-malignant conditions because some somatic block is highly likely.

A technique for percutaneous radiofrequency upper thoracic sympathectomy has been described by Yarzebski and Wilkinson (1987). It is a difficult procedure and has been superseded by endoscopic surgical techniques (Malone et al 1986), thoracoscopic sympathectomy being very successful in the treatment of hyperhidrosis (Byrne et al 1990, Gordon & Collin 1994). Interpleural block is an alternative way of producing unilateral sympathetic block of the arm, and Reiestad and colleagues (1989) used this technique to give daily injections of 3 ml

bupivacaine 0.5% with epinephrine through an indwelling catheter. Finally, a thoracic epidural infusion can be used to produce sympathetic as well as somatic block.

### Complications

There is a significant risk of complications, including *pneumothorax, subarachnoid injection, somatic nerve injury* and *somatic nerve block.*

## Splanchnic nerve block

### Anatomy (Fig. 21.3)

The greater, lesser and least splanchnic nerves cross the lateral side of the body of $T_{12}$ as they sweep forward to penetrate the diaphragm and form the coeliac plexus. The pleura lies lateral, and the crura of the diaphragm anterior, to the nerves. The pleura is attached posteriorly to the vertebral bodies and creates a well-defined compartment (Boas 1983).

### Technique

The patient should lie prone. Under image intensifier control the lateral end of the transverse process of $L_1$ is identified. The needle is inserted just lateral to it, and is directed to pass beneath the twelfth rib on to the side

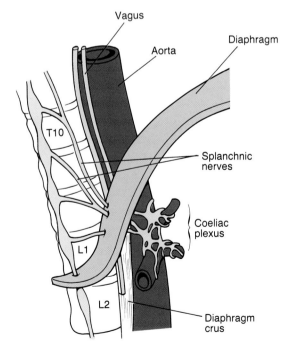

**Fig 21.3** Position of the splanchnic nerves and coeliac plexus. Note that the latter lies more anterior than the sympathetic chain

of the body of $T_{12}$. The needle is manoeuvred, in the lateral view, until the tip is just posterior to the anterior edge of the vertebra. Injection of contrast should show that the spread of dye is limited anteriorly and inferiorly by the crus of the diaphragm, and posteriorly by the attachment of the pleura to the vertebrae.

*Choice of solution*
Up to 15 ml of either bupivacaine 0.5% or phenol 6% can be injected using constant radiographic monitoring. Volumes as small as 3 ml have been used.

*Complications*
A *pneumothorax* may be produced if the needle is not kept close to the side of the body of $T_{12}$, and both intrathecal and epidural injection may occur.

## Coeliac plexus block

*Anatomy* (Figs 21.3 & 21.4)
The coeliac plexus, the largest of the prevertebral plexuses, is formed by the union of the greater ($T_5$–$T_{10}$), lesser ($T_{10}$–$T_{11}$) and least ($T_{12}$) splanchnic nerves with the coeliac branch of the right vagus. It therefore contains

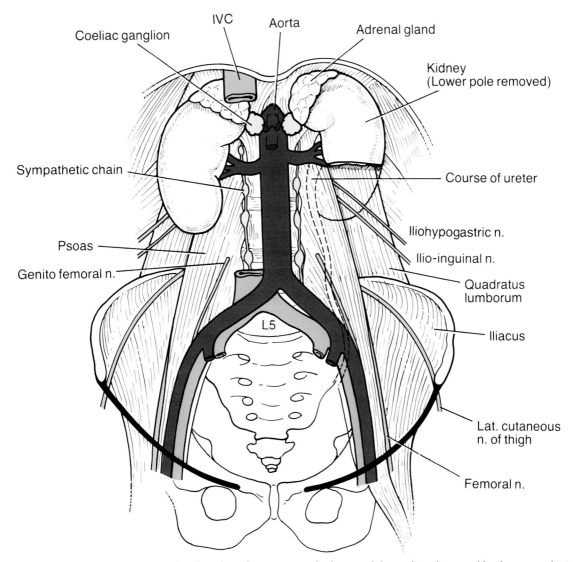

**Fig 21.4** View of posterior abdominal wall to show the position and relations of the coeliac plexus and lumbar sympathetic chain

both sympathetic and parasympathetic fibres. There are usually two semilunar-shaped ganglia at the level of the lower part of the twelfth thoracic and the upper part of the first lumbar vertebrae. The ganglia lie in the retroperitoneal tissue, between the suprarenal glands, posterior to the stomach, pancreas and the left renal vein, anterior to the crura of the diaphragm, and mainly anterolateral to the aorta. The kidneys are in close relationship. The ganglia surround the origin of the coeliac and superior mesenteric arteries and bilateral spread of the solution is necessary to ensure a complete block.

In the classic retrocrural technique, first described by Kappis in 1919, two needles are positioned posterior to the crura of the diaphragm. The solution may only block the splanchnic nerves or may follow the aorta through the diaphragm to reach the coeliac plexus as well. However, the needle must penetrate the diaphragm and lie 1–2 cm anterior to the front of the vertebral body to be certain of reaching the whole of the coeliac plexus. This is easier on the right side, but the needle is likely to encounter the aorta on the left. A combined approach has been described involving a right transcrural injection and a left retrocrural injection (Brown & Moore 1988).

### Technique

The patient is positioned prone on the X-ray table. The spinous process and transverse processes of the first lumbar vertebra are identified using the image intensifier, and a point is marked 6–7 cm lateral to the spine making sure that it is inferior to the transverse processes and the twelfth rib (Fig. 21.5). The skin and deeper tissues are infiltrated with local anaesthetic before a 15 cm, 20 g needle is inserted at the marked point and directed towards the side of the body of $L_1$ (Fig. 21.6). The needle is likely to damage the kidney if the insertion point is more than 7.5 cm lateral to the spine (Moore et al 1981). The needle is advanced slightly cephalad and at about 60° to the coronal plane.

Once contact has been made with the vertebral body the needle is guided anteriorly, monitored in the lateral view. The needle tip should be kept close to the vertebral body until it lies at the anterior edge of the body. A second needle is inserted on the opposite side. The coeliac plexus lies more anterior than the sympathetic chain so the right needle should be advanced to lie about 1–2 cm anterior to the vertebral body, the left a little less because of the presence of the aorta. An anteroposterior X-ray view at this stage should show the

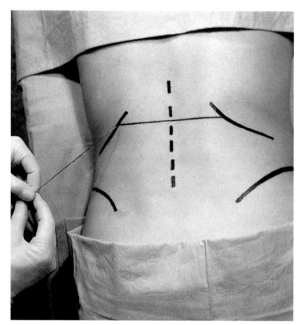

**Fig 21.5** Landmarks and needle alignment (patient supine, pictured from above) for coeliac plexus block. The posterior spines of $T_5$–$T_{12}$ have been marked

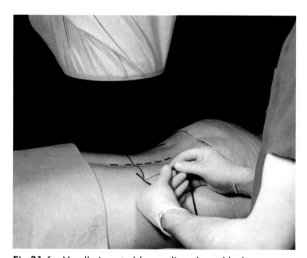

**Fig 21.6** Needle inserted for coeliac plexus block

needle points situated medial to the lateral edge of the vertebra (Fig. 21.7). Injection of contrast solution should demonstrate spread in the longitudinal axis without any lateral or posterior extension. Careful aspiration tests should precede the injection, which should be very easy; resistance suggests that the needle tip lies in the wrong place. A small volume of local anaesthetic should be injected before the alcohol because the latter can produce considerable discomfort.

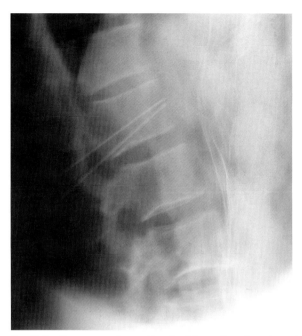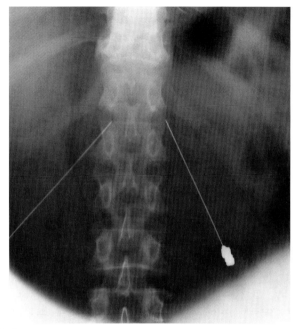

**Fig 21.7** Correct needle position for bilateral coeliac plexus block

A single-needle, transaortic approach has been described by Ischia and colleagues (1983). The needle is inserted on the left side and positioned to ensure that its point is in the middle of the coeliac plexus. In a modified version of this technique, the needle is inserted as for the standard approach and advanced until a characteristic 'click' and aspiration of blood confirm that the tip is in the aorta. The needle is then advanced through the anterior aortic wall. The point must lie in an area of very low resistance to injection, and not in the wall of the aorta. This technique is only recommended if difficulties are encountered when the standard approach is used for a neurolytic plexus block in a patient with cancer.

It is claimed that the use of CT scanning (Fig 21.8) improves the safety and effectiveness of coeliac plexus block (Filshie et al 1983, Brown & Moore 1988). Lieberman and Waldman (1990) used a CT-guided, single-needle transaortic approach and injected only 12 ml of neurolytic solution. Although Kirvela and colleagues (1992) have described the advantages of using ultrasonic guidance for both lumbar sympathetic and coeliac plexus block, Rathmell and colleagues (2000) have concluded that the best imaging modality for coeliac plexus block has yet to be determined.

The procedure can be performed in the lateral position if the patient is unable to lie prone, and the

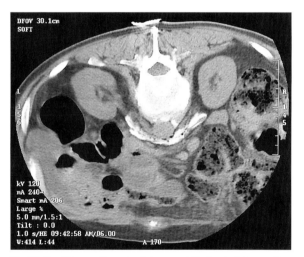

**Fig 21.8** CT scan through abdomen at the level of the coeliac plexus. Note the dye lying in the plane anterior to the aorta

single-needle, ultrasound-guided, anterior approach is also an option for such patients. It is claimed that this technique reduces the risk of neurological complications because the needle is never near the spinal cord or spinal arteries (Montero-Matamala et al 1989).

## Choice of solution

Diagnostic and therapeutic local anaesthetic injections may be performed with up to 20 ml of plain

**303**

bupivacaine 0.25% on each side. Depot preparations of steroid can be added for chronic pancreatitis, although the value of this remains unproven (Kennedy 1983). For a neurolytic block, up to 20 ml of alcohol 50% is injected on each side. Absolute alcohol can be diluted with bupivacaine 0.25%. Repeated aspiration tests must be performed and the dispersion of the contrast solution observed. Brown and Moore (1988) advocate the injection of larger volumes because they claim that standard ones result frequently in incomplete neurolysis and inadequate pain relief. Phenol can be used in smaller volumes of 5–10 ml per side.

### Complications

*Hypotension* is an almost inevitable consequence, and it can persist for many days after a neurolytic block, so coeliac plexus block is contraindicted in hypovolaemic patients. *Diarrhoea* is also a common complication.

*Paraplegia* has been reported. The needles or neurolytic solution may cause damage to, or spasm of, the spinal blood vessels, particularly the artery of Adamkiewicz, the largest artery supplying the lumbar spinal cord (Davies 1993). Other *neurological sequelae* may follow spread of neurolytic solution to the lumbar somatic nerves, and inadvertent epidural or intrathecal injection may cause major problems.

Either the needle or the neurolytic solution may damage other adjacent structures such as the aorta, the coeliac and superior mesenteric arteries, the pleura, the thoracic duct or the kidneys. Finally, *failure of ejaculation* is a significant risk so neurolytic blocks must be avoided in young males or any man unwilling to accept the risk of this side-effect.

Davies (1993) reviewed 2730 neurolytic coeliac plexus blocks and estimated that major complications (paraplegia with or without loss of sphincter function) happened once every 683 blocks. A meta-analysis by Eisenberg and colleagues (1995) reported local pain in 96%, diarrhoea in 44%, hypotension in 38% and major neurological complications such as weakness or paraesthesia in 1% of patients.

## Lumbar sympathetic block

### Anatomy (Figs 21.4 & 21.9)

The lumbar sympathetic trunk is situated in the retroperitoneal connective tissue anterior to the vertebral bodies and the medial margin of psoas muscle. The aorta and the inferior vena cava are anterior relations,

the genitofemoral nerve lies laterally on psoas, and the kidney and ureter are posterolateral in position. All the sympathetic fibres pass through or synapse at the $L_2$ ganglion, so in theory a block at the upper level of $L_3$ should abolish all the sympathetic supply to the lower limb, but opinions differ over the number of levels which need to be injected to produce optimal lower limb sympathectomy. Boas (1983) reviewed 500 patients and was unable to demonstrate any difference between single level injection ($L_2$ or $L_3$), double level injection ($L_2$ & $L_3$, or $L_3$ & $L_4$) or triple level injections ($L_2$, $L_3$ & $L_4$), although Walsh and colleagues (1984) reported over 400 cases, and claimed that triple level injection produced the best results. Umeda and colleagues (1987) studied 19 cadavers and concluded that the optimal site was level with either the lower third of the $L_2$ vertebral body or the upper third of $L_3$. A single level injection is safer and faster to perform, and the spread of solution can be observed with the image intensifier. If it is insufficient, the injection can be repeated at an adjacent level.

Usually, four pairs of lumbar arteries arise from the aorta and wind around the upper four lumbar vertebral bodies, deep to the sympathetic trunks and under the tendinous arches which give origin to psoas. The arteries are often accompanied by lumbar veins which may form plexiform networks. All of these vessels are vulnerable to penetration by needles.

### Technique

The injection can be performed with the patient prone, or in a lateral position. The patient and the

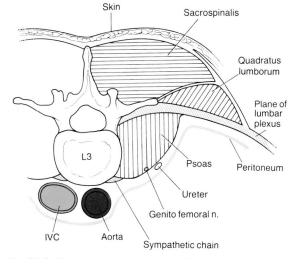

**Fig 21.9** Transverse section through $L_3$ to show the position and relations of the lumbar sympathetic chain

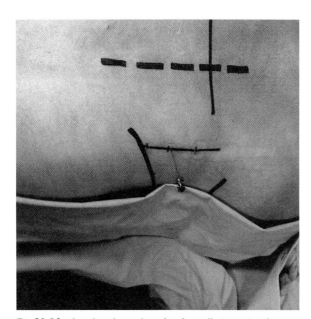

**Fig 21.10** Landmarks and angle of needle insertion for lumbar sympathectomy at the level of $L_3$

various anatomical landmarks are more stable in the prone position, and bilateral blocks can be performed more easily. Thus, the lateral position is reserved for the patient who cannot lie prone.

The prone approach is essentially the same for splanchnic nerve block, coeliac plexus block, lumbar sympathetic block at any level and block of the superior hypogastric plexus. The needle can be inserted at any lumbar level. Blocks for the lower limb (e.g. for peripheral vascular disease) usually target $L_3$ and $L_4$, but a block at $L_1$ is indicated for renal pain. Mandl (1947) described the classical approach, which depended upon needle contact with the transverse process to gauge depth. A more lateral approach, designed to avoid the transverse process, was described by Reid and colleagues (1970) and can be used with an image intensifier so that the needle misses this obstacle.

**Prone position** The spinous process of $L_3$ is identified with the image intensifier and a point marked 7–10 cm lateral to it, and midway between the transverse processes of $L_3$ and $L_4$ (Fig. 21.10). It is essential to ensure that the transverse process will not obstruct the passage of the needle, otherwise correct placement will be difficult or even impossible. The skin and deeper tissues are infiltrated with local anaesthetic; a 15 cm, 20 g needle is inserted at the point marked and is then directed towards the side of the body of $L_3$. The needle

should be at approximately 60° to the coronal plane, and some practitioners find it helpful to rotate the image intensifier to 60° as well, so that the needle is inserted along the direction of the X-ray view. Once contact is made with the vertebral body, the needle is manoeuvred anteriorly, monitored in the lateral view. The needle tip should remain close to the vertebra and its final position should be level with the anterior edge of the vertebral body (Fig. 21.11). A characteristic 'click' is often felt as the needle passes through the psoas fascia. An anteroposterior X-ray at this stage should show that the needle tip lies midway between the lateral edge of the vertebral body and the spinous process.

Injection of contrast solution should demonstrate linear spread in the longitudinal axis alone without any lateral or posterior extension (Fig. 21.11). Injection into psoas muscle produces a characteristic pattern which radiates inferolaterally away from the vertebral body. Occasionally, the contrast medium will be 'whisked' away in a small vessel, even though aspiration tests were negative. If the pattern of spread from the initial level of injection is satisfactory, then all the solution should be injected at that level. If the spread is not entirely satisfactory it may be possible to use a small volume at that level and to repeat the procedure at vertebral levels above or below. The same needle can usually be partially withdrawn, then redirected on to the adjacent vertebra. If difficulty is encountered, a second needle should be inserted at the appropriate level.

For an injection at $L_1$ the insertion point should not be more than 7.5 cm lateral to the spinous process. Insertion should be at the level of the $L_1$–$L_2$ interspace with the needle directed slightly cephalad to reach the side of the body of $L_1$.

**Lateral position** Very little modification in technique is needed for the lateral position. The major problem is positioning the patient so that the X-rays are truly anteroposterior and lateral. Once the patient is accurately positioned the procedure is basically as described for the prone position.

**Continuous block** A catheter can be inserted into the prevertebral area and a continuous sympathetic block maintained by an infusion of local anaesthetic (Betcher et al 1953). Some authors recommend a prognostic block for up to 5 days as a prerequisite to neurolytic block (Breivik et al 1998). Such an infusion may be

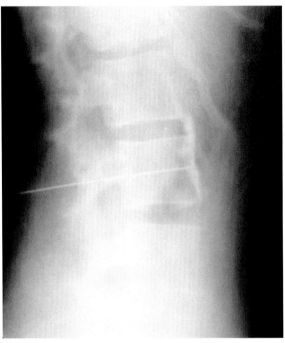
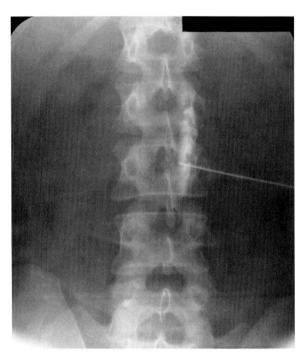

**Fig 21.11**  Films taken after completion of injection for lumbar sympathectomy. Note how the dye has spread longitudinally from the single injection point

indicated in young patients when there is doubt about the long-term effect of a chemical sympathectomy. CT-guided single-needle techniques have been described, and some authors claim that they offer advantages (Dondelinger & Kurdziel 1984, Redman et al 1986).

### Choice of solution

A diagnostic block requires a small volume which has been precisely placed: 2–5 ml of bupivacaine 0.5% at each level should suffice. Therapeutic local anaesthetic injections of 5–10 ml bupivacaine 0.5% may be given at a single level. Neurolytic injections should be made with aqueous phenol 6%, or a stronger solution, dissolved in X-ray contrast medium. A volume of about 2–5 ml is usually satisfactory, but recommendations range from 1 to 10 ml (Boas 1983, Walsh et al 1984). The needle should be flushed with local anaesthetic before withdrawal to avoid leaving a track of phenol through the more superficial tissues. Radiofrequency lumbar sympathectomy has been described (Rocco 1995).

### Complications

Major complications such as inadvertent injection of phenol into the vertebral canal, the peritoneal cavity or a blood vessel should not occur with a correct technique performed under radiographic control. Similarly, damage by the needle or neurolytic solution to the kidney, renal pelvis, ureter and intervertebral discs should also be avoidable. Injury to blood vessels in the posterior abdominal wall is not uncommon, but a significant retroperitoneal haematoma is unlikely in a patient with normal coagulation. However, phenol damage to blood vessels may explain some otherwise unaccountable neurological complications (Clarke 1984).

*Mild backache* is common and is likely to be more severe if neurolytic solution is deposited inadvertently in the posterior abdominal wall. Destruction of sympathetic fibres may cause a characteristic cramp-like or burning pain and dysaesthesia in the anterior thigh – so-called '*sympathalgia*' (Boas 1983, Kramis et al 1996) – which may also follow surgical sympathectomy (Tracy & Cockett 1957). *Neuropathic pain* may be caused by spread of phenol to the genitofemoral nerve where it lies on psoas. Occasionally, other somatic nerves may be damaged by the needle or by injected phenol. Treatment of both sympathalgia and neuritis may include carbamazepine or amitriptyline and TENS, but these are not always immediately effective and the patient will need to be reassured that remission should occur over a period of several weeks.

The vasodilatation produced by sympathectomy may result in *hypotension*, especially in the elderly or after bilateral blocks. Blood pressure should be monitored for at least 2 hours after the procedure and the patient supervised during mobilisation in case there is postural hypotension. Hypotension usually responds quickly to elevation of the legs so vasopressors or intravenous fluids are required rarely. *Intravascular 'steal'* may occur after sympathectomy in arteriosclerotic patients and result in diversion of blood from compromised distal vessels into the more proximal or less diseased circulation.

*Failure of ejaculation* is a real risk after bilateral block and this risk must be explained to male patients (Baxter & O'Kafo 1984).

## Superior hypogastric plexus block

### Anatomy
The superior hypogastric plexus, which innervates pelvic viscera, is situated retroperitoneally in front of the lower third of the fifth lumbar vertebra and the upper third of the first sacral segment.

### Technique
The method has been described by both Plancarte and colleagues (1990a) and Leon-Casasola and colleagues (1993). The $L_4/L_5$ interspace is identified and bilateral needle entry points are marked 5–7 cm lateral to the midline at that level. Using the same general principles as for a lumbar sympathectomy, the two needles are inserted to lie anterolateral to the $L_5/S_1$ interspace. If aspiration reveals blood at this stage, Leon-Casasola and colleagues (1993) recommend that the needle be advanced further until aspiration of blood ceases. Injected contrast solution should remain anterior to the $L_5/S_1$ interspace. For a diagnostic block 8–10 ml bupivacaine 0.25% is injected through each needle. For a neurolytic block 8 ml aqueous phenol is injected on each side. Waldman and colleagues (1991) described a modified technique for superior hypogastric block using a single needle and CT guidance.

## Ganglion impar

Plancarte and colleagues (1990b) described a technique for presacral block of the ganglion impar for intractable perineal pain associated with cancer. The injection is performed with a bent needle inserted just anterior to the tip of the coccyx and then directed to the front of the sacrococcygeal junction under X-ray guidance. After a test dose of 4 ml of local anaesthetic, 4–10 ml phenol at 6% or 10% concentration can be injected.

## Intravenous regional sympathetic blocks

Intravenous regional sympathetic block is a development of intravenous regional anaesthesia. It is a simple and relatively inexpensive technique which involves the injection of a drug into an exsanguinated limb isolated from the circulation by a tourniquet. Guanethidine (Hannington-Kiff 1974) is the drug most frequently used in the UK. Guanethidine blocks the re-uptake of norepinephrine and depletes stores in the postganglionic nerve terminals. Complete repletion takes up to 10 days, but the effect of the block may last much longer. Other drugs which have been used include ketanserin (Davies et al 1987, Hanna & Peat 1989), bretylium (Ford et al 1988, Hord et al 1992), reserpine (Lief et al 1987), labetalol (Parris et al 1987), ketorolac (Vanos et al 1992), hydralazine, methyldopa, clonidine, and droperidol.

The effects on peripheral sympathetic mechanisms of bretylium, guanethidine and bethanidine were recorded as long ago as 1963 (Cooper et al 1963, Ardill et al 1967), but the mode of action of intravenous regional sympathetic blocks in pain management is not well understood. The effects are not confined to the sympathetic nervous system (Loh et al 1980). The final result may be influenced by the solution in which the active drug is dissolved, the tourniquet pressure and/or the ischaemic period (Glynn et al 1981, McKain et al 1983, Casale et al 1992). When used to treat painful conditions a series of intravenous blocks may produce relief of longer duration than repeated sympathetic chain block (Ericksen 1981, Bonelli et al 1983).

However, Jadad and colleagues (1995) conducted a systematic review of intravenous regional sympathetic blocks for patients with a diagnosis of RSD and were only able to find a total of seven randomised controlled trials. Guanethidine was used in four of these and none showed a significant effect on the pain of RSD. Two reports, one of ketanserin and one of bretylium, with only 17 patients in total, showed some advantage of the blocks over control. Jadad and colleagues then conducted their own randomised double-blind crossover study of these blocks with guanethidine in 16 patients with RSD. The trial was stopped prematurely because of the severity of side-effects, but no significant difference was found between guanethidine and placebo on any of the outcome measures. Ramamurthy and colleagues (1995) performed a randomised controlled trial and reported that guanethidine was no better than saline.

### Technique

Firm scientific guidelines do not exist, so there is wide variation in recommendations from different centres and the choices are made on a purely empirical basis. The technique is essentially the same as for intravenous regional anaesthesia for surgery. Sedation may be necessary before the tourniquet is inflated and, if the limb is particularly sensitive, exsanguination by elevation rather than compression is advised. The injection of the solution may cause a burning pain, possibly related to the release of catecholamines by the guanethidine. Most practitioners keep the tourniquet inflated for 15–20 minutes. Reactive hyperaemia follows release of the tourniquet and blood pressure should be monitored carefully. Prolonged hypotension may require active treatment (Sharpe et al 1987).

It is not possible to give firm guidelines on the optimal frequency or the total number of blocks if a series is planned, but an interval of 1 week between blocks is often used. It would seem pointless continuing beyond 3–4 blocks if no benefit were apparent, although some authors disagree. If the blocks produce short-term pain relief, that period should be used for physiotherapy and exercise.

### Choice of solution

For an arm, guanethidine 10–20 mg in up to 40 ml of preservative-free prilocaine or lidocaine 0.5% is used, and for a leg 20–30 mg guanethidine in up to 50 ml of prilocaine or lidocaine.

The recommended dose of bretylium is 1–1.5 mg kg$^{-1}$ in the same volume of prilocaine or lidocaine. Prilocaine should not be used in doses greater than 600 mg because of the risk of significant methaemoglobinaemia.

### Complications

*Prolonged hypotension, bradycardia and dizziness* may be very troublesome (Sharpe et al 1987, Jadad et al 1995). *Pain on injection* may occur despite the use of prilocaine or lidocaine. Onset may be immediate or it may develop while the tourniquet is inflated. Occasionally, the presenting condition is exacerbated and the patient returns the next day with a painful, red, swollen hand or foot. In this case the block should not be repeated.

### Conclusion

Many questions remain over the continued use of intravenous regional techniques for sympathetic block (Blanchard et al 1990, Jadad et al 1995, Kingery 1997). Are the techniques really no better than placebo? Which drug is best? Which carrier solution is best? What is the optimal interval between blocks and for how long should treatment be continued? Are the techniques superior to simple somatic block or superior to sympathetic ganglion block? Great care must be exercised with the use of these blocks until reliable evidence is available.

## References

Ali NMK 1995 Does sympathetic ganglionic block prevent postherpetic neuralgia? Regional Analgesia 20: 227–233

Ardill BL, Bhatnagar VM, Fentem PH 1967 Intravenous administration of drugs for obtaining regional adrenergic block. Cardiovascular Research 1: 233–240

Arner S 1991 Intravenous phentolamine test: diagnostic and prognostic use in reflex sympathetic dystrophy. Pain 46: 17–22

Baxter AD, O'Kafo BA 1984 Ejaculatory failure after chemical sympathectomy Anesthesia and Analgesia 63: 770–771

Betcher AM, Bean G, Casten DF 1953 Continuous procaine block of paravertebral sympathetic ganglions: observations on one hundred patients. Journal of the American Medical Association 151: 288–292

Blanchard J, Ramamurthy S, Walsh N, Hoffman J, Schoenfeld L 1990 Intravenous regional sympatholysis: a double blind comparison of guanethidine, reserpine, and normal saline. Journal of Pain and Symptom Management 5: 357–361

Boas RA 1983 The sympathetic nervous system and pain. In: Swerdlow M (ed) Relief of intractable pain, pp 215–237. Elsevier, Amsterdam

Boas RA 1998 Sympathetic nerve blocks: in search of a role. Regional Anesthesia and Pain Medicine 23: 292–305

Bonelli S, Conoscente F, Movilia PG, Rostelli L, Francucci B, Grossi E 1983 Regional intravenous guanethidine versus stellate ganglion blocks in reflex sympathetic dystrophy: a randomised trial. Pain 16: 297–307

Breivik H, Cousins MJ, Lofstrom BJ 1998 Sympathetic neural blockade of upper and lower extremity. In: Cousins MJ, Bridenbaugh PO (eds) Neural blockade. 3rd edn, pp 411–447. Lippincott-Raven, Philadelphia

Bristow A, Foster JMG 1988 Lumbar sympathectomy in the management of rectal tenesmoid pain. Annals of the Royal College of Surgeons of England 70: 38–39

Brown DL, Moore DC 1988 The use of neurolytic celiac plexus block for pancreatic cancer: anatomy and technique. Journal of Pain and Symptom Management 3: 206–209

Brown DL, Bulley CK, Quiel EL 1987 Neurolytic celiac plexus block for pancreatic cancer pain. Anesthesia and Analgesia 66: 869–873

Byrne J, Walsh TN, Hederman WP 1990 Endoscopic transthoracic electrocautery of the sympathetic chain for palmar and axillary hyperhidrosis. British Journal of Surgery 77: 1040–1049

Casale R, Glynn C, Buonocore M 1992 The role of ischaemia in the analgesia which follows Bier's block technique. Pain 50: 169–175

Charlton JE 1990 Reflex sympathetic dystrophy: non-invasive methods of treatment. In: Stanton-Hicks M, Janig W, Boas RA (eds) Reflex sympathetic dystrophy, pp 151–164. Kluwer, Boston

Clarke IMC 1984 Nerve blocks. Clinics in Oncology 3: 181–193

Cooper CJ, Fewings JD, Hodge RL, Whelan RF 1963 Effects of bretylium and guanethidine on human hand and forearm vessels and on their sensitivity to noradrenaline. British Journal of Pharmacology 21: 165–173

Davies DD 1993 Incidence of major complications of neurolytic coeliac plexus block. Journal of the Royal Society of Medicine 86: 264–266

Davies JAH, Beswick T, Dickson G 1987 Ketanserin and guanethidine in the treatment of causalgia. Anesthesia and Analgesia 66: 575–576

Defalque RJ 1984 Axillary versus stellate ganglion blocks for reflex sympathetic dystrophy of the upper extremity. Regional Anesthesia 9: 35

Dondelinger R, Kurdziel JC 1984 Percutaneous phenol neurolysis of the lumbar sympathetic chain with computed tomography control. Annals of Radiology 27: 376–379

Eisenberg E, Carr DB, Chalmers TC 1995 Neurolytic celiac plexus block for treatment of cancer pain: a meta-analysis. Anesthesia and Analgesia 80: 290–295

Eriksen S 1981 Duration of sympathetic blockade. Stellate ganglion versus regional guanethidine block. Anaesthesia 36: 768–771

Filshie J, Golding S, Robbie DS 1983 Unilateral computerised tomography guided coeliac plexus block: a technique for pain relief. Anaesthesia 38: 498–503

Ford SR, Forrest WH, Eltherington L 1988 The treatment of reflex sympathetic dystrophy with intravenous regional bretylium. Anesthesiology 68: 137–140

Geurts JWM, Stolker RJ 1993 Percutaneous radiofrequency lesion of the stellate ganglion in the treatment of pain in upper extremity reflex sympathetic dystrophy. The Pain Clinic 6: 17–25

Gleim M, Maier C, Melchert U 1995 Lumbar neurolytic sympathetic blockades provide immediate and long-lasting improvement of painless walking distance and muscle metabolism in patients with severe peripheral vascular disease. Journal of Pain and Symptom Management 10: 98–104

Glynn CJ, Basedow RW, Walsh JA 1981 Pain relief following postganglionic sympathetic blockade with i.v. guanethidine. British Journal of Anaesthesia 53: 1297–1302

Gordon A, Collin J 1994 Thoracoscopic sympathectomy. European Journal of Vascular Surgery 8: 247–248

Gordon A, Zechmeister K, Collin J 1994 The role of sympathectomy in current surgical practice. European Journal of Vascular Surgery 8: 129–137

Hanna MH, Peat SJ 1989 Ketanserin in reflex sympathetic dystrophy. A double-blind placebo controlled cross-over trial. Pain 38: 145–150

Hannington-Kiff JG 1974 Intravenous regional sympathetic block with guanethidine. Lancet i: 1019–1020

Hardy PAJ, Wells JCD 1987 Stellate ganglion blockade with bupivacaine: effect of volume on extent of sympathetic blockade. British Journal of Anaesthesia 59 933P–934P

Hogan QH 1993 The sympathetic nervous system in post-herpetic pain. Regional Anesthesia 18: 271–273

Hogan QH, Erickson SJ, Haddox JD, Abram SE 1992 The spread of solutions during stellate ganglion block. Regional Anesthesia 17: 78–83

Hord AH, Rooks MD, Stephens BO, Rogers HG, Fleming LL 1992 Intravenous regional bretylium and lidocaine for treatment of reflex sympathetic dystrophy: a randomised, double blind study. Anesthesia and Analgesia 74: 818–821

Ischia S, Luzzani A, Ischia A, Faggion S 1983 A new approach to the neurolytic celiac plexus block: the transaortic technique. Pain 16: 333–341

Jadad AR, Carroll D, Glynn CJ, McQuay HJ 1995 Intravenous regional sympathetic blockade for pain relief in reflex sympathetic dystrophy: a systematic review and a randomised double-blind crossover study. Journal of Pain and Symptom Management 10: 13–20

Kennedy SF 1983 Celiac plexus steroids for acute pancreatitis. Regional Anesthesia 8: 39–40

Kingery WS 1997 A critical review of controlled clinical trials for peripheral neuropathic pain and complex regional pain syndromes. Pain 73 123–139

Kirvela O, Svedstrom E, Lundblom N 1992 Ultrasonic guidance of lumbar sympathetic and coeliac plexus block. A new technique. Regional Anesthesia 17: 43–46

Kozin F 1992 Reflex sympathetic dystrophy: a review. Clinical and Experimental Rheumatology 10: 401–409

Kramis RC, Roberts WJ, Gillette RG 1996 Post-sympathectomy neuralgia: hypothesis on peripheral and central mechanisms. Pain 64: 1–9

Leon-Casasola OA de, Kent E, Lema MJ 1993 Neurolytic superior hypogastric plexus block for chronic pelvic pain associated with cancer. Pain 54: 145–151

Lieberman R, Waldman SD 1990 Celiac plexus neurolysis with the modified transaortic approach. Radiology; 175: 274–276

Lief PA, Reisman R, Rocco A, McKay W, Kaul A, Benfell K 1987 IV regional guanethidine vs. reserpine for pain relief in reflex sympathetic dystrophy (RSD): a controlled, randomised, double-blind, crossover study. Pain Supplement 4: 398

Loh L, Nathan PW, Schott GD, Wilson PG 1980 Effects of regional guanethidine infusion in certain painful states. Journal of Neurology, Neurosurgery and Psychiatry 43: 446–451

McCallum MID, Glynn CJ 1986 Intercostal neuralgia following stellate ganglion block. Anaesthesia 41: 850–852

McKain CW, Urban BJ, Goldner JL 1983 The effects of intravenous regional guanethidine and reserpine. Journal of Bone and Joint Surgery 65A: 808–811

McLachlan EM, Janig W, Devor M, Michaelis M 1993 Peripheral nerve injury triggers noradrenergic sprouting within dorsal root ganglia. Nature 363: 543–546

Malmqvist L-A, Bengtsson M, Bjornsson G, Jorfeldt L, Lofstrom JB 1987 Sympathetic activity and haemodynamic variables during spinal analgesia in man. Acta Anaesthesiologica Scandinavica 31: 467–473

Malone PS, Cameron AEP, Rennie JA 1986 Endoscopic thoracic sympathectomy in the treatment of upper limb hyperhidrosis. Annals of the Royal College of Surgeons England 68: 93–94

Mandl F 1947 Paravertebral Block. Heinemann, London

Manriquez RG, Pallares V 1978 Continuous brachial plexus block for prolonged sympathectomy and control of pain. Anesthesia and Analgesia 57: 128–130

Mercadante S 1993 Celiac plexus block versus analgesics in pancreatic cancer pain. Pain 52: 182–192

Merskey H, Bogduk N 1994 (eds) Classification of chronic pain, 2nd edn, pp 40–43. IASP Press, Seattle

Montero-Matamala, AM, Lopez FV, Sanchez JLA, Bach LD 1989 Percutaneous anterior approach to the coeliac plexus using ultrasound. British Journal of Anaesthesia 62: 637–640

Moore DC, Bash WH, Burnett LL 1981 Celiac plexus block: a roentgenographic, anatomic study of technique and spread of solution in patients and corpses. Anesthesia and Analgesia 60: 369–379

Nikolajsen L, Jensen TS 2001 Phantom limb pain. British Journal of Anaesthesia 87: 107–116

Owen-Falkenberg A, Olsen KS 1992 Continuous stellate ganglion blockade for reflex sympathetic dystrophy. Anesthesia and Analgesia 75: 1041–1042

Parris WCV, Harris R, Lindsay K 1987 Use of intravenous regional labetalol in treating resistant sympathetic dystrophy. Pain Supplement 4: 399

Plancarte R, Amescua C, Patt RB, Aldrete JA 1990a Superior hypogastric plexus block for pelvic cancer pain. Anesthesiology 73: 236–239

Plancarte R, Amescua C, Patt RB et al 1990b Presacral blockade of the ganglion of Walther (ganglion impar). Anesthesiology 73: A751

Purcell-Jones G, Justins DM 1988 Delayed contralateral sympathetic blockade following chemical sympathectomy – a case history. Pain 34: 61–64

Racz GB, Holubec JT 1989 Stellate ganglion neurolysis. In: Racz GB (ed) Techniques of neurolysis, pp 133–144. Boston, Kluwer

Raja SN, Treede R-D, Davis KD, Campbell JN 1991 Systemic alpha-adrenergic blockade with phentolamine: a diagnostic test for sympathetically maintained pain. Anesthesiology 74: 691–698

Ramamurthy S, Hoffman J, the Guanethidine Study Group 1995 Intravenous regional guanethidine in the treatment of reflex sympathetic dystrophy/causalgia: a randomised double-blind study. Anesthesia and Analgesia 81: 718–723

Rathmell JP, Gallant JM, Brown DL 2000 Computed tomography and the anatomy of celiac plexus block. Regional Anesthesia and Pain Management 25: 411–416

Redman DRO, Robinson PN, Al-Kutoubi MA 1986 Computerized tomography guided lumbar sympathectomy. Anaesthesia 41: 39–41

Reid W, Watt JK, Gray TG 1970 Phenol injection of the sympathetic chain. British Journal of Surgery 57: 45–50

Reiestad F, McIlvaine WB, Kvalheim L, Stokke T, Pettersen B 1989 Interpleural analgesia in treatment of upper extremity reflex sympathetic dystrophy. Anesthesia and Analgesia 69: 671–673

Rocco AG 1995 Radiofrequency lumbar sympatholysis. The evolution of a technique for managing sympathetically maintained pain. Regional Anesthesia 20: 3–12

Schott GD 1998 Interrupting the sympathetic outflow in causalgia and reflex sympathetic dystrophy. British Medical Journal 316: 792–793

Schutzer SF, Gossling HR, Connecticut F 1984 The treatment of reflex sympathetic dystrophy syndrome. Journal of Bone and Joint Surgery 66A(4) 625–629

Sharpe E, Milaszkiewicz R, Carli F 1987 A case of prolonged hypotension following intravenous guanethidine block. Anaesthesia 42: 1081–1084

Tracy GD, Cockett FB 1957 Pain in the lower limb after sympathectomy. Lancet i: 12–14

Umeda S, Arai T, Hatano Y 1987 Cadaver anatomic analysis of the best site for chemical lumbar sympathectomy. Anesthesia and Analgesia 66: 643–646

Vanos DN, Ramamurthy S, Hoffman J 1992 Intravenous regional block using ketorolac: preliminary results in the treatment of reflex sympathetic dystrophy. Anesthesia and Analgesia 74: 139–141

Waldman SD, Wilson WL, Kreps RD 1991 Superior hypogastric block using a single needle and computed tomography guidance: description of a modified technique. Regional Anesthesia 16: 286–287

Walker SM, Cousins MJ 1997 Complex regional pain syndromes: including 'reflex sympathetic dystrophy' and 'causalgia'. Anaesthesia and Intensive Care 25: 113–125

Walsh JA, Glynn CJ, Cousins MJ, Basedow RW 1984 Blood flow, sympathetic activity and pain relief following lumbar sympathetic blockade or surgical sympathectomy. Anaesthesia and Intensive Care 13: 18–24

Wang JK, Johnson KA, Tucker GT 1985 Sympathetic blocks for reflex sympathetic dystrophy. Pain 23:13–17

Wettervik C, Claes G, Drott C et al 1995 Endoscopic transthoracic sympathectomy for severe angina. Lancet 345: 97–98

Woolf CJ, Mannion RJ 1999 Neuropathic pain: aetiology, symptoms, mechanisms and management. Lancet 353: 1959–1964

Wu CL, Marsh RH, Dworkin RH 2000 The role of sympathetic nerve blocks in herpes zoster and postherpetic neuralgia. Pain 87: 121–129

Yarzebski JL, Wilkinson HA 1987 $T_2$ and $T_3$ sympathetic ganglia in the adult human: a cadaver and clinical radiographic study and its clinical application. Neurosurgery 339–341

# 22. Regional anaesthesia for day-care surgery

## H B J Fischer

*'Local anaesthesia should be used on as many day patients as possible; alone, with sedation or with general anaesthesia. It maintains the best balance between effectiveness and side effects for postoperative analgesia. If it can be used, use it.'*

(Rudkin 1997)

During the last decade, there has been sustained growth in the number of patients undergoing day surgery as advances in anaesthesia and surgery have enabled a greater variety of procedures to be performed safely and effectively. Up to 50% of elective surgery is now performed in purpose-designed day-stay or ambulatory surgery units (Commission on Provision of Surgical Services 1992). With such large numbers of patients undergoing routine surgery the working practices of day units must be geared to proper selection of suitable patients, efficient management of the operating time and the rapid restoration of the patients to 'street fitness' in order that they are discharged home with the minimum of postoperative morbidity. In well-run units, the unplanned admission of patients to an inpatient bed after surgery should be no more than 2–3% of total activity (Gold et al 1989), and many units manage a lower incidence than this.

The major causes of unplanned admission that relate to anaesthesia are postoperative nausea and vomiting (PONV), uncontrolled pain and delayed recovery from general anaesthesia. Systemic opioids are associated with an increased incidence of all three causes of morbidity. In order to minimise or avoid their use, non-steroidal anti-inflammatory drugs (NSAIDs), oral preparations of compound analgesic drugs and oral opioids are often used in combination, but they may be inadequate for controlling early postoperative pain.

## GENERAL CONSIDERATIONS
### Role of regional anaesthesia

Regional anaesthesia is employed increasingly as the main technique because it improves the efficiency of a day surgery unit, decreases unplanned admission rates and reduces costs (Dexter & Tinker 1995). An unplanned overnight stay in an acute hospital bed can double the cost of a surgical procedure.

*Pain control*
Ineffectual pain control is often the primary reason for delayed discharge and, because surgeons perform increasingly complex surgery on a day-stay basis, effective pain management becomes both more important and more difficult to achieve. Regional anaesthesia can provide a quality and intensity of analgesia, especially in the early postoperative period, which is unsurpassed by any other analgesic regimen (Report of the Working Party on Pain after Surgery 1990). Not only is the analgesia of regional anaesthesia superior to that attainable with opioids, but it is also free from their side-effects – PONV, sedation and dysphoria.

*Postoperative nausea and vomiting (PONV)*
PONV is very common, with an incidence of up to 30% after general anaesthesia (Watcha & White 1992), and up to 40% after opioid administration (Campell 1990); it is often the most important factor in delayed discharge after day surgery (Green & Jonsson 1993). Regional anaesthesia is associated with a minimal risk of PONV (Bridenbaugh 1983), provided that side-effects such as hypotension and bradycardia are avoided, and that the surgical technique is modified to avoid stimulation outside the area of the regional block. Such stimulation

is an important cause of morbidity in procedures such as inguinal hernia repair where traction on the spermatic cord can produce visceral pain due to peritoneal stimulation, resulting in nausea and hypotension despite a fully functional inguinal field block.

### Postoperative sedation and dysphoria

Whether regional anaesthesia is used as the sole technique, or with minimal intravenous sedation or in combination with light general anaesthesia, patients demonstrate earlier recovery compared to general anaesthesia alone. Opioid requirements are reduced so there is less sedation. The patients, therefore, spend less time in the post-anaesthetic recovery area, require nursing care for a shorter period and can mobilise and co-operate with the physiotherapist at an earlier stage (Wallace et al 1994).

### Discharge time

The combination of decreased pain scores, minimal PONV and less postoperative sedation allows for earlier tolerance of oral intake and mobilisation. Several studies have demonstrated significant reduction in the time to discharge after a variety of procedures (Brown et al 1993, Flanaghan et al 1994, D'Alessio et al 1995).

### Nursing workload

The demands on nursing time in the immediate recovery phase after surgery are reduced, allowing the nursing staff to concentrate on ensuring that the patients' analgesic requirements and other post-discharge needs are properly met.

## Patient preparation

There are no set rules by which to determine the most appropriate regional technique for a particular surgical procedure and, similarly, the choice between a regional technique alone, or with sedation or a light general anaesthetic is a matter for the particular team involved.

On the day of admission, the detailed discussion of the role of regional anaesthesia for an individual patient is the responsibility of the anaesthetist concerned, but much of the groundwork can be done beforehand. For example, the surgeon can discuss the possible use of regional anaesthesia with the patient in the outpatient clinic. Many day-care surgery units have nurse-managed preoperative assessment clinics and, subject to agreed guidelines, suitable regional anaesthetic techniques can also be discussed with the patient at this stage.

Patients should receive the same written instructions regarding preoperative restriction of fluids and food as patients undergoing general anaesthesia – except for the most minor procedures. Inadequate local anaesthesia, an unco-operative patient, surgical complications and other unforeseen factors may necessitate the use of a general anaesthetic, so the stomach should be empty preoperatively.

Patients are more amenable to remaining awake during surgery if the prevailing atmosphere within the unit is geared towards the use of regional anaesthesia as a routine. Explanation and reassurance can begin during the process of admission with emphasis on the positive benefits of early recovery, fewer side-effects and that first cup of tea or coffee. In the operating theatre the patient is entitled to a degree of privacy and dignity while the block is performed, and warmth and comfortable support for the head and other pressure areas is appreciated. Conversation between members of staff should be limited to matters relating to the patient and the operation. Patients like to be informed about the progress of surgery and some may need to be distracted with quiet, gentle conversation, but incessant talking soon becomes irritating and does nothing to promote a relaxed atmosphere. With the increasing use of video technology, many patients enjoy the chance to watch the operation, while the surgeon can describe the nature of their problem as the operation proceeds.

Appropriate written information, packs of oral analgesics to take home, and efficient back-up facilities in the event of postoperative complications must be provided to ensure that the full benefits of regional anaesthesia are realised.

## Use of regional anaesthesia by surgeons

Although anaesthetists perform the majority of formal local anaesthetic techniques, some of the simpler blocks are suitable for use by surgeons, either as the sole anaesthetic technique or as a supplement to general anaesthesia (Table 22.1).

However, all but the most minor techniques carry the risk of systemic toxicity from overdose or inadvertent intravascular injection, so surgeons must be properly trained in the safe use of local anaesthetic drugs and in the recognition and treatment of systemic toxicity if they use these techniques with no anaesthetist present. Full resuscitation facilities and patient monitoring equipment must be immediately available and formal

**Table 22.1** Suitable local anaesthetic techniques for use by surgeons

| Regional anaesthesia technique | Surgical procedure |
| --- | --- |
| Topical drops, gels and cream | Eye surgery, urology |
| Wound irrigation/wound edge infiltration | Skin incisions, superficial surgery |
| Infiltration field blocks | Breast biopsy/surgery, inguinal hernia |
| Intraarticular injection | Arthroscopy of knee, elbow |
| Intraperitoneal instillation | Laparoscopic sterilisation |
| Discrete nerve block under direct vision | Spermatic cord, carpal tunnel |
| Peribulbar/retrobulbar/sub-Tenons | Cataract surgery |
| Intravenous regional | Forearm (and foot) surgery |

**Table 22.2** Regional blocks for day-care surgery

| Surgical procedure | Regional anaesthetic technique |
| --- | --- |
| Minor head and neck | Infiltration, discrete nerve blocks |
| | Superficial cervical plexus |
| Upper limb orthopaedic/plastic surgery | Brachial plexus block |
| | Peripheral nerve blocks – elbow/wrist/hand |
| | Intravenous regional anaesthesia |
| | Suprascapular nerve |
| Lower limb orthopaedic/plastic surgery | Lumbar plexus |
| | Spinal/epidural |
| | Peripheral nerve block – femoral/sciatic/popliteal ankle/foot |
| Lower abdominal cavity (laparoscopic) | Spinal/epidural |
| Thoraco-abdominal wall (breast, hernia) | Paravertebral |
| | Infiltration/field block |
| Urogenital: male external genitalia | Inguinal canal block/penile/scrotal infiltration |
| female genitalia | Caudal/pudendal nerve/infiltration |

arrangements for an anaesthetist to attend if necessary should be in place.

## REGIONAL TECHNIQUES FOR DAY-CARE SURGERY

The demands on day-care anaesthesia are increasing as new surgical procedures allow more major cases to be undertaken. Not only the complexity, but also the duration, of day-care surgery is increasing, and it is now considered reasonable to undertake major gynaecological, orthopaedic and general surgical procedures (White 2000). Effective and skilfully applied methods of pain management are required if these patients are to recover rapidly and be discharged safely. Upper and lower limb and peripheral nerve blocks are now used routinely, so it is possible to perform major arthroscopic surgery such as anterior cruciate ligament reconstruction and shoulder joint decompression on a day care basis. Table 22.2 lists some suitable techniques.

Many of the regional blocks described in the preceding chapters are suitable for day-care surgery, although some modification to the standard descriptions may be necessary to restrict the duration and, particularly, the extent of the block so that any associated sensory and motor dysfunction is kept to a minimum, consistent with effective analgesia. For minor surgery, a long-lasting peripheral nerve block can provide all the analgesia necessary, but after more major surgery a balanced analgesia regimen will be required.

## Upper limb surgery (see Ch. 14)

### Brachial plexus block
Administration of 0.5% bupivacaine will produce analgesia and residual motor weakness in excess of 12 hours, but this is usually inappropriate for surgery distal to the elbow. It is therefore preferable to use a short-acting agent such as prilocaine or lidocaine at 1.5–2%, so that the block, while providing adequate anaesthesia for the surgery and tourniquet, will regress within 2–4 hours and allow rapid recovery of shoulder

315

and elbow function. The axillary approach to the plexus has minimal effect on shoulder function as well as having a lower risk of serious side-effects, so it is popular for day-care surgery.

An alternative means of prolonging postoperative analgesia without prolonging the accompanying motor block is to use adjuvant drugs such as opioid or clonidine. Morphine 3 µg kg$^{-1}$, added to a mixture of lidocaine 1% and bupivacaine 0.5%, increases the duration of analgesia from 11 to 21 hours (Bazin et al 1997). Clonidine has a dose-dependent effect on both analgesia and anaesthesia; 0.1–0.4 µg kg$^{-1}$ of clonidine in 1% mepivacaine prolongs analgesia, and doses of 0.5–1.5 µg kg$^{-1}$ prolong both analgesia and anaesthesia (Singelyn et al 1996). As long as the dose of morphine or clonidine is within the stated limits, systemic side-effects do not occur because absorption from the brachial plexus is slow.

### Peripheral nerve blocks

Blocks at the elbow or wrist can provide prolonged analgesia distal to the elbow after hand or forearm surgery, which forms the large majority of day-care surgery to the upper limb. Six peripheral nerves (ulnar, median, radial, lateral medial and posterior cutaneous nerves of forearm) can be blocked separately or in combination at the elbow according to surgical requirements, and three nerves can be blocked at the wrist (ulnar, median and radial). Blocking the nerves distal to the brachial plexus restricts the area of block to the site of surgery, so prolonged postoperative analgesia is obtained with minimal motor and sensory dysfunction. If a tourniquet is required, patients will usually tolerate it for a brief period, but if surgery is likely to last longer than about 20 minutes, a light general anaesthetic or a short-duration brachial plexus block may be necessary.

### Intravenous regional anaesthesia (see Ch. 14)

This technique may be considered for minor surgery distal to the elbow if a tourniquet is to be used. It is easy and quick to perform and ensures a rapid return of limb function before discharge. Its main drawback is the lack of residual analgesia once the tourniquet is deflated and this may necessitate the use of local infiltration of the wound site by the surgeon.

### Intra-articular injections

These can provide some analgesia after shoulder joint arthroscopy.

### Suprascapular nerve block

This is an alternative technique which provides excellent analgesia for shoulder arthroscopy or joint manipulation and intra-articular steroid injection. The superior approach (Pinnock et al 1996) to the suprascapular nerve, using a peripheral nerve stimulator and an insulated short-bevel needle, has a high success rate and avoids the risk of pneumothorax associated with the posterior approach. The block is easier to perform when the patient is supine, rather than sitting, with the head turned slightly away from the side of injection (Fig. 22.1). The posterior border of the clavicle is traced laterally until the angle formed with the trapezius muscle, over the medial border of the acromioclavicular joint, is identified. A 7 cm, 22 g insulated needle is inserted at this point and aimed towards the contra-lateral nipple in the horizontal plane, or very slightly posterior to it. Stimulation of the supraspinatus muscle, which abducts the shoulder, should be apparent at a depth of 3–4 cm. The suprascapular nerve is stimulated at its point of exit from the suprascapular notch, and if the needle is inserted too deeply it will impinge on the medial border of the notch.

## Lower limb surgery (see Ch. 15)

### Femoral and sciatic nerve blocks

These provide extensive sensory, motor and sympathetic block which can last up to 24 hours if bupivacaine 0.5–0.75% is used. For major surgery to the knee, such as anterior cruciate ligament reconstruction, this may be beneficial if appropriate care can be guaranteed after discharge. A shorter duration of 6–10 hours is obtainable with lidocaine 2%.

### Popliteal block

This is preferable if surgery is restricted to below the knee. The block is limited to the calf and foot and, if it is combined with subcutaneous infiltration of the saphenous nerve, all the lower leg is anaesthetised, while the hip and knee joints are unaffected.

### Ankle blocks

These are an important component of anaesthesia for surgery to the foot, especially block of the posterior tibial nerve which provides analgesia to the whole of the sole of the foot. The five nerves supplying the foot (sural, tibial, superficial and deep peroneal and saphenous) can be blocked in combination according to the site of surgery; it should not be necessary to

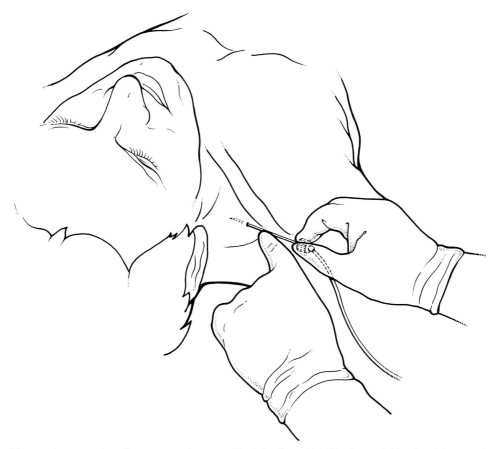

**Fig 22.1** The superior approach to the suprascapular nerve. The index finger identifies the medial border of the acromioclavicular joint and the needle is inserted in the horizontal plane. (From CA Pinnock, HBJ Fisher & RP Jones, 1996 with permission)

block them all unless extensive surgery is planned in which case a combination of saphenous nerve and popliteal block at the knee is more appropriate. Patients should be warned against mobilising or weight-bearing on a foot which has been blocked until sensation has fully returned.

*Intra-articular block of the knee*

This block is ideal for day-care arthroscopic surgery. It produces no motor or sensory deficit so patients can mobilise immediately afterwards. In addition, the quality of analgesia is sufficient to provide adequate pain control after quite major surgery, such as partial meniscectomy and debridement of synovium or cartilage. Under strict aseptic conditions, up to 30 ml of 0.5% bupivacaine with 1:200 000 epinephrine is injected under the medial border of the patella. This should be performed at least 20 minutes before surgery and can easily be done in the ward area of the day unit. The addition of 1–2 mg of morphine has been shown to increase the duration of analgesia, though some studies have failed to confirm this (see Kalso et al 1997 for review). The addition of clonidine 150 μg has the same effect as morphine in prolonging the duration and improving the quality of analgesia (Gentili et al 1997).

The block is usually combined with a light general anaesthetic, but can be entirely adequate as the sole anaesthetic technique if combined with subcutaneous injections of local anaesthetic to the sites of the arthroscope portals and if a tourniquet is not required. Some surgeons prefer to avoid preoperative intra-articular injection, citing the risks of infection or needle trauma within the joint. Close attention to detail and proper discussion about the benefits of establishing the block preoperatively should allay any concerns. The practice of the surgeon injecting, at the end of surgery, a variable concentration and volume of local anaesthetic, most of which escapes immediately through the portals, leads to inadequate analgesia and should be actively discouraged.

## The trunk (see Ch. 13)

### Inguinal field block

This is used extensively for inguinal herniorraphy, varicocoele surgery, orchidopexy and other urogenital surgery. It is important to identify carefully the fascia of the external oblique muscle and then the internal oblique muscle so that local anaesthetic is injected around the iliohypogastric and the deeper ilioinguinal nerve in the correct tissue planes. A short-bevel needle makes identification of the planes easier and reduces the risk of injecting the local anaesthetic too deep and accidentally blocking the femoral nerve. To improve the quality of analgesia, the spermatic cord should be blocked separately and this can be done either by percutaneous injection of 5 ml of local anaesthetic into the inguinal canal prior to surgery, or by the surgeon infiltrating the cord when the inguinal canal is opened. Because of the risk of femoral nerve block, patients should only be mobilised after formal assessment has demonstrated equal motor power in the quadriceps muscles and equal straight-leg raising ability in both legs.

### Regional anaesthesia for laparoscopy

Laparoscopy remains a common cause of unplanned overnight admission because of inadequate analgesia, nausea and vomiting. This is especially true of fallopian tube surgery where the pain is mainly visceral and often requires systemic opioids which, although effective, increase the likelihood of overnight admission due to sedation or nausea. Subserosal injection of 2–3 ml local anaesthetic into the cornual end of the fallopian tube, mesenteric injection of 5 ml of local anaesthetic at the point of application of the clips or rings, topical application of local anaesthetic gel to the clips and topical instillation of local anaesthetic solution directly on to the tubes have all been associated with a reduction in postoperative pain levels, but regional anaesthesia alone is not invariably successful without additional balanced analgesia. Instillation of dilute local anaesthetic into the peritoneal cavity has been tried for a variety of laparoscopic procedures, but with variable effect on postoperative pain, and infiltration of the instrument portals produces little, if any, benefit.

As an alternative to general anaesthesia, lumbar epidural anaesthesia has been used successfully for many years in some institutions. Reduced anaesthetic complications and earlier hospital discharge have been claimed (Bridenbaugh 1983).

## Central neural block

Caudal blocks are widely used in day-care surgery, particularly in children (see Ch. 19), and after urogenital, anorectal and lower limb procedures. In a number of countries spinal and lumbar epidural block has been popular in day surgery for many years although their use in Great Britain and Ireland is limited. This geographic discrepancy is more to do with social, cultural and professional factors than the techniques themselves, and there is extensive evidence that central neural blocks are safe, effective and well tolerated when used routinely for day surgery (Bridenbaugh & Soderstrom 1979). The increasing use of unilateral peripheral blocks may reduce the need for central blocks for lower limb procedures, and lumbar paravertebral block may be more appropriate for unilateral anaesthesia of the trunk than a lumbar epidural. On the other hand, as laparoscopic surgery becomes more widely performed as a day-care procedure, lumbar epidural block may be used more frequently.

### Caudal anaesthesia (see Ch. 12)

As well as being indicated for the operations mentioned above, caudal block can also be useful in circumstances where peripheral nerve block is impractical. The analgesia achievable with local anaesthetic alone (e.g. bupivacaine 0.25%) lasts 3–4 hours, but may be increased by the addition of fentanyl 100 µg or clonidine 150 µg. The main disadvantages are the residual motor weakness and visceral dysfunction which may delay mobilisation and the return of bladder control.

### Lumbar epidural and spinal anaesthesia

These methods are used in day-care surgery for abdominal and lower limb surgery and have a number of benefits, including superior analgesia, lower cost, earlier discharge and fewer side effects compared with general anaesthesia. They are usually easy to perform and, if a spinal is used, the quicker onset, more predictable anaesthesia and shorter recovery time result in minimal delay between patients. Table 22.3 compares the benefits and drawbacks of spinal and epidural block for lower abdominal and lower extremity surgery in the adult when lidocaine 2% is used as the local anaesthetic.

*Spinal anaesthesia* of sufficient intensity to allow surgery may not permit early ambulation postoperatively. On the other hand, the duration of action may be inadequate if a short-acting local anaesthetic or low-dose bupivacaine

**Table 22.3** Comparative details of spinal and epidural anaesthesia for day-care surgery

| Feature | Spinal | Epidural |
|---|---|---|
| Onset time | Rapid – a few minutes | Up to 20 minutes |
| Quality of anaesthesia | Predictable, dense | Unpredictable, normally adequate |
| Duration of anaesthesia | 60–90 minutes (50–70 mg 2% lidocaine) | 90–120 minutes (20 ml 2% lidocaine) |
| Time to complete regression | 110–150 minutes | Up to 210 minutes |
| Time to discharge | Within 5 hours | Within 5 hours |
| Complications | PDPH (onset may be delayed) Visceral disturbance Orthostatic hypotension Transient neurological symptoms | Delayed surgery Orthostatic hypotension Risk of dural puncture Visceral disturbance |

or ropivacaine is used (Mulroy & Wills 1995, Tarkkila et al 1997, Liam et al 1998, Gautier et al 1999).

Spinal lidocaine, prilocaine or low-dose bupivacaine have been advocated for day-care surgery (Mulroy & Wills 1995). They are reliable, with a rapid onset and similar discharge rates to a general anaesthetic, but without the residual sedation and higher incidence of nausea or vomiting. Some favour the combined spinal–epidural (CSE) technique because it enables a very small dose of intrathecal drug to be used and the block can be extended with epidural increments (Urmey et al 1995).

Spinal anaesthesia for day-care surgery may cause:

- Residual motor block and lack of proprioception of the lower limbs;
- Urinary retention;
- Postdural puncture headache (Pittoni et al 1995, Corbey et al 1997, Lambert et al 1997, Despond et al 1998, Spencer 1998);
- Transient neurologic symptoms (Corbey & Bach 1998, Henderson et al 1998).

## Complications

*Postdural puncture headache (PDPH)* after spinal anaesthesia occurs more frequently in day-care patients than the equivalent population of inpatients (Flaatten & Raeder 1985). The reasons for this are not clear as there seems to be no association with early mobilisation, and the high incidence may simply reflect a younger population of patients. In females under 40 years of age, the incidence is unacceptably high with 25–26 g needles – up to 40% – but with 27 g or pencil-point type needles the incidence is much lower for both sexes, especially in the over-40 age groups, and is typically less than 1% (Halpern & Preston 1994).

*Backache* may occur after spinal anaesthesia and may be due to stretching of anaesthetised ligaments and joints during surgery. It is more common when the patient has been placed in the lithotomy position. The patient should be positioned carefully, and abnormal postures should not be allowed because the protective effect of pain will have been removed.

*Transient neurological symptoms (TNS)*, formerly called transient radicular irritation (TRI), is a current concern in day-care surgery (Corbey & Bach 1998). It is a transient radicular pain or dysaesthesia which radiates to the buttocks and legs, and is thought to be due to musculoskeletal strain rather than neurotoxicity. It is not dependent on dose, concentration or osmolality, but seems to occur mostly with 5% hyperbaric lidocaine. It is usually short lived, but the patient should be warned of backache which may last a few days before it resolves spontaneously (Hampl et al 1995).

## Balanced analgesia

For major day-care surgery, regional anaesthesia is an important component of perioperative pain management, but may be insufficient as a sole technique. For inguinal herniorraphy (Ding & White 1995), laparoscopic sterilisation (Eriksson et al 1996), laparoscopic cholecystectomy (Kapur 1996) and arthroscopic anterior cruciate ligament reconstruction (Reuben et al 1998), all of which are now performed on a day-care basis, a balanced (multimodal) analgesia technique is required to manage the different acute pain mechanisms. Although there is a degree of flexibility about the precise components, a typical regimen would consist of the following:

1. Oral paracetamol, 1 g given 1 hour preoperatively
2. An oral NSAID given 1 hour preoperatively (e.g. ibuprofen 400 mg)

3. A small dose of short-acting opioid (fentanyl or alfentanil) should be included if general anaesthesia is used
4. Appropriate local anaesthetic block with a long-acting local anaesthetic
5. Postoperative paracetamol and NSAID prescribed 'regularly', not 'as required'
6. Oral opioids (e.g. dihydrocodeine 30 mg 4-hourly as required) in addition to regular paracetamol and NSAID.

## Postoperative and post-discharge care

One of the major benefits of regional anaesthesia, either as the sole anaesthetic technique or in combination with a light general anaesthetic, is a more rapid attainment of 'street fitness' than with general anaesthesia alone, and the day-care system must be geared to take advantage of this. The patient should meet the following discharge criteria when regional anaesthesia is used alone or combined with general anaesthesia or sedation:

- Full restoration of mental function
- Able to tolerate oral fluids and light diet
- Full recovery of motor, sensory and proprioceptive function (central blocks)
- Recovery of bladder function
- Support and protection of areas with residual analgesia/anaesthesia (peripheral block)
- Effective sequential analgesia established.

### Block regression

After spinal or epidural anaesthesia, regression of the upper and lower segmental sensory levels of the block and formal assessment of motor power and proprioception should be recorded. Patients can mobilise safely without orthostatic hypotension or motor weakness if perineal sensation is normal, proprioception of the great toe is perceived correctly and motor function of the lower limbs has fully recovered. Adjuvant drugs such as fentanyl and clonidine can prolong the duration of analgesia of central and peripheral nerve blocks without increasing the duration of the local anaesthetic effect, and they are increasingly being used in day-care patients.

### Urinary function

Bladder control can be disturbed by urogenital or inguinal surgery with both general and regional anaesthesia. The incidence of urinary retention following central neural block with short-acting drugs is low and may be no higher than the incidence following general anaesthesia. It is customary to keep patients in the unit until they can void spontaneously, but adults without risk factors for retention, and children, may be discharged home before they void provided that there are clear guidelines about what to do if voiding becomes a problem. Risk factors for retention include a previous history, pelvic and urological surgery, perioperative bladder catheterisation, and spinal or epidural anaesthesia with long-acting local anaesthetic drugs or opioids (Marshall & Chung 1999).

### Protection of the anaesthetised area

Peripheral blocks of the extremities may last 12 hours or more, during which time the affected area must be protected from inadvertent damage from pressure due to immobility, thermal injury or ischaemic injury from casts or dressings applied too tightly. The upper limb should be supported in a sling until shoulder and elbow function has fully recovered, and patients with lower limb blocks should not bear weight until full motor, sensory and proprioceptive function has returned. Brachial plexus blocks produce widespread effect, but

---

**Table 22.4** Regional anaesthesia patient information leaflet

You have had a local anaesthetic nerve block for pain control after your operation. While the area is numb or heavy and difficult to control you should follow the instructions below until the feeling and muscle power has returned to normal. This could take up to … hours

1. Avoid knocking or pressing the affected area
2. Protect it from heat, pressure and tight clothing
3. Avoid putting weight on an affected leg/foot or trying to use your hand/arm
4. Elevate the affected arm/leg when resting. When sitting or lying, rest your arm on your chest in the support provided/elevate your leg with a pillow under the calf on the bed or a footstool. Avoid draping heavy blankets over your leg/foot
5. Take the pain-killing tablets regularly as prescribed even if you are not in much pain. This should prevent the onset of severe pain as feeling returns to your wound
6. As feeling and muscle power return, gently exercise the affected area but avoid straining the muscles
7. Contact the Day Surgery Unit or the duty anaesthetist at the hospital if you have any concerns about your nerve block. (Telephone number ………………….)

for forearm and hand surgery discrete nerve blocks at the elbow offer prolonged analgesia below the elbow and leave the protective reflexes of the shoulder and elbow joints in tact. Femoral and sciatic nerve blocks produce extensive anaesthesia of very long duration which, although useful in special circumstances, may be excessive for routine lower limb surgery. Although popliteal fossa blocks and ankle/foot blocks affect a smaller area, the patient must not bear weight until the block has regressed fully. A simple information leaflet about local anaesthetic techniques, prepared for patients and their carers, is shown in Table 22.4.

### Sequential analgesia
The quality of analgesia produced by regional anaesthesia is usually excellent, so the onset of pain as the block wears off can be unexpected, unpleasant and distressing. The patient should be prescribed adequate sequential analgesia to prevent this. An adequate supply of oral analgesics must be provided, with written as well as oral instructions to take the drugs 'regularly' rather than 'as necessary'; administration of the first dose should be timed, so that adequate plasma concentrations are achieved before the block wears off. For example, after repair of an inguinal hernia under field block with 0.5% bupivacaine, the patient can expect 6–8 hours of postoperative analgesia. Within the first hour or so of recovery, the patient should be able to take a drink and a light diet with 400 mg of ibuprofen (or equivalent NSAID); a second dose 6 hours later should provide adequate sequential analgesia to coincide with the regression of the block.

The patient and the carer should be fully informed about the action to be taken after discharge, should the analgesia be inadequate or other complications of anaesthesia occur. A 24-hour contact telephone number must be available and specific advice given on the discharge instruction sheet. If central neural block has been used, a telephone call from the anaesthetist on the second or third postoperative day will enable any delayed post-spinal headache or back pain to be recorded and suitable advice given.

## CONCLUSIONS
Regional anesthesia techniques offer a number of significant advantages to patients undergoing day-care surgery, in particular the provision of effective pain control without the sedation, nausea and vomiting associated with the use of systemic opioids. Many of the peripheral blocks are simple, safe and effective, and are suitable for both surgeons and anaesthetists to perform after appropriate training. More complex techniques such as brachial plexus, major lower limb and central neural blocks also have a role where suitable systems are in place to ensure that the benefits of the blocks are fully realised and that the patient is managed safely before and after discharge.

## References
Bazin JE, Massoni C, Bruelle P et al 1997 The addition of opioids to local anaesthetics in brachial plexus block: the comparative effects of morphine, buprenorphine and sufentanil. Anaesthesia 52: 858–862

Bridenbaugh LD 1983 Regional anesthesia for outpatient surgery. A summary of 12 years experience. Canadian Anaesthesia Society Journal 30: 548–552

Bridenbaugh LD, Soderstrom RM 1979 Lumbar epidural block anesthesia for outpatient laparoscopy. Journal of Reproductive Medicine 23: 85–86

Brown AR, Weiss R, Greenberg C et al 1993 Interscalene block for shoulder arthroscopy: comparison with general anaesthesia. Arthroscopy 9: 295–300

Campbell WI. 1990 Analgesic side effects and minor surgery: which analgesics for minor day case surgery? British Journal of Anaesthesia 64: 617–620

Commission on the Provision of Surgical Services 1992 Guidelines for day case surgery. Royal College of Surgeons of England, London

Corbey MP, Bach AB. 1998 Transient radicular irritation (TRI) after spinal anaesthesia in day-care surgery. Acta Anaesthesiologica Scandinavica 42: 425–429

Corbey MP, Bach AB, Lech K, Frorup AM. 1997 Grading of severity of postdural puncture headache after 27-gauge Quincke and Whitacre needles. Acta Anaesthesiologica Scandinavica 41: 779–784

D'Alessio JG, Rosenblum M, Shea KP et al 1995 A retrospective comparison of interscalene block and general anesthesia for ambulatory surgery shoulder arthroscopy. Regional Anesthesia 20: 62–68

Despond O, Meuret P, Hemmings G 1998 Postdural puncture headache after spinal anaesthesia in young orthopaedic outpatients using 27-g needles. Canadian Journal of Anaesthesia 45: 1106–1109.

Dexter F, Tinker JH 1995 Analysis of strategies to decrease postanesthesia care costs. Anesthesiology 82: 94–101

Ding Y, White PF 1995 Post-herniorrhaphy pain in outpatients after pre-incision ilioinguinal–iliohypogastric nerve block during monitored anaesthesia care. Canadian Journal of Anaesthesia 42: 12–15

Eriksson H, Tenhunen A, Kortilla K 1996 Balanced analgesia improves recovery and outcome after outpatient tubal ligation. Acta Anaesthesiologica Scandinavica 40: 151–155

Flaatten H, Raeder J 1985 Spinal anaesthesia for outpatient surgery. Anaesthesia 40: 1108–1111

Flanagan JFK, Edkin B, Spindler K 1994 3 in 1 femoral nerve block following ACL reconstruction allows predictably earlier discharge and significant cost savings Anesthesiology 81: A950

Gautier PE, De Kock M, Van Steenberge A et al 1999 Intrathecal ropivacaine for ambulatory surgery. Anesthesiology 91: 1239–1245

Gentili M, Houssel P, Osman M et al 1997 Intraarticular morphine and clonidine produce comparable analgesia but the combination is not more effective. British Journal of Anaesthesia 79: 660–661

Gold BS, Kitz DS, Lecky JH, Neuhaus JM 1989 Unanticipated admission to hospital following ambulatory surgery. Journal of the American Medical Association 262: 3008–3010

Green G, Jonsson L 1993 Nausea: the most important factor in determining length of hospital stay after ambulatory anesthesia. A comparative study of isoflurane and/or propofol techniques. Acta Anaesthesiologica Scandinavica 37: 742–746

Halpern S, Preston R 1994 Postdural puncture headache and spinal needle design. Metaanalyses. Anesthesiology 81: 1376–1383

Hampl KF, Schneider MC, Ummenhofer W, Drewe J 1995 Transient neurologic symptoms after spinal anaesthesia. Anesthesia and Analgesia 81: 1148–1153

Henderson DJ, Faccenda KA, Morrison LM. 1998 Transient radicular irritation with intrathecal plain lignocaine. Acta Anaesthesiologica Scandinavica 42: 376–378

Kalso E, Tramer M, Carroll D et al 1997 Pain relief from intraarticular morphine after knee surgery: a qualitative systematic review. Pain 71: 642–651

Kapur PA. 1996 Preoperative multimodal analgesia facilitates recovery after ambulatory laparoscopic cholecystectomy. Anesthesia and Analgesia 82: 44–51

Lambert DH, Hurley RJ, Hertwig L, Datta S 1997 Role of needle gauge and tip configuration in the production of lumbar puncture headache. Regional Anesthesia 22: 66–72

Liam BL, Yim CF, Chong JL 1998 Dose response study of lidocaine 1% for spinal anaesthesia for lower limb and perineal surgery. Canadian Journal of Anaesthesia 45: 45–50

Marshall S, Chung F 1999 Discharge criteria and complications after ambulatory surgery. Anesthesia and Analgesia 88: 508–517

Mulroy MF, Wills RP 1995 Spinal anesthesia for outpatients: Appropriate agents and techniques. Journal of Clinical Anesthesiology 7: 622–627

Pinnock CA, Fischer HBJ, Jones RP 1996 Superior approach to the suprascapular nerve. In: Peripheral Nerve Blockade, Pinnock CA, Fischer HBJ (eds) pp 116–117. Churchill Livingstone, Edinburgh

Pittoni G, Toffoletto F, Cacarella G, Zanette G, Giron GP 1995 Spinal anesthesia in outpatient knee surgery: 22-gauge versus 25-gauge Sprotte needle. Anesthesia and Analgesia. 81: 73–79

Report of the Working Party on Pain after Surgery 1990 The Royal College of Surgeons of England and the College of Anaesthetists, London, p 20

Reuben SS, Steinberg RB, Cohen MA et al 1998 Intraarticular morphine in the multimodal analgesic management of postoperative pain after ambulatory anterior cruciate ligament repair. Anesthesia and Analgesia 86: 374–378

Rudkin GE 1997 Pain management in the adult day surgery patient. In: Millar JM, Rudkin GE, Hitchcock M (eds) Practical anaesthesia and analgesia for day surgery, pp 89–105. Bios Scientific Publishers, Oxford

Singelyn FJ, Gouverneur J-M, Robert A 1996 A minimum dose of clonidine added to mepivacaine prolongs the duration of analgesia and anaesthesia after axillary plexus block. Anesthesia and Analgesia 83: 1046–1050

Spencer HC 1998 Postdural puncture headache: what matters in technique? Regional Anesthesia and Pain Medicine 23: 374–379

Tarkkila P, Huhtala J, Tuominen M 1997 Home-readiness after spinal anaesthesia with small doses of hyperbaric 0.5% bupivacaine. Anaesthesia 52: 1157–1160

Urmey WF, Stanton J, Peterson M, Sharrock NE 1995 Combined spinal–epidural anesthesia for outpatient surgery: dose–response characteristics of intrathecal isobaric lidocaine using a 27-gauge Whitacre spinal needle. Anesthesiology 83: 528–534

Wallace DA, Carr AJ, Loach AB et al 1994 Day case arthroscopy under local anaesthesia. Annals of the Royal College of Surgeons of England 76: 330–331

Watcha MF, White PF 1992 Postoperative nausea and vomiting. Its etiology, treatment and prevention. Anesthesiology 77: 162–184

White PF 2000 Ambulatory anesthesia advances into the new millenium. Anesthesia and Analgesia 90: 1234–1235

# 23. Regional anaesthesia in the elderly patient

## B T Veering

The elderly population, particularly those aged 85 and over, continues to increase rapidly in every developed country, leading to a progressive growth in the number of surgical interventions in this age group. Knowledge of age-related changes in anatomy and physiology is important for the selection of an optimal anaesthetic regimen, and regional techniques are chosen frequently in such patients, especially during orthopaedic, genitourinary, gynaecological, cataract and hernia surgery. However, their use raises some general points which, while not exclusive to the elderly, apply particularly to them.

## GENERAL CONSIDERATIONS
### Preservation of consciousness

*Advantages* Properly performed regional anaesthesia leaves consciousness unimpaired and minimises the disorientation and confusion (see later) which may follow a general anaesthetic. It also allows the patient to act as his or her own monitor and communicate with attendant staff. Thus, a diabetic patient can recognise and report the symptoms of hypoglycaemia, and distress during transurethral resection of the prostate can give early warning that bladder irrigation fluid has entered the circulation. Although some elderly patients are apprehensive about being conscious during surgery, the majority are remarkably phlegmatic about it, and they often appreciate that the presence of intercurrent disease, which is so common in this age group, may increase the risk of general anaesthesia.

*Disadvantages* The elderly find it very difficult to lie still on a hard operating table for a long time, and considerable discomfort may develop in those parts of the body not affected by the block. Joints stiffen and bony prominences, being less well covered, are at risk of skin breakdown. Special care should be given to these pressure areas if a regional block has rendered them insensitive or immobile. In addition, deafness, or the mental slowing which accompanies old age, impairs the communication which is so essential during the performance of the block and throughout surgery.

## Anatomical changes

Distortion, such as curvature or rotation of the spine, can make central blocks difficult to perform. Intervertebral spaces may be narrowed, ligaments may be calcified, and osteophytes are often present. Limitation of abduction at the shoulder joint may make the axillary approach to the brachial plexus difficult or impossible.

At the cellular level, one-third of myelinated fibres have disappeared from peripheral nerves by the age of 90.

## Physiological changes

Changes in body composition, hepatic blood flow and hepatic mass that occur with normal ageing may have an impact on the rate and extent of the systemic absorption, distribution, metabolism and excretion of local anaesthetics (Yoshikawa 1986). The increase in body fat with age may result in greater volumes of distribution of lipophilic local anaesthetics (Greenblatt et al 1982). Hepatic blood flow declines with age (Wynne et al 1989, 1990), so there is decreased clearance of local anaesthetics with a high hepatic extraction ratio, such as lidocaine and mepivacaine. There is also a gradual decline in hepatic mass, and consequently, the clearance of local anaesthetics with relatively low hepatic extraction ratios (which are mostly dependent upon metabolising hepatic enzyme activity) may also decrease with age.

This chapter focuses on the issues relating to the impact of age on the pharmacodynamics and pharmacokinetics of central neural block.

## CENTRAL NEURAL BLOCK

### Factors which modify central neural block

Changes in anatomy, physiology and pharmacokinetics may directly or indirectly alter certain aspects of central neural block in elderly patients. Decline in the neurone population within the spinal cord and in peripheral nerves, deterioration of myelin sheaths and connective tissue barriers, a decrease in the size of nerve fibres, and slowing of conduction velocity, especially in motor nerves, contribute to altered nerve block characteristics after epidural and subarachnoid administration of local anaesthetics (Bromage 1978, Ferrer-Brechner 1986). These factors are accelerated by arteriosclerosis (Bromage 1978). Furthermore, changes occur in the lumbar and thoracic spine; for example, elderly patients often have a dorsal kyphosis and a tendency to flex the

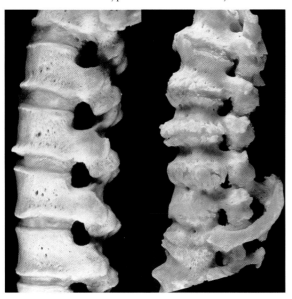

**Fig 23.1** Blocking of the intervertebral foramina by osteoarthritic changes. On the left, part of the thoracolumbar spine is seen in lateral view of a 32-year-old man and, on the right, of a 92-year-old man. Notice the disposition of the intervertebral foramina. (From Bullough PG, Boachie-Adjei O 1988 *Atlas of spinal diseases*. J B Lippincott, Philadelphia, with permission)

hips and knees because of osteoarthritis and cartilage calcification, and the intervertebral foramina are narrowed by sclerosis and calcification (Fig. 23.1). Degenerative disc and joint changes result in distortion and compression of the epidural space; the dura becomes more permeable to local anaesthetics because of a significant increase in the size of the arachnoid villi, and there is an associated reduction in volume and an increase in the specific gravity of cerebrospinal fluid (CSF) (Greene 1981, May et al 1990). All these factors contribute to an increased sensitivity to local anaesthetics.

## Advantages of central neural block

Epidural or spinal anaesthesia has advantages compared with general anaesthesia for surgical procedures performed commonly in the elderly. Intraoperative blood loss is reduced in patients undergoing hip replacement surgery, probably due to a reduction in central venous pressure (Hole et al 1980, Ferrer-Brechner 1986, Sharrock 1978). Several studies have shown that when regional anaesthesia is employed, there is a significantly lower incidence of thromboembolic events, and this is associated with lower morbidity and mortality (Hole et al 1980) due, probably, to a combination of increased blood flow to the lower extremities, favourable changes in coagulation and fibrinolysis, and inhibition of platelet aggregation. Compared with general anaesthesia, epidural (Lundh et al 1983) and spinal anaesthesia (McKenzie et al 1980) result in less deterioration in acid–base status during and after the operation. Catley and colleagues (1985) demonstrated that when regional anaesthesia (either epidural anaesthesia or intercostal nerve block) is used for post-operative pain control, it has a greater margin of safety in terms of respiratory side-effects than the continuous intravenous administration of morphine.

Continuous epidural catheter techniques provide safe and excellent postoperative analgesia in elderly patients. In addition, epidural and spinal anaesthesia is associated with a reduction in postoperative negative nitrogen balance and an amelioration of endocrine stress responses to surgery, particularly in operations on the lower abdomen and lower extremities (Kehlet 1989). Data suggest that the cortisol response is increased in elderly patients, whereas other responses may be similar to those of younger patients (Hakanson et al 1984).

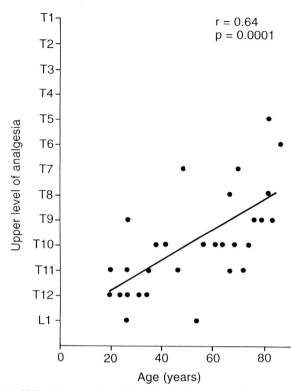

**Fig 23.2** The upper level of analgesia increases with age after epidural administration of bupivacaine. (From Veering BT, Burm AG , Van Kleef JW, Hennis PJ, Spierdijk J 1987 Epidural anaesthesia with bupivacaine: effects of age on neural blockade and pharmacokinetics. *Anesthesia and Analgesia* 66: 589–594)

## Clinical aspects of epidural anaesthesia

Age influences the spread of local anaesthetic in the epidural space, but discrepancies exist among studies. Some investigators found a slight increase in the extent of analgesic spread with age after administration of a fixed volume of a local anaesthetic agent (Fig. 23.2) (Park et al 1982, Veering et al 1987a, 1992, Nydahl et al 1991) and, more specifically, Hirabayashi and Shimizu (1993) found that age was associated with a higher upper level of analgesia after the thoracic epidural administration of a fixed dose. Others found the influence of age on the dose–effect relationship to be variable (Sharrock 1978, Anderson & Cold 1981).

Increased epidural compliance and decreased epidural resistance (considered to be due to degeneration of fatty tissue within the epidural space), increased residual epidural pressure, and progressive sclerotic closure of the intervertebral foramina with advancing age may all contribute to enhanced spread in the elderly (Bromage 1978, Hirabayashi et al 1990).

The onset time to maximal caudal spread has been reported to decrease with age (Veering et al 1987a, 1992), so surgery in areas innervated by these segments can be started sooner in older than in younger patients. In addition, a more rapid onset and enhanced intensity of motor block has been demonstrated.

Epinephrine is used frequently as a test for intravascular injection. Elderly patients may have a reduced responsiveness to a given dose of epinephrine (Guinard et al 1995), because the beta-receptor affinity for adrenergic agonists is diminished (Vestal et al 1979).

Lumbar epidural anaesthesia with lidocaine stimulates the ventilatory response to hypercapnoea to the same degree as in young patients (Sakura et al 1995) and does not affect the resting ventilation parameters such as minute ventilation and tidal volume. It therefore appears to be a safe technique in elderly patients.

## Clinical aspects of spinal anaesthesia

Spinal anaesthesia permits the use of small doses of local anaesthetic agents with minimal risk of systemic toxicity. Other advantages of spinal anaesthesia over epidural anaesthesia are a visible indication of successful needle placement, rapid onset and profound analgesia. Studies on possible correlations between age and onset, duration and spread of analgesia following subarachnoid administration of a local anaesthetic are confusing because of the variation in the types and doses of local anaesthetic agents used, and the differences in the baricity of the injected solutions. Some investigators found no effect of age on nerve block characteristics with a hyperbaric solution of tetracaine (Park et al 1975, Tuominen et al 1987), whereas Dohi and colleagues (1979) reported a prolongation of motor block with age, and Boss and Schuh (1993) found that an isobaric solution of 2% mepivacaine produced a slightly higher level of sensory analgesia.

Glucose-free (plain) bupivacaine is slightly hypobaric at body temperature, but the effect of age on the maximal height of analgesia is marginal (Pitkanen et al 1984, Veering et al 1987b). The complete, profound, long-lasting motor block and the increased duration of analgesia with glucose-free bupivacaine in elderly patients provide satisfactory conditions for orthopaedic

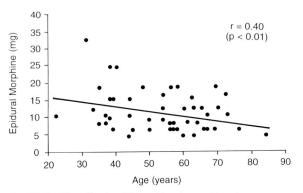

AGE vs 24 HOUR EPIDURAL MORPHINE DOSE

r = 0.40
(p < 0.01)

**Fig 23.3** The effective 24-h epidural morphine dose decreases with age after abdominal hysterectomy. (From Ready LB, Chadwick HS, Ross B 1987 Age predicts effective epidural morphine dose after abdominal hysterectomy. *Anesthesia and Analgesia* 66: 1215–1218)

**Table 23.1** Age-related changes in the pharmacokinetics of lidocaine

| Route | Change | Reference |
|---|---|---|
| i.v. | $\downarrow$CL, $\leftarrow$ V, $\uparrow$ $t_{1/2z}$ (male) $\leftarrow$ CL, $\leftarrow$ V, $\leftarrow$ $t_{1/2z}$ (female) | Abernethy et al 1983 |
| i.v. | $\leftarrow$ CL, $\uparrow$ V, $\uparrow$ $t_{1/2z}$ | Nation et al 1977 |
| i.v. | $\leftarrow$ CL, $\leftarrow$ V, $\uparrow$ $t_{1/2z}$ $\downarrow$ fu | Cusson et al 1985 |
| Caud | $\leftarrow$ $C_{max}$, $\leftarrow$ $t_{max}$, $\leftarrow$ AUC | Freund et al 1984 |
| Epi | $\leftarrow$ $C_{max}$, $\leftarrow$ $t_{max}$, $\downarrow$ CL | Bowdle et al 1986 |
| Epi | $\leftarrow$ $C_{max}$, $\leftarrow$ $t_{max}$ | Finucane et al 1987 |

$\leftarrow$ = no change; $\uparrow$ = increase; $\downarrow$ = decrease.
i.v. = intravenous; Caud = caudal; Epi = epidural.
CL = total plasma clearance; V = volume of distribution;
$t_{1/2z}$ = terminal half-life; $C_{max}$ = peak concentration; $t_{max}$ = time to
$C_{max}$; fu = unbound fraction; AUC = area under the curve.

procedures in the lower limbs. Glucose-free and hyperbaric bupivacaine solutions result in increased duration of analgesia at the $T_{12}$ dermatome, and this gives more time for operations in the lower abdominal or inguinal region. With hyperbaric bupivacaine the level of analgesia increases with age (Racle et al 1988, Veering et al 1988, 1991a). Injection of hyperbaric bupivacaine at the $L_4/L_5$ interspace instead of the $L_3/L_4$ interspace does not influence the final height of block (Veering et al 1996).

## Epidural and spinal analgesia with opioids

Intrathecal and epidural opioids are administered in order to prolong postoperative analgesia, and older patients show an increased responsiveness to them (Kaiko et al 1982). A reduction in the requirements of epidural morphine in older patients has been reported and is thought to be due to relatively high concentrations of morphine in the cerebrospinal fluid (Fig. 23.3) (Ready et al 1991).

Spinal anaesthesia with bupivacaine in combination with fentanyl decreases pain intensity in the immediate postoperative period and does not alter the mental state of geriatric patients receiving pre- and intraoperative benzodiazepines for sedation (Fernandez-Galinski et al 1996), but 25 µg of spinal fentanyl does induce oxygen desaturation and pruritus. On the other hand, in unpremedicated elderly patients, spinal anaesthesia with bupivacaine and 25 µg fentanyl induces no decrease in oxygen saturation (Varrassi et al

1992). Caution should be used when intraspinal opioids are administered to elderly patients and extra vigilance is required to detect unpredictable sedation or respiratory depression (Gustafsson et al 1982).

## Pharmacokinetic aspects

Blood concentrations of local anaesthetics are of clinical importance with respect to their systemic toxicity. These concentrations are dependent upon vascular uptake (absorption) from the extravascular injection site and systemic disposition (distribution into the blood stream and elimination from the body). Knowledge of the absorption rate is important, as this affects the duration of the nerve block.

Most data on the effect of age on the pharmacokinetics of lidocaine are available after intravenous administration (Table 23.1). The plasma elimination half-life of lidocaine is prolonged in the elderly (Nation et al 1977, Abernethy & Greenblatt 1983, Cusson et al 1985). This change is secondary to either an increase in the apparent volume of distribution or a decrease in clearance. The greater percentage of body fat contributes to the greater volume of distribution, and Abernethy and Greenblatt (1983) showed a male-specific decline in clearance with advancing age. However, Cusson and colleagues (1985) found no change in either the clearance or the volume of distribution. After a single epidural dose of lidocaine, the peak plasma concentrations are unaffected by age (Freund et al 1984, Bowdle et al 1986, Finucane et al 1987), but the terminal half-life is prolonged and the clearance is decreased.

**Table 23.2** Age-related changes in the pharmacokinetics of bupivacaine

| Route | Change | Reference |
|---|---|---|
| Caud | ← $C_{max}$, ← $t_{max}$, ← AUC | Freund et al (1984) |
| Epi | ↑ $C_{max}$, ← $t_{max}$, ↓ CL, ↑ $t_{1/2z}$ | Veering et al (1987) |
| Epi | ← $F_1$ ← $t_{1/2a1}$ ← $F_2$, ← $t_{1/2a2}$ | Veering et al (1992) |
| Spin | ← $C_{max}$, ↑ $t_{max}$, ↓ CL ← $t_{1/2z}$ | Veering et al (1988) |
| Spin | ↑ $C_{max}$, ← $t_{max}$, ↓ CL, ↑ $t_{1/2z}$ | Veering et al (1987) |
| Spin | ← $F_1$ ← $t_{1/2a1}$ ← $F_2$, ↓ $t_{1/2a2}$ | Veering et al (1991) |

← = no change; ↑ = increase; ↓ = decrease.
Caud = caudal; Epi = epidural; Spin = spinal.
$C_{max}$ = peak concentration; $t_{max}$ = time to $C_{max}$; $F_1$ = fraction of dose absorbed during the fast absorption process; CL = total plasma clearance; AUC = area under the curve; $t_{1/2z}$ = terminal half-life; $F_2$ = fraction of dose absorbed during the slow absorption process; $t_{1/2a1}$ = fast absorption half-life; $t_{1/2a2}$ = slow absorption half life.

This may lead to increased accumulation of lidocaine with continuous epidural infusions, or with intermittent bolus doses.

Studies which have evaluated the effects of age on the pharmacokinetics of bupivacaine after subarachnoid and epidural administration are summarised in Table 23.2. The peak plasma concentrations of bupivacaine and the corresponding times to peak after epidural administration do not seem to change with age (Veering et al 1987a, 1992, Freund et al 1984). The terminal half-life increases whereas the total plasma clearance of bupivacaine decreases after both epidural and subarachnoid administration (Veering et al 1987a, b, 1991a, 1992). The consequences of reduced clearance of bupivacaine will be most apparent during continuous block when it is probable that plasma concentrations will rise to higher levels, with consequent reduction in the safety margin. Infusion rates and bolus doses may therefore need to be adjusted. This should not necessarily affect the quality of block because of the increased sensitivity to bupivacaine in older patients.

Because bupivacaine exhibits a relatively low hepatic extraction ratio, the observed age-related decline in clearance is more likely to be due to a change in the drug-metabolising hepatic enzyme activity or serum protein binding than to an alteration in liver blood flow. However, age has not been shown to affect the protein binding of bupivacaine (Veering et al 1991a), so the decline in clearance is best explained by a decrease in hepatic enzyme activity. Whether this is due to decreased activity of the hepatic enzymes *per se* or to a reduction in the size of the liver remains to be clarified.

In order to evaluate the pharmacokinetics of bupivacaine in the elderly, a stable isotope method has been used (Burm et al 1988). After epidural and subarachnoid administration, bupivacaine shows a biphasic absorption profile: a rapid initial phase followed by a much slower phase (Veering et al 1991b, 1992, Burm et al 1988). The initial fast absorption rate is a reflection of the high initial concentration gradient and the vascularity of the epidural space. The slower second absorption phase is believed to be due to slow uptake of local anaesthetics sequestered in the epidural fat.

The systemic absorption of bupivacaine after subarachnoid administration is also biphasic. The initial absorption is much slower than after epidural administration, because the subarachnoid space is less well perfused than the epidural space. However, the mean absorption of bupivacaine after subarachnoid administration is shorter in elderly patients because of a faster late absorption rate (Veering et al 1991b). In view of this, one might expect a shorter duration of spinal anaesthesia in older patients, but this has not been demonstrated.

The results of absorption studies confirm that elderly patients are more sensitive to both epidural and subarachnoid bupivacaine. This is more likely to be due to changes in pharmacodynamics than to impairment of vascular absorption.

## Disadvantages of central neural block

### Technical difficulty
The techniques of spinal and epidural anaesthesia are more difficult in the elderly because of the anatomical changes already described, so there is always a chance of failure.

### Postdural puncture headache
This is the most common complication of spinal anaesthesia. Although it is largely related to the size of the needle, the incidence decreases with age, possibly because decreased elasticity of the tissues allows less stretching of the dura mater, so that less CSF leaks from the subarachnoid space (Gielen 1989).

327

## Hypotension

Untreated hypotension, secondary to sympathetic nerve block, leading to relative hypovolaemia and decreased venous return, can be highly detrimental to the elderly patient, and it is especially harmful to those with limited cardiac reserve. Normal ageing is associated with a reduction in the heart rate response to hypotension that is mediated by the baroreceptor reflex, so elderly patients may not respond with the same degree of sympathetic activity as younger patients (Duke et al 1976). Carpenter and colleagues (1992) found that high levels of sensory anaesthesia and increasing age appeared to be the two main risk factors for the development of hypotension. Decreased cardiac reserve, structural changes in the arterioles and changes in the autonomic nervous system with increasing age may play a role. Transthoracic electrical bioimpedance studies of subarachnoid block in elderly patients (53–96 years) revealed that systolic blood pressure decreased by 25% as early as 6–9 minutes after the block (Critchley et al 1994). Cardiac output was unaffected because a decrease in stroke index in the more severe cases of hypotension was compensated for by an increase in heart rate. The higher the block, the more aggressive was the treatment required.

***Treatment of hypotension*** Opinions on managing hypotension in elderly patients during spinal and epidural anaesthesia range from the administration of moderate volumes of intravenous fluid to the use of vasopressors. Administration of ephedrine prophylactically with a fluid preload, usually about 7 ml kg$^{-1}$, has been recommended (Critchley 1996). It should be emphasised, however, that rapid preloading constitutes a potential risk in older patients with limited cardiac reserve, and hypotension commonly follows spinal anaesthesia in normovolaemic elderly patients undergoing elective procedures, irrespective of whether or not any fluid is given (Buggy et al 1997). Since the potential for exaggerated cardiovascular changes during a subarachnoid block is directly related to the height of the block, one of the most effective methods of preventing hypotension is to avoid a high sensory block. Unfortunately, injection at the $L_4/L_5$ interspace offers no advantage in this respect compared with injection at $L_3/L_4$ (Veering et al 1996).

The incidence and severity of hypotension can be reduced by the use of incremental injections of local anaesthetic solutions. This allows the level of block to be controlled more easily. The technique can be applied to continuous spinal (CSA), continuous epidural and combined spinal epidural anaesthesia (CSE), and it is useful for minimising hypotension, not only when the initial block is being established, but also throughout the subsequent course of the anaesthetic. Favarel-Garrigues and colleagues (1996) found that when small, titrated doses of hyperbaric bupivacaine were injected by a CSA technique, haemostability was better than single-dose spinal anaesthesia in elderly patients. When haemodynamic stability is critically important, CSE or CSA may be the technique of choice for lower abdominal or lower limb surgery in the elderly.

## Confusion

Prompt and complete postoperative recovery of mental function to the preoperative state is particularly important in elderly patients if mental faculties are already compromised by age-related disease or drug therapy. Elderly surgical patients are prone to postoperative confusion or delirium, both of which are non-specific symptoms of central nervous system dysfunction. Postoperative confusion, transient fluctuations of consciousness and mood, and severe disruption of sleep within the first week after surgery is particularly common in elderly orthopaedic patients (Gustafson et al 1988, Williams-Russo et al 1992). In most cases, recovery of cognitive function is prompt and complete within one week. Neither the choice of anaesthetic technique nor the method employed for the management of postoperative pain appears to be an important determinant of postoperative confusion.

The mechanism of postoperative confusion following orthopaedic surgery and other operations is probably multi-factorial (Moller et al 1998). Sensitivity to benzodiazepines and anticholinergic drugs is increased in elderly people, and even the relatively sparing use of intravenous sedation may delay the rapid recovery of mental function which otherwise occurs after regional anaesthesia (Chung et al 1989). The altered mental state, which persists for more than a week after surgery, is most common in older patients with a preoperative history of psychiatric disturbance, particularly clinical depression.

## Hypothermia

Hypothermia (a decrease in core temperature) is common in patients undergoing surgery with epidural and spinal anaesthesia. Elderly patients may be especially at risk because low core temperature may not trigger protective vasomotor responses, so their responses to hypothermia may be delayed or less efficient than in younger subjects. Vassilieff and colleagues (1995) have shown that elderly patients have a lower shivering threshold than younger patients during spinal anaesthesia. This is probably because their low core temperature may not initiate autonomic protective responses. Shivering is potentially a serious problem because the elderly have a higher incidence of ischaemic heart disease and may not be able to tolerate the increased oxygen demands associated with the shivering state.

In elderly patients body temperature is reduced by general anaesthesia to a greater degree than by epidural anaesthesia when the operating room temperature is cold, but this difference is not significant when the temperature is relatively warm. The time required for postoperative rewarming to restore body temperature to normal also appears to increase directly with advancing age.

## Regional versus general anaesthesia: outcome studies

Three outcome studies have shown that a combined general/epidural anaesthetic technique followed by continuous epidural analgesia is associated with a beneficial effect on coagulation in patients undergoing vascular reconstruction of the lower extremity. Such patients are mostly elderly and generally have accompanying cardiovascular or other disorders (Tuman et al 1991, Christopherson et al 1993, Rosenfeld et al 1993). Compared with general anaesthesia, epidural anaesthesia is associated with a reduction in graft occlusion so it may be advantageous for this population.

Discrepancies exist between studies which have evaluated early mortality (within 1 month) in elderly patients, after major orthopaedic surgery under either regional (epidural or spinal) or general anaesthesia. Some investigators found a lower mortality rate after spinal than after general anaesthesia (McLaren et al 1978, McKenzie et al 1980), whereas others found no such difference (Wickstrom et al 1982, Valentin et al 1986, Sutcliffe 1994). The reduction in early mortality may be related to a decreased incidence of deep venous thrombosis. Long-term studies of morbidity and mortality (2 months to 1 year) show little difference between regional and general anaesthesia (Wickstrom et al 1982, McKenzie et al 1980, Sutcliffe 1994).

Age-related disease, as opposed to old age *per se*, is primarily responsible for the progressive increase in morbidity and mortality of elderly surgical patients. Factors other than the choice of anaesthesia may be crucial for long-term survival.

## CONCLUSION

Elderly patients are more sensitive to local anaesthetic agents. They develop slightly higher levels of sensory and motor block after epidural and spinal anaesthesia and are also at somewhat greater risk of arterial hypotension due to acute sympathetic block. Regional anaesthesia offers several advantages to elderly patients because it provides postoperative analgesia with minimal sedative side-effects, although intrathecal opiates may produce significant respiratory depression in this age group. Epidural and spinal anaesthesia reduce the incidence of thromboembolic complications in elderly patients, especially after orthopaedic or lower extremity vascular surgery.

Most controlled trials have failed to demonstrate that regional anaesthesia or general anaesthesia is clearly superior in terms of outcome in elderly patients. General anaesthesia and spinal anaesthesia appear to be equally safe for patients with a hip fracture. The probability of a serious pulmonary or haemodynamic complication after surgery in elderly patients, as in young adults, is largely determined by the nature of the surgery and by the patient's physical state. Many individual controlled studies comparing regional anaesthesia to general anaesthesia have lacked the statistical power to provide a conclusive answer as to which gives the better outcome in terms of morbidity and mortality.

However, a recent meta-analysis (Rodgers et al 2000) supports more widespread use of central neural block. Overall mortality was reduced by about one-third in patients who received a central block either with or without concomitant general anaesthesia. A block reduced the risk of deep venous thrombosis by 44%, pulmonary embolism by 55%, transfusion requirements by 50%, pneumonia by 39% and respiratory depression by 59%. There were also reductions in myocardial infarction and renal failure. Further research is required to determine whether these advantages are due solely to the benefits of the block or are due in part to avoidance of general anaesthesia. The meta-analysis reviewed all controlled trials before 1997 and included all types of surgery in adults, including many elderly patients. It is likely that the benefits of using central neural block in the elderly at least match these figures, though an elderly subgroup was not specifically analysed.

A continuous evaluation of the clinical and pharmacological aspects of regional anaesthesia in elderly patients remains necessary. Regional anaesthesia should be carefully considered as a potentially safer option when anaesthesia for the elderly is required.

# References

Abernethy DR, Greenblatt DJ 1983 Impairment of lidocaine clearance in elderly male subjects. Journal of Cardiovascular Pharmacology 5: 1093–1096

Anderson S, Cold GE 1981 Dose responses studies in elderly patients subjected to epidural analgesia. Acta Anaesthesiologica Scandinavica 25: 279–281

Boss EG, Schuh FT 1993 Der Einfluss des Lebensalters auf die Ausbreitung der Spinalanasthesie mit isobarem Mepivacain 2%. Anaesthesist 42: 162–168

Bowdle TA, Freund PR, Slattery JT 1986 Age dependent lidocaine pharmacokinetics during lumbar peridural anesthesia with lidocaine hydrocarbonate or lidocaine hydrochloride. Regional Anesthesia 11: 123–127

Bromage PR 1978 Epidural analgesia. WB Saunders, Philadelphia

Buggy D, Higgins P, Moran C, O'Brien D, O'Donovan F, McCarroll M 1997 Prevention of spinal anesthesia-induced hypotension in the elderly: comparison between preanesthetic administration of crystalloids, colloids and no prehydration. Anesthesia and Analgesia 84: 106–110

Burm AGL, Van Kleef JW, Vermeulen NPE, Olthof G, Breimer DD, Spierdijk J 1988 Pharmacokinetics of lidocaine and bupivacaine following subarachnoid administration in surgical patients: simultaneous investigation of absorption and disposition kinetics using stable isotopes. Anesthesiology 69: 584–592

Catley DM, Thornton C, Jordan C, Lehane JR, Royston D, Jones JG. 1985 Pronounced, episodic oxygen desaturation with ventilatory pattern and analgesic regimen. Anesthesiology 63: 20–28

Carpenter RL, Caplan RA, Brown DL, Stephenson C, Wu R 1992 Incidence and risk factors for side effects of spinal anesthesia. Anesthesiology 76: 906–912

Christopherson R, Beattie C, Meinert CL et al 1993 Perioperative Ischemia Randomized Anaesthesia Trial Study Group: Perioperative morbidity in patients randomized to epidural or general anaesthesia for lower extremity vascular surgery. Anesthesiology 79: 422–434

Chung FF, Chung A, Meier RH, Lautenschlaeger E 1989 Comparison of perioperative mental function after general anaesthesia and spinal anaesthesia with intravenous sedation. Canadian Journal of Anaesthesia 36: 382–387

Critchley LAH 1996 Hypotension, subarachnoid block and the elderly patient. Anaesthesia 51: 1139–1143

Critchley L H, Stuart JC, Short TG, Gin T 1994 Haemodynamic effects of subarachnoid block in elderly patients. British Journal of Anaesthesia 73: 464–470

Cusson J, Nattel S, Matthews C, Talajic M, Lawand S 1985 Age-dependent lignocaine disposition in patients with acute myocardial infarction. Clinical Pharmacology and Therapeutics 37: 381–386

Dohi S, Naito H, Takahashi T 1979 Age-related changes in blood pressure and duration of motor blockade in spinal anaesthesia. Anesthesiology 50: 319–323

Duke PC, Wade JG, Hickey RF, Larson CP 1976 The effects of age on baroreceptor reflex function in man. Canadian Journal of Anaesthesia 23: 111–114

Favarel-Garrigues JF, Sztark F, Petitjan ME, Thicoïpé M, Lassié P, Dabadie P 1996 Hemodynamic effects of spinal anaesthesia in the elderly: single dose versus titration through a catheter. Anesthesia and Analgesia 82: 312–316

Fernandez-Galinski D, Rué M, Moral V, Castells C, Puig MM 1996 Spinal anaesthesia with bupivacaine and fentanyl in geriatric patients. Anesthesia and Analgesia 83: 537–541

Ferrer-Brechner T 1986 Spinal and epidural anaesthesia in the elderly. Seminars in Anesthesiology V: 54–61

Finucane BT, Hammonds WD, Welch MB 1987 Influence of age on vascular absorption of lidocaine from the epidural space. Anesthesia and Analgesia 66: 843–846

Freund PR, Bowdle TA, Slattery JT, Bell LR 1984 Caudal anesthesia with lidocaine or bupivacaine: plasma local anesthetic concentration and extent of sensory spread in old and young patients. Anesthesia and Analgesia 63: 1017–1020

Gielen M 1989 Postdural headache (PDPH). A review. Regional Anesthesia 14: 101–106

Greenblatt DJ, Sellers EM, Shader RI 1982 Drug disposition in old age. New England Journal of Medicine 306: 1081–1108

Greene N M 1981 Physiology of spinal anaesthesia, 3rd edn, p 5. Williams and Wilkins, Baltimore

Guinard J P, Mulroy M F, Carpenter R L 1995 Aging reduces the reliability of epidural epinephrine test doses. Regional Anesthesia 20: 193–195

Gustafsson LL, Schildt B, Jacobsen KJ. 1982 Adverse effects of extradural and intrathecal opiates: report of a nationwide survey in Sweden. British Journal of Anaesthesia 54: 479–486

Gustafsson Y, Beggren D, Bannström B et al 1988 Acute confusional states in elderly patients treated for femoral neck fracture. Journal of the American Geriatric Society 36: 525–530

Hakanson E, Rutberg H, Jorfeldt L, Wiklund L 1984 Endocrine and metabolic responses after standardized moderate surgical trauma: Influence of age and sex. Clinical Physiology 4: 461–473

Hirabayashi Y, Shimizu R 1993 Effect of age on extradural dose requirement in thoracic extradural anaesthesia. British Journal of Anaesthesia 71: 445–446

Hirabayashi Y, Shimizu R, Matsuda J, Inoue S 1990 Effect of extradural compliance and resistance on spread of extradural analgesia. British Journal of Anaesthesia 65: 508–513

Hole A, Terjesen T, Breivik H 1980 Epidural versus general anaesthesia for total hip arthroplasty in elderly patients. Acta Anaesthesiologica Scandinavica 24: 279–287

Kaiko RF, Wallenstein SL, Rogers AG 1982 Narcotics in the elderly. Medical Clinics of North America 66: 1079–1089

Kehlet H 1989 Surgical stress: the role of pain and analgesia. British Journal of Anaesthesia 63: 189–195

Lundh R, Hedenstierna G, Johansson H 1983 Ventilation–perfusion relationship during epidural analgesia. Acta Anaesthesiologica Scandinavica 27: 410–416

May C, Kaye JA, Atack JR, Shapiro MB, Friedland RP, Rapoport SI 1990 Cerebrospinal fluid production is reduced in healthy aging. Neurology 40: 500–503

McKenzie PJ, Wishart HY, Dewar KMS, Gray J, Smith G 1980 Comparison of the effects of spinal anaesthesia and general anaesthesia on postoperative oxygenation and perioperative mortality. British Journal of Anaesthesia 52: 49–55

McLaren AD, Stockwell MC, Reid VT 1978 Anaesthetic techniques for surgical correction of fractured neck of femur. A comparative study of spinal and general anaesthesia in the elderly. Anaesthesia 33: 10–14

Moller JT. Cluitmans P. Rasmussen LS et al 1998 Long-term postoperative cognitive dysfunction in the elderly. International Study of Post-Operative Cognitive Dysfunction (ISPOCD) 1 study. The Lancet 351: 857–861

Nation RL, Triggs EJ, Selig M 1977 Lignocaine kinetics in cardiac patients and aged subjects. British Journal of Clinical Pharmacology 4: 439–448

Nydahl PA, Philipson L, Axelsson K, Johansson JE 1991 Epidural anesthesia with 0.5% bupivacaine: influence of age on sensory and motor blockade. Anesthesia and Analgesia 73: 780–787

Park WY, Balingit PE, Macnamara TE 1975 Effects of patient age, pH of cerebrospinal fluid and vasopressors on onset and duration of spinal anesthesia. Anesthesia and Analgesia 54: 455–458

Park WY, Balingit PE, Macnamara TE 1982 Age and the epidural dose response in adult man. Anesthesiology 56: 318–332

Pitkänen M, Haapaniemi L, Tuominen M, Rosenberg PH 1984 Influence of age on spinal anaesthesia with isobaric 0.5% bupivacaine. British Journal of Anaesthesia 56: 279–264

Racle JP, Benkhadra A, Poy JY, Gteizal B 1988 Spinal analgesia with hyperbaric bupivacaine: influence of age. British Journal of Anaesthesia 60: 508–514

Ready LB, Chadwick HS, Ross B 1987 Age predicts effective epidural morphine dose after abdominal hysterectomy. Anesthesia and Analgesia 66: 1215–1218

Ready LB, Loper KA, Nessley M, Wild L 1991 Postoperative epidural morphine is safe on surgical wards. Anesthesiology 75: 452–456

Rodgers A, Walker N, Schug S et al 2000 Reduction of postoperative mortality and morbidity with epidural or spinal anaesthesia: results from overview of randomised trials. British Medical Journal 321: 1493–1497

Rosenfeld BA, Beattie C, Christopherson R et al 1993 Perioperative Ischemia Randomized Anaesthesia Trial Study Group: The effects of different anesthetic regimen on fibrinolysis and the development of postoperative arterial thrombosis. Anesthesiology 79: 435–443

Sakura S, Saito Y, Kosaka Y 1995 The effects of epidural anesthesia on ventilatory response to hypercapnia and hypoxia in elderly patients. Anesthesia and Analgesia 82: 306–311

Sharrock N E 1978 Epidural anesthetic dose response in patients 20 to 80 years old. Anesthesiology 49: 425–428

Sutcliffe A J 1994 Mortality after spinal and general anaesthesia for surgical fixation of hip fractures. Anaesthesia 49: 237–240

Tuman KJ, McCarthy RJ, Marck RJ, Delaria GA, Patel RV, Ivankovick AD 1991 Effects of epidural anaesthesia and analgesia on coagulation and outcome after major vascular surgery. Anesthesia and Analgesia 73: 696–670

Tuominen M, Pitkänen M, Doepel M, Rosenberg PH 1987 Effects of age and body mass on subarachnoid anaesthesia with tetracaine. Acta Anaesthesiologica Scandinavia 31: 474–478

Valentin N, Lumhott B, Jensen JS, Hejgaard J, Kreiner S 1986 Spinal or general anaesthesia for surgery of the fractured hip? A prospective study of mortality in 578 patients. British Journal of Anaesthesia 58: 284–291

Varrassi G, Celleno D, Capogna G et al 1992 Ventilatory effects of subarachnoid fentanyl in the elderly. Anaesthesia 47: 558–562

Vassilieff N, Rosencher N, Sessler DI, Conseiller C 1995 Shivering threshold during spinal anaesthesia is reduced in elderly patients. Anesthesiology 83: 1162–1166

Veering BT, Burm AGL, Van Kleef JW, Hennis PJ, Spierdijk J 1987a Epidural anaesthesia with bupivacaine: effects of age on neural blockade and pharmacokinetics. Anesthesia and Analgesia 66: 589–594

Veering BT, Burm AGL, Van Kleef JW, Hennis PJ, Spierdijk J 1987b Spinal anaesthesia with glucose-free bupivacaine: effects of age on neural blockade and pharmacokinetics. Anesthesia and Analgesia 66: 965–970

Veering BT, Burm AGL, Spierdijk J 1988 Spinal anaesthesia with hyperbaric bupivacaine: effects of age on neural blockade and pharmacokinetics. British Journal of Anaesthesia 60: 187–194

Veering BT, Burm AGL, Gladines MPRR, Spierdijk J 1991a Age does not influence the serum protein binding of bupivacaine. British Journal of Clinical Pharmacology 32: 501–503

Veering BT, Burm AGL, Vletter AA, Van den Hoeven RAM, Spierdijk J 1991a The effect of age on the systemic absorption and systemic disposition of bupivacaine after subarachnoid administration. Anesthesiology 74: 250–257

Veering BT, Burm AGL, Vletter AA, Van den Heuvel RPM, Onkenhout W, Spierdijk J 1992 The effect of age on the systemic absorption and systemic disposition of bupivacaine after epidural administration. Clinical Pharmacokinetics 22: 75–84

Veering BT, Ter Riet PM, Burm AGL, Stienstra R, Van Kleef JW 1996 Spinal anaesthesia with hyperbaric 0.5% bupivacaine in elderly patients: effect of the site of injection on the spread of analgesia. British Journal of Anaesthesia 77: 1–4

Vestal RE, Wood AJJ, Shand DG 1979 Reduced beta-adrenoceptor sensitivity in the elderly. Clinical Pharmacology and Therapeutics 26: 181–188

Wickstrom J, Holmberg J, Stefansson T 1982 Survival of female geriatric patients after hip fracture surgery. A comparison of 5 anaesthetic methods. Acta Anaesthesiologica Scandinavica 26: 607–614

Williams-Russo P, Urquhart RN, Sharrock NE, Charlson ME 1992 Post-operative delirium: predictors and prognosis in elderly orthopedic patients. Journal of the American Geriatric Society 40: 759–767

Wynne HA, Cope LH, Mutch E et al 1989 The effect of age upon liver volume and apparent liver blood flow in healthy man. Hepatology 9: 297–301

Wynne HA, Goudevenos J, Rawlins MD, James OFW, Adams PC, Woudhouse KW 1990 Hepatic drug clearance: the effect of age using indocyanine green as a model compound. British Journal of Clinical Pharmacology 30: 634–637

Yoshikawa TT 1986 Physiology of aging: impact on pharmacology. Seminars in Anesthesiology V: 8–13

# Index

## A

Abdominal surgery, 189
Abducent nerve, 243
Ab fibres, 26, 29, 30
Abscesses, epidural, 16, 135, 163–164, 278
Absorption profile of bupivacaine, elderly patients, 327
Accumulation, 55–56
Acidosis, 54
Action potentials, 37–39
  compound, 21–22, 23
  ectopic discharges, 30
Acute pain nurses, 157
Acute pain services, audit, 289
Acute pain teams, 156–157
Ad fibres, 25, 26
Adjuvants, 72–73
  see also specific drugs
Adrenaline see Epinephrine
Adrenoceptor agonists see
  Clonidine; Vasopressors
Afferent neurones, primary, 23–25
Age
  drug kinetics, 52, 57
  epidural anaesthesia, 150
  postdural puncture headache, 135
  see also Elderly patients
Air
  loss of resistance, 146–147, 276
  test, caudal block, 173–174
Air embolism, 276
Akinesia, eye, 241, 244, 247
Alcohol, 297
Alkalinisation, 72–73
Allergic reactions, 68, 81, 98
Allodynia, 29, 295
  $\alpha_1$-acid glycoprotein, 53
  $\alpha_2$-adrenergic agonists see
  Clonidine
Ambulation

after central block, 105, 158
  see also Mobility
Amethocaine, 4
  gel, 31, 271
Amide local anaesthetic agents, 43, 70–72
  clearance, 55
  drug interactions, 68
  kinetics, 67
  systemic absorption, 50
Amino acids, neurotransmitters, 27
Amputation, sympathetic block, 294
Amylocaine, 4
Anaesthetic rooms, 91
Anaesthetists, 18, 85
Analgesia (systemic), 11, 97, 105, 175, 321
Anal surgery, 189
Anaphylaxis, management, 98
Anastomosis breakdown
  incidence, 17
  postoperative signs, 160
Anatomy
  assessment, 93
  see also Variants
Angina, sympathetic block, 294
Ankle, nerve supply, 213
Ankle block, 224–225, 285, 316–317
Annuli fibrosi, 116
Anomalies see Variants
Antecubital fossa, 206, 207
Anterior ethmoidal nerve, 230, 235
Anterior longitudinal ligament, 116
Anterior spinal artery, 120
  syndrome, 136
Anterolateral spinothalamic tract, 28
Antiarrhythmic agents, ion channel
  block, 43
Anticoagulants
  eye block, 243
  obstetrics, 259

valve prostheses, 258
  see also Coagulopathies
Anticonvulsants, 69
Antiplatelet agents, 83
Anus, surgery, 189
Anxiolysis, 13, 159–160
Aortic stenosis, 78
Aortocaval compression, 252–253, 262
Apnoea
  neonates, 278–279
  spinal anaesthesia, 134
Arachnoiditis, 135
Arrhythmias, 66, 270
Arteries
  epidural space, 120–121
  spinal cord, 120
  damage at coeliac plexus block, 304
  sympathetic block, 293–294
Arterio-venous admixture,
  pulmonary blood flow, 12
Arteriovenous fistula, haemodialysis, 80
Arthroscopy, knee joint, 226, 317
Ascending pathways, 28
Aseptic techniques, 94, 127–128
Aspiration tests, 67, 68, 97, 274–275
Aspirin, 83, 84
Assistants, 91
Asthma, sympathetic block, 14
Atelectasis, 12, 17
Atherosclerosis, 293
Atlas, 113
Atropine, 102
Audit, postoperative care, 287–290
Auriculotemporal nerve, 231, 237
Australia, audit, 288
Autonomic fibres, pain, 23
Autonomic hyperreflexia, 79–80
Average Rectified Electromyography, 153

Awake intubation, 238–239
Axillary block, 193, 197, 203–205
   children, 271, 272
   day surgery, 316
   elderly patients and, 323
Axillary nerve, 197
   axillary block, 203
Axis, 113
Axons, 25, 36–37

## B

Backache, 106, 135
lumbar sympathetic block, 306
   obstetrics, 252, 261
   spinal anaesthesia, 319
Bacteraemia, 81
Balanced anaesthesia, 6, 155, 319–320
Balloon method, epidural puncture, 147
Barbotage, 130
Baricity, 130
   elderly patients and, 325–326
   see also Hyperbaric solutions
Benoxinate, 244
Benzocaine, 42, 70, 73
Benzodiazepines, 69, 87, 98
b-adrenergic block, 78
Bevels, needles, 92–93
   head and neck, 234
   spread of epidural block, 151–152
Bicarbonate, local anaesthetic agents, 72–73
Bier, A., central blocks, 4
Bier's block see Intravenous regional anaesthesia
Bisulphites, 45–46, 69, 164
Bladder
   catheterisation, 105, 163
   preoperative emptying, 86
Bleeding diatheses see Coagulopathies
Block packs, 92
Blood flow
   renal, 12–13
   toxicity, 66
Blood loss, 17
Blood patches, dural, 162
Blood vessels, peripheral nerves, 35

Bloody tap
   sacral epidural injection, 173
   see also Intravascular injection
Bolus injections, epidural anaesthesia, 157, 158
Bone, needle damage, 93
Bowel surgery, 14
Brachial plexus, 193–197
   sheath, 197
Brachial plexus block, 193–205
   accidental, 299
   day surgery, 315–316
   drug kinetics, 51
   postoperative pain control, 285–286
   see also Axillary block
Bradycardia, 99
   atropine for, 102
   total spinal block, 261
Brain damage, 136
Breast cancer surgery, paravertebral block, 185
Breech delivery, vaginal, 258
Bretylium, 307, 308
Bromage scales, 153
Bronchospasm, sympathetic block, 14
Buccal nerve, 231, 236
Buck's fascia, 187, 188
Bupivacaine
   applications
      brachial plexus block, 198, 199
      caudal block, 175
      epidural anaesthesia, 153–154, 277–278
      inguinal field block, 187
      intercostal nerve block, 181
      interpleural block, 183
      obstetrics, 256, 257
      spinal anaesthesia, 131
   cardiotoxicity, 43, 71
   children, 269, 271
   chirality and properties, 45
   clinical aspects, 71, 73
   elderly patients, 327
   eye surgery solutions, 244
   historical aspects, 6
   intravenous regional anaesthesia and, 208
   kinetics, 50, 51, 55
   metabolites, 57

physicochemical properties, 41, 44, 45
   protein binding, 67
   toxicity, 50, 160–161
Burettes, 157
Burke, W., 4
Butyrophenones, 87

## C

Caesarean section, 261–263
   heart disease, 258
   lidocaine, 256
   respiratory disease, 259
Caffeine, 135, 162
Cancer pain
   neuropathy, 295
   sympathetic block, 294
Carbonated local anaesthetic agents, 72
Cardiac arrest
   audit results, 289
Cardiac failure
   drug interactions, 69
   drug kinetics, 58
Cardiac output
   drug kinetics, 66, 67
Cardiovascular disease
   lower limb blocks, 214
   obstetrics, 258
   sympathetic block for, 293–294
Cardiovascular system
   morbidity, 16
   obstetrics, 258
   pregnancy see Aortocaval compression
   sympathetic block, 13–14, 99
   for cardiac pain, 294
   sympathetic effects, 12
   toxicity, 65–66, 270
      bupivacaine, 43, 71
   stereo-isomers compared, 45
Carotid arteries
   accidental injection, 98
   surgery to, 234, 239
Catecholamines
   neuropathic pain, 294
   see also Epinephrine
Catheters, 93
   continuous sciatic block, 227

epidural, 141
caudal anaesthesia, 175, 275–276
children, 276–277
complications, 163
insertion, 145
level of tip, 155, 157
Tuohy needles and, 140
unilateral block and, 255
removal, haematoma, 82
spinal anaesthesia, 133, 287
Cauda equina syndrome, 69, 135
Caudal block, 169–176
children, 274–276
day surgery, 318
drug kinetics, 51
haemorrhoidectomy, advantages, 11
labour, 253–254
Causalgia, 295
Cell bodies, neurones, 25
Central nervous system
pain, 21, 28–29
stress response to surgery, 15
toxicity, 65
Central sensitisation, 30
Cephalad angulation 148, 150, 155
Crawford needle, 140
paramedian approach, 147–149
Cerebrospinal fluid, 122–123
diffusion into, 49
identification, 144
leakage
children, 276
see also Postdural puncture headache
lumbar puncture, 129
pressure, 123
specific gravity, 130
Cervical nerves, 233, 237–238
Cervical plexus, 233
Cervical spine
epidural space, 150
vertebrae, 112–113
CES see Cauda equina syndrome
C fibres, 25, 26, 36, 269
Challenge testing, allergy, 68
Chassaignac's tubercle, 237
Chemosis, 248
Children, 269–282

drug kinetics, 52, 57, 269
midazolam, 87
Chirality, 44–45
kinetics, 49, 51, 55
Chloroprocaine, 4
clinical aspects, 70, 73
nerve damage, 45, 69, 257
obstetrics, 257
Cholinesterase, 67, 68
Chronic pain
brain changes, 29
paravertebral block, 183
see also Cancer pain; Neurolytic blocks
Chronic renal failure, 52, 80
Ciliary ganglion, 241
Cinchocaine, 4
Circumflex humeral nerve see Axillary nerve
Cirrhosis, drug kinetics, 58
Claudication, 293–294
Clearance, 55
in elderly patients, 326–327
Clonidine
brachial plexus block, 199, 316
children, 279
epidural anaesthesia, 159, 257
intra-articular block, knee, 317
spinal anaesthesia, 131
Coagulopathies, 81–84
contra-indication to sympathetic block, 295–296
obstetrics, 259
Cocaine, 3–4, 70, 73, 235
Coeliac plexus, 179
neurolytic block, 294, 301–304
Colic, postoperative, 160
Colon see Bowel surgery
Combination drug regimens
epidural anaesthesia, 159
see also Balanced anaesthesia
Combined spinal epidural anaesthesia, 133
Caesarean section, 262
day surgery, 319
elderly patients, 328
obstetrics, 255–256
Common peroneal nerve, 216, 220

Compartments, epidural, 121–122, 123
Compartment syndrome, children, 278
Complex regional pain syndromes, 295
Complications, 9–10
obstetrics, 260–261
Compound action potentials, 21–22, 23
Compression neuropraxia, 278
Computed tomography, coeliac plexus block, 303
Concha, anaesthesia, 238
Conduction blocks, 40–43
dynamics, 45–46
onset times, 69–70, 96
Confusion, elderly patients, 328
Conjunctiva, injections, 244
Consciousness, preservation, 10–11
Consent, epidural anaesthesia in obstetrics, 251
Continuous methods
axillary block, 272
brachial plexus block, 205
caudal block, 175
epidural anaesthesia
children, 277–278
elderly patients, 324, 328
labour, 254–255
perioperative, 155–156
plasma concentrations, 55–56
postoperative, 158
tissue toxicity, 69
lower limb blocks, 226–227
lumbar sympathetic block, 305–306
spinal anaesthesia, 5, 11, 15, 133, 260, 328
stellate ganglion block, 299
wound infiltration, 285
Contiplex D catheter, 227
Contrast medium, lumbar sympathetic block, 305
Conus medullaris, puncture, 135
Convulsions, 65, 270
audit results, 289
drug kinetics, 54
management, 98, 270

Core/mantle concept, 199
Corning, L., 4
Coronary blood flow, 78
Crawford needle, 140, 141
Cricothyroid puncture, 238–239
CSEA *see* Combined spinal epidural anaesthesia
Cytochrome P450 enzymes, 57, 58

**D**
Data collection, for audit, 288
Day surgery, 313–322
Deconvolution analysis, systemic absorption, 50
Deep cervical plexus, 233
    block, 237
    carotid endarterectomy, 239
Deep peroneal nerve, 225
Deep sedation, 102–103
Density (solutions), 129–130
Density of motor block, 153
Dental practice, 10
Depolarisation, 37–39
Dermatomes, 23, 24
    'mismatches', 157
    upper limb, 195
Descending fibres
    children, 269
    diffuse noxious inhibitory control, 28
    pain modulation, 25
Descriptors, stereo-isomers, 44–45
Dextrans, 73
Diabetes mellitus
    drug kinetics, 58
    eye block, 244
    obstetrics, 258
    regional anaesthesia, 11, 80
Diagnostic sympathetic blocks, 296
Diamorphine
    epidural anaesthesia, 158–159
    children, 278
    subarachnoid, 287
Diarrhoea, coeliac plexus block, 304
Diclofenac, premedication, 87
Differential nerve block, 46
Diffuse noxious inhibitory control, 28
Diffusion barriers, 45
Digital nerve blocks

fingers, 208
    toes, 225–226
Dihydrocodeine, 320
Dihydroergotamine, 102
Doctors, postoperative pain and, 283
Dorsal horns, spinal cord, 25, 30
Dorsal nerve of penis, 187
Dosages
    brachial plexus block, 198–199
    caudal block, 174–175
    children, 271
    caudal block, 275
    epidural anaesthesia, 277–278
    epidural anaesthesia, 151
    spinal anaesthesia, 130, 131
    toxicity, 66, 68, 95
'Double barrel' needles, 256
'Doughty' technique, 147
Dressings, over epidural catheters, 145, 146
Droperidol, 87
Drug interactions, 58, 68–69
Drying agents, 238
Dural blood patches, 162
Dural puncture
    accidental, 161–162, 173, 260, 276
    *see also* Lumbar puncture
Dura mater, 118
    elderly patients, 324
    inferior extremity, 169
Durations
    epidural anaesthesia, 152, 153
    spinal anaesthesia, 130–131
    surgery, 85

**E**
Ear, 238
Ectopic discharges, 30
Education of patient, 283, 284
Ejaculation failure
    coeliac plexus block, 304
    lumbar sympathetic block, 307
Elbow, nerve blocks at, 206–207
Elderly patients, 323–332
    epidural anaesthesia, 151
    dosage, 324–329
    premedication, 87

Elimination half-lives, 55
    children, 57, 269
    elderly patients, 326
    patient variables, 57–58
EMLA *see* Eutectic mixture of local anaesthetics
Enantiomers, 44
Endocrine response to surgery, 9, 12–13, 14–15, 324
Endoneurium, 35
Endorphins, 27
Endoscopic transthoracic sympathectomy, 294
Endotracheal intubation (awake), 238–239
Enoxaparin, 82
Ephedrine, 101, 163, 253
Epidural anaesthesia, 31, 139–167
    abdominal surgery, 189
    accidental cervical, 201, 299
    Caesarean section, 262–263
    cardiac disease, 78
    cervical, 233–234
    children, 274, 276–278
    clinical profile, 152–154
    complications, 16
    day surgery, 318, 319
    diffusion to CSF, 49
    discontinuing, 161
    drug kinetics, 51, 52
    elderly patients, 151, 324–329
    haematomas, 16, 82–84, 106, 135, 162–163
    historical aspects, 5
    laparoscopy, 318
    management, 154–161
    nerve damage, 45–46, 164–165
    obstetrics, 261
    obstetrics, 254–256, 262–263
        contra-indications, 259–260
        incomplete block, 260, 263
    onset times, 96, 152–154, 325
    postoperative pain control, 156–161, 288–287
    ropivacaine, 55–56
    sacral *see* Caudal block
    *vs* spinal anaesthesia, sympathetic block, 14
    spread from lumbar plexus, 217

systemic absorption, 50
systemic infections, 81
test doses, 97–98, 145–146, 155, 255
*see also* Thoracic epidural anaesthesia
Epidural fat, 120
Epidural haematoma, 162–163
Epidural pressure, 123, 150–151
    pregnancy, 123, 252
    use in epidural puncture, 147
Epidural space, 117–118, 120–122, 144–145, 150, 252
Epidural veins, 120, 121
Epinephrine, 72
    for anaphylaxis, 98
    brachial plexus block, 199
    caudal block, 175
    children, 270
    elderly patients, 325
    epidural anaesthesia, 14, 153, 154
    intercostal nerve block, 181
    knee arthroscopy, 226
    on local anaesthetic kinetics, 52
    nerve damage, 164
    overdose, 98
    prophylactic, 101
    spinal anaesthesia, 131
    test doses, 67–68, 146
Epineurium, 35, 36
Equipment
    epidural anaesthesia, 139–142
    children, 276–277
    testing, 141–142
    regional anaesthesia, 92–93
    *see also* Catheters; Needles
Erdtman, H., 4
Ester local anaesthetic agents, 43, 67, 68, 70
Ether spray (Richardson), 2
Etidocaine
    clinical aspects, 72, 73
    kinetics, 51, 55
    metabolites, 57
    physicochemical properties, 41
    protein binding, 67
Eutectic mixture of local anaesthetics (EMLA), 31, 57, 73, 271
Excitatory neurotransmitters, 40

Excretion, 54–55
Explanations to patient, 86, 320, 321
Exsanguination, IVRA, 210
External nasal nerve, 230, 234
Eye blocks, 241–250

**F**
Facial nerve, 232, 243
Failures of regional anaesthesia, 85, 95, 96–97
    obstetrics, 260, 263
Fainting *see* Vaso-vagal reactions
Fallopian tube surgery, 318
Fascia iliaca compartment block
    dosage in children, 271
    *see also* Three-in-one block
Fasting, preoperative, 86
    day surgery, 314
    eye block, 244
Felypressin, 72
Femoral nerve, 216, 218
    three-in-one block, 219–220
Femoral nerve block
    day surgery, 316
    dosage in children, 271
    drug kinetics, 51
    at hip, 217, 218
    induction time, 215
Fentanyl
    epidural anaesthesia, 159, 255, 257
    children, 278
    spinal anaesthesia, 131, 287
    elderly patients, 326
Fetus, 59
    prilocaine, 71
Filters, epidural anaesthesia, 141
Fluid loading, 100–101, 253
    elderly patients, 328
    for sympathetic blocks, 297
Forceps delivery, spinal anaesthesia, 262
Freud, S., 3
Frontal nerve, 229

**G**
Gag reflex, 238
Ganglion impar block, 307
Gastric lavage, 55

Gastrointestinal obstruction, 10
Gastrointestinal tract
    morbidity, 17
    spinal anaesthesia, 134
    sympathetic block, 14
    sympathetic effects, 12
Gate control theory of pain, 21, 26
General anaesthesia
    avoidance, 9
    morbidity, 16, 17–18
    neonates, apnoea, 278–279
    regional anaesthesia, 11, 91–92, 103, 155
    Caesarean section, 263
    cardiovascular effects, 100
    children, 270
Genes, pain sensitisation, 30
Genitofemoral nerve
    genital branch, 185, 188
    neuropathic pain, 306
Glass syringes, 93, 140–141
Glaucoma, 249
Globe perforation, 248
Glossopharyngeal nerve and block, 232, 238
Gloves, 94
Glucose, on solution baricity, 130
Glutamate, 27, 30
Glycopyrrolate, 238
Gowns, 94
G-protein coupled receptors, 27
Grafting, vascular, 329
Great auricular nerve block, 238
Greater occipital nerve, 233, 238
Greater sciatic foramen, 222
Guanethidine, 307–308

**H**
Haematomas, 106
    vertebral canal, 16, 82–84, 106, 135, 162–163
Haemodialysis, AV fistula, 80
Haemorrhage
    eye block, 248
    postoperative, 160
    *see also* Blood loss
Haemorrhoidectomy, caudal block, 11
Hall, R., 4

Halothane
  epinephrine, 154
  local anaesthetic clearance, 58
Halsted, W., 4
Hanging drop method, 147
Headache, 16, 106, 126, 134–135
  *see also* Postdural puncture
    headache
Head and neck, 229–240
Head-down tilt, 134
Height, epidural anaesthesia,
  dosage, 151
Heparin, 83
  aspirin and, 84
  *see also* Low-molecular-weight
    heparin
Hepatectomy, drug kinetics, 58
Hepatitis, drug kinetics, 58
Herniorrhaphy *see* Inguinal
  herniorrhaphy
Herpes zoster, 295
High dependency units, postoperative
  epidural anaesthesia, 156
Hip joint
  nerve supply, 213
  postoperative analgesia, 227
  prostheses, bladder catheterisation
    and infection, 163
Histamine, surgical stress, 13
Historical aspects, 1–8
Horner's syndrome, 201, 296, 299
Hyaluronidase, 73, 244
Hyoscine hydrobromide, 160
Hyperalgesia, 29, 269, 295
Hyperbaric solutions, 130
  bupivacaine
    Caesarean section, 262
    spinal anaesthesia in children,
      279
  lidocaine, adverse effects, 106
Hypercapnia, 54
Hyperhidrosis, 294
Hypobaric solutions, 130
Hypoglossal nerve, 233
Hypospadias repair, 188
Hypotension, 10
  beneficial effects, 100
  coeliac plexus block, 304
  elderly patients, 328

epidural anaesthesia, 150, 163
  thoracic, 150
general anaesthesia and, 103
ischaemic heart disease, 77
lumbar sympathetic block, 307
obstetrics, 253, 260, 263
physiology, 13–14
postoperative, 104–105
treatment, 98, 99–102, 160
Hypothermia, 103–104, 328–329
Hypovolaemia
  abdominal surgery, 189
  on drug kinetics, 52
  pregnancy, 253
  sympathetic block, 99–100
    contra-indication, 296
Hysterectomy, epidural anaesthesia,
  dosage, 155

**I**

Ibuprofen, 87
Ileus, regional anaesthesia on
  incidence, 17
Iliohypogastric nerve
  anterior cutaneous branch, 185
  block in children, 272
Ilio-inguinal nerve, 185
  block in children, 272
Imaging
  coeliac plexus block, 303
  paravertebral block, 183
  sympathetic blocks, 297
    lumbar, 305, 306
Immobile needle sets, 95, 96, 197
Immunosuppression, by surgery,
  13, 15
Incontinence, sympathetic block, 14
Inco-ordinate uterine action, 259
Induction, regional anaesthesia, 91
  *see also specific blocks*
Induction rooms, 91
Infections, 80–81
  epidural abscesses, 16, 135,
    163–164, 278
Inferior dental nerve, 231, 236
  carotid endarterectomy, 239
Inferotemporal component, orbital
  block, 245, 246
Infiltration anaesthesia, 31

Caesarean section, 261
  perineal block, 253
  wounds, 271, 285
Inflammatory soup, 30
Infraclavicular block, 197
Infraorbital foramen, 232
Infraorbital nerve, 230, 236
Infratrochlear nerve, 229–230, 234
Infusions *see* Continuous methods
Inguinal field block, 185–187, 318
Inguinal herniorrhaphy, 189
  children, local anaesthetic
    dosage, 271
  epidural anaesthesia, dosage, 155
  nausea, 314
  paravertebral block, 185
Inhalational anaesthetic agents,
  epinephrine and, 154
Inhalational analgesia, labour, 251
Inhibitory neurotransmitters, 40
Insulated needles, 94
Intensity of central block, 262
Intensive care units, postoperative
  epidural anaesthesia, 156
Intercostal nerve block, 179–182
  abdominal surgery, 189
  children, 271, 272
  drug kinetics, 51, 52
  postoperative pain control, 286
Intercostal nerves, 177
Intercostal neuralgia, stellate
  ganglion block, 299–300
Intercostobrachial nerve block, 204
Interleukin-II, surgical stress, 13
Intermittent positive pressure
  ventilation, epidural anaesthesia
  and, 100
Interpleural block, 182–183, 286
  children, 272–273
  drug kinetics, 52
  sympathetic block, 300
Interscalene block, 193, 197,
  199–201
Interspinous ligaments, 116
Intervertebral discs, 116–117
Intervertebral foramina, 117, 120
Intervertebral joints, 115–117
Intestinal obstruction, epidural
  anaesthesia, 10

Intra-articular block, knee joint, 226, 317
Intracranial hypotension, spontaneous, 134
Intradermal test doses, 81
Intraneural injection, 95
Intravascular injection
  accidental, 66, 233
  caudal block, 274–275
  prevention, 67–68, 97
  test doses for, 97 98, 146
  see also Venous puncture
Intravenous cannulae see Venous cannulae
Intravenous induction agents, for convulsions, 98
Intravenous phentolamine testing, 296
Intravenous regional anaesthesia, 193, 208–210
  day surgery, 316
  drug kinetics, 52, 66
  lower limb, 226
Intravenous regional sympathetic blocks, 307–308
Introducer needles, 128
Ion channels, 37–40
  sodium channel block, 40, 42–43
Ionotropic receptors, 27
Ischaemic heart disease, 77–78
  epidural anaesthesia, 163
  regional anaesthesia, 16
IVRA see Intravenous regional anaesthesia

**K**

Ketamine
  epidural, children, 279
  premedication, 87
Ketanserin, 307
Kidney
  local anaesthetic agents, excretion, 54–55
  surgery
  choice of block, 189
  effects, 12–13
  see also Chronic renal failure
Kinetics, local anaesthetic agents, 49–63, 66–67

children, 269
elderly patients, 323–324, 326–327
Knee joint
  arthroscopy, 226, 317
  nerve supply, 213
  replacement, bladder catheterisation and infection, 163
Knotting, epidural catheters, 163
Koller, C., 3–4

**L**

Labelling regulations, 45
Labour
  epidural anaesthesia, 254–256
  pain pathways, 251–252
Lacrimal nerve, 230, 235
Laminae (of Rexed), 26, 27
Laparoscopy, 318
  inguinal herniorrhaphy, 187
Large dense core vesicles, 25
Larynx, anaesthesia, 238–239
Lateral approach, lumbar puncture, 128
Lateral cutaneous nerve of forearm, 207
Lateral cutaneous nerve of thigh, 216, 217–219
Lateral position
  caudal block, 171
  lumbar puncture, 126
Lesser occipital nerve, 233, 238
Levels
  epidural catheter tip, 155, 157
  epidural puncture, 142, 155
  lumbar puncture, 130
Levobupivacaine
  brachial plexus block, 198
  chirality, 45
  clinical aspects, 71–72, 73
  obstetrics, 256
  spinal anaesthesia, 131
Lidocaine
  brachial plexus block, 198, 199
  caudal block, 175
  clinical aspects, 70, 73
  elderly patients, 326
  epidural anaesthesia, 153
  eye surgery solutions, 244

historical aspects, 4–5
hyperbaric, adverse effects, 106
intravenous regional anaesthesia, 209
kinetics, 51, 55
metabolites, 56, 57
obstetrics, 256
physicochemical properties, 41, 44
protein binding, 67
skin incision, concentrations, 73–74
spinal anaesthesia, 131
Ligaments
  intervertebral, 115–117
  sacrococcygeal, 171, 274
Ligamentum flavum, 116, 121, 150
Lignocaine see Lidocaine
Limbs see Lower limb; Upper limb
Lingual nerve, 231, 236
Lipid solubility, 44
Liposomal encapsulation, 49–50
Liposuction, drug absorption, 52
Liver
  disease, drug kinetics, 58
  local anaesthetic clearance, 55
  cardiogenic shock, 67
  drugs on, 58
  elderly patients, 323–324, 327
Loading see Fluid loading
Local anaesthetic agents
  additives, 72–73
  administration methods, 30–31
  allergic reactions, 68, 81, 98
  antiplatelet action, 69
  children, 269–271
  drug interactions, 58, 68–69
  drug profiles, 69–72
  epidural anaesthesia, 153–154
  eye surgery, 244
  mixtures, 74
  physicochemical properties, 40–42
  preparations, 86
  structure–activity relationships, 43–45
  toxicity see Cardiovascular system, toxicity; Myotoxicity; Neurological complications
  see also Kinetics
Lofgren, N., 4–5

Log-books, training, 289
Lorazepam, premedication, 87
Loss of resistance
  to air, 146–147, 276
  to saline, 144
Lower limb
  anaesthesia, 213–228
  children, 272
  day surgery, 316–317
  postoperative pain control, 286
  weakness, epidural anaesthesia, 15, 16
Low-molecular-weight heparin, 83
  obstetrics, 259
  vertebral canal haematoma, 82
Lumbar plexus, 216
Lumbar plexus blocks, 216–217
  continuous, 227
  postoperative pain control, 286
Lumbar puncture, 125, 126–129
  levels, 130
  postoperative management, 135
  see also Postdural puncture headache
Lumbar sympathetic block, 304–307
Lumbar vertebrae, 114
Lumbosacral plexus, 213, 214
Lung
  on drug kinetics, 53, 67
  function see Pulmonary function

Magnesium, antagonism, 262
Magnetic resonance imaging
  epidural space, 121
  sacrum, 171
Malignant hyperthermia, 81
Mandibular branch, facial nerve, 232
Mandibular nerve, 231, 236–237
Masks, 94
Mastectomy, paravertebral block, 185
Maxillary nerve, 230, 235, 236
Mean segmental duration profile, epidural anaesthesia, 152, 153
Mechanical measurement of isometric muscle force, 153
Medial angulation, paramedian approach, 149
Medial cutaneous nerve of forearm, block, 207

Median nerve, 197
  block at elbow, 206–207
  block at wrist, 207, 208
Meninges, spinal, 117–118
Meningitis, 81
Mental foramen, 232, 236–237
Mental nerve, 231, 236–237
Mepivacaine
  clinical aspects, 70, 73
  kinetics, 50, 51, 55
  metabolites, 57
  physicochemical properties, 41
  protein binding, 67
  spinal anaesthesia, 131
Meta-analysis, regional anaesthesia vs general anaesthesia, elderly patients, 329–330
Metabisulphite, 45–46, 69, 164
Metabolism
  children, 269
  effects of surgery, 13, 14–15
Metabolites, local anaesthetic agents, 56–57
Metabotropic glutamate receptors (mGluRs), 27
Metastases, epidural anaesthesia and, 165
Methaemoglobinaemia, 57, 71, 98–99
Methoxamine, 101–102
Methylene blue, 71, 99
Microcatheters, 133
Midazolam, children, 87
Midline approaches
  epidural anaesthesia, 142
  lumbar puncture, 127–128
Midline strands, epidural, 121–122
Mid-thoracic spinal block, 132
Midwives, epidural anaesthesia, 255
Minimally invasive surgery
  inguinal herniorrhaphy, 187
  intercostal nerve block, 181
  see also Laparoscopy
Minimum local analgesic concentration, 257
Mixtures, local anaesthetic agents, 74
MLAC (minimum local analgesic concentration), 257
Mobility
  labour, 254, 255, 256

  see also Ambulation
Modulation of pain, 28–29
Monitoring, 103–104
  sympathetic block induction, 297
Moore, J., nerve compression, 1, 2
Morbidity, regional anaesthesia on, 16–18
Morphine
  brachial plexus block, 316
  early experiments, 2
  epidural anaesthesia, 158, 278
  spinal anaesthesia, 131, 287
Motor block, 15
  brachial plexus block, 199
  density, 153
  epidural in labour, 255
  postoperative, 160
Multidose vials, 86
Multimodal anaesthesia see Balanced anaesthesia
Multimodal care, 284
Multiple pregnancy, delivery, 258
Multiple sclerosis, 79, 259
μ opioid receptors, 27–28
Muscle cone, orbit, 241
Muscle disease, 81
Muscle relaxation see Motor block; Neuromuscular blockers
Musculocutaneous nerve ($C_5$–$C_7$)
  and block, 195, 197, 204
  axillary block, 203
Myelin sheaths, 36, 37
Myocardial infarction, hypotension, 77
Myopia, 248
Myotoxicity, eye block, 248

### N

Naloxone, children, dosage, 278
Nasal cavity anaesthesia, 235
Nasal component, orbital block, 247
Nasociliary nerve, 229–230
Nausea
  postoperative, 16, 106–107
  day surgery, 313–314
  spinal anaesthesia, 134
Neck see Cervical spine; Head and neck
Needles, 92–93

caudal block, 172–173, 174
  children, 274
  epidural anaesthesia, 139–140
    children, 276
  insertion, 142–144
  head and neck, 234
  immobile sets, 95, 96, 197
  insertion, 95
  *see also* Lumbar puncture
  insulated, 94
  introducer, 128
  spinal, 128–129
  upper limb blocks, 205
    brachial plexus, 197
Needle-through-needle method, 256
Neonates
  elimination half-lives, 57
  pain, 269
  phenytoin for arrhythmias, 270
  postoperative apnoea, 278–279
Neostigmine, bowel surgery, 14
Nerve block *see* Conduction blocks; Differential nerve block
Nerve compression (Moore), 1, 2
Nerve fibres, 21–22, 23, 36–37
  differential block, 46
Nerve impulses, 37–40
  *see also* Conduction blocks
Nerve roots, 35–36, 119, 120
Nerve stimulators, 94, 198
  lumbar plexus block, 217
  sciatic block, 220–222
  upper limb blocks, 205
Neurological complications, 69, 79–80, 105–106
  audit results, 289
  brachial plexus block, 199
  chloroprocaine, 45, 69, 257
  compression neuropraxia, 278
  epidural anaesthesia, 45–46, 164–165, 261
  optic nerve damage, 248
  spinal anaesthesia, 135
  tourniquet injury, 210
  upper limb blocks, 206
Neurolytic blocks, 296–297
  coeliac plexus, 294, 301–304
  stellate ganglion, 299

Neuromuscular blockers
  for convulsions, 98
  epidural anaesthesia and, 155
Neurones, 25
Neuropathic pain
  genitofemoral nerve, 306
  sympathetic block, 294–295
Neuropathy, peripheral, 80
Neuropeptides, 27–28
Neurotransmitters, 25, 27
  diffuse noxious inhibitory control, 28
  mechanisms, 40
Neurotrophins, 25
Nitrous oxide, 97
*N*-methyl-D-aspartate (NMDA) receptors, 27
  antagonists *see* Ketamine
Nociceptin, 28
Nociceptors, 23, 24–25
  sensitisation, 29
Non-steroidal anti-inflammatory drugs (NSAIDs)
  balanced anaesthesia, 319, 320
  postoperative, 159, 321
  premedication, 87
Nucleus pulposus, 116–117
Nurses
  day surgery, 314
  postoperative pain and, 283

## O

Obersteiner–Redlich zones, 35–36
Obesity, 80
  drug kinetics, 57
  epidural anaesthesia, 148, 151
  lateral cutaneous nerve of thigh block, 219
Obstetrics
  multiple sclerosis, 79
  prilocaine and, 71
  regional anaesthesia, 10, 251–267
  *see also* Ropivacaine, obstetrics
Obstruction, gastrointestinal, epidural anaesthesia, 10
Obturator nerve block, 219, 227
Occipitoposterior position, persisting, analgesia, 257
Oculomotor nerve, 241–243

Onset times
  conduction blocks, 69–70, 96
  epidural anaesthesia, 96, 152–154
  elderly patients, 325
  lower limb anaesthesia, 215–216
Ophthalmic nerve, 229–230, 234–235, 241
Opioid peptides, 27
Opioid receptors, 27–28
  neonates, 269
Opioids
  balanced anaesthesia, 320
  brachial plexus block, 199, 316
  day surgery and, 313
  epidural anaesthesia, 158–159
  children, 278
  elderly patients, 326
  obstetrics, 257
  postoperative pain control, 287
  intravenous regional anaesthesia and, 209
  with local anaesthetic agents, 73
  premedication, 87
  spinal anaesthesia, 131, 326
  systemic, 159
Optic nerve damage, 248
Orbit, 241–243
Orbital regional block, 244–248
Orphanin FQ (nociceptin), 28
Osmolality, CSF, 130
Outcome studies, regional anaesthesia *vs* general anaesthesia, elderly patients, 329
Oxygen therapy, 101

## P

Packs, sterile, 92
Paediatrics *see* Children
Pain, 21–33
  children, 269
  injection sites, 106
  labour, pathways, 251–252
  postoperative, 283–290
  recurrence, 160
  prevention *vs* relief, 156
  psychology, 13
  on pulmonary function, 12
  quality of relief, audit, 290
  *see also* Cancer pain; Chronic pain

Pain services
 audit, 289
 *see also* Acute pain teams
Pancreas, pain
 interpleural block, 182
 *see also* Coeliac plexus
Paracervical block, 253
Paracetamol, 319, 320
Paraesthesiae, 93
 brachial plexus block, 199
 interscalene block, 201
 subclavian perivascular block,
  202–203
Paramedian approaches
 epidural anaesthesia, 147–149
 children, 277
 Crawford needle, 140
 thoracic, 150
Paraplegia, coeliac plexus block,
 304
Parasympathetic system
 pain, 23
 supply to trunk, 178
Paravertebral block, 183–185
 children, 273
 postoperative pain control, 286
 somatic, 31
Paravertebral space, 184
Patient-controlled epidural
 analgesia, 255
Patients, attitudes to postoperative
 pain, 283
Pedicles, vertebrae, 111
Pelvis, sympathetic supply, 179
Pencil point needles, 128, 261
Penile block, 187–188
 children, 271, 272
Perforation, globe, eye block, 248
Peribulbar block, 241, 245, 246
Perineal block
 ganglion impar block, 307
 infiltration anaesthesia, 253
 *see also* Saddle block
Perineurium, 35, 36
Perioperative epidural infusion,
 155–156
Peripheral nerve blocks, 31
 children, 271–273
 day surgery, 316–317

postoperative pain prevention, 285
 trunk, 185–188
 upper limb, 193, 205–208
Peripheral nerve endings, 23–25, 40
Peripheral nerves, 35–48
 anatomy, 22–23
 core/mantle concept, 199
 role in pain, 21–25
Peripheral neuropathy, 80
Peripheral sensitisation, 30
Peripheral vascular disease,
 sympathetic block for, 293–294
Persisting O-P position, 257
Pharmacokinetics *see* Kinetics
Pharyngeal branch, vagus nerve,
 232–233
Phasic block, 42–43
Phenol, 297
Phentolamine, testing, 296
Phenylephrine, 101, 102, 253
 spinal anaesthesia, 131
Phenytoin, for arrhythmias in
 neonates, 270
Phrenic nerve, 201, 233, 299
Pia mater, 118
p$K_a$ values, local anaesthetic agents,
 43–44
Placental transfer, local anaesthetic
 agents, 58–59
Plasma concentrations, local
 anaesthetic agents, 49, 50–51
 children, 270
 elderly patients, 326–327
 protein binding, 53–54
 toxicity, 50, 66
Plasticity, nervous system, 21, 29
Platelets
 local anaesthetic agents on, 69
 pulmonary trapping, 12
 vertebral canal haematoma and,
  83
Pleurodesis, 181
Plexus of Batson, 120, 121
Plica mediana dorsalis, 121
Pneumonia, regional anaesthesia
 on incidence, 17
Pneumothorax, 102
 intercostal nerve block
 incidence, 182

prevention, 181
 interpleural block, 183
 stellate ganglion block, 299
 subclavian perivascular block, 203
Popliteal fossa block, 223–224, 316
Positioning of patient, 104
 axillary block, 204
 Caesarean section, 262
 caudal block, 171
 epidural anaesthesia, 142
 eye block, 244
 intercostal nerve block, 180
 interscalene block, 200
 lumbar puncture, 126–127
 lumbar sympathetic block,
  304–305
 postoperative, 105
 ulnar nerve block, 206
 *see also* Posture
Postdural puncture headache, 106,
 126, 134–135, 162
 day surgery, 319
 elderly patients, 327
 obstetrics, 260, 261
Posterior cutaneous nerve of
 forearm, 207
Posterior cutaneous nerve of thigh,
 220
Posterior longitudinal ligament,
 116, 121
Posterior spinal artery, 120
Postoperative period, 9, 11, 104–107
 convalescence, 17
 day surgery, 313–314, 320–321
 elderly patients, 324
 lower limb anaesthesia, 227
 lung function, 79
 minor complications, 15–16
 neonatal apnoea, 278–279
 pain, 160, 283–290
 plasma drug concentrations, 53,
  55–56
 ropivacaine, 154
 *see also* Epidural anaesthesia,
  postoperative
Posture
 drug kinetics, 58
 epidural anaesthesia, infusions,
  157

epidural pressure, 150
hypotension, 101
spread of epidural block, 151
spread of spinal block, 130
*see also* Positioning of patient
Potassium, 37–39
Pre-eclamptic toxaemia, 257–258
spinal anaesthesia for Caesarean
section, 262
Pre-emptive analgesia, 31–32
Pregnancy
drug kinetics, 58
epidural pressure, 123, 252
epidural space, 252
Preloading *see* Fluid loading
Premature infants, delivery, 258
Premedication, 86–87
Preoperative assessment, 77–84
day surgery, 314
eye block, 243–244
Preoperative visits, 86–87, 283
Preservatives, 45–46, 72, 164
Pressure
cerebrospinal fluid, 123
paravertebral space, 184
*see also* Epidural pressure
Pressure areas, 323
Prilocaine
brachial plexus block, 198, 199
caudal block, 175
chirality and properties, 45
clinical aspects, 70–71, 73
epidural anaesthesia, 153
inguinal field block, 187
intravenous regional anaesthesia,
209
kinetics, 51, 55
methaemoglobinaemia, 57, 71,
98–99
physicochemical properties, 41, 44
protein binding, 67
Primary afferent neurones, 23–25
Procaine, 4, 41, 70, 73
Prognostic sympathetic blocks, 296
Prone position, 10–11
caudal block, 171
Propofol, 85, 239
Propranolol, on local anaesthetic
clearance, 58

Prostaglandins
peripheral nerve endings, 40
renal sympathetic effects, 12–13
Protection of anaesthetised areas,
320–321
Protein binding, local anaesthetic
agents, 44, 53–54, 67
Protocols, epidural anaesthesia
management, 160
Proxymetacaine, 244
Pruritus, opioids, 158, 287
Psoas compartment block, 216–217
Psoas major muscle, 216
contrast medium injection, 305
Psychiatric illness, 81
Psychology, pain, 13
Pterygopalatine fossa, 236
Ptosis, 245
Pudendal nerve block, 253
Pulmonary blood flow, sympathetic
effects, 12
Pulmonary function, 79
elderly patients, 325
intercostal nerve block, 182
motor block, 102
spinal anaesthesia, 134
sympathetic block, 14
sympathetic effects, 12
Pulmonary morbidity, 17
respiratory distress, spinal
anaesthesia, 263
Pulse oximetry,
methaemoglobinaemia, 99

**Q**
Quality of care, 284, 287–290
Quincke, H.I., 4
Quincke needles, 128

**R**
Race, drug kinetics, 58
Racemic mixtures, 44
Radial nerve, 197
block at elbow, 207
block at wrist, 207, 208
Radiofrequency upper thoracic
sympathectomy, 300
Radiology *see* Imaging
Rami communicantes, 178

Receptors
neurotransmitters, 27
*see also* Opioid receptors
Rectus muscles, eye, 241
Recurrent laryngeal nerve and
block, 201, 233, 299
Referred pain, 23
Reflex sympathetic dystrophy, 295,
297
Regional anaesthesia, monitoring
of, 104
Regression, central anaesthesia,
130–131, 320
Remifentanil, carotid
endarterectomy, 239
Renal failure *see* Chronic renal failure
Respiratory depression, epidural
opioids, children, 278
Respiratory disease, 78–79
obstetrics, 259, 263
Respiratory distress, spinal
anaesthesia, 263
Respiratory system *see* Pulmonary
function
Resting potential, 37, 39
Resuscitation, facilities, 85–86
Retention *see* Urinary retention
Retrobulbar block, 241
Retrocrural technique, coeliac
plexus block, 302
Re-usable needles, 93
Rexed's laminae, 26, 27
Richardson, B.J., 2
Risk levels, vertebral canal
haematoma, 83–84
Ropivacaine, 139
brachial plexus block, 198, 199
caudal block, 175
chirality and properties, 45
clinical aspects, 71, 73
epidural anaesthesia, 154, 263
children, 278
epinephrine with, 52
kinetics, 50, 55
metabolites, 57
obstetrics, 71, 256
minimum local analgesic
concentration, 257
physicochemical properties, 41

postoperative 55–56
protein binding, 67
spinal anaesthesia, 131
toxicity, *vs* plasma concentration, 50

**S**

Sacral cornua, 274
Sacral epidural anaesthesia *see* Caudal block
Sacral hiatus, 169, 171
Sacrococcygeal ligament, 171, 274
Sacrum, 114–115, 169–171
Saddle block
  epidural anaesthesia, 151
  spinal anaesthesia, 132
Saline
  epidural infusion, 162
  epidural puncture technique, 144–145
  *see also* Fluid loading
Saltatory conduction, 39, 40
Saphenous nerve
  block, 224
  at ankle, 224–225
  tourniquets and, 216
Scalene muscles, 195
  *see also* Interscalene block
Schwann cells, 25, 36, 37
Sciatic block
  continuous, 227
  day surgery, 316
  drug kinetics, 51
  at hip, 220–223
  induction time, 215
  popliteal block, 223–224, 316
Sedation, 85, 102–103
  carotid endarterectomy, 239
  eye block, 244
  inadequate conduction block, 97
  regional block induction, 91–92
  requirement for, 11
  sympathetic blocks, 297
Segmental dose requirement, 150
Segmental latency profiles, 152
Sensitisation to pain, 29–30
Septum posticum, 119–120
Sequence rule notation, 44–45
Sequential analgesia, 321

Sex difference, elimination half-lives, 57
Shaving, 94
Shivering, elderly patients, 329
Shoulder joint, suprascapular nerve block, 316
Sickle cell disease, 81
Simpson, J.Y., 1
Sitting position, 126–127
Skin
  graft harvesting, 217, 218
  incisions, lidocaine concentrations, 73–74
  innervation
    head and neck, 230
    lower limb, 213, 215
    upper limb, 195
  marking, 91
  temperature tests, 296
  topical anaesthesia *see* Eutectic mixture of local anaesthetics
Societies of regional anaesthesia, 6
Sodium, 37–39
Sodium bicarbonate, local anaesthetic agents, 72–73
Sodium channel block, 40, 42–43
Specific gravity, 129–130
Spermatic cord, 318
Sphenopalatine ganglion block, 235
Sphygmomanometer cuffs, 209
Spinal anaesthesia, 31, 125–138
  abdominal surgery, 189
  accidental, 161–162, 201, 237, 260–261, 299
  adverse report (1950), 6
  Caesarean section, 262
  children, 278–279
  complications, 134–136
  day surgery, 318–319
  drug kinetics, 52
  ease of administration, 10
  elderly patients, 324–329
  *vs* epidural anaesthesia, sympathetic block, 14
  haematomas, 16, 82–84, 106, 135, 162–163
  head and neck surgery and, 233–234

indications and contraindications, 125–126
  postoperative opioids, 287
  respiratory distress, 263
  side-effects, 133–134
  spread of block, 129–130, 131
  elderly patients, 325–326
  tissue toxicity, 69
  *see also* Continuous methods, spinal anaesthesia
Spinal cord
  anatomy, 118–120
  injury, 79–80
  coeliac plexus block, 304
  pain transmission, 25–28
  puncture, 135
Spinal needles, 128–129
Spinal stenosis, 165
Spine *see* Vertebral column
Spinothalamic tract, anterolateral, 28
Splanchnic nerves, 179, 300–301
Spontaneous intracranial hypotension, 134
Spread of block
  caudal block, 175
  epidural anaesthesia, 150–152, 252, 325
  intercostal nerve block, 181
  paravertebral block, 184, 273
  spinal anaesthesia, 129–130, 131
  elderly patients, 325–326
Sprotte needles, 128
Standards, for audit, 288
Stellate ganglion, 178–179, 297–300
Stereo-isomers, 44–45
Sternocleidomastoid muscle, 238
Steroids, depot, coeliac plexus, 304
Stimulators *see* Nerve stimulators
Street fitness, 320
Subarachnoid anaesthesia *see* Spinal anaesthesia
Subarachnoid injection, test doses for, 97–98
Subarachnoid space, 118–120, 125
  cranial nerves, spread of local anaesthetics, 233
Subatmospheric pressure *see* Epidural pressure

Subclavian perivascular block, 193, 197, 201–203
Subconjunctival anaesthesia, 248
Subcostal incisions, 181
Subcostal nerve, 185
Subdural compartment, spine, 118
Subdural haematoma, 135
Substance P, 27, 30
Substantia gelatinosa, 26
Sub-Tenon's fascia block, 241, 248–249
Sufentanil, spinal anaesthesia, 131
Sumatriptan, 162
Superficial cervical plexus, 233
    block, 238
    carotid endarterectomy, 239
Superficial peroneal nerve, 224
    ankle block, 225
Superior hypogastric plexus block, 307
Superior laryngeal nerve, 233, 239
Superotemporal component, orbital block, 247–248
Supraclavicular nerves, 233
Supraorbital foramen, 232
Supraorbital nerve, 229, 234
Suprascapular nerve block, 316, 317
Supraspinous ligament, 116
Supratrochlear nerve, 229, 234
Sural nerve, 220
    ankle block, 225
Surgeons
    in anaesthetic rooms, 91
    regional anaesthesia by, 5, 9, 314–315
    view of regional anaesthesia, 85
Sustentaculum tali, 225
Sweat production, tests, 296
Sympathalgia, 306
Sympathetic block, 11–14, 134
    adverse effects, 99–102
    coronary blood flow, 78
    physiology, 13–14
    therapeutic, 293–311
Sympathetic blocking drugs, 307
Sympathetic nervous system
    pain, 23
    supply to trunk, 177, 178–179
Syringes, 2, 3, 93

epidural anaesthesia, 140–141
Systemic absorption, 50–52
    intercostal nerve block, 181
Systemic analgesia, 11, 97, 105, 175, 321
Systemic disposition, local anaesthetic agents, 53–59, 66–67
Systemic toxicity, 9–10, 65–68
    acidosis, 54
    children, 269–270
    paravertebral block, 273
    epidural anaesthesia in labour, 260
    eye block, 248
    interpleural block, 183
    intravenous regional anaesthesia, 210
    lower limb anaesthesia, 215
    management, 97–98
    plasma concentrations, 50, 66
    in postoperative period, 160–161

T
T cells, surgery on, 13
Temazepam, premedication, 87
Test doses
    allergy, 81
    children, 270
    epidural anaesthesia, 97–98, 145–146, 155, 255
    epinephrine, 67–68, 146
    for intravascular injection, 97–98, 146
Testing of regional anaesthesia, 95–96
Tetracaine
    clinical aspects, 70, 73
    spinal anaesthesia, 131, 279
Thoracic epidural anaesthesia, 149–150
    adverse effects, 99–100
    catheter from sacral puncture, 276
    ischaemic heart disease, 78
Thoracic nerves, 177
    subcostal nerve, 185
Thoracic surgery
    choice of block, 188
    intercostal nerve block, 181

Thoracic sympathetic block, 300
Thoracic vertebrae, 113–114
Thoracoscopic sympathectomy, 300
Three-in-one block, 219–220
    see also Fascia iliaca compartment block
Thromboembolic complications, regional anaesthesia on, 14, 17, 69, 84
Tibial nerve, 220
    ankle block, 225
Tilt, head-down, 134
Tissue distribution, local anaesthetic agents, 54, 67
Tissue toxicity, eye block, 248
Toes
    digital nerve blocks, 225–226
    mid-tarsal block, 285
Topical anaesthesia, 31
    awake intubation, 238–239
    children, 271
    eye, 244, 248
    nasal cavity, 235
    skin see Eutectic mixture of local anaesthetics
Top-ups, epidural, 255, 260
Total spinal block, 161–162, 260–261
Tourniquets, 105–106
    intravenous regional anaesthesia, 209
    compression injury, 210
    lower limb, 226
    lower limb operations, 215, 216
Toxicity see Cardiovascular system, toxicity; Myotoxicity; Neurological complications; Systemic toxicity
Toxins, potential for local anaesthesia, 46–47
Tracheal intubation (awake), 238–239
Training, log-books, 289
Tramadol, 278
Transaortic approach, coeliac plexus block, 303
Transarterial technique, axillary block, 204

Transient neurological symptoms (TNS), 136, 319

Transurethral surgery, 11, 189

Transverse cervical nerve, 233

Transverse myelitis, 135

Trauma, regional anaesthesia, 10

Trigeminal ganglion, 229, 234

Trigeminal nerve, 229–232
blocks, 234–237

Trochlear nerve, 243

Trunk, regional anaesthesia, 177–192, 318

Tuffier's line, 127

Tuohy needle, 140

Twin pregnancy, delivery, 258

Two-interspace method, combined spinal epidural anaesthesia, 255–256

Two-segment regression time, 153

**U**

Ulnar nerve, 197
block at elbow, 206
block at wrist, 207

Unilateral spinal anaesthesia, 133

Unilateral spread, epidural anaesthesia, 260

Upper limb, 193–211
day surgery, 315–316
postoperative pain control, 285–286

Upper lumbar block, spinal anaesthesia, 132

Urinary retention, 16, 105
day surgery, 320
epidural anaesthesia, 163
morphine, 158
spinal anaesthesia, 134

Urogenital tract, sympathetic supply, 179

Use-dependent block, 42–43

Uterus
inco-ordinate action, 259
pain pathways, 251–252
scars, 260

**V**

Vagus nerve, 232–233
auricular branch block, 238

Valvular heart disease
prostheses, obstetrics, 258
sympathetic block, 14, 78

Variants (anatomical)
contra-indication to sympathetic block, 296
sacrum, 169–171
vertebral column, 115

Vascular disorders, sympathetic block for, 293–294

Vascular grafting, 329

Vasoactivity, local anaesthetics, 65
kinetics, 51
stereo-isomers, 45

Vasoconstrictors
in local anaesthetic solutions, 72
spinal anaesthesia, 131

Vasopressors
postoperative monitoring, 104
pregnancy, 253
prophylactic, 101
therapeutic, 101–102

Vaso-vagal reactions (fainting), 11
stellate ganglion block, 299
sympathetic block, 14

Veins, epidural, 120, 121

Venous cannulae
continuous anaesthesia
brachial plexus, 205
caudal, 175
intravenous regional anaesthesia, 209

Venous puncture, accidental
epidural anaesthesia, 162–163
*see also* Intravascular injection

Venous return, reduction, 100

Ventilation (IPPV), 100

Ventricular fibrillation, 66, 71

Vertebrae, 111–114

Vertebral arteries, accidental injection, 98, 201, 237

Vertebral canal, 111–124
anatomy, 111–122

haematomas, 16, 82–84, 106, 135, 162–163

Vertebral column, 111–115
elderly patients, 323, 324
movement, 117
previous surgery, 259

Very low birth weight, interpleural block, 273

Viral hepatitis, drug kinetics, 58

Visceral pain, 23
sympathetic block, 294

Voltage-gated ion channels, 37–40
*see also* Sodium channel block

Volume expansion *see* Fluid loading

Volumes of distribution, 53, 54
elderly patients, 323

Volume transmission, neuropeptides, 27

Vomiting, 16, 106–107, 134, 313–314

**W**

Ward care
acute pain nurses, 157
postoperative epidural anaesthesia, 156

Warfarin, 83

Weaning off epidural anaesthesia, 161

Weight, epidural anaesthesia, dosage, 151

Whitacre needles, 128

'Whoosh test', 174

Wind up, 30

Wood, A., 2, 3

Wounds
infiltration anaesthesia, 271, 285
postoperative pain, 283

Wrist, peripheral nerve blocks at, 207–208

**Z**

Zoster, 295

Zygomaticofacial nerve, 230, 236

Zygomaticotemporal nerve, 230, 236